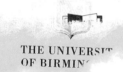

THE UNIVERS~
OF BIRMIN~

SECOND OPINION
AN INTRODUCTION TO HEALTH SOCIOLOGY

SECOND EDITION

SECOND OPINION
AN INTRODUCTION TO HEALTH SOCIOLOGY

Edited by JOHN GERMOV

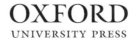

OXFORD

UNIVERSITY PRESS

OXFORD
UNIVERSITY PRESS

253 Normanby Road, South Melbourne, Victoria 3205, Australia

Oxford University Press is a department of the University of Oxford.
It furthers the University's objective of excellence in research, scholarship,
and education by publishing worldwide in

Oxford New York

Auckland Bangkok Buenos Aires Cape Town Chennai
Dar es Salaam Delhi Hong Kong Istanbul Karachi Kolkata
Kuala Lumpur Madrid Melbourne Mexico City Mumbai Nairobi
São Paulo Shanghai Taipei Tokyo Toronto

OXFORD is a trade mark of Oxford University Press
in the UK and in certain other countries

National Library of Australia
Cataloguing-in-Publication data:

Germov, John
Second opinion: an introduction to health sociology.

2nd ed.
Bibliography.
Includes index.
ISBN 0 19 551369 X. $2305 7653$.

1. Social medicine—Australia. 2. Health—Social aspects—Australia.
3. Sociology, Medicine. 4. Social medicine. I. Germov, John.

306.4610994

Typeset by OUPANZS
Printed through Bookpac Production Services, Singapore

Foreword

The publication of the second edition of *Second Opinion: An Introduction to Health Sociology* is a clear mark of the success of the first edition. It is a well-researched collection with many virtues, including being well organised, written in accessible language, up-to-date and well geared to the needs of students through use, not only of more traditional teaching/learning techniques, but also through engagement with the new capacities afforded by the web. The book is not only aimed to equip readers for the next stage of academic work, though it aims to do this effectively. Its focus is also on developing reflective practices within the health and allied professions and thus fostering a reflective citizenry with sociological imagination.

In a user-friendly manner, the contributors to this volume introduce the theories, concepts and issues that are needed to equip students of health sociology. Learning to think sociologically inevitably involves coming to grips with new forms of conceptual analysis. The feedback from both students and teachers suggests that students generally find that this book provides the support they need to develop the necessary analytic skills. The chapters are well staged with a range of teaching aids, including clearly defined terms and challenging and appropriate questions for class discussion; useful appendices on key health sociology resources and tips on effective use of the web for research; and a book web site that provides access to relevant web sites and supplementary material, and that solicits feed-back. Such feedback from the first edition has informed the development of this volume.

My pleasure in being associated, in this very small way, with this enterprise is not only linked to the qualities of the book. It has a historical element to it as well. I have been around universities since the very beginning of sociology as a formally named discipline in Australia. Of course many people were thinking and theorising sociologically before that time, but many academics were not convinced that this was academically legitimate, let alone an indispensable approach for illuminating social issues. In the 1970s John Powles was attempting to introduce health sociology to the medical students at Monash University. He was seriously hampered, not only by the subject matter's lack of credibility, but also by a severe lack of Australian resource material. At that time, most sociologists had to rely on overseas material to teach their students. He and others like him would have greatly benefited, in those early years, from *Second Opinion*, and from the store of primary research data and secondary literature that is available today. That I am introducing a second edition of the book underscores the vitality that health sociology has achieved in Australia over the last three decades.

A strong health sociology in Australia with a strong public voice is crucial if there are to be good policies and services and thus good health outcomes. The importance of the social context for health and well-being is nowhere more starkly reflected than in relation to the health of Indigenous Australians. This is being constantly underscored by reports suggesting that rather than improving, the statistics relating to the health of Indigenous Australians are becoming more alarming. This is discussed specifically in chapter 6 of this book where it is made abundantly clear how, without addressing people's specific social circumstances, the mere offering of technical health services will always be ineffectual. This message underlies the whole of this book and indeed health sociology generally.

Health remains a high priority for Australian citizens, and they are increasingly expressing concern about economic policies that lead to cuts in funding to public services, including health. This concern is heightened because of increased longevity, which clearly calls for more and better, rather than less, provision of services. The complex issues involved in increased privatisation and reduced government activity are canvassed in relation to many specific issues in the chapters of this volume, and the issues surrounding health insurance are directly addressed in chapter 13.

The key broad health issues that are currently on the political agenda are also discussed in the book. This is a mark of the range of expertise of the contributors and a clear indication of the book's relevance and sensitivity to student interests and needs. This also makes it valuable to a wider audience than the target readership of introductory students. Genetic engineering, euthanasia, healthism, multicultural approaches, community health, alternative health practice, and women's and men's health are just some of the important, politically prominent issues dealt with. The book also offers a valuable analysis of the complex occupational issues that are ever present for doctors, nurses, and allied professionals—issues that explicitly affect cross-professional relationships.

This book is extremely well pitched for its readership, whose reactions will continue to be monitored and heeded through the web site. It thus provides an accessible introduction to the social issues within which health is embedded and the conceptual and analytic skills for understanding these issues. I recommend *Second Opinion* to all those readers—old hands as well as novices—who want an up-to-date, well-written, information-packed, and politically sensitive account of these issues, and hope you will find it as useful and rewarding as I have.

Lois Bryson
Emeritus Professor of Sociology
University of Newcastle and RMIT University
January 2002

Contents

Preface to the Second Edition   ix
Acknowledgments   xii
Contributors   xiii
Abbreviations   xvii

Introduction: Health Sociology and the Social Model of Health   **1**

1   Imagining Health Problems as Social Issues   3
John Germov

2   Theorising Health:
Major Theoretical Perspectives in Health Sociology   28
John Germov

3   Researching Health:
Methodological Traditions and Innovations   49
Douglas Ezzy

**Part 1: The Social Production and Distribution of
Health and Illness**   **65**

4   Class, Health Inequality, and Social Justice   67
John Germov

5   Gender and Health   95
Dorothy Broom

6   Indigenous Health: The Perpetuation of Inequality   112
Dennis Gray and Sherry Saggers

Part 2: The Social Construction of Health and Illness   **133**

7   Ethnicity, Health, and Multiculturalism   135
Roberta Julian

8   The Medicalisation of Deviance   155
Sharyn L. Roach Anleu

9   The Body, Medicine, and Society   180
Deborah Lupton

10   Health Promotion Dilemmas   195
Katy Richmond

11 The Human Genome Project:
A Sociology of Medical Technology   215
Evan Willis

12 Ageing, Dying, and Death as the Twenty-first
Century Begins   231
Maureen Strazzari

**Part 3: The Social Organisation of Health Care:
Professions, Politics, and Policies**   **255**

13 Power, Politics, and Health Care   257
Helen Belcher

14 Challenges to Medical Dominance   283
John Germov

15 Nursing and Sociology: An Uneasy Relationship   306
Deidre Wicks

16 Alternative Medicine   325
Gary Easthope

17 In Search of Profession: A Sociology of Allied Health   343
Lauren Williams

18 Community Health Services in Australia   365
Fran Baum

Conclusion: Future Directions in the Social Model of Health   **389**

19 Citizenship and Health as a Scarce Resource   391
Bryan S. Turner

20 Health Sociology and Your Sociological Imagination   407
John Germov

Appendix 1: Key Web Sites, Books, and Journals   413
Appendix 2: Tips on Web Use, and Referencing the
Web and this Book   423
Glossary   425
References   439
Index   472

Preface to the Second Edition

Second Opinion aims to introduce students to the field of health sociology through an accessible yet authoritative overview of key debates, research findings, and theories. The second edition expands on the successful format of the first with a new introductory section, new chapters and updated material, and new features added in response to feedback from lecturers and students. Since the book is designed to be used as a teaching text, each chapter contains:

- an overview section that begins with a series of questions and a short summary of the chapter to grab the reader's interest and to encourage a questioning and reflective approach to the topic
- key terms (concepts and theories) are highlighted in bold in the text and defined in separate margin paragraphs as well as appearing in a glossary at the end of the book
- summary of main points
- discussion questions
- further investigation questions: essay-style questions new to this edition
- further reading and recommended chapter-specific web sites.

What's new?

All of the chapters have been revised in terms of the latest available statistics, research findings and references to bring the text completely up to date with current developments in the field. Specifically, the second edition of *Second Opinion* includes:

- **New introductory section:** the new introductory part of the book includes a substantially revised introductory chapter that clearly maps out the social model of health in contrast to the biomedical model, situating it in a historical framework of public health, social medicine, and the new public health, as well as introducing the sociological perspective via the sociological imagination template.
- **New chapters:** theories in health sociology by John Germov, on health research methods by Douglas Ezzy, and community health by Fran Baum.
- **New material:** on issues such as evidence-based medicine, Divisions of General Practice, clinical governance, corporatisation, new public health, social medicine, the latest developments in health insurance policy, and a substantially updated chapter on class-based health inequalities that addresses the research of Wilkinson, Marmot, and colleagues as

well as individual behaviour/lifestyle debates and the issue of social capital.

- **New pedagogic features—Further investigation section and web resources:** a Further investigation section of essay-style questions as well as chapter-specific web sites have been added to all chapters.
- **New appendices:**
  - **Appendix 1:** A completely updated and expanded list of relevant web sites, books, and journals
  - **Appendix 2:** Provides student tips on the critical use of web resources, how to reference the web, and how to reference chapters in this book.
- **New *Second Opinion* web site:** <www.oup.com.au/cws/germov> a new professionally designed web site provides access to:
  - Relevant web sites, online journals, and databases accessible via the web
  - Supplementary reading material accessible in pdf format from the Oxford University Press back catalogue that can be set as extra student reading or as further resources for assignments
  - Downloadable PowerPoint slides of all diagrams and tables in the book.
- **New Teaching Manual and Test Bank of Multiple-choice Questions:** to support the text a rewritten Teaching Manual is available, which includes short tutorial exercises in the form of 'icebreakers' for each chapter to facilitate student discussion as well as a test bank of multiple-choice questions. The Teaching Manual is available free of charge from the publisher for those using the book as a course text.

Structure and content of the book

The structure and content of the book assumes no prior knowledge of sociology and is intended for undergraduate students. The book is structured to provide a solid foundation in health sociology as well as mapping out the key dimensions of the social model of health. The book is divided into the following parts:

- Introduction: Health Sociology and the Social Model of Health
- Part 1: The Social Production and Distribution of Health and Illness
- Part 2: The Social Construction of Health and Illness
- Part 3: The Social Organisation of Health Care: Professions, Politics, and Policies
- Conclusion: Future Directions in the Social Model of Health.

The Introduction part provides the foundation for understanding the sociological contribution to studying health and illness. The first chapter explains the development of the social model of health, reviews critiques of the biomedical model, and provides an overview of the sociological imagination and how it can be used to analyse health issues. Chapters 2 and 3 are new to this edition, and specifically address the main theoretical perspectives and methodological debates in health sociology. Part 1 concerns the social production and distribution of health and illness in terms of class, gender, and Aboriginality. Part 2, on the social construction of health and illness, covers debates about changing conceptions of health and illness and the power to define someone or some condition as healthy or unhealthy, normal or abnormal through chapters on ethnicity and health, the medicalisation of deviance, the sociology of the body, health promotion, the new genetics, and ageing, death and dying. Part 3 of the book examines the political features of the Australian health system, focusing on health professions (medicine, nursing, and allied health and alternative therapies) and health policies (debates and policies over health funding, health insurance, and community health) that fundamentally shape how health care is organised, delivered, and utilised. The conclusion points to new directions in the social model of health in terms of a focus on citizenship rights and capabilities, as well as outlining additional issues for students to consider in further developing their sociological imagination.

Suggestions, comments, and feedback

I am very interested in receiving feedback on the book and suggestions for future editions. You can contact me at: <John.Germov@newcastle.edu.au>

John Germov
University of Newcastle
January 2002

Acknowledgments

A book such as this is a team effort and once again I thank all of the contributors for producing chapters of high quality and consistency, and for making my job as editor a pleasurable one. Kind thanks to my dear friend and colleague Lauren Williams for being a constant source of help and advice on my writing, ensuring its conceptual clarity and sensitivity to the work of health professionals. Thanks also to Helen Belcher for her willingness to provide invaluable feedback on drafts of various chapters, and to Annette Murphy for her expert indexing. From the first edition my continuing gratitude to Lois Bryson and Deidre Wicks who provided advice throughout the evolution of the book for which I am forever in their debt. My publishers, Jill Henry and Debra James, who have been a constant source of support, insight, and professionalism. Thanks also to Steve Campitelli for his illustrations and to the editor Tim Fullerton and the designers Anitra Blackford and Racheal Stines. And finally a special note of appreciation to Sue Jelovcan for her support, patience, and good humour during the production of this book.

The author and publisher are grateful to the following copyright holders for granting permission to reproduce various extracts and figures in this book: Australian Institute of Health and Welfare for permission to reproduce figure from C. Mathers, T. Vos, and C. Stevenson, *The Burden of Disease and Injury: Summary Report*, Australian Institute of Health and Welfare, Canberra, 1999, p. 25, fig. 14; University of Queensland Press for permission to reproduce figure from D. Gordon, *Health, Sickness and Society*, University of Queensland Press, Brisbane, 1976, p. 186, fig. 19; Beacon Press for the extract from R. Hubbard and E. Wald, *Exploding the Gene Myth*, Beacon Press, Boston, 1993; Simon Kneebone for his kind permission to allow the use of his cartoon on p. 327. Every effort has been made to trace the original source of all material reproduced in this book. Where the attempt has been unsuccessful, the author and publisher would be pleased to hear from the copyright holder concerned to rectify any omission.

Contributors

Fran Baum is Head of Department and Professor of Public Health at Flinders University, Adelaide, and Foundation Director of the South Australian Community Health Research Unit. She is also Immediate Past National President of the Australian Public Health Association. She has eighteen years' experience of health-promotion research, planning, and evaluation. She has been involved with Australian Healthy Cities initiatives since their inception in the 1980s and regularly undertakes consultancies for the World Health Organisation on Healthy Cities projects in South East Asia and the Pacific region. Professor Baum has a PhD from the University of Nottingham. She has published more than a hundred articles, numerous reports, edited two books, and written one herself. Her publications relate to aspects of research and evaluation in community health, theories of health promotion, political economy of health, qualitative public health research, Healthy Cities, and more recently, social capital and health promotion. Her most recent book is a comprehensive textbook *The New Public Health: An Australian Perspective* (1998).

Helen Belcher is a lecturer in health sociology in the School of Social Sciences at the University of Newcastle. She has a background in nursing, and lectures nurses and health professionals. Her research interests include health policy and religion. She is currently undertaking PhD research on the topic 'Health Insurance and the Catholic Church: Mission or Politics?'.

Dorothy Broom is a senior fellow at the National Centre for Epidemiology and Population Health (NCEPH), Australian National University (ANU), where she is involved in research on inequalities in health, the relationship between work and family health, and gendering health. She also supervises PhD candidates who have diverse interests. She was formerly Convenor of Women's Studies at ANU, and is the author of a number of articles and books, including *Damned If We Do: Contradictions in Women's Health Care* (1991) and *Double Bind: Women Affected by Alcohol and Other Drugs* (1994). In 1993 she was named Canberra Woman of the Year for distinguished service to the Australian Capital Territory's women's movement and to women's health. In 1994 she was made a Member of the Order of Australia for services to women and women's health.

Gary Easthope is an associate professor in the School of Sociology and Social Work at the University of Tasmania. He has eclectic research interests and has published books, articles, and chapters on the topics of education, social research methods, ethnicity and health, disability, the wilderness movement, drug use, and heritage sailing as well as writing about alternative medicine both in a book (*Healers and Alternative Medicine*, 1986) and, more recently, in sociological and medical journals. He is a joint editor, with colleagues in Australia and England, of a book that looks at Complementary and Alternative Medicine (CAM) in the USA, Canada, England, Australia, and New Zealand to be published by Routledge in 2003.

Douglas Ezzy is a lecturer in sociology at the University of Tasmania. Doug's books include *Qualitative Research Methods: A Health Focus* (1999) with Pranee Rice, *Narrating Unemployment* (2002), and *Qualitative Analysis* (2002). His research is inspired by a desire to understand how people make meaning and find dignity in their lives. He has published articles on research methodology, unemployment and mental health, the meaning of work, living with HIV/AIDS, and contemporary witchcraft.

John Germov is a senior lecturer in sociology in the School of Social Sciences at the University of Newcastle. John is President of The Australian Sociological Association (TASA) and has been a member of its Executive Committee since 1995, establishing the TASA web site and e-mail discussion list. Recent books include: *Get Great Marks for Your Essays* (2000), and with Lauren Williams: *Surviving First Year Uni* (2001), *Get Great Information Fast* (1999), and *A Sociology of Food and Nutrition: The Social Appetite* (1999). His research interests include health policy, the professions, managerialism, sociology of management, education, sociology of food, gender and body image.

Dennis Gray is an associate professor at the National Drug Research Institute, Curtin University, where he manages the Indigenous Australian Research Program. As a researcher, consultant, and administrator, he has worked in the area of Aboriginal health for more than twenty years. With Sherry Saggers, he has co-written *Aboriginal Health and Society: The Traditional and Contemporary Struggle for Better Health* (1991) and *Dealing with Alcohol: Indigenous Usage in Australia, New Zealand and Canada* (1998).

Roberta Julian is a senior lecturer in the Department of Sociology at the University of Tasmania where she lectures on migrants in Australian society. Her research interests focus on the social construction of identity, gender, refugee settlement, and multiculturalism in the Australian context. She has jointly written (with Gary Easthope) two chapters in the area of health and ethnicity: 'Migrant Health' in Carol Grbich (ed.), *Health in Australia* (1999), and 'Mental Health and Ethnicity' in Michael Clinton and Sioban Nelson (eds), *Mental Health and Nursing Practice* (1996).

Deborah Lupton is a professor of sociology and cultural studies at Charles Sturt University. She has authored or co-authored several books on the sociocultural aspects of medicine and public health, including

Medicine as Culture (1994), *The Imperative of Health* (1995), *The New Public Health* (1996) (with Alan Petersen), and *Television, AIDS and Risk* (1997) (with John Tulloch). Her latest books are *Risk* (1999) and the edited volume *Risk and Sociocultural Theory: New Directions and Perspectives* (1999).

Katy Richmond is a senior lecturer in sociology at La Trobe University. She has written on women in employment, women and deviance, homosexuality in prisons, and women and health. Her current research is on Aboriginal women's health. She was a founding member of TASA's Women's Section and was president of the Association in 1991–92. Her teaching has been in the areas of work, gender, and the sociology of deviance and social control.

Sharyn L. Roach Anleu is an associate professor in the Department of Sociology at Flinders University, and immediate past president of the Australian Sociological Association. She is one of three editors of the *Journal of Sociology* and is the author of *Law and Social Change* (2000) and three editions of *Deviance, Conformity and Control* (1999). She recently collaborated with Kathy Mack on a national study of guilty plea negotiations in Australia, which has resulted in numerous publications. She has also published articles on the legal regulation of new reproductive technologies, women lawyers, and the legal profession. Sharyn and Kathy are currently engaged in a national study of magistrates and their courts in Australia.

Sherry Saggers is an associate professor in the School of International, Cultural and Community Studies, and Program Director, Institute for the Service Professions, Edith Cowan University. Her contributions have included work on Indigenous health and social life, women's work and childcare, and social evaluation. With Dennis Gray, she has published widely on Indigenous health, including *Aboriginal Health and Society: The Traditional and Contemporary Struggle for Better Health* (1991) and *Dealing with Alcohol: Indigenous Usage in Australia, New Zealand and Canada* (1998).

Maureen Strazzari is a lecturer in the School of Social Sciences at the University of Newcastle. Her research interests are reflected in chapter 12, on ageing, death, and dying. By and large, these interests emerged as a result of previously held positions in the Migrant Health Unit of the Hunter Area Health Service, firstly as Health Education Officer and then as Ethnic Aged Services Coordinator. Currently her research is focused on completing a PhD thesis on the subject of euthanasia.

Bryan Turner is a professor of sociology at the University of Cambridge. His research interests are in the sociology of citizenship with special reference to voluntary associations and social capital in Britain and Australia, the sociology of the body where he is conducting research (with Steven Wainwright) on injury and retirement among ballet dancers in the Royal Ballet Company, and the sociology of generations where he is doing research on postwar cultural change. He is the founding editor of three journals: *Citizenship Studies, Body & Society* (with Mike Featherstone), and *Journal of Classical Sociology* (with John O'Neill). His most recent publication, with Chris Rojek, is *Society & Culture: Principles of Scarcity and Solidarity* (2001).

Deidre Wicks is an honorary associate (formerly senior lecturer) in the School of Social Sciences at the University of Newcastle. Her research interests include work on gender and healing, vegetarianism, and an on-going involvement in the Women's Health Australia project, a longitudinal study on women's health. Her most recent publication is *Nurses and Doctors at Work: Rethinking Professional Boundaries* (1999).

Lauren Williams is a lecturer in the Bachelor of Health Science course in nutrition and dietetics at the University of Newcastle. She holds tertiary qualifications in science, dietetics, and social science. Her research interests include weight change at menopause and gendered dieting. Lauren is an accredited practising dietitian who stills works in private practice and who has also worked in the health system, predominantly in community and public health nutrition. She has been involved in the Dietitians Association of Australia, since 1986, serving as national vice-president in 1995–96.

Evan Willis is a professor of sociology and Head of Humanities and Social Sciences at the Albury/Wodonga Campus of La Trobe University. His research interests are in medical technology assessment, chronic illness and the quality of life, as well as the social consequences of increasing societal polarisation.

Abbreviations

ABS	Australian Bureau of Statistics
ACTU	Australian Council of Trade Unions
AGPS	Australian Government Publishing Service
AIDS	acquired immune deficiency syndrome
AIHW	Australian Institute of Health and Welfare
AMA	Australian Medical Association
ATR	Australian Torts Reports
ATSIC	Aboriginal and Torres Strait Islander Commission
BMA	British Medical Association
BRW	*Business Review Weekly*
DAA	Dietitians Association of Australia
DHFS	Department of Health and Family Services
DNA	deoxyribonucleic acid
DRS	Doctors Reform Society
DSM	*Diagnostic and Statistical Manual of Mental Disorders*
DSM-IV	Fourth edition of *Diagnostic and Statistical Manual of Mental Disorders*
EBM	evidence-based medicine
ECG	electrocardiogram
ELSI	ethical, legal, and social implications (of the Human Genome Project)
EPAC	Economic Planning and Advisory Council
GDP	gross domestic product
GP	general practitioner
HGH	human growth hormone
HGP	Human Genome Project
HIC	Health Issues Centre
HIV	human immunodeficiency virus
HMSO	Her Majesty's Stationery Office
IHP	individualist health promotion
IVF	*in vitro* fertilisation
MPH	Masters of Public Health
NACCHO	National Aboriginal Community Controlled Health Organisation
NAHS	National Aboriginal Health Strategy
NAMI	National Alliance for the Mentally Ill
NCEPH	National Centre for Epidemiology and Population Health
NDU	Nursing Development Unit
NEB	Nurses Education Board
NESB	non-English-speaking background

NHS	National Health Strategy (Australia) or National Health Service (United Kingdom)
OECD	Organization for Economic Cooperation and Development
OHS	occupational health and safety
PDA	Private Doctors Association
PDD	premenstrual dysphoric disorder
PMS	premenstrual syndrome
pni	psychoneuroimmunology
RAFI	Rural Advancement Foundation International
RCTs	randomised control trials
RSI	repetitive strain injury
SCHP	structuralist-collectivist health promotion
SDL	sexual division of labour
SES	socioeconomic status
TASA	The Australian Sociological Association
WHO	World Health Organization

Introduction

Health Sociology and the Social Model of Health

The health of the people is really the foundation upon which all their happiness and all their powers as a state depend.

Benjamin Disraeli

We live in a health-obsessed age. We are bombarded with messages from health authorities, health professionals, and fitness gurus to 'do this' and 'don't do that'. Everywhere we turn we are urged to take individual responsibility for our health. Yet amid this ruckus we hear very little about the social origins of disease or our social responsibility to address the living and working conditions that impact on our health—this is where a sociological second opinion can help.

It is often said that it is wise to get a second opinion. We seek second opinions about a whole range of things, but why do we need a second opinion about health and illness? What could sociology have to offer? And what is sociology anyway? This book sets out to answer these questions and show the relevance and importance of sociology to the study of health and illness. We all have a basic idea of what a medical opinion entails, even if we do not always fully understand it. A sociology of health and illness, or health sociology, offers a different perspective—a second opinion—by focusing on the social determinants that make us well or unwell.

At the heart of health sociology is a belief that many health problems have social origins. Therefore, the focus of health sociology is not on medical treatment or individual cures for health problems. Health sociology asks you to step outside the square, to look beyond medical opinions to the way society is organised. While individuals suffer ill-health and require health care, some of the causes and cures can often lie in the social context in which they live and work. Health, illness, and the health care system are by-products of the way a society is organised. This book shows you how the social, cultural, economic, and political features of society affect an individual's chance of health and illness.

This introductory part of the book provides an overview of health sociology: what it is, its major theoretical perspectives and the types of health research it draws upon. Specifically, the Introduction consists of three chapters:

* Chapter 1 examines the social determinants of health, highlights the limitations of medical approaches and introduces the social model of health. It also explains what is distinctive about the perspective of sociology and how it can be applied to explain health problems.
* Chapter 2 explores the main theoretical perspectives used in health sociology.
* Chapter 3 outlines some of the key issues and debates encountered by sociologists when researching health.

1

Imagining Health Problems as Social Issues

John Germov

Overview

* *What social patterns of health and illness exist?*
* *What is the social model of health and how does it differ from the medical model?*
* *What is sociology and how can it be used to understand health problems?*

This chapter introduces you to the sociological perspective and how it can be used to understand a wide range of health issues. While conventional approaches to health and illness focus on the biology and behaviour of individuals, health sociology focuses on the social determinants of health and illness such as the influence of living and working conditions. Health sociologists look for social patterns of illness, such as the different health statuses between women and men, the poor and the wealthy, or the Indigenous and White populations, and seek social, rather than biological or psychological, explanations. Throughout this chapter you are introduced to examples of how health and illness can be analysed sociologically by using a social model of health that views health problems as social issues.

Key terms

agency	gender/sex	social institutions
biological determinism	health promotion	social model of health
biomedical model	lifestyle choices	social structure
biopsychosocial model	new public health	sociological imagination
Cartesian dualism	public health	specific aetiology
class	'race'	state
ecological model	reductionism	structure/agency debate
epidemiology/social	risk factors	victim-blaming
epidemiology	social construction	
ethnicity	social Darwinism	

Introduction: the social context of health and illness

If we are ill we tend to seek medical opinions and treatments to make us well. When we think of health and illness it is difficult not to conjure up images of doctors in white coats and high-tech hospitals. Our personal experience of illness means that we tend to view it in an individualistic way—as a product of bad luck, poor lifestyle or genetic fate. As individuals we all want quick and effective cures when we are unwell and thus we turn to medicine to help. Yet this is only part of the story.

Health and illness is also a social experience. For example, even the highly individualised and very personal act of suicide occurs within a social context. In 1998, of the 2683 suicide-related deaths in Australia, more than 80% were male, with the highest rates occurring between the ages of 20 and 39 (AIHW 2000). In fact, the social patterning of suicide was first highlighted in the late nineteenth century by the sociologist Émile Durkheim (1858–1917). While Durkheim acknowledged individual reasons for a person committing suicide, he found that suicide rates varied between countries and between different social groups within a country. The social context of health and illness can be clearly seen when we compare the life-expectancy figures of various countries. As we all know, life expectancy in the least developed countries is significantly lower than that in industrially developed and comparatively wealthy countries such as Australia and the USA. For example, the average life expectancy of people living in the least developed countries of the world is approximately 52 years. This is 20 to 30 years less than that for developed countries such as Australia, which has an average life expectancy of 78 years (WHO 1998). As Table 1.1 shows, life expectancy varies among developed countries as well. Therefore, the living conditions of the country in which you live can have a significant influence on your chances of enjoying a long and healthy life.

By international standards, Australia ranks high on the life-expectancy scale. However, this is not due to any distinct biological advantage in the Australian gene pool, but is rather a reflection of our distinctive living and working conditions. We can make such a case for two basic reasons. First, life expectancy can change in a short period of time, and in fact it did increase for most countries during the twentieth century. For example, Australian life expectancy has increased by more than 20 years since 1910 (AIHW 2000), which is too short a timeframe for any genetic improvement to occur in a given population. Second, data compiled over decades of immigration shows that the health of migrants comes to reflect that of their host country over time, rather than their country of origin. The longer migrants live in their new country, the more their health mirrors that of the local population (Marmot 1999). While the average

Australian life-expectancy figure is comparatively high, it is important to distinguish between different social groups within Australia. Life expectancy figures are crude indicators of population health and actually mask significant health inequalities among social groups within a country. For example, in Australia those in the lowest socioeconomic group have the highest rates of illness and premature death, use preventative services less and have higher rates of illness-related behaviours such as smoking (AIHW 1999, 2000; NHS 1992). Furthermore, as Table 1.1 shows, Aboriginal Australians have a life expectancy almost 20 years less than that of White Australians. In fact, the current life expectancy of Aboriginal Australians is closer to that of 'Australians born at the beginning of the twentieth century' (AIHW 2000, p. 208).

Table 1.1 Life expectancy

Country	Life expectancy	
	Men	Women
Australia	75.9	81.5
Aboriginal Australians	56.9	61.7
Canada	75.2	81.2
France	73.9	81.9
Germany	73.3	79.8
Italy	74.3	80.7
Japan	77.0	83.6
Malaysia	69.3	74.1
New Zealand	73.4	79.1
Philippines	63.1	66.7
Russian Federation	58.3	71.7
Sweden	76.5	81.5
United Kingdom	74.3	79.5
USA	72.5	78.9

Source: Adapted from AIHW (2000); WHO (1999)

Health sociology concerns the study of such social patterns of health and illness. It provides a second opinion to the conventional medical view of illness derived from biological and psychological explanations, by exploring the social context of health and illness—the social, economic, cultural, and political features of society that influence why some groups of people get sicker and die sooner than others. To find answers to why health inequalities exist, we need to look beyond the individual and investigate the social origins of illness.

The social origins of illness: social medicine and public health

Recognition of the social origins of health and illness can be traced to the mid nineteenth century, with the development of 'social medicine' (coined by Jules Guérin in 1848) or what more commonly became known as **public health** (sometimes referred to as social

public health/public health infrastructure Public policies and infrastructure to prevent the onset and transmission of disease among the population, with a particular focus on sanitation and hygiene, such as clean air, water, and food, and immunisation. Public health infrastructure refers specifically to the buildings, installations, and equipment necessary to ensure healthy living conditions for communities and populations.

health or preventative medicine). At this time, infectious diseases such as cholera, typhus, smallpox, diphtheria, and tuberculosis were major killers for which there were no cures and little understanding of how they were transmitted. During the 1800s, a number of people such as Rene Villermé (1782–1863), Rudolph Virchow (1821–1902), John Snow (1813–58), Edwin Chadwick (1800–90), and Friedrich Engels (1820–95) established clear links between infectious diseases and poverty (Porter 1997; Rosen 1972).

Engels, Karl Marx's collaborator and patron, in *The Condition of the Working Class in England* (1958/1845), made a strong case for the links between disease and poor living and working conditions as an outcome of capitalist exploitation. He used the case of 'black lung', a preventable lung disease among miners, to make the point that 'the illness does not occur in those mines which are adequately ventilated. Many examples could be given of miners who moved from well-ventilated to badly ventilated mines and caught the disease. It is solely due to the colliery owners' greed for profit that this illness exists at all. If the coalowners would pay to have ventilation shafts installed the problem would not exist' (1958/1845, p. 281). Engels also noted the differences in the death rates between labourers and professionals, claiming that the squalid living conditions of the working **class** were primarily responsible for the disparity, stating that 'filth and stagnant pools in the working class quarters of the great cities have the most deleterious effects upon the health of the inhabitants' (1958/1845, p. 110).

In 1854, a cholera epidemic took place in Soho, London. John Snow, a medical doctor, documented cases on a city map and investigated all of the 93 deaths that had occurred within a well-defined geographical area. After interviewing residents he was able to establish that people infected with cholera had sourced their water from the same public water pump in Broad Street. Snow came to the conclusion that the water from the pump was the source of cholera, and at his insistence, the pump's handle was removed and the epidemic ceased (Snow 1936/1855; Rosen 1972; Porter 1997; McLeod 2000). This case is famous for being one of the earliest examples of the use of **epidemiology** to understand and prevent the spread of disease.

Virchow, often remembered in medical circles for his study of cellular biology, also made a clear case for the social basis of medicine, highlighting its preventative role when he claimed '[m]edicine is a social science, and politics nothing but medicine on a grand scale … if medicine is really to accomplish its great task, it must intervene in political and social life … The improvement of medicine would eventually prolong human life, but improvement of social conditions could achieve this result even more rapidly and successfully' (cited in Rosen 1972, p. 39 and Porter 1997, p. 415).

class (or social class) A position within a system of structured inequality based on the unequal distribution of power, wealth, income, and status. Class membership is determined by three characteristics: ownership and control of scarce economic resources; ownership of marketable skills and qualifications; and wage labour. People who share a social-class position typically share similar life chances.

epidemiology/ social epidemiology The statistical study of patterns of disease in the population. Originally focused on epidemics, or infectious diseases, it now covers non-infectious conditions such as stroke and cancer. Social epidemiology is a sub-field aligned with sociology that focuses on the social determinants of illness.

state A term used to describe a collection of institutions, including the parliament (government and Opposition political parties), the public-sector bureaucracy, the judiciary, the military, and the police.

Virchow was a significant advocate for public health care and argued that the **state** should act to redistribute social resources, particularly to improve access to adequate nutrition. Therefore, social medicine and the public health movement grew from recognition that the social environment played a significant role in the spread of disease (Porter 1997; Rosen 1972). In other words, the infectious diseases that afflicted individuals had social origins that necessitated social reforms to prevent their onset (see Waitzkin 1983 and Rosen 1972 for informative histories of social medicine and Porter 1997 for a very readable history of medicine in general).

In Britain, Chadwick was a key figure in the development of the first Public Health Act (1848) based on his 'sanitary idea'— that disease could be prevented through improved waste disposal and sewerage systems, particularly by removing cess pools of decomposing organic matter from densely populated areas, as well as the introduction of high-pressure flushing sewers, and food hygiene laws to protect against food adulteration. Public health legislation in Australia was first introduced in Victoria in 1854, largely mirroring the British Act, with other colonies following suit (Reynolds 1995). In Australia and elsewhere, public health approaches were resisted by many doctors who viewed them as unscientific and as potentially undermining the need for medical services (Porter 1997; Waitzkin 1983). Such views had some popularity given the dominant *laissez-faire* political philosophy of the time, which supported only minor state intervention in economic and public affairs. Nonetheless, investment in public health was made, perhaps because infectious disease knew no class barriers (that is, it was worth spending money on the poor to prevent the spread of disease to the rich!).

Despite the influence of social medicine and the success of public health measures, health care would develop in an entirely different direction. The insights of social medicine would be cast aside for almost a century as the new science of biomedicine gained ascendancy.

The rise of the biomedical model

In 1878 Louis Pasteur (1822–96) developed the germ theory of disease, whereby illness was caused by germs infecting organs of the human body: a model of disease that became the foundation of modern medicine. Robert Koch (1843–1910) refined this idea through the doctrine of 'specific aetiology' (meaning specific cause of disease) through 'Koch's postulates': a set of criteria for proving that specific bacteria caused a specific disease (Dubos 1959; Capra 1982). The central idea was that specific micro-

biomedicine/biomedical model
The conventional approach to medicine in Western societies. It diagnoses and explains illness as a malfunction of one of the body's biological mechanisms. The biomedical approach of most health services focuses on the treating of individuals, and generally ignores social, economic, and environmental factors.

organisms caused disease by entering the human body through air, water, food and insect bites (Porter 1997). This mono-causal model of disease, which came to be known as the medical or **biomedical model**, became the dominant medical paradigm by the early 1900s. While early discoveries led to the identification of many infectious diseases, there were few effective cures. However, one of the earliest applications of the scientific understanding of infectious disease was the promotion of hygiene and sterilisation procedures, particularly in surgical practice, to prevent infection through the transmission of bacteria (Capra 1982). Until the early 1900s, it had been common practice to operate on patients without a concern for hygiene or the proper cleaning and sterilisation of equipment, resulting in high rates of post-operative infection and death following surgery.

The biomedical model is based on the assumption that each disease or ailment has a specific cause that physically affects the human body in a uniform and predictable way, meaning that universal 'cures' for people are theoretically possible. It involves a mechanical view of the body as a machine made up of interrelated parts, such as the skeleton and circulatory system. The role of the doctor is akin to a body mechanic identifying and repairing the broken part/s (Capra 1982). Throughout the twentieth century medical research, training, and practice increasingly focused on attempts to identify and eliminate specific diseases in individuals, and thus moved away from the perspective of social medicine and its focus on the social origins of disease (Najman 1980).

Before the development of medical science, quasi-religious views of health and illness were dominant, whereby illness was connected with sin, penance and evil spirits. Therefore, the 'body as machine' metaphor represented a significant turning-point away from religious notions towards a secular view of the human body. Until this time, the dominant view was to conceive the body and soul as a sacred entity beyond the power of human intervention. However, the influence of scientific discoveries, particularly through autopsies that linked diseased organs with symptoms before death, as well as Pasteur's germ theory, eventually endorsed a belief in the separation of body and soul. In philosophical circles, this view came to be known as mind/body dualism and is sometimes referred to as **Cartesian dualism** after the philosopher René Descartes (1590–1650). Descartes, famous for the saying 'I think therefore I am', suggested that while the mind and body interacted with one another, they were separate entities. Therefore, the brain was part of the physical body while the mind (the basis of individuality) existed in the spiritual realm and was apparent evidence of a god-given soul. Such a distinction provided the philosophical justification for secular interventions on the physical

Cartesian dualism Also called mind/body dualism and named after the philosopher Descartes, it refers to a belief that the mind and body are separate entities. This assumption underpins medical approaches that view disease in physical terms and thus ignore the psychological and subjective aspects of illness.

body in the form of medical therapies. Since the body was merely a vessel for the immortal soul or spirit, medicine could rightly practise on the body while religion could focus on the soul (Capra 1982; Porter 1997). The assumption of mind/body dualism underpinned the biomedical model, whereby disease was seen as located in the physical body, and thus the mind, or mental state of a person, was considered unimportant.

The limits of medicine

While the biomedical model represented a significant advance in understanding disease and resulted in beneficial treatments, it has come under significant criticism from both within medicine and from a range of social and behavioural disciplines like sociology and psychology. The major criticism is that the biomedical model underestimates the complexity of health and illness, particularly by neglecting social and psychological factors. The range of criticisms made of the biomedical model can be grouped under the following terms and phrases and are discussed in turn below:

- the fallacy of specific aetiology
- objectification and medical scientism
- **reductionism** and **biological determinism**
- interventionist bias
- **victim–blaming**.

reductionism The belief that all illnesses can be explained and treated by reducing them to biological and pathological factors.

The idea of a specific cause for a specific disease, specific aetiology, only applies to a limited range of infectious diseases. As early as the 1950s, Rene Dubos (1959, p. 102) argued that 'most disease states are the indirect outcome of a constellation of circumstances rather than the direct result of single determinant factors'. Furthermore, Dubos noted that not all people exposed to an infectious disease contracted it. For example, we may all come into contact with someone suffering from a contagious condition like the flu, but only a few of us will get sick. Therefore, disease causation is more complex than the biomedical model implies and is likely to involve multiple factors such as physical condition, nutrition, and stress, which affect an individual's susceptibility to illness (Dubos 1959).

biological determinism The unproven belief that people's biology determines their social, economic, and health statuses.

victim-blaming The process whereby social inequality is explained in terms of individuals being solely responsible for what happens to them in relation to the choices they make and their assumed psychological, cultural, and/or biological inferiority.

The biomedical model, underpinned by mind/body dualism and a focus on repairing the 'broken' parts of the machine-like body, can lead to the objectification of patients. Since disease is viewed only in physical terms, as something that can be objectively observed, treating 'it' takes primacy over all other considerations, and patients may become objectified as 'diseased bodies' or 'cases' rather than treated as unique individuals with particular needs. This form of criticism often underpins claims of doctors' poor interpersonal and communication skills. Such a situation is also related to what Fritjov Capra (1982) calls 'medical scientism', that is, a reverence for scientific methods of measurement and observation as the most superior form of knowledge about understanding and treating disease. Therefore, patients' thoughts, feelings and subjective experiences of illness are considered 'unscientific' and are mostly dismissed.

A further criticism of medicine is its reductionism. The development of medical science has led to an increasing focus on smaller and smaller features of human biology for the cause and cure of disease—from organs to cells to molecules and most recently to genes. By reducing its focus on disease at the biological, cellular and genetic level, medicine has ignored or downplayed the social and psychological aspects of illness. In concentrating on the pathology within an individual body, the patient and their suffering is divorced from their social environment, and the disease treated as if it occurred in a social vacuum. Not only does this marginalise the importance of social support networks, it also ignores the role played by social factors such as poverty, poor working conditions and discrimination in affecting an individual's physical and mental health.

A related outcome of reductionism has been an ever-growing number of medical specialities, such as cardiologists (heart specialists) and ophthalmologists (eye specialists), based on the assumption that each body part and function can be treated almost in isolation from the others. Such an approach has fuelled the search for 'magic bullet' cures, resulting in huge expenditure on medical drugs, technology and surgery. It has also led to a curative and interventionist bias in medical care, often at the expense of prevention and non-medical alternatives.

Reductionism can also lead to biological determinism: a form of social Darwinism that assumes people's biology causes or determines their inferior social, economic, and health status. Biological determinism underpins most elitist, racist, and sexist beliefs. For example, some people argue that the poor are poor because they are born lazy and stupid. Such views have often been used to justify slavery and exploitation of Blacks, women, children, and workers in general; it is a very convenient 'explanation', particularly when those at the top of the social ladder espouse it. When people argue that social or health inequalities are biologically determined, the implication is that little can or should be done to change them. Although such beliefs have no scientific validity, they have not vanished from our society and can be found as the basis of so-called 'commonsense' views of the world.

A final criticism of the biomedical model is its tendency towards victim-blaming through the individualisation of health problems (Ryan 1971) because it locates the cause and cure of disease as solely within the individual. As Capra states, '[i]nstead of asking why an illness occurs, and trying to remove the conditions that lead to it, medical researchers try to understand the biological mechanisms through which the disease operates, so that they can then interfere with them' (1982, p. 150).

Therefore, the individual body becomes the focus of intervention, and health and illness become primarily viewed as an individual responsibility. A preoccupation with treating the individual has the potential to legitimate a victim-blaming approach to illness, either in the form of genetic fatalism (your poor health is the result of poor genetics) or as an outcome of poor **lifestyle choices**. By ignoring the social context of health and illness and locating primary responsibility for illness within the individual, there is little acknowledgment of social responsibility, that is, the need to ensure healthy living and working environments.

The critique of the biomedical model above has necessarily been a generalisation and does not imply that all doctors work from within the confines of this model. In fact, many of the criticisms of the model have come from those within the medical profession itself. While it is now widely accepted that the causes of illness are multi-factorial, it is still fair to claim that the biomedical model remains the dominant influence over medical training and practice to this day.

lifestyle choices/factors The decisions people make that are likely to impact on their health such as diet, exercise, smoking, alcohol, and other drugs. The term implies that people are solely responsible for choosing and changing their lifestyle.

Rediscovering the social origins of health and illness

Thomas McKeown (1976, 1979, 1988), a doctor and epidemiologist, was one of the earliest authors to expose the exaggerated role of medical treatment in improving population health. McKeown argued that the medical profession and governments had overestimated the influence of medical discoveries on improvements in life expectancy during the twentieth century. McKeown (1976, 1979) found that mortality (death) from most infectious diseases had declined before the development of effective medical treatments, meaning that improvements in life expectancy were not substantially due to medical intervention. Similar findings have been reported by McKinlay and McKinlay (1977) for the USA, and Gordon (1976) and Lawson (1991) in Australia. Figure 1.1 provides a graphic example of this, showing the declining rate of tuberculosis for Australia, which occurred before effective medical treatment. The same trend occurred in the UK and the USA in the period given. Graphs for most infectious diseases tell a similar story, aside from vaccination against smallpox and polio, indicating that the contribution of medicine to population-level improvements in life expectancy appear to have been minor.

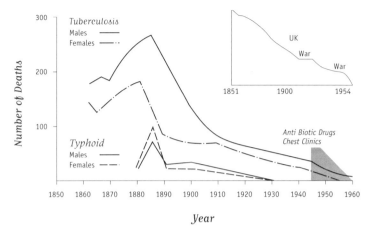

Figure 1.1 Decline in tuberculosis death rates for Australia

Source: Gordon (1976); after graph by H. Silverstone, Department of
Social and Preventive Medicine, University of Queensland.
Data from H. O. Lancaster and others.

McKeown (1979) suggests that the major reasons for the
increase in life expectancy were not due to medical treatments, but
rather to rising living standards, particularly improved nutrition,
which increased people's resistance to infectious disease. While
McKeown's work highlighted the importance of social, non-
medical interventions for improving population health, S. Szreter
(1988, p. 37) provides a more complex argument. He suggests that
rather than the '"invisible" hand of rising living standards', it was
the state's redistribution of economic resources that increased life
expectancy through improved working conditions and a range of
public health measures such as improved public housing, food
regulation, education, and sanitation reforms.

While it is impossible to determine the exact contribution of
public health measures, rising living standards, and medicine to
improving population health, the significance of McKeown's
work and subsequent findings has been to highlight the importance of addressing the social origins of health and illness. As
McKeown states, 'there is need for a shift in the balance of effort,
in recognition that improvement in health is likely to come in
future … from modification of the conditions which lead to disease, rather than from intervention in the mechanism of disease
after it has occurred' (1979, p. 198).

It is important to note that McKeown himself was not anti-
medicine, but wanted to reform medical practice so that it focused
on prevention of what he saw were the new threats to health:
'personal behaviour', as evidenced through smoking, alcohol consumption, drug taking, diet and lack of exercise. Therefore, he still
viewed health care in individualistic terms, by focusing preventative
efforts at the level of modifying the behaviour of individuals.

Lifestyle and risk: from risk-taking to risk-imposing factors

risk factors Conditions that are thought to increase an individual's susceptibility to illness or disease such as abuse of alcohol or smoking.

Since McKeown's work, there has been considerable growth in preventative efforts aimed at individuals, particularly in the form of identifying **risk factors** exhibited by individuals. While the notion of 'lifestyle diseases' or 'diseases of affluence' is a clear indication of the social origins of health and illness, many preventative efforts in the form of **health promotion** have tried to reform the individual rather than pursue wider social reform (ignoring the fact that diseases of affluence affect the least affluent much more). By solely targeting risk-taking individuals, there is a tendency to victim-blaming by ignoring the social determinants that give rise to risk-taking in the first place, such as stressful work environments, the marketing efforts of corporations, and peer group pressure (see chapter 10). As Michael Marmot (1999, p. 1) incisively puts it, there is a need to understand the 'causes of the causes'. In other words, rather than just focus on risk-taking individuals, there is also a need to address 'risk-imposing factors' and 'illness-generating social conditions' (Ratcliffe et al. 1984; Waitzkin 1983)—the social, cultural, economic, and political features of society that create unhealthy products, habits, and lifestyles.

health promotion Any combination of education and related organisational, economic, and political interventions designed to promote behavioural and environmental changes conducive to good health. This promotion may cover a variety of strategies, including legislation, health education, community development, advocacy, and so on. Health promotion has usually, however, been restricted to interventions focusing on the behavioural end of the spectrum.

There is no denying the significant role medicine has played in the treatment of illness, particularly in trauma medicine, palliative care, and general surgery, as well as the prevention of illness through immunisation. Thus the expertise of doctors lies in treating individuals once they are ill. Yet the reductionist focus of the biomedical model on individual pathology has obscured the social origins of illness. The World Health Organization effectively acknowledged this limitation of the model in 1946, when it included in its constitution the now-famous holistic definition of health as 'a state of complete physical, mental and social well-being and not merely the absence of disease or infirmity' (WHO 1946). This often-quoted definition implies that a range of biological, psychological, and social factors determine health. Furthermore, health is conceptualised as 'not merely the absence of disease', but rather in the positive sense of 'well-being'. While this definition has been criticised for its utopian and vague notion of 'complete well-being', it is of symbolic importance because it highlights the need for a broader approach to health than the biomedical model alone can deliver.

biopsychosocial model This model is an extension of the biomedical model. It is a multi-factorial model of illness that takes into account the biological, psychological, and social factors implicated in a patient's condition. Like the biomedical model, it focuses on the individual patient for diagnosis, explanation, and treatment.

ecological model A model of health, derived from the field of human ecology, that suggests that the environmental impacts of urban and rural settlements, including industry, technology, education, and culture, are linked to quality of life.

The widespread recognition of the biomedical model's limitations, from those within and outside the medical profession, have led to the development of a variety of multi-factorial models, such as the **biopsychosocial model** (Engel 1977, 1980; Cooper et al. 1996), web of causation (MacMahon & Pugh 1970), and the **ecological model** (Hancock 1985) (see Box 1.1). While these models represent a significant advance on the biomedical model in acknowledging the multiple and social determinants of health, to greater and lesser degrees they remain focused on health interventions aimed at the individual, particularly through lifestyle/behaviour modification and health education. It has been the **social model of health**, the most notable of which has been the **new public health** approach, that has substantially been responsible for highlighting the social determinants of health and proposing health interventions at the population and community level (Waitzkin 1983; Ashton and Seymour 1988; Baum 1998).

social model of health A model of health that focuses on social determinants such as the social production, distribution, and construction of health and illness, and the social organisation of health care. It directs attention to the prevention of illness through community participation and social reforms that address living and working conditions.

new public health A social model of health linking 'traditional' public health concerns, which focus on physical aspects of the environment (clean air and water, safe food, occupational safety through legislation), with the behavioural, social, and economic factors that affect people's health. The model is supported by a social movement that emphasises primary prevention, participation, and primary health care.

Box 1.1 Models of health

The number of health models that have been proposed by various authors from a range of disciplines is exhaustive. For this reason the models listed here are those most commonly found in the literature. Moreover, for the sake of simplicity and brevity, they are generalisations. There is also a vast array of 'alternative' models of health, such as acupuncture and homoeopathy, which are covered in detail in chapter 16.

Biomedical model

The biomedical model is the traditional approach to medicine in Western societies. Illness is diagnosed and explained as a malfunction of one of the body's biological systems. The model focuses on fixing these problems by treating individuals, particularly through surgery and drug therapy.

Biopsychosocial model

This model is an extension of the biomedical model. It is a multi-factorial model of illness that takes into account the biological, psychological, and social factors implicated in a patient's condition. Like the biomedical model, it focuses on the individual for diagnosis and treatment.

Web of causation

The web of causation approach is an epidemiological model of illness that views disease as the result of a complex web of interweaving risk factors between the agent (e.g. a virus), the host (the individual in which the disease manifests), and the environment (e.g. unhygienic living conditions). The model is derived from statistical studies of disease at the population level, which are used to identify risk factors to focus on prevention efforts aimed at the level of the individual.

Ecological model

The ecological model is derived from the broad field of human ecology, which studies the interrelationship of human interaction, social organisation, and the natural environment. It relates the quality of life to the development of ecological resources at a population level, in terms of addressing the environmental impact of urban and rural settlements, industry, technology, and culture.

New public health

A social model of health that links the 'traditional' public health concerns of sanitation, hygiene, and clean air and water, with the social, cultural, behavioural, and politico-economic factors that affect people's health. It directs attention to the prevention of illness through community participation and social reforms that address living and working conditions.

A sociological second opinion: the social model of health

The social model of health, sometimes referred to as the new public health approach, focuses attention on the societal level of health determinants and health intervention. The two terms are used interchangeably by some authors, but have different disciplinary origins, with the new public health approach arising from the health sciences (particularly public health), and the social model drawn primarily from the field of health sociology. Some new public health approaches arising from the health sciences have been criticised by sociologists for an over-reliance on individualistic solutions in practice (see Petersen & Lupton 1996; Lupton 1995; and chapter 10). However, there are significant examples of sociologically informed approaches that can make it problematical to draw distinctions between the two terms (see especially Baum 1998; Beaglehole & Bonita 1997). Nonetheless, for our purposes we will keep the distinction between the two and use the term the social model of health, as it better reflects the unique theories, research methods and modes of analysis of health sociology discussed in this book.

The social model of health has been used as a general umbrella term to refer to approaches that focus on the social determinants of health and illness (see Broom 1991; Gillespie & Gerhardt 1995). As Dorothy Broom (1991, p. 52) states, 'the social model locates people in social contexts, conceptualises the physical environment as socially organised, and understands ill health as a process of interaction between people and their environments.' It is one of the aims of this book to map out in more detail what a social model of health entails. Table 1.2 contrasts the key features of the biomedical model with the social model to highlight the different focus, assumptions, benefits, and limitations of each. It is important to emphasise that the social model does not deny

Table 1.2 A comparison of biomedical and social models of health: key characteristics

	Biomedical model	*Social model*
Focus	Individual focus: acute treatment of ill individuals	Societal focus: living and working conditions that affect health
	Clinical services, health education, immunisation	Public health infrastructure/legislation, social services, community action, equity/access issues
Assumptions	Health and illness are objective biological states	Health and illness are social constructions
	Individual responsibility for health	Social responsibility for health
Key indicators of illness	Individual pathology	Social inequality
	Hereditary factors, sex, age	Social groups: class, gender, 'race', ethnicity, age, occupation, unemployment
	Risk factors	Risk-imposing/illness-inducing factors
Causes of illness	Gene defects and micro-organisms (viruses, bacteria)	Political/economic factors: distribution of wealth/income/ power, poverty, level of social services
	Trauma (accidents)	Employment factors: employment and educational opportunities, stressful and dangerous work
	Risk-taking behaviour/lifestyle	Cultural factors (values, traditions), prejudice/ discrimination (racism, sexism, homophobia)

the existence of biological or psychological aspects of disease that manifest in individuals, or deny the need for medical treatment. Instead, it highlights that health and illness occur in a social context and that effective health interventions, particularly preventive efforts, need to move beyond the medical treatment of individuals. In exposing the social origins of illness, it necessarily implies that a greater balance between individual and social interventions is required, since the vast majority of health funding continues to be directed towards medical intervention. Therefore, the social model is not intended as a replacement for the biomedical model, but rather coexists alongside it.

The biomedical model focuses on the level of the individual for the cause and cure of disease by attempting to address pathology and/or modify behaviour, assuming the individual is solely responsible for their health. The social model assumes health is a social responsibility by examining the social determinants on individuals' health status and health-related behaviour. Therefore, while the biomedical model concentrates on treating disease and risk-taking among individuals, the social model focuses on societal factors that are risk-imposing or illness-inducing (for

gender/sex This term refers to the socially constructed categories of feminine and masculine (the cultural values that dictate how men and women should behave), as opposed to the categories of biological sex (female or male).

	Biomedical model	Social model
Intervention	Cure individuals via surgery and pharmaceuticals	Public policy
	Behaviour modification (non-smoking, exercise, diet)	State intervention to alleviate health and social inequalities
	Health education and immunisation	Community participation, advocacy and political lobbying
Goals	Cure disease, limit disability and reduce risk factors to prevent disease in individuals	Prevention of illness and reduction of health inequalities to aim for an equality of health outcomes
Benefits	Addresses disease and disability of individuals	Addresses the social determinants of health and illness
	Prevention of disease through immunisation	Highlights the need for preventative measures that often lie outside the scope of the health system
Criticisms	Disease focus leads to lack of preventive efforts	Utopian goal of equality leads to unfeasible prescriptions for social change
	Reductionist: ignores the complexity of health/illness	Over-emphasis on the harmful side effects of medical approaches
	Fails to take into account social origins of health/illness	Proposed solutions can be complex and difficult to implement in the short term
	Medical opinions can reinforce victim-blaming	Sociological opinions can under-estimate individual responsibility and psychological factors

ethnicity Sociologically, the term refers to a shared cultural background, which is a characteristic of all groups in society. As a policy term, it is used to identify migrants who share a culture that is markedly different from that of Anglo-Australians. In practice, it often refers only to migrants from non-English-speaking backgrounds (NESB migrants).

'race' A term without scientific basis that uses skin colour and facial features to describe allegedly biologically distinct groups of humans. It is a social construction that is used to categorise groups of people and usually infers assumed (and unproven) intellectual superiority or inferiority.

example, toxic pollution, stressful work, discrimination, peer pressure), and in particular highlights the health inequalities suffered by different social groups based on class, **gender**, **ethnicity**, **'race'**, and occupation, to name a few. What should be clear from the comparison offered in Table 1.2 is that health issues have a number of dimensions.

The social model logically implies that any attempts to improve the overall health of the community need to address overall living and working conditions such as poverty, employment opportunities, working conditions, and cultural differences. The social model gives equal priority to the prevention of illness along with the treatment of illness and aims to alleviate health inequalities. Such issues necessitate community participation and state interventions that include social services and public policies (such as workplace safety and pollution controls), which lie outside the strict confines of the health system or individuals' control. It must be acknowledged that this makes the interventions proposed by advocates of the social model more complex and difficult to achieve, given their broad thrust, long-term implications and need for intersectoral collaboration.

The three main dimensions of the social model of health

The social model arose as a critique of the limitations and misapplications of the biomedical model, such as its inability to effectively explain and address health inequalities experienced by various social groups (for example Indigenous groups and those in poverty). Sociological research and theorising that underpins the social model of health has comprised three main dimensions or themes that are reflected in the structure of this book:

1 **The social production and distribution of health and illness**: highlights that many illnesses from which individuals suffer are socially produced, that is, they are an outcome of certain living and working conditions. For example, illnesses arising from exposure to hazardous work practices are often beyond an individual's control and therefore need to be addressed at a societal level, such as through occupational health and safety legislation. Furthermore, there is an unequal social distribution of health, whereby some social groups suffer higher rates of morbidity and mortality. Therefore, a focus on the social production and distribution of health examines the role that living and working conditions can play in causing and alleviating illness.

2 **The social construction of health and illness**: refers to how definitions of health and illness can vary between cultures and change over time, whereby what is considered a disease in one culture or time period may be considered normal and healthy elsewhere and at other times. For example, homosexuality was once considered a psychiatric disorder despite the lack of scientific evidence of pathology. It is no longer medically defined as a disorder, but nonetheless is an example of how cultural beliefs, social practices and social institutions shape, or construct, the ways in which health and illness are understood. Therefore, notions of health and illness are not necessarily objective facts or static states, but can be **social constructions** that reflect the culture, politics and morality of a particular society at a given point in time.

social construction/ constructionism Refers to the socially created characteristics of human life based on the idea that people act-ively construct reality, meaning it is neither 'natural' nor inevitable. Therefore, notions of normality/abnormality, right/ wrong, and health/illness are subjective human creations that should not be taken for granted.

3 **The social organisation of health care**: concerns the way a particular society organises, funds and utilises its health services. A central focus of study has been the dominant role of the medical profession, which has significantly shaped health policy and health funding to benefit its own interests, largely to the detriment of nursing, allied, and alternative health practitioners. Unequal relationships between the health professions can prevent the efficient use of health resources and the optimal delivery of health care to patients.

How can sociology help? Using a sociological imagination

As individuals we are brought up to believe that we control our own destinies, especially our health. It is simply up to each individual to 'do what they wanna do and be what they wanna be'. However, this belief ignores the considerable influence of society. Sociology makes us aware that, individually, we cannot ignore the social conditions that influence our lives. We are social animals and are very much the product of our environment, from the way we dress to the way we interact with one another, we are all influenced by the **social structure**, or the way social life is organised. Social structure is a key sociological concept that refers to the social patterns or recurring arrangements that we experience in our daily lives (from cultural customs to **social institutions**). The idea of social structure serves to remind us of the social or human-created aspects of life, in contrast to purely random events or products of nature (López & Scott 2000). In other words, the social structure is a product of human action and interaction.

The social structure can be likened to the human skeleton. The various parts of the body—the muscles, heart, lungs, and other organs—need the frame of the skeleton to exist and function. If we think of society as having a skeleton that links its parts together, we begin to understand the concept of social structure. Figure 1.2 is a

social structure The recurring patterns of social interaction through which people are related to each other, such as social institutions and social groups.

social institutions Formal structures within society—such as health care, government, education, religion, and the media—that are organised to address identified social needs.

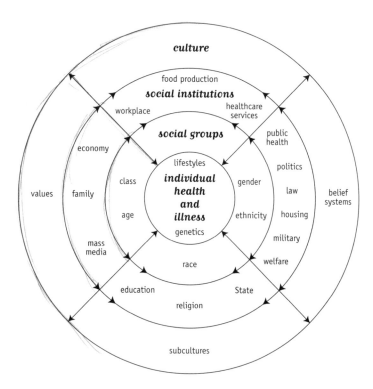

Figure 1.2 The social skeleton: the interplay of structure and agency

'social skeleton' and shows the basic features of the social structure of which we are all a part. It represents a way of conceptualising the key elements of how our society is organised or structured. The various parts of the social skeleton are interrelated (as the two-way arrows indicate). For example, the type of economy we have has influenced our culture and our political system. Religion, through marriage and the family, has significantly influenced the structure of our personal relationships. Therefore, understanding the structure of society enables us to examine the social influences on our personal behaviour and our interactions with others.

Social institutions (such as the media, health care, government, and education) are formal structures within society that are set up to address identified social needs. Social groups form as a result of the way that these social institutions are structured. For example, social classes emerge from the economic system; culture, laws, and education influence male and female roles, and attitudes to people who may look or act differently from the majority (Indigenous and ethnic groups, for example). Other social relationships also form, such as those between doctors and patients, teachers and students, parents and children, or employers and employees. While the social structure has a great influence on us all it is not fixed in one shape for eternity and recent history has shown it can be subject to significant change. The two-way arrows in Figure 1.2 are used to indicate that we exercise **agency** in our daily lives and in doing so can influence the way society is structured. The interplay between structure and agency along the various layers of the social skeleton are the subject matter of sociology.

agency The ability of people, individually and collectively, to influence their own lives and the society in which they live.

Is society to blame? Introducing the structure/agency debate

To what extent are we products of society? How much influence do we have over our lives? Are we solely responsible for our actions or is society to blame? These questions represent a key debate in sociology, often referred to as the **structure/agency debate**. There is no simple resolution to this debate, but it is helpful to view structure and agency as interdependent, that is, humans shape and are simultaneously shaped by society. In this sense, structure and agency are not 'either/or' propositions in the form of a choice between constraint and freedom, but are part of the interdependent processes of social life. Therefore, the social structure should not automatically be viewed in a negative way, as only serving to constrain human freedom, since in many ways the social structure enables us to live, by providing health care, welfare, education, and work. As Charles Wright Mills (1916–62) maintained, an individual 'contributes, however minutely, to the shaping of this society and to the course of its history, even as he is made by society and by its historical push and shove' (1959, p. 6). What

structure/agency debate A key debate in sociology over the extent to which human behaviour is determined by social structure.

is particularly interesting in this quote, is that Mills was clearly a product of the 'historical push and shove' of his social structure, as he uses the masculine 'he' to refer to both men and women—a usage now seen as dated and sexist.

Peter Berger long ago warned against depicting people as 'puppets jumping about on the ends of their invisible strings' (1966, p. 140). If we use the 'all the world's a stage and we are mere actors' analogy, we could liken life to a theatre in which we all play our assigned roles (father, mother, child, labourer, teacher, student, and so on). Whether it is how we are dressed as we walk down the street or how we present ourselves at a funeral, customs and traditions dictate expected modes of behaviour. In this sense we are all actors on a stage. Yet we have the scope to consciously participate in what we do. We can make choices about whether simply to act, or whether to modify or change our roles and even the stage on which we live our lives.

Although we are born into a world not of our making and in countless ways our actions and thoughts are shaped by our social environment, we are not simply 'puppets on strings'. Humans are sentient beings, that is, we are self-aware and thus have the capacity to think and act individually and collectively to change the society into which we are born. Structure and agency may be in tension, but they are interdependent, that is, one cannot exist without the other. Sociology is the study of the relationship between the individual and society; it examines how human behaviour both shapes and is shaped by society, or how 'we create society at the same time as we are created by it' (Giddens 1986, p. 11).

The sociological imagination: a template for doing sociological analysis

What is distinctive about the sociological perspective? In what ways does it uncover the social structure that we often take for granted? How is sociological analysis done? The American sociologist C. Wright Mills answered such questions by using the phrase the '**sociological imagination**' to describe the distinctive feature of the sociological perspective. The sociological imagination is 'a quality of mind that seems most dramatically to promise an understanding of the intimate realities of ourselves in connection with larger social realities' (Mills 1959, p. 15). According to Mills, the essential aspect of thinking sociologically, or seeing the world through a sociological imagination, is making a link between 'private troubles' and 'public issues'.

As individuals, we may experience personal troubles without realising they are shared by other people as well. If certain problems are shared by groups of people, they may have a common cause and be best dealt with through some form of social, or collective, action.

sociological imagination A term coined by Charles Wright Mills to describe the sociological approach to analysing issues. We see the world through a sociological imagination, or think sociologically, when we make a link between personal troubles and public issues.

In the late 1960s the phrase 'the personal is political' became popular in the women's liberation movement. The phrase encapsulates
the sociological imagination by linking women's personal experiences to wider social and political issues. For example, issues of
sexism, discrimination, domestic violence, and access to childcare
and contraception were traditionally regarded as 'personal troubles'
and often considered taboo topics not fit for public discussion, leaving many women to suffer individually in silence. However, these
personal problems were, and in some cases continue to be, shared
by many women and can only be addressed through public debate
and social reforms, such as equal pay, sex discrimination legislation,
and equal-opportunity policies. As Mills (1959, p. 226) states, 'many
personal troubles cannot be solved merely as troubles, but must
be understood in terms of public issues ... public issues must be
revealed by relating them to personal troubles.'

The Australian sociologist Evan Willis (1999) suggests that the
sociological imagination consists of four interrelated parts: historical, cultural, structural and critical. This four-part sociological
imagination template is an effective way to understand how to
think and analyse in a sociological way. The four parts of the
sociological imagination template are:

1   historical factors: how the past influences the present
2   cultural factors: how our culture impacts on our lives
3   structural factors: how particular forms of social organisation
    shape our lives
4   critical factors: how we can improve on what exists.

Figure 1.3 represents the sociological imagination template as
a diagram that is easy to remember. Anytime you want to sociologically analyse a topic, simply picture this diagram in your mind.

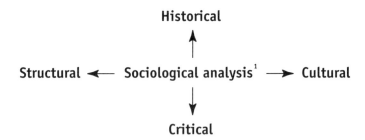

Figure 1.3 The sociological imagination template

Sociological analysis involves applying these four aspects to
the issues or problems under investigation. For example, a sociological analysis of why manual labourers have a shorter life

---

1   Derived from Willis 1999.

expectancy would examine how and why the work done by manual labourers affects their health by investigating:

1 historical factors: to understand why manual workplaces are so dangerous
2 cultural factors: such as the cultural value of individual responsibility
3 structural factors: such as the way work is organised, the role of managerial authority, the rights of workers, and the role of the state
4 critical factors: such as alternatives to the status quo (increasing the effectiveness of occupational health and safety legislation, for instance).

By using the four parts of the sociological imagination template, you begin to 'do' sociological analysis. It is worth highlighting at this point that the template simplifies the process of sociological analysis. When analysing particular topics, it is more than likely that you will find that the parts overlap with one another, making them less clear-cut than the template implies. It is also probable that for some topics, parts of the template will be more relevant and prominent than others—this is all to be expected. The benefit of the template is that it serves as a reminder of the sorts of issues and questions a budding sociologist should be asking. In fact it is the intention of the structure and content of this book to apply the sociological imagination to the key dimensions of the social model of health outlined earlier. To help develop your own sociological imagination further, attempt the exercise in Box 1.2.

Box 1.2 Developing your sociological imagination: a sociological autobiography

Apply the four parts of the sociological imagination template to explain the person you have become. In other words, write a short sociological autobiography by briefly noting the various things that have influenced you directly or indirectly in terms of what you believe and how you behave.

- **Historical factors**: how has your family background, or key past events and experiences, shaped the person you are?
- **Cultural factors**: what role have cultural background, traditions and belief systems played in forming your opinions and influencing your behaviour?
- **Structural factors**: how have various social institutions influenced you?

> • **Critical factors**: have your values and opinions about what you consider important changed over time? Why/why not?
> What insights can you make from this autobiographical application of the sociological imagination?

Conclusion

Question: What do you get when you cross a sociologist with a member of the Mafia?

Answer: An offer you can't understand.

Giddens 1996, p. 1

A common accusation made of sociology is that it is just common-sense dressed up in unnecessary jargon. The subject matter of sociology is familiar, and as members of society it is easy to think we should all be experts on the subject. It is this familiarity that breeds suspicion and sometimes contempt. All disciplines have specialist concepts to help classify their subject matter and sociology is no different. Sociological concepts, such as those you have been introduced to in this chapter, are used to impose a sense of intellectual order on the complexities of social life; they are a form of academic shorthand to summarise a complex idea in a word or phrase.

As this chapter has shown, to understand the complexity of health and illness, we need to move beyond biomedical approaches and incorporate a social model of health. Sociology enables us to understand the links between our individual experiences and the social context in which we live, work and play. With a sociological imagination, seeing health problems as social issues can be a healthy way of opening up debate on a range of topics previously undiscussed.

Summary of main points

- Much of health sociology has arisen as a critique of the dominance of the medical profession and its biomedical model.
- Health sociology examines social patterns of health and illness, particularly various forms of health inequality, and seeks to explain them by examining the influence of society. When groups of people experience similar health problems, there are likely to be social origins that require social action to address them.
- Health sociology challenges individualistic and biological explanations of health and illness through a social model of health

that involves three key dimensions: the social production and distribution of health, the social construction of health and the social organisation of health care.

- The sociological imagination, or sociological analysis, involves four interrelated features—historical, cultural, structural, and critical—which can be applied to understand health problems as social issues.

Discussion questions

1 Why did the insights of social medicine/public health approaches have such a limited influence over the development of modern medicine? What have been some of the consequences of the dominance of biological explanations for our understanding of health and illness?

2 What are the key features of the biomedical model? What are the advantages and limitations of the model?

3 What are the key features of the social model? What are the advantages and limitations of the model?

4 In what ways is illness a product of the social structure? Refer to the 'social skeleton' in Figure 1.2 and give examples in your answer.

5 In 1946, the World Health Organization defined health as 'a state of complete physical, mental and social well-being and not merely the absence of disease or infirmity'. Why might some groups regard this definition as 'radical' and utopian? Who might these groups be? What do you think of the definition?

6 Choose a health problem of interest to you and apply the socio-logical imagination template by briefly noting any key points that come to mind under the four parts of the template.

Further investigation

1 Why has the biomedical model been the dominant influence on our understanding and treatment of health problems?

2 If illness is not simply a matter of bad luck, bad judgment or bad biology, in what ways can a sociological imagination help us to understand the social origins of illness?

Further reading and web resources

General introductions to sociology

Beilharz, P. & Hogan, T. (eds) 2002, *Social Self, Global Culture: An Introduction to Sociological Ideas*, 2nd edn, Oxford University Press, Melbourne.

Bessant, J. & Watts, R. 2002, *Sociology Australia*, 2nd edn, Allen & Unwin, Sydney.

Jureidini, R. & Poole, M. (eds) 2000, *Sociology: Australian Connections*, 2nd edn, Allen & Unwin, Sydney.

Najman, J. M. & Western, J. S. (eds) 2000, *A Sociology of Australian Society*, 3rd edn, Macmillan, Melbourne.

van Krieken, R., Smith, P., Habibis, D., McDonald, K., Haralambos, M., & Holborn, M. 2000, *Sociology: Themes and Perspectives*, 2nd Australian edn, Longman, Sydney.

Willis, E. 1999, *The Sociological Quest*, 3rd edn, Allen & Unwin, Sydney.

Introductions to health sociology

Clarke, A. 2001, *The Sociology of Healthcare*, Prentice-Hall, Essex.

Freund, P. E. S. & McGuire, M. B. 1999, *Health, Illness, and the Social Body: A Critical Sociology*, 3rd edn, Prentice Hall, Englewood Cliffs, NJ.

George, J. & Davis, A. 1998, *States of Health: Health and Illness in Australia*, 3rd edn, Addison Wesley Longman, Melbourne.

Grbich, C. (ed.) 1999, *Health in Australia: Sociological Concepts and Issues*, 2nd edn, Longman, Sydney.

Lupton, G. M. & Najman, J. M. (eds) 1995, *Sociology of Health and Illness: Australian Readings*, 2nd edn, Macmillan, Melbourne.

Advanced readings

Albrecht, G. L., Fitzpatrick, R., & Scrimshaw, S. C. (eds) 2000, *Handbook of Social Studies in Health and Medicine*, Sage, London.

Annandale, E. 1998, *The Sociology of Health and Medicine: A Critical Introduction*, Polity Press, Cambridge.

Berger, P. & Luckmann, T. 1967, *The Social Construction of Reality*, Penguin, Harmondsworth.

Berkman, L. F. & Kawachi, I. (eds) 2000, *Social Epidemiology*, Oxford University Press, New York.

Bird, C., Conrad, P., & Fremont, A. M. (eds) 2000, *Handbook of Medical Sociology*, 5th edn, Prentice Hall, New Jersey.

Capra, F. 1982, *The Turning Point: Science, Society and the Rising Culture*, Simon & Schuster, Great Britain.

Charmaz, K. & Paterniti, D. A. (eds) 1999, *Health, Illness and Healing: Society, Social Context and Self—An Anthology*, Roxbury Publishing, Los Angeles.

Cockerham, W. C., Glasser, M., & Heuser, L. S. (eds) 1998, *Readings in Medical Sociology*, Prentice Hall, New Jersey.

Davey, B., Gray, A., & Seale, C. (eds) 2001, *Health and Disease: A Reader*, 3rd edn, Open University Press, Buckingham.

Eckersley, R., Dixon, J., & Douglas, J. (eds) 2001, *The Social Origins of Health and Well-being*, Cambridge University Press, Melbourne.

Heller, T., Muston, R., Sidell, M., & Lloyd, C. (eds) 2001, *Working for Health*, Open University Press/Sage, London.

Marmot, M. & Wilkinson, R. G. (eds) 1999, *Social Determinants of Health*, Oxford University Press, Oxford.

Najman, J. 1980, 'Theories of disease causation and the concept of general susceptibility', *Social Science & Medicine*, vol. 14A, pp. 231–7.

Petersen, A. & Waddell, C. (eds) 1998, *Health Matters*, Allen & Unwin, Sydney.

Scambler, G. 2002, *Health and Social Change: A Critical Theory*, Open University Press, Buckingham.

Scambler, G. & Higgs, P. (eds) 1998, *Modernity, Medicine and Health*, Routledge, London.

Turner, B. 1995, *Medical Power and Social Knowledge*, 2nd edn, Sage, L.

White, K. 1991, 'The sociology of health and illness: A trend report', *Cn.*
　　Sociology, vol. 39, no. 2, pp. 1–115.

White, K. 2001, *An Introduction to the Sociology of Health and Illness*, Sage,
　　London.

Web sites

Second Opinion web site:
　　<www.oup.com.au/cws/germov>
Australian Institute of Health & Welfare: <www.aihw.gov.au>
ESocHealth—Health Section of The Australian Sociological Association:
　　<www-sph.health.latrobe.edu.au>
Medical Sociology Group of the British Sociological Association:
　　<www.britsoc.org.uk/about/medsoc.htm>
Medical Sociology Section of the American Sociological Association:
　　<www.kent.edu/sociology/asamedsoc/>
Public Health Virtual Library: <www.ldb.org/vl/index.htm>
A Social Health Atlas of Australia: <www.publichealth.gov.au/atlas.htm>
Society for Social Medicine: <www.socsocmed.org.uk>
World Health Organization: <www.who.org>

2

Theorising Health

Major Theoretical Perspectives in Health Sociology

John Germov

Overview

* *What is theory?*
* *Why is theory necessary?*
* *What are the main theoretical approaches in health sociology?*

This chapter provides an overview of the main theoretical perspectives in health sociology: functionalism, Marxism, feminism, Weberianism, symbolic interactionism and post-structuralism/postmodernism. It draws out the key features, assumptions, and concepts of these different theoretical approaches. The chapter aims to provide an appreciation of what theory is and the reasons why it is important. Differences between theoretical perspectives are discussed, particularly with reference to the structure/agency debate and the different questions addressed by various perspectives. The chapter ends with a plea for theoretical pluralism and a caution against confusing perspectives with specific theories.

Key terms

agency	ideal type	social construction
biological determinism	McDonaldisation	social control
biomedical model	medical-industrial complex	social structure
capitalism	meta-narratives	socialism/communism
class	patriarchy	sociological imagination
commodification of health care	pluralism	stigma
deviance	rationalisation	structure/agency debate
emotional labour	sexual division of labour	theory
feminism	sick role	total institutions
functional prerequisites	socialisation	women's health movement
gender	social closure	

Introduction: what is theory and why do we need it?

theory A system of ideas that uses researched evidence to explain certain events and to show why certain facts are related.

A **theory** is an explanation of how things work and why things happen. Theories allow us to make sense of our world—they provide answers to the 'how' and 'why' questions of life—by showing the way certain facts are connected to one another. We often think of theory as somehow divorced from reality, but we actually make use of theories every day of our lives. For example, when some people suggest that violence on television or in the lyrics of popular music may lead to increased acts of violence in the wider community, they are espousing a theory of why things happen.

It is not uncommon to hear people espouse their everyday opinions or theories for the differences between women and men, rich and poor, black and white, heterosexuals and homosexuals, to name but a few. Such theories can influence how people relate to one another, how tolerant they are of others, and whether they support social policies and laws aimed at addressing various forms of discrimination and inequality. So, rightly or wrongly, people have opinions or theories about how and why social life is the way it is.

Perhaps it is because of our familiarity with the subject matter of sociology—the study of social life and human behaviour—that it is not unusual to be a little sceptical of sociological theories. Whereas many of us don't understand the theories of chemistry and physics, we tend to accept them because they often have practical applications such as medicinal drugs and technologies. Yet at first glance sociological theories (or social theories for short) appear to be impractical and seem to overly complicate a world we already know much about (Craib 1992). Everyday opinions such as those noted above, however, are usually based on little detailed evidence and unacknowledged prejudices. What sets social theories apart from everyday opinions is that they attempt to explain social life by presenting a logical, detailed, and coherent account derived from systematically researched evidence.

Theoretical perspectives in health sociology: an overview

> The Answer to the Great Question Of … Life, the Universe and Everything … Is … Forty-two.
>
> Adams 1979, p. 135

As the above quote from *The Hitch-Hiker's Guide to the Galaxy* implies, the search for a 'theory of everything' is likely to be a futile task. Even if we could construct a theory that explains every imaginable event, issue, or action, would its complexity mean we could never really understand it? A theory attempts to simplify reality and generalise its common and related features relevant to the topic at hand. The sheer variety of social life and the diversity of human behaviour mean that there is no single sociological 'theory of everything'. As Fritjov Capra puts it, '[a]ll scientific theories are approximations to the true nature of reality ... each theory is valid for a certain range of phenomena. Beyond this range it no longer gives a satisfactory description of nature, and new theories have to be found to replace the old one, or, rather, to extend it by improving the approximation' (1982, p. 93).

As you read the chapters of this book and consult the wider literature, you will quickly become aware that there are many different and sometimes opposing social theories on a topic. While the **sociological imagination** outlined in chapter 1 is the core of a sociological approach, there are significant differences of opinion over how to put it into practice. Over the years, many social theories have been developed and advocated by sociologists, making it frustrating for those new to sociology to steer a course through the maze of theories that exist. One way to navigate through this theory maze is to start by grouping them into the following six main theoretical perspectives or frameworks:

sociological imagination A term coined by Charles Wright Mills to describe the sociological approach to analysing issues. We see the world through a sociological imagination, or think sociologically, when we make a link between personal troubles and public issues.

- structural functionalism
- Marxism
- Weberianism
- symbolic interactionism
- feminism
- post-structuralism/postmodernism.

Theoretical perspectives are a form of shorthand to group similar theories of society together. Within each perspective there exist many individual theories developed by different writers, but they all tend to share the core features of the particular perspective. Any attempt to group theories in this way necessarily involves simplification by focusing on the similarities within the one perspective, at the expense of the differences between specific theories. For example, many Marxist theorists today would disagree with some of Karl Marx's ideas, but they would nonetheless still share the core assumptions and principles of a Marxist perspective.

One of the main distinctions between perspectives is the purpose or the questions they address. For example, some authors are concerned with explaining social order, others with explaining social inequality, and others with understanding and promoting social change. While these concerns often overlap, they have caused considerable debate among sociologists about the appropriate uses of sociological knowledge. Some perspectives, such as functionalism, attempt to understand society as it currently exists and do not take part in advocating how social life ought to be.

Other perspectives seek to use sociological knowledge to promote social change. For example, Marxist and feminist perspectives propose alternatives to present social arrangements to overcome social and economic inequalities.

Another distinction between theoretical perspectives is the level of analysis in relation to the **structure/agency debate**. Whereas we can imagine that the natural world exists without our presence, it is difficult to imagine that a society could exist without humans (Giddens 1997). Therefore, humans collectively 'make' society through their daily social interactions and through the social institutions they create, support, reproduce, and reform. It is this interplay between **social structure** and human **agency** that sociologists seek to understand, by exploring how people are shaped by, or shape, social life in particular circumstances. Despite this, there is continuing disagreement among sociologists over the extent to which individuals are shaped or can shape the social structure. Some theoretical perspectives lean more towards the structure side of the debate and others more to the agency side.

As Figure 2.1 shows, sociological perspectives can be depicted along a structure–agency continuum, with structuralist approaches at one end and agency approaches at the other. Structuralist approaches assume that social structures like the economic and political system shape individual and group behaviour, that is, that they determine the type of person you are: how you think, feel, and act, as well as your chances of health, wealth, and happiness. Agency approaches maintain that society is fundamentally the product of individuals acting socially or collectively to make the society in which they live. These perspectives focus on small-scale aspects of social interaction, such as that which occurs in a classroom between a teacher and students or between health professionals and patients, rather than focusing on the education or health system as a whole.

structure/agency debate A key debate in sociology over the extent to which human behaviour is determined by social structure.

social structure The recurring patterns of social interaction through which people are related to each other, such as social institutions and social groups.

agency The ability of people, individually and collectively, to influence their own lives and the society in which they live.

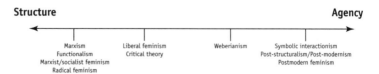

Figure 2.1 Theoretical perspectives along the structure–agency continuum

For our purposes here it is important to realise that most sociological theories fall between these two extremes. Few authors writing within any of the perspectives completely deny the roles that social structure or individuals play in any given social situation; nevertheless a bias to one side of the continuum is usually displayed.

Key features of major theoretical perspectives

Table 2.1 summarises the key features of the major theoretical perspectives in health sociology and how they apply to health issues 'at a glance'. Greater detail on each perspective is provided in the remainder of the chapter.

Table 2.1 The major theoretical perspectives in health sociology

Theoretical perspective	Key theorists	Key concepts	Focus of analysis	Health example
Structural functionalism	Émile Durkheim Talcott Parsons Robert Merton Jeffrey Alexander	value consensus functional prerequisites sick role	Structuralist focus: shows how various parts of society function to maintain social order	The 'sick role' (social expectations of how doctors and patients should behave) exposes the management of illness as a social experience
Marxism	Karl Marx Friedrich Engels Vincente Navarro Howard Waitzkin Lesley Doyal Bob Connell	class conflict capitalism medical-industrial complex commodification of health care	Structuralist focus: shows how the unequal distribution of scarce resources in a capitalist society is based on class division and highlights 'who benefits' and who is disadvantaged	Analyses the links between class and health status, and between class, medical power, and profit-maximisation
Weberianism	Max Weber George Ritzer Magali Larson Anne Witz Bryan Turner	bureaucracy ideal type rationalisation McDonaldisation	Combines a primary focus on agency, with structuralist tendencies: shows how the increasing regulation of social life takes place and may stifle human creativity; also explains the multiple forms of social inequality and social conflict	Examines how health professionals are increasingly subject to regulation and managerial control, producing greater efficiency and uniformity in health care delivery, but potentially decreasing the effectiveness of patient care
Symbolic interactionism	George H. Mead Erving Goffman Herbert Blumer Howard S. Becker Anselm Strauss	the self labelling theory stigma total institutions negotiated order	Agency focused: emphasises how individual and small-group interaction construct social meaning in everyday settings to	Uncovers how and why certain forms of behaviour are treated as deviance, exposing the stigma, negative

continued

Theoretical perspective	Key theorists	Key concepts	Focus of analysis	Health example
Symbolic interactionism			construct and change social patterns of behaviour	consequences, and biased treatment of social groups whose behaviour is deemed 'abnormal' (e.g. homosexuality)
Feminism	Germaine Greer Ann Oakley Sylvia Walby Naomi Wolf Susan Bordo	patriarchy gender sexual division of labour	Consists of a range of strands that are either structuralist or agency focused; seeks to explain and address the unequal position of women in society	Exposes sexism, biological determinism, and gender inequality in health research, theory, and treatment
Post-structuralism/ Post-modernism	Michel Foucault David Armstrong Nicholas Fox Rosemary Pringle Elizabeth Grosz	discourse panopticon bio-power power-knowledge surveillance	Agency focused: critiques theories based on universal truths and structuralist assumptions; concentrates on subjectivity, diversity, and fragmentation	Examines how certain discourses of normality and panoptic effects serve to discipline and control various social groups

Functionalism (or structural functionalism)

Émile Durkheim (1858–1917), Talcott Parsons (1902–79), and Robert Merton (1910–) are the key theorists of structural functionalism, which is more commonly known simply as functionalism. Popular in the USA, this perspective studies the way social structures function to maintain social order and stability. Functionalism focuses on large-scale social processes and is based on the assumption that a society is a system of integrated parts, each of which have certain 'needs' (or **functional prerequisites**) that must be fulfilled for social order to be maintained. Hence, functionalists study various parts of society to understand how they interrelate and function to promote social stability.

Functionalism is sometimes referred to as 'consensus theory' because of its concentration on how social order is reached and maintained in society. In viewing society as a social system of related parts, functionalism has been particularly influential in organisational studies and public policy analysis, where it is often referred to as 'systems theory'. For example, it is not uncommon to find descriptions of the health system as consisting of inputs, outputs, processes, and roles (for a contemporary example, see Duckett 2000). While such an approach can be useful for describing the basic operation of the health system, it neglects the influence of political and economic interests, power struggles

functional prerequisites
A debated concept based on the assumption that all societies require certain functions to be performed for them to survive and maintain social order. Also known as functional imperatives.

based on professional rivalries, and personality clashes, all of which make the health system less consensual, ordered, or 'systematic' than a functionalist perspective would depict. Critics of functionalism also highlight its conservative tendencies (due to its focus on social stability and consensus) and hence its difficulties in accounting for social conflict and social change (Ritzer 1996). Since the 1980s, some theorists such as Jeffrey Alexander (1947–) have attempted to address many of these criticisms through the development of the perspective of 'neo-functionalism' (see Alexander 1985, 1998).

The functionalist analysis of health care has been primarily influenced by the work of Parsons (1951), who viewed the health of individuals as a necessary condition of a stable and ordered society. He conceptualised illness as a form of **deviance**, that is, he viewed it as stopping people from performing various social roles, such as paid work and caring for children, which were essential to the functioning of society. In Parsons's terms, 'health is intimately involved in the functional pre-requisites of the social system … too low a general level of health, too high an incidence of illness, is dysfunctional … because illness incapacitates the effective performance of social roles' (1951, p. 430).

For Parsons, illness disrupted the normal functioning of society, and thus it was important that the sick were encouraged to seek expert help, so that they returned to health and could perform their social roles. This was achieved through the **sick role**, that is, the social expectations that dictated how an individual sick person was meant to act and be treated.

According to Parsons, the sick role involves a series of rights and responsibilities. Once sick, it is the right of individuals to be exempted from their normal social roles such as those of the parent, employee or student. This exemption from performing their duties is legitimated by medical diagnosis and treatment. For example, students regularly have to provide medical certificates to support their case for not performing their student roles of turning up to class or submitting work on time(!). A further right of the sick person is that since illness is generally beyond an individual's control, they are not held personally responsible and should be able to rely on others to care for them while they are ill. However, the sick person also has certain responsibilities. For example, they are expected to seek medical assistance and comply with the recommended treatment. Moreover, they are obliged to recover and resume their normal social duties.

The 'sick role' concept directs attention to the social nature of the illness experience and focuses attention on the doctor–patient relationship. However, the importance of the concept also lies in the many critiques it has inspired as a result of its limited application to

deviance Behaviour or activities that violate social expectations about what is normal.

sick role A concept used by Talcott Parsons to describe the social expectations of how sick people are expected to act and of how they are meant to be treated.

biomedicine/biomedical model
The conventional approach to medicine in Western societies. It diagnoses and explains illness as a malfunction of one of the body's biological mechanisms. The biomedical approach of most health services focuses on the treating of individuals, and generally ignores social, economic, and environmental factors.

capitalism An economic system based on the private ownership of the means of production.

socialism/communism Political ideology with numerous variations, but generally refers to the creation of societies in which private property and wealth accumulation are replaced by state ownership and distribution of economic resources. Communism represents a utopian vision of society based on communal ownership of resources, cooperation, and altruism to the extent that social inequality and the state no longer exist. Both terms are often used interchangeably to refer to societies ruled by a communist party.

chronic, terminal and permanently disabling conditions, as well as its uncritical acceptance of the role of the medical profession and its neglect of the limitations of the **biomedical model** (see chapter 1).

Marxism

The term Marxism refers to a wide body of theory and political policies based on the writings of Karl Marx (1818–83) and Friedrich Engels (1820–95). Marx was a philosopher, economist, and sociologist. He was also politically active, and since his death his writings have not only inspired many sociologists, but have also laid the foundations for numerous political movements around the world. Marxism, also known as 'conflict theory', asserts that society is dominated by a conflict of interest between two social classes: the bourgeoisie (the capitalist class) and the proletariat (the working class) derived from the economic system of **capitalism**. The influence and contribution of Marxism in sociology is widespread, but the perspective's core concern remains class analysis, especially its emphasis on class conflict as the defining feature of social life and the catalyst of social change (towards its desired goal of **socialism/communism**).

To add to the definitional confusion, some conflict theorists such as Randall Collins (1975), while acknowledging a debt to Marx, no longer consider themselves Marxist, since they have abandoned communism and have incorporated other forms of social conflict, such as that engendered in various organisational settings and among a range of social movements (such as youth, environmental and anti-nuclear movements). Much of Marx's theory has been reinterpreted and modified, and is now often referred to as neo-Marxism. Critical theory is one such neo-Marxist approach, in which a diverse group of theorists (such as Herbert Marcuse, Jurgen Habermas, and Douglas Kellner) produced critiques of communist regimes (which were influenced by Marxism), emphasised the importance of culture in comparison with the economy, and merged psychoanalysis with Marxism (Ritzer 1996).

The Marxist perspective of health and illness, reflected in the contemporary writings of Howard Waitzkin (1983, 2000), Lesley Doyal (1979), Vicente Navarro (1976, 1986), Evan Willis (1989b), and Bob Connell (1988), focuses on the role of the medical profession and the impact of working and living conditions in capitalist society and how these contribute to illness. In particular, Marxist perspectives have highlighted that the exploitation of workers and the pursuit of profit can create dangerous work environments and poor living conditions, resulting in higher mortality and morbidity rates among the working class (see chapter 4).

Marxist analyses of health care tend to focus on the professional power of doctors to serve class interests by placing profit-maximisation above access to optimal health care. Navarro and Waitzkin have been strong critics of the medical profession's individualistic focus and their continued reliance on the biomedical model. By locating the cause and treatment of illness in individuals and ignoring what Waitzkin (1983, 2000) calls 'illness-generating social conditions', the medical profession is viewed as performing an ideological function by masking the real causes of illness and thereby supporting the capitalist system. According to Navarro (1986, p. 35), in capitalist societies the influence of work on health 'is of paramount importance' since workers 'have no control over their work and, thus, over their lives, including their health'. In the Australian context, there has been significant research documenting workplace health hazards (see Mayhew & Petersen 1999; Quinlan 1993, 1988; Willis 1994).

Australian sociologists Evan Willis (1989b) and Bob Connell (1988) have highlighted the profit-orientation and entrepreneurial ethos of the medical profession and its tendency to align itself with upper-class interests. For example, a significant section of the medical profession opposes forms of public health provision, as exemplified by the Australian Medical Association's (AMA) continued opposition to the Medicare system (see chapters 13 and 14). Furthermore, fee-for-service, self-regulation, and the suppression of competition from other health practitioners (see Willis 1989b) are indicative of medicine's alignment with 'the economic and ideological patterns of capitalism' (Connell 1988, p. 214). According to Connell, this has resulted in a commonality of lifestyles and interests between doctors and the upper class so that 'doctors as a group ... have particular political and economic interests they do not share with most of their patients: interests in maintaining a sharp division of labour in health care, in a substantial amount of public ignorance about health, and in seeing that self-help arrangements for health care remain marginal or ineffective' (1988, p. 214).

A further area of interest for Marxist authors has been the entry of large profit-oriented corporations into the health sector, often referred to as the **medical–industrial complex**, a term originally coined by Navarro and colleagues (see Navarro 1998) and popularised by Arnold S. Relman (1980). The medical–industrial complex highlights the **commodification of health care**, whereby health is increasingly viewed as a commodity from which profit can be made, the pursuit of which may clash with meeting the health needs of individuals and the wider community. Connell (1988) among others cautions against the vast growth and influence of profit-oriented medical industries, such as drug companies, pathology and radiology clinics, private health insurance companies, private nursing homes, and private hospitals. While Australians have universal access to public health care

medical-industrial complex

The growth of profit-oriented medical companies and industries, whereby one company may own a chain of health services, such as hospitals, clinics, and radiology and pathology services.

commodification of health care

Treating health care as a commodity to be bought and sold in the pursuit of profit maximisation.

through Medicare, some groups seek to undermine the system, despite its overwhelming public support (see chapter 13). This has been an especially important insight in the USA, which has a significantly under-funded public health system, whereby more than 40 million Americans have no public or private health cover (Hehir 1996; Callahan 1990).

Weberianism

Max Weber (1864–1920) (pronounced 'vay-ber')[1] ranks along with Marx as one of the most influential theorists in sociology. Weber (1968/1921) produced a theory of society that acknowledges the way in which people both shape and are shaped by the social structure. Weber's writings are extensive, but his major contributions concern his analysis of bureaucracy and his account of power and social inequality through the concepts of class, status, and party. Like Marx, Weber viewed class as important and believed that social conflict was a defining characteristic of increasingly complex societies. Rather than two basic classes as in Marx's theory, Weber also considered the middle classes as important, which he saw as consisting of those occupational groups with qualifications and skills that provided them with market advantages (higher wages, prestige, and better working conditions) over those in manual occupations. Not only did the diversity of social classes lay the basis for various forms of collective action to protect and expand group interests, laying the basis for social conflict, Weber suggested that in addition to class inequality, status groups and parties were also a source of group formation and social inequality.

Status groups reflect cultural and sometimes legally conferred privileges, social respect, and honour. They are usually based on membership of specific professional, ethnic and religious groups, and members tend to share common interests and lifestyles. Status group membership is often restricted through what Weber termed a process of **social closure**. While class and social status tend to be closely related, they need not be. Moreover, other groups, or parties in Weber's terms, could also serve the basis for collective interests and social inequality. Parties refer to groups attempting to wield power and include political parties, associations such as unions and professional bodies, as well various interest/pressure groups.

social closure A term first used by Max Weber to describe the way that power is exercised to exclude outsiders from the privileges of social membership (in social classes, professions, or status groups).

Examples of Weberian approaches to social inequality can be found in the work of Australian authors such as Sol Encel (1970) and Ron Wild (1978, 1974). In the health sector, Robert Alford's (1975) work on the competing interest groups is often cited. He argues that health policy and the delivery of health care are a compromise between three main vested interest groups: professional

---

1   I would like to acknowledge a debt to Bessant and Watts (2002) for their insights in conveying the pronounciations of author surnames.

rationalisation The standardisation of social life through
rules and regulations (see also
McDonaldisation).

ideal type A concept originally
devised by Max Weber to refer to
the abstract or pure features of
any social phenomenon.

McDonaldisation A term coined
by George Ritzer to refer to the
standardisation of work processes
by rules and regulations. It is
based on increased monitoring
and evaluation of individual performance, akin to the uniformity
and control measures used by
fast-food chains.

monopolists (doctors), corporate rationalists (public and private
sector managers), and equal health advocates (various patient-
rights groups). Alford, like many Weberians, acknowledges that
some groups (such as doctors) are clearly dominant and exercise
more power, but nonetheless maintains that other groups can and
do exert influence (see chapters 13 and 14).

Another strand of Weber's work concerned the process of
rationalisation, which he considered was the over-arching trend
in society, epitomised by the growth of bureaucracy. Weber
(1968/1921) predicted the 'future belongs to bureaucratisation'
(p. 1401) and described an **ideal type** bureaucratic organisation
as having a highly specialised and hierarchical division of labour
bounded by formal rules and regulations (see Weber 1968/1921,
pp. 221–3). For Weber, bureaucracies were an effective response to
social complexity and democracy by attempting to eliminate
fraud, mismanagement, and inefficiency through conformity to
standardised procedures. Despite what he saw as the significant
benefits of bureaucracy, he feared that social life would be so governed by objective and informal rules that people would become
entrapped by an 'iron cage' of regulations that would limit their
creativity and individuality.

Weberian analyses of health tend to focus on health professions
and the health bureaucracy. Prominent theorists include Magali
Sarfati Larson (1977), Anne Witz (1992), Bryan Turner (1995,
1987), and George Ritzer (1993). Ritzer updates Weber's idea of
rationalisation and suggests that the fast food industry (rather than
bureaucracy) represents an intensified model of rationalisation,
which he terms **McDonaldisation**. For example, medical practice
is increasingly subject to regulations and performance indicators so
that health care becomes predictable and uniform (just like a fast
food restaurant). Ritzer's argument extends Weber's concept of the
'iron cage', whereby the introduction of performance indicators
that are motivated by cost factors alone may make health professionals more consistent in their treatment, but may also
dehumanise interaction with patients and lessen the flexibility and
quality of care provided (see chapter 14).

Symbolic interactionism

Symbolic interactionism is associated with key theorists such as
George Herbert Mead (1863–1931), Charles Cooley (1864–1929),
Howard Becker (1928–), Erving Goffman (1922–82), Anselm
Strauss (1916–96), and Herbert Blumer (1900–87), who coined the
term in 1937. The perspective arose as a reaction against structuralist approaches such as structural functionalism, which tends to
view humans as simply responding to external influences. Instead,
symbolic interactionists focus on agency and how people construct,

interpret, and give meaning to their behaviour through interaction with others. The core philosophical assumption is that humans create reality through their actions and the meanings they give to them. Therefore, society is the cumulative effect of human action, interaction, and interpretation, and these are more significant than social structures, hence the focus of the perspective. Symbolic inter-actionism has a number of strands, such as ethnomethodology (see Garfinkel 1967) and phenomenology (see Schutz 1972/1933; Berger & Luckmann 1967). Its emphasis on the **social construc-tion** of reality has influenced many other perspectives, such as cultural studies and postmodernism (Ritzer 1996).

social construction/constructionism Refers to the socially created characteristics of human life based on the idea that people act-ively construct reality, meaning it is neither 'natural' nor inevitable. Therefore, notions of normality/abnormality, right/wrong, and health/illness are subjective human creations that should not be taken for granted.

Symbolic interactionism provides a theoretical bridge between sociology and psychology by concentrating on small-scale social interaction and how this impacts on an individual's identity or image of themselves (often referred to as 'the self' or 'self-concept'). Cooley's (1964/1906) term 'the looking-glass self' encapsulates this approach, whereby the reactions of others influence the way we see ourselves and thus how we in turn behave. For example, if people regularly tell you that you are attractive and intelligent, this reaction can impact on what you believe and how you behave.

Symbolic interactionism emphasises that health and illness are perceived subjectively, and are social constructions that change over time and vary between cultures. Therefore, what is considered an illness is socially defined and passes through a social lens that reflects the culture, politics, and morality of a particular society at a particular point in time. Such a viewpoint has been used to great effect by interactionist theorists to expose many medical practices and opinions that are based on social (or moral), rather than biological, factors. Many interaction studies have also focused on patients' subjective experience of illness, interactions between patients and health professionals, and interactions among health professionals (especially between doctors and nurses). However, here we will briefly discuss the contributions of Becker and Goffman, both of whom significantly influenced the field of health sociology.

Becker (1963) argues that deviance is created through social interaction when certain behaviours or groups of people are labelled as deviant by social institutions such as the police, the courts, and mental health authorities. According to Becker, 'deviance is not a quality of the act a person commits, but rather a consequence of the application by others of rules and sanctions to an offender. The deviant is one to whom that label has suc-cessfully been applied; deviant behaviour is behaviour that people so label' (1963, p. 9).

Labelling theory examines the effect that being labelled deviant has for the individual concerned. Such an approach draws attention

social control Mechanisms that aim to induce conformity, or at least to manage or minimise deviant behaviour.

stigma A physical or social trait, such as a disability or a criminal record, that results in negative social reactions such as discrimination and exclusion.

total institutions A term used by Erving Goffman to refer to institutions such as prisons and asylums in which life is highly regulated and subjected to authoritarian control to induce conformity.

to how and why certain behaviours and groups of people are labelled deviant. For example, in the 1960s, Black people involved in street protests or 'race riots' in the USA were 'labelled' as exhibiting deviant, abnormal, and even pathological behaviour. Labelling theory exposed the way that medicine (in this case psychiatry) could be used as an instrument of **social control** to constrain the actions of 'difficult' social groups (see chapter 8 and Roach Anleu 1999).

Goffman (1961, 1963) examined **stigma** and focused attention on what he termed **total institutions** such as asylums. According to Goffman, a person becomes stigmatised when they possess an attribute that negatively affects social interaction. He identified three forms of stigma: physical deformity, individual characteristics (mental disorder), and 'tribal' factors (based on 'race', ethnicity, and religion). In his terms, these resulted in tainted or 'spoiled identities', whereby social interaction was affected by negative traits associated with the particular stigma. For example, people may react to someone with a physical disability through outright discrimination or may treat him or her as if they were also mentally incompetent. A person diagnosed as having suffered from schizophrenia may be treated as (and often called) a 'schizophrenic' as if it was the sole characteristic of who they were, whereby the stereotype associated with the condition over-rides the actual personality, actions, and achievements of the individual concerned.

Goffman's (1961) analysis of institutionalisation (the incarceration of people for some form of treatment or sanction) focused on the experience from the perspective of the 'inmates'. His observations of the interaction between inmates and institutional staff reflected the overt and covert forms of power relationships imbued in what he termed the 'total institution'. While such institutions served to impose highly regimented and authoritarian forms of conformity on inmates, often to the detriment of their personal and health needs, they also resulted in a hidden 'underlife' through which people kept a sense of their individual identity by resisting or undermining authority in secret ways (see also Scheff 1966). Goffman's insights on the negative affects of institutionalisation have had a wide impact, which can be seen in fictional works such as *One Flew Over the Cuckoo's Nest*. Excellent discussions of deviance can be found in Sharyn Roach Anleu's (1999) *Deviance, Conformity and Control* and Peter Conrad and John Schneider's (1992) *Deviance and Medicalisation: From Badness to Sickness*.

Feminism

Feminist perspectives in sociology first arose in the 1960s and were primarily aimed at addressing the neglect of gender issues and in some cases blatant sexism of traditional sociological theories, exposing that most mainstream sociology was in fact 'male-stream' (Abbott & Wallace 1997). Women's experiences as

feminism/feminist A broad social and political movement based on a belief in equality of the sexes and the removal of all forms of discrimination against women. A feminist is one who makes use of, and may act upon, a body of theory that seeks to explain the subordinate position of women in society.

patriarchy A system of power through which males dominate households. It is used more broadly by feminists to refer to society's domination by patriarchal power, which functions to subordinate women and children.

women's health movement A term used broadly to describe attempts to address sexism in medicine by highlighting the importance of gender in health research and treatment. Achievements include women's health centres and the National Women's Health Policy.

sexual division of labour This refers to the nature of work performed as a result of gender roles. The stereotype is that of the male breadwinner and the female home-maker.

emotional labour Refers to the use of feelings by employees as part of their paid work. In health care, a key part of nursing work is caring for patients, often by providing emotional support.

workers, partners, carers, or victims of abuse were rarely studied or theorised about. For example, most traditional theories of social class excluded the study of women and concentrated on fathers and sons, rather than mothers and daughters. Furthermore, some approaches perpetuated sexist assumptions about the role of women in society, such as Parsons's view of women as perform-ing 'expressive roles' in society, fulfilling the 'function' of providing emotional care and support of men and families. Hence, feminist perspectives addressed the question 'What about the women?' and focused on social inequality between women and men.

Feminism is a broad social and intellectual movement that addresses many issues from a range of academic disciplines. Germaine Greer (1967), Kate Millet (1977), Rosemary Pringle (1998), Sylvia Walby (1990), Sandra Bartky (1998), and Naomi Wolf (1990) are some of the many prominent feminist theorists. There are many 'feminisms', most of which can be grouped into four 'schools of thought':
- liberal feminism
- radical feminism
- socialist and Marxist feminism
- post-structuralist feminism/post-feminism (postmodern feminism).[2]

Abbott and Wallace (1997), Beasley (1999), Wearing (1996), and Tong (1998) provide comprehensive introductions to feminist perspectives.

Despite the diversity of approaches, feminist perspectives all highlight the importance of **patriarchy**. Feminists argue that the social structure is patriarchal, with social institutions such as the legal, health, and education systems, as well as the wider culture, reflecting sexist values and supporting the privilege of men. They challenge biological assumptions about women's nature, high-lighting that gender is a social construction and identifying gender-role socialisation and sex discrimination as keys to under-standing inequality between the sexes.

Feminist perspectives of health care have underpinned the **women's health movement** and have drawn attention to:
- the **sexual division of labour** in health care, particularly the historical role of women healers, the subordination of female-dominated professions such as nursing, the performance of **emotional labour**, the role of women as informal carers out-side the health system, and the effect of the increasing entry of women into the medical professions (Ehrenreich & English 1973, 1974, 1979; Pringle 1998; Broom 1991; Hothschild 1979; Gibson & Allen 1993; Wicks 1999)

---

2   There are also other versions of feminism such as ecofeminism, Freudian feminism, and psychoanalytic feminism, which focuses on 'race' and ethnicity.

biological determinism The
unproven belief that people's
biology determines their social,
economic, and health statuses.

- sexism and **biological determinism** in health care, particularly medical research and treatment, according to which much health research has been conducted on men and extrapolated to women, and women's specific health concerns have been under-researched or falsely assumed to be the result of their menstrual cycles (that is, women as 'helpless victims of their hormones') (Barrett & Roberts 1978; Woodward et al. 1995)
- unwarranted and sometimes harmful interventions in the management of pregnancy, childbirth, contraception, reproductive technology, and gynaecological disorders (Oakley 1980; Frankfort 1972; Doyal 1995; Annandale & Clarke 1996)
- the issues of sexuality, rape, and domestic violence as key health issues requiring the need for appropriate health policies and specialised training of health workers (Abbott & Wallace 1997; Doyal 1995)
- body image and eating disorders (Bartky 1998; Wolf 1990; Bordo 1993; Williams & Germov 1999).

Today feminist perspectives and concerns are a central feature of sociology and health sociology in particular. Feminism has exposed the sexism and biological determinism of medical approaches, and facilitated increasing attention on women's health rights in terms of health research, funding, and the provision of appropriate services (see chapter 5).

Post-structuralism and postmodernism

The terms post-structuralism and postmodernism[3] are often used interchangeably (Ritzer 1997), and even though distinctions can be made between the two, for our purposes we will focus on their similarities and treat them as one (and for simplicity only use the term postmodernism). Postmodernism arose in the 1980s and reflects a diverse range of social theories from many academic disciplines, making it difficult to categorise or treat systematically. However, to greater or lesser degrees, most social theorists who fall under the umbrella of postmodernism share the following key assumptions:

- The rejection of universal truths about the world, instead suggesting that reality is a social construction. Therefore, all theoretical perspectives (whether they be in the natural, health, or social sciences) reflect the vested interests of one group or another and thus all knowledge is merely a claim to truth, reflecting the subjectivity of those involved.

meta-analysis and meta-narratives The 'big picture' analysis that frames and organises observations and research on a particular topic.

- The rejection of grand theories or **meta-narratives**: postmodern perspectives are critical of structuralist perspectives such as functionalism and Marxism that suggest there is an

---

3 The use of either term usually reflects a particular author's preference; however, some authors who are considered postmodern theorists dispute the validity of the term or any attempt to generalise about postmodernism. The spelling of the terms also varies slightly, with some authors preferring to use a hyphen: 'post-modernism'.

over-riding logic of social organisation. They dispute the existence or importance of unifying trends and structural determinants such as functional prerequisites, class conflict, patriarchy, or rationalisation.

* Since no perspective is neutral and there are no universal structural determinants of social life, postmodernists focus on how truth claims about the world are socially constructed. Thus, there is no single reality or ultimate truth, only versions or interpretations of what is 'real', 'true', 'normal', 'right', or 'wrong'. Postmodernists adopt a pluralist approach and claim that social life is characterised by fragmentation, differentiation, and subjectivity, reflecting people's difference in terms of their culture, lifestyle, and vested interests. Such a perspective supports tolerance of diversity, but can imply that 'almost anything goes'.

The main social theorists are Michel Foucault (pronounced 'Foo-co'), Jean-Francois Lyotard (pronounced 'Leo-tar'), Jean Baudrillard (pronounced 'Bo-dree-ar'), Fredric Jameson, Barry Smart, Mike Featherstone, Charles Lemert, Stephen Seidman, and David Harvey—most of whom are not actually sociologists, but have nonetheless produced social theories. In sociology, the work of Foucault (1926–84) has had the most influence, especially his historical work on asylums, prisons, and hospitals, which uncovered how knowledge and power are used to regulate and control various social groups.

Foucault's (1979) conceptualisation of the panopticon as a metaphor for his theory of surveillance and social control has been a key legacy of his work. The panopticon (all-seeing place) was developed by Jeremy Bentham in the eighteenth century as an architectural design for a prison, consisting of a central observation tower surrounded by circles of cells so that every cell could be observed simultaneously. According to Foucault:

> All that is needed, then, is to place a supervisor in a central tower and to shut up in each cell a madman, a patient, a condemned man, a worker, or a schoolboy ... [resulting in] a state of consciousness and permanent visibility that assures the automatic functioning of power ... in short, that the inmates should be caught up in a power situation of which they themselves are the bearers (1979, p. 200–1).

Therefore, control could be maintained by the assumption of being constantly under surveillance, so that individuals subjected to the disciplinary gaze were 'totally seen without ever seeing, whilst the agents of discipline see everything, without ever being seen' (Foucault 1979, p. 202). The idea that social control of people's behaviour can be exerted in such an indirect and self-induced way has been a significant insight. For example, the wide promotion of the thin ideal of female beauty in Western societies results in panoptic effects whereby many women perceive themselves to be under constant body surveillance and undergo numerous disciplined activities in an attempt to conform to the pressure to be thin (see Williams & Germov 1999).

Postmodernism has significantly influenced feminist perspectives, with the strand of postmodern feminism (or post-feminism) being developed by a diverse range of authors such as Rosemary Pringle, Michelle Barrett, Elizabeth Grosz, Sandra Bartky, and Judith Butler. Postmodern feminism focuses on agency and subjectivity, exploring 'difference' among women in terms of class, religion, 'race', and ethnicity. As Poovey states:

> All women may currently occupy the position 'woman' . . . but they do not occupy it in the same way. Women of colour in a white ruled society face different obstacles than do white women, and they may share more important problems with men of colour than with their white 'sisters' . . . consolidating all women into a falsely unified 'woman' has helped mask the operations of power that actually divide women's interests as much as unite them (1988, p. 59).

Postmodern feminists stress that women use their agency to mediate, resist, and in some cases overcome patriarchy (see Weedon 1987; Bartky 1990; Barrett & Phillips 1992; Pringle 1995; McNay 1992; Butler 1990). In her book *Sex and Medicine*, Rosemary Pringle (1998) explores the impact that increasing numbers of female doctors are having on the organisation and delivery of health care. While not discounting the patriarchal basis of the medical profession, Pringle shows how female doctors are making a difference, and while 'struggles go on at a local level and outcomes vary' (1998, p. 222), their efforts have been primarily responsible for establishing the viability of women's health centres and addressing sexism in medical practice.

For introductions to postmodern approaches to health, particularly influenced by Foucault, see the work of David Armstrong (1983), Nicholas Fox (1993), Rosemary Pringle (1998), and an edited collection by Alan Petersen and Robyn Bunton (1997). For a very short introduction to the field, see Lupton (1998), and for an alternative view, see Chapman (1998).

Conclusion

Despite the differences between the theoretical perspectives discussed here, the distinctions between specific social theories produced by individual authors are likely to be less clear-cut. As Bessant and Watts state (1999, p. 34), sociologists 'constantly "hover" between and in and out of different traditions', and specific social theories are not 'as neat or coherent' as grouping them into theoretical perspectives implies. While sociologists generally align themselves with particular perspectives, they tend to be in less disagreement than the differences between perspectives might imply. This is partly due to the fact that sociologists attempt to incorporate the insights of a range of perspectives into their specific social theory.

While the existence of so many perspectives can be challenging, new theories and perspectives are likely to continue to emerge. Social theories change over time as society itself changes and new knowledge, ideas, and capabilities emerge. This is as true of natural sciences as it is of the social sciences. In response to social change and the development of new insights, theories are regularly modified, reinterpreted and even rejected. Furthermore, some theories defy easy categorisation, for example those of Ulrich Beck (1992) and Anthony Giddens (1984, 1991), and these have not been specifically discussed here for this reason, even though they are often grouped into the increasingly diverse category of critical theory.

It is worth noting that the theoretical perspectives presented in this chapter are more complex than can be discussed here. Furthermore, no attempt has been made to evaluate the theoretical perspectives, a feature beyond the scope of this introductory chapter (see the Further reading and web resources section for recommended sources in this regard). However, the aim has been to convey a basic understanding of some of the main assumptions, concepts, and approaches to explain the differences between perspectives and the insights they offer, and help lay the foundations of understanding for various sociological theories you will encounter in this text and the wider literature.

At this point it is important to sound a note of caution about the use and critique of sociological theories. This chapter began by using the framework of theoretical perspectives as a useful form of shorthand to convey the types of theories sociologists have developed. There is a danger then that when attempting to evaluate how well a specific social theory fits the evidence, the mistake is made of critiquing the general perspective to which the theory belongs, rather than assessing the insights of the specific theory itself. This is not an argument to ignore the various limitations of theoretical perspectives that many authors have exposed, but rather to warn against falling into the trap of dismissing a theory because it is allegedly guilty of all the sins of the perspective to which it is associated. A much healthier approach to adopt is a position of theoretical pluralism, that is, to accept that many theories have something to offer, even though you may have a preference for a certain theoretical perspective. Because different theoretical perspectives often address different levels of analysis and different issues, and attempt to find answers to varied questions, they should be viewed as *potentially* complementary rather than *automatically* oppositional (Turner 1995). It is up to you to judge how well a particular *theory* fits the researched evidence, based on your wider reading.

Summary of main points

- Sociologists seek to interpret their findings by to offering a 'how' and/or 'why' explanation—a theory—for what they seek to understand.
- However, there is often disagreement over which 'how' and 'why' explanations, or social theories, best explain certain aspects of social life. Just as there are people with different opinions, there are sociologists who offer different theories to explain social life.
- One way to understand the range of social theories that exist is to group them into six main theoretical perspectives: functionalism, Marxism, Weberianism, symbolic interactionism, feminism, and post-structuralism/postmodernism.
- Differences between the theoretical perspectives are based on a range of philosophical assumptions and levels of focus, which direct attention to particular aspects of social life and how they should be investigated.
- The use of theoretical perspectives over-simplifies the reality of social theorising, so that some sociologists may adopt different theoretical positions according to the topic under study or may incorporate the insights of other perspectives into their own social theory.
- Therefore, a specific social theory should not necessarily be discarded by being accused of the limitations of the theoretical perspective to which it belongs. While it is important to be aware of the underlying assumptions and limitations of theoretical perspectives, a specific social theory should always be evaluated on its merit.

Discussion questions

1 Which theoretical perspective most appeals to you? Why?
2 What are some of the limitations of adopting one theoretical perspective and ignoring others? (Provide examples in your answer.)
3 Which perspectives focus their attention on studying the interactions between health professionals and patients?
4 Marxist theorists suggest that health care is being increasingly commodified in Australia. In what ways? What factors do other perspectives highlight as important influences on health?

5   What insights into health issues and health care have feminist perspectives exposed?
6   Are postmodern perspectives anti-establishment or a new form of conservatism?

Further investigation

1   Choose two of the perspectives discussed in this chapter and examine the similarities and differences in their approach to studying health and illness.
2   'The sick role is no longer applicable to the experience of illness and health care in a postmodern world.' Discuss.

Further reading and web resources

Health sociology texts

Albrecht, G. L., Fitzpatrick, R., & Scrimshaw, S. C. (eds) 2000, *Handbook of Social Studies in Health and Medicine*, Sage, London.

Annandale, E. 1998, *The Sociology of Health and Medicine: A Critical Introduction*, Polity Press, Cambridge.

Bird, C., Conrad, P., & Fremont, A. M. (eds) 2000, *Handbook of Medical Sociology*, 5th edn, Prentice Hall, New Jersey.

Bury, M. R. 1986, 'Social constructionism and the development of medical sociology', *Sociology of Health & Illness*, vol. 8, no. 3, pp. 137–69.

—— 1998, 'Postmodernity and health' in G. Scambler & P. Higgs (eds), *Modernity, Medicine and Health*, Routledge, London, pp. 137–69.

Chapman, S. 1998, 'Postmodernism and public health', *Australian and New Zealand Journal of Public Health*, vol. 22, no. 3, pp. 403–5.

Cheek, J., Shoebridge, J., Willis, E., & Zadoroznyj, M. 1996, *Society and Health: Social Theory for Health Workers*, Longman Australia, Melbourne.

Cockerham, W. C., Glasser, M., & Heuser, L. S. (eds) 1998, *Readings in Medical Sociology*, Prentice Hall, New Jersey.

Conrad, P. & Schneider, J. 1992, *Deviance and Medicalisation: From Badness to Sickness*, 2nd edn, Temple University Press, Philadelphia.

Doyal, L. 1979, *The Political Economy of Health*, Pluto, London.

Fox, N. J. 1993, *Postmodernism, Sociology and Health*, Open University Press, Buckingham.

Lupton, D. 1998, 'A postmodern public health?', *Australian and New Zealand Journal of Public Health*, vol. 22, no. 2, pp. 3–5.

Morris, D. 1998, *Illness and Culture in the Postmodern Age*, University of California Press, Berkeley.

Petersen, A. & Bunton, R. (eds) 1997, *Foucault, Health and Medicine*, Routledge, London.

Roach Anleu, S. L. 1999, *Deviance, Conformity and Control*, 3rd edn, Longman, Melbourne.

Scambler, G. & Higgs, P. (eds) 1998, *Modernity, Medicine and Health*, Routledge, London.

Turner, B. 1995, *Medical Power and Social Knowledge*, 2nd edn, Sage, London.

—— 1982, 'The government of the body: medical regimes and the rationalisation of diet', *British Journal of Sociology*, vol. 33, no. 2, pp. 254–69.

White, K. 1991, 'The sociology of health and illness: a trend report', *Current Sociology*, vol. 39, no. 2, pp. 1–115.

General social theory books

Abbott, P. & Wallace, C. 1997, *An Introduction to Sociology: Feminist Perspectives*, 2nd edn, Routledge, London.

Beck, U. 1992, *Risk Society: Towards a New Modernity*, Sage, Thousand Oaks, Calif.

Berger, P. & Luckmann, T. 1967, *The Social Construction of Reality*, Penguin, Harmondsworth.

Craib, I. 1992, *Modern Social Theory*, 2nd edn, Harvester Wheatsheaf, London.

—— 1997, *Classical Social Theory*, Oxford University Press, Oxford.

Cuff, E. C., Sharrock, W. W., & Frances, D. W. 1998, *Perspectives in Sociology*, 4th edn, Routledge, London.

Lemert, C. (ed.) 1997, *Social Theory: The Multicultural and Classic Readings*, Westview, Oxford.

May, T. 1996, *Situating Social Theory*, Open University Press, Buckingham.

Ritzer, G. 1997, *Postmodern Social Theory*, McGraw-Hill, New York.

—— 1996, *Sociological Theory*, 4th edn, McGraw-Hill, New York.

Tong, R. P. 1998, *Feminist Thought: A Comprehensive Introduction*, 2nd edn, Allen & Unwin, Sydney.

Walby, S. 1990, *Theorizing Patriarchy*, Blackwell, Oxford.

Wearing, B. 1996, *Gender: The Pain and Pleasure of Difference*, Addison Wesley Longman, Melbourne.

Web sites

Dead Sociologists Society:
  <http://raven.jmu.edu/~ridenelr/DSS/ INDEX.HTML>
Sociology Timeline from 1600 by Ed Stephan:
  <www.ac.wwu.edu/~stephan/timeline.html>
Sociosite: <www.pscw.uva.nl/sociosite/>

3

Researching Health

Methodological Traditions and Innovations

Douglas Ezzy

Overview

* *What are the limitations of the major research methods used in bio-medical studies such as evidence-based medicine, randomised control trials, and epidemiology?*
* *In what way do health sociologists address some of these limitations through qualitative approaches to the study of health and illness?*
* *What are some recent innovations in qualitative methods?*

Health research includes a number of different methodologies. In this chapter we examine the limitations of the dominant research methods used in biomedical studies of health and illness, which tend to emphasise individualistic approaches to health. In contrast, epidemiological and qualitative methodologies informed by a sociological perspective recommend health policy responses that are more focused on social, cultural, and public health factors.

Key terms

autoethnography
biomedical model
epidemiology
ethnography
evidence-based medicine
  (EBM)
positivism
purposive sampling

qualitative research
quantitative research
randomised control trials (RCTs)
research methods
risk factors
rigour

Introduction

research methods Procedures used by researchers to collect and investigate data.

The **research methods** of health sociology are still profoundly shaped by biomedical research. Though the field of health sociology publishes its own journals and is increasingly contributing to health policy debates, the biomedical model still strongly influences research into health issues. This is reflected by its dominance in the field of 'scientific' research, which covers nearly all aspects of health and illness. Although biomedical research methods such as **randomised control trials** (**RCTs**) are not part of health sociology's research methods, it is essential for health sociologists to understand their logic, and the consequences of the theoretical and political baggage they carry with them. The first section of this chapter discusses randomised control trials, evidence-based medicine, and the more public-health-oriented epidemiological research methods. The second section provides an overview of traditional **qualitative research**, introducing the distinctive logic of qualitative methods rather than discussing any particular tradition in detail. Third, recent innovations in qualitative methods are briefly outlined, pointing to the value of experimentation in methodologies.

qualitative research Research that focuses on the meanings and interpretations of the participants.

positivism Research methods that attempt to study people in the same way that physical scientists study the natural world by focussing on quantifiable and directly observable events.

The positivist tradition

Positivist research methodologies attempt to study the world through standardised procedures, uninfluenced by politics, subjectivity, or culture. Positivist methodologies such as randomised control trials and epidemiological surveys have proved to be very powerful methods for examining the efficacy of various treatments and identifying the risk factors associated with particular diseases. However, positivist methodologies are not very useful for examining meanings, interpretations, and the experience of illness. Positivist research is typically considered to be more important than other forms of research and, as a consequence, the cultural and interpretive dimensions of social life are often inadequately researched and understood. Further, supporters of positivist methodologies pretend that politics does not influence the research process, and as a consequence, are often blind to the power of the particular interest groups that these research methodologies serve.

randomised control trials (RCTs) A biomedical research procedure used to evaluate the effectiveness of particular medications and therapeutic interventions. 'Random' refers to the equal chance of participants being in the experimental or control group (the group to which nothing is done and is used for comparison), and 'trial' refers to the experimental nature of the method. It is often mistakenly viewed as the best way to demonstrate causal links between factors under investigation, but privileges biomedical over social responses to illness.

Randomised control trials

Randomised control trials are a powerful way of demonstrating the efficacy of drugs and other biomedical interventions for diseases. An excellent example of an RCT is provided by Hetzel (1995), who describes a trial of the injection of iodised oil for the prevention of cretinism in Papua New Guinea during the 1970s. The trial established that the children of mothers who had received a dose of iodine did not give birth to cretin infants, whereas women who had not received the iodine continued to produce children with cretinism. The trial was 'randomised' in the sense that whether a person received an iodine injection was decided randomly. This prevents the biasing influence of doctors, for example, choosing to give the medication to people whom they think may be more likely to benefit. It is a 'controlled' trial in the sense that a comparison group of people, who do not receive the medication but who are drawn from the same social group, are included in the trial. The benefit of the medication is then assessed by comparing the two groups, in which the only difference is whether they received the medication or not. RCTs are important because they allow cherished beliefs to be disproved. For example, the drug clofibrate was initially thought to be beneficial because it significantly reduced the level of cholesterol in the blood. It was used extensively to treat high cholesterol until an RCT demonstrated that, on the contrary, it increased mortality (Sackett 1981).

Richards (1988) provides an excellent account of the social and political nature of RCTs. She makes the strong claim that '[t]he randomised controlled clinical trial, no matter how tightly organized and evaluated, can neither guarantee objectivity nor definitively resolve disputes over contentious therapies or technologies' (Richards 1988, p. 686). She also provides a detailed analysis of the use of RCT to test the efficacy of vitamin C as a cancer treatment. Two rival medical clinics were involved in examining the efficacy of vitamin C. One clinic argued for the value of vitamin C, not as a drug to kill cancer cells, but as a supplement to support the immune system's own suppression of the cancer tumours. However, the rival clinic was funded to conduct the trials, and evaluated the therapeutic value of vitamin C using criteria drawn from comparable trials of cytotoxic drugs. Not surprisingly, vitamin C was found to be ineffective. 'They made no attempt to evaluate the efficacy of vitamin C … and ignored or were unaware of the available information on the physicology of vitamin C which should have been taken into account in the design of their study' (Richards 1988, p. 672). Richards shows how the conduct of the published RCTs was clearly influenced by the theoretical and professional perspectives of the scientists involved.

However, as noted by Richards, the most telling criticism of the debate over vitamin C is that the clinic advocating the value of vitamin C was prevented from publishing further research, and was not given the opportunity to comment on the existing studies already published. This puts paid to the myth of disinterested and open scientific discussion. Richards (1988, p. 672) concludes,

biomedicine/biomedical model
The conventional approach to medicine in Western societies. It diagnoses and explains illness as a malfunction of one of the body's biological mechanisms. The biomedical approach of most health services focuses on the treating of individuals, and generally ignores social, economic, and environmental factors.

'If the orthodox claim of the inefficacy of vitamin C in cancer treatment prevails … it will *not* be as the result of agreement or consensus brought about by the disinterested application of impersonal rules of experimental procedure' (original emphasis). She provides a further analysis that suggests a direct, or indirect, influence of big business with vested interests in maintaining control over expensive treatments and preventing the use of widely available, relatively cheap alternatives. 'The institution of medicine has a great deal invested in the perpetuation of the myth of objective evaluation. It underpins the cognitive and social authority of its practitioners and legitimates powerful vested interests, not only in medicine, but in society at large' (Richards 1988, p. 686).

This criticism of one RCT does not, of course, demonstrate that all RCTs are unreliable. However, it does demonstrate that political and theoretical interests are inherent in the conduct of medical and health research. This is one of the central insights of the application of sociological theory to **biomedical** research methodology.

Evidence-based medicine (EBM)

evidence-based medicine (EBM)
An approach to medicine arguing that all clinical practice should be based on evidence from randomised control trials (RCTs) to ensure the effectiveness and efficacy of treatments.

Evidence–based medicine (EBM) is an extension of the privileging of RCTs, arguing that clinical practice should be based on evidence from RCTs, rather than other forms of evidence that are thought to be potentially more biased, and therefore less effective. However, both RCTs and EBM are not as universally applicable and objective as they are claimed. Both are infused with political and theoretical biases that are unavoidable. While they are useful and rigorous within the parameters for which they are designed, they become problematic when it is forgotten, or ignored, that they cannot be used to assess all aspects of health and illness, particularly those relating to social, cultural, and interpretative dimensions of illness.

The underlying worldview that privileges RCTs as the 'gold standard' against which all other methodologies must be assessed, results in a failure to properly research, or understand, the dimensions of health and illness that cannot be studied utilising RCTs. It is difficult and quite unusual, for example, to conduct randomised control trials of the effects of clean water, or of poverty, or of international debt repayments on the health of people. The rhetoric of RCTs and EBM focuses on the individual. There is little analysis of the social and cultural variables that profoundly shape the distribution of disease in contemporary society (White & Willis 1988). As such, EBM and RCTs do not represent the radical paradigm shift they are vaunted to be by their advocates. Rather, they are an extension of the positivist, individualistic, politically driven model of science that has informed most of modern medical practice.

Similarly, RCTs are not a particularly useful way of under-standing, for example, how people maintain hope during illness, or of how people adjust to life after serious illness. The privileging of RCTs implicitly devalues the social and cultural aspects of the experience of illness. Can people be understood by just studying their bodies? The problematic nature of this somatic fundamental-ism is clearest in the treatment of 'diseases' such as depression and mental illness, where huge sums of money are expended on new drugs, but by comparison relatively little research has been con-ducted on the social and cultural dimensions. It is not difficult to see the political interests of drug companies and doctors in pro-ducing this imbalance in research, and as a consequence in treatment. Similarly, children in the USA are fifty times more likely to be diagnosed with attention deficit hyperactivity disorder than children in Britain and France, but the individualistic medical dis-ease model means that the cultural and social factors that might generate these differences are rarely examined (Reid et al. 1993). Instead, research focuses on the efficacy of various drug treatments, or on locating the problem in the individual's biology, and is dom-inated by RCTs as a research methodology.

Epidemiology and public health research

In public health research, epidemiological surveys have been used to perform a similar function, becoming the 'scientific' standard. **Epidemiology** examines the distribution of diseases, and tries to identify the specific nature of the **risk factors** associated with the development of the disease. Epidemiological surveys are typically very large, and aim to generate statistically representative samples that can be used to generalise the findings to the general popul-ation. The aim is to identify risk factors that can then be targeted in both prevention and treatment of the disease (Daly et al. 1997).

Epidemiological surveys can be powerful tools for examining the distribution of a disease, and planning the nature of the response to it. For example, when the AIDS epidemic first came into public consciousness, prevention efforts were focused on the entire popul-ation, with the memorable and psychically scarring image of the grim reaper in television advertising to encourage people to practise safe sex. However, epidemiological research soon demonstrated that in Australia the main risk groups were sexually active homosexual men and injecting drug users. This meant that prevention campaigns could be targeted on these groups, making more effective use of resources and greatly increasing the effectiveness of the prevention campaigns. Australia still has a very low level of HIV/AIDS infec-tion, and this is largely a consequence of being well informed by epidemiological research, and having effective prevention policies in place, including safe-sex campaigns and needle exchanges.

epidemiology/social epidemiology The statistical study of patterns of disease in the population. Originally focused on epidemics, or infectious diseases, it now covers non-infectious conditions such as stroke and cancer. Social epidemiology is a sub-field aligned with sociology that focuses on the social determinants of illness.

risk factors Conditions that are thought to increase an individ-ual's susceptibility to illness or disease such as abuse of alcohol or smoking.

Nevertheless, epidemiological research still privileges the aspects of social life that can be measured and statistically summarised. For example, in the excellent research paper by the National Health Strategy (NHS) *Enough to Make You Sick*, an impressive variety of statistical evidence is utilised to demonstrate that 'On almost every measure, the health of Aborigines is poorer than the health of non-Aborigines' (NHS 1992, p. 86). The report convincingly demonstrates the effect of social structural factors on Aboriginal health, such as unemployment, poor education and housing, and lack of public infrastructure. However, it further suggests that these problems are a product of 'other factors such as dispossession, alienation and racism' (NHS 1992, p. 97). Yet, there is little evidence provided for this explanation since these are cultural and interpretative factors that are difficult to quantify. Although the authors of the report are insightful enough to indicate the significance of these factors, they are unable to demonstrate them with epidemiological and survey data. The study of these factors requires a different methodology that explicitly examines people's meanings and interpretations.

The qualitative tradition

The logic, theoretical framing, and practice of qualitative methods are fundamentally different to those of the statistical approach of the positivist tradition. This is both its strength and its weakness. It is a strength because qualitative methods enable an examination of the meanings and interpretations of illness that are inaccessible to traditional statistical methods. It is a weakness because positivist 'scientific' methods and rhetoric still dominate in the spheres of policy making, research funding, and the publishing of academic journals. Consequently, qualitative research, and many aspects of life that are only brought to light using qualitative methods, are routinely ignored and undervalued.

quantitative research Research that focuses on the collection of statistical data.

Qualitative methods are different to **quantitative methods** in two ways. First, qualitative researchers examine meanings. They explicitly examine how people interpret or make sense of their illness experience. Statistics reduces interpretations and evaluations to scales and numerical values. Qualitative researchers are interested in the stories, the ways that people make sense, and the way social interaction changes these meanings.

Second, qualitative methods typically use a very different sampling strategy. Good statistical studies attempt to draw representative samples, so that if 10 per cent of the sample report something, the researchers can be confident that 10 per cent of the wider population will experience the same thing. The objective of qualitative sampling is not to make statistical generalisation, but to

purposive sampling Refers to the selection of units of analysis to ensure that the processes involved are adequately studied, and where statistical representativeness is not required.

generalise about the nature of the experience. This is called **purposive sampling**. The aim is to be able to describe the processes, meanings, and interpretations that lie behind the different aspects of the experience. For example, in my study of mental health and unemployment, I describe the different types of stories that lead some people to report feeling depressed after losing a job and other people to report feeling much better about themselves (Ezzy 2000b). Survey research has already established that about one-third of people who lose their job report feeling better, and two-thirds report feeling worse. My sample of unemployed people was not drawn randomly, to ensure statistical representativeness, but purposively, to ensure that I interviewed enough people from both groups so that the processes that lead to depression or hope were clearly understood. That is to say, the sample was chosen purposively to ensure that the different types of meanings of unemployment were properly understood, rather than to ensure that they statistically represented the more general population of unemployed people (for a more detailed explanation see Rice & Ezzy 1999, chapter 2).

Similarly, Kathy Charmaz (1994) takes the basic statistical observation that men contract more serious and life-threatening chronic illnesses than women, and asks, what is it that is distinctive about the experience of illness for men? She is not interested in the statistical distribution of the illness of the men she studies. Rather, she examines the meanings, interpretations, and identity dilemmas that are characteristic of the men's illness experiences. The focus is on describing the social processes, not the statistical distributions. Charmaz asks her research questions in this way: 'What is it like to be an active, productive man one moment, and a patient who faces death the next? What is it like to change one's view of oneself accordingly? Which identity dilemmas does living with continued uncertainty pose for men? How do they handle them? When do they make identity changes? When do they try to preserve a former self?' (Charmaz 1994, p. 271). Notice the structure of the questions. They are not about the distribution of illness experience, but about the process of making sense of illness; they explore meanings and interpretations. Only qualitative methods can answer these sorts of questions.

Charmaz (1994) shows how masculine identities tend to be active and problem-solving, emphasising personal power, autonomy, and bravery in the face of danger. When dealing with illness, these masculine identity strategies allow men to develop some distinctive coping strategies, but also prevent them from developing others. The emphasis on active problem-solving facilitates the recreation of new identities to replace those lost as a consequence of chronic illness. However, if it proves difficult to find a new active identity, the men find it difficult to develop and feel comfortable with identities that are less autonomous and less active. If satisfying alternative identities cannot be found, this can increase the likelihood of depression.

An excellent example of the tension between statistical methods and qualitative methods is provided by Boston's (1999) study of palliative care nurses. In Canada a workload-measurement statistical system had been implemented by nursing administrators. Under this system all aspects of the nurses' work were quantified in an attempt to plan nursing requirements and to increase efficiency of services. Based on a qualitative study using 50 long interviews, Boston shows that this attempt to objectively quantify and systematise nurses' work fails to deal with the nature of nursing care required in a multicultural environment. The problem that Boston identifies is not simply that the workload measurement system has insufficient categories to cover the wide range of tasks that nurses consider part of their work. Rather, Boston argues that it is impossible to quantify many aspects of nursing practice that involve intuitive and personalised ways of dealing with patients in a culturally complex environment. In particular, dealing with patients from diverse cultural backgrounds requires taking time to learn, understand, and accommodate culturally distinct responses to terminal illness, diagnosis, and rituals associated with death and dying. These processes are extremely difficult to quantify. As a consequence: 'that subjective "inner" knowledge, which necessarily involves prioritising cultural concerns, is left to "fall between the cracks" ' (Boston 1999, p. 151). In short, statistical, categorical, and deductive methodologies for assessing and studying nursing practice miss many of the central tasks that nurses perform.

Evaluating the quality of research

The criteria for what constitutes 'good' research also significantly change between quantitative and qualitative methods. In survey research, studies are designed to be valid (to accurately reflect what is being studied) and reliable (or repeatable, and subsequently verifiable). In contrast, qualitative researchers typically prefer to describe good research as 'rigorous'. Surely, you might ask, qualitative research should also aim to be valid and reliable? However, the problem with these terms is that they ignore the way in which social life is a product of interpretative processes. Qualitative researchers tend to prefer to use the term **rigour** to avoid the positivist overtones of the terms validity and reliability. The aim of rigorous research is to closely scrutinise the meanings and interpretations of the people being studied (Lincoln 1995). People's meanings change with time, and depending on who they

rigour A term used by qualitative researchers to describe trustworthy research that carefully scrutinises and describes the meanings and interpretations given by participants.

are talking to. Qualitative methods try to explicitly engage with the fluidity of meanings and interpretations rather than avoiding them, as is attempted by quantitative research.

For example, the experience of living with HIV/AIDS in Australia was very different in the 1980s and early 1990s to what it was in the late 1990s. This was due to a number of factors, including the discovery of some at least partially effective treatments in 1996, a move away from a culture of fear, and declining death rates. This means that it is impossible to assess the reliability of research conducted in the early 1990s, such as Adam and Sears's (1996) excellent study of the experience of living with HIV. Although there are many similarities, living with HIV/AIDS is profoundly different today, as a consequence of the new treatments. It would be impossible to repeat their study (and test its reliability) because meanings and interpretations have changed. Further, the aim of qualitative research is not to accurately measure meanings (validity); rather it is to closely scrutinise these meanings, locating them in the complexity of the culture of which they are a part. Adam and Sears do this well, using extensive extracts from their interviews, focusing on the processes through which meanings are constructed, and demonstrating how the interpretative and subjective aspects of social life are formed. Meaning and the interpretative process are integral to qualitative methods, and rigorous research explicitly engages with this interpretative process.

Kavanagh and Broom (1997) provide an example of a qualitative study of women's understanding of an abnormal cervical smear-test result, drawing on long interviews with Australian women. Previous research has demonstrated a statistical link between an abnormal cervical smear result and psychological and sexual difficulties of various kinds. Kavanagh and Broom describe the experiences of the women during their interaction with the healthcare services that may contribute to these difficulties. In particular they show how the interaction during the medical encounter often created fear, and did not allow for the development of trust or for the women to gain an understanding of what was happening to them. While the women wanted to participate in decisions about their treatment, they found this difficult because doctors provided little information during the consultation and did not encourage them to ask questions. They conclude that 'the inherent power structure of medical practice combined with time pressures often make it difficult for doctors to give the detailed information and reassurance patients need when a diagnosis is distressing or when investigation and treatment are strange and upsetting' (Kavanagh & Broom 1997, p. 1388). Their qualitative methodology allowed them to examine the experiences and interpretations the women gave to the medical encounter. This, in turn, can be used to make sense of the statistically observed relationships. However, only a qualitative methodology can identify these interpretative processes, and as a consequence, suggest changes to the medical interaction that might alleviate them.

Analysis and reporting of qualitative research

Similarly, for qualitative research the structure of analysis and the nature of research reports are quite different to statistical studies. The analysis process does not aim to follow correct procedures to produce objective results, although good procedure is important. Rather, qualitative analysis methodologies such as thematic analysis (Kellehear 1993), grounded theory (Strauss & Corbin 1990), narrative analysis (Riessman 1993), and cultural studies (Alasuutari 1995) all aim to analyse data by interpreting them. The process of interpretation can be described, but it cannot be systematised. This difference is clearest in the computer packages developed to assist qualitative data analysis. These computer packages *do not* analyse the qualitative data for the researcher. Rather, they assist the analysis through sophisticated search, coding, and filing mechanisms (Rice & Ezzy 1999). It is impossible to automate the process of qualitative data analysis, as can be done with statistics, because the process of interpretation and understanding is central to the analytic process. Similarly, qualitative research reports are difficult to produce as short summaries similar to those that appear in many medical journals. The reason for this is that the heart of qualitative research is in the detail. It aims to provide *understanding* of the meanings, the details that shape why people do what they do. To do this well requires long quotations and careful explanation of cultural and social context.

Orona (1990) provides one of the clearest accounts of the process of analysing qualitative data using a grounded theory methodology. She emphasises the role of uncertainty and the exploratory nature of the analytic process. She describes how she read and re-read her interviews so that she became immersed in the world of her participants. This process of imaginative participation is at the heart of good qualitative research. In this way it is possible to genuinely listen, hear, and be transformed by the voice of participants, and as a consequence, to discover new understandings. Orona emphasises the need to embrace uncertainty, to explore, and to use her intuition and creativity as part of the analysis process. As she immersed herself in her data she began to see patterns and relationships, and began to build a theory of the experience of identity loss during Alzheimer's disease, which was the focus of her research.

This explicit engagement with personal subjectivity and the interpretative process may sound far from 'scientific'. However, the alternative is to pretend that you can avoid the interpretative process. Qualitative researchers are increasingly arguing that it is impossible to avoid the role of subjectivity in the research process. The aim is not to avoid subjectivity, but to allow the researcher to engage in a dialogue with the participants in their research (Lincoln 1995). Rigorous qualitative research aims to genuinely hear the voice of the participants. To do so requires engaging in a dialogue in which we are honest about the influence of our own subjectivity on the research process.

Future directions: qualitative innovators

While qualitative research is increasingly becoming an accepted methodology, it is typically understood as a poor cousin to the 'stronger' statistical methods such as surveys and RCTs. However, some qualitative researchers are pushing their methodology even further away from the theory and practice of the positivist tradition. Influenced by the arguments of postmodernists, cultural studies, and hermeneutics, these practitioners argue for the explicit incorporation of politics and the subjectivity of the researcher into the research process, the need to experiment with less formal writing styles such as poetry and performance, and a greater degree of engagement of participants in the research process (Lincoln 1995; Denzin 1997).

These qualitative innovations, of course, are deeply disturbing to those who espouse the more traditional methodologies. Some researchers still try to portray qualitative research as a 'scientific' method, and apply all the rhetoric and terms of the statistical methods to qualitative research (Green 1998). They believe that qualitative researchers should be objective, distancing themselves from their research, that the research should be validated and reliable, and that the report should not contain any account of the researcher's subjective experience, but be politically neutral, and written in standard scientific format. The problem with this attempt to make qualitative methods 'scientific' is that it devalues the central process that qualitative methods aim to examine—the process of interpretation. While qualitative methods can be moulded to fit this scientific worldview, researchers are increasingly arguing that such an approach is deceptive, and does not produce research that is as useful, insightful, respectful, or as politically appropriate as it could be (Denzin 1997; Ezzy 2001).

Estroff (1995) draws on her study of chronic illness to demonstrate that qualitative interviews are not events in which objective information is gathered from subjects. People do not have 'objective' unchanging stories of events that they carry around in their heads and that a qualitative research can simply 'gather' like measurements.

Rather, people shape and change their story, often unconsciously, to fit the particular interactive context. Interviews are moments of the co-creation of narratives (Estroff 1995). To pretend otherwise is to deceive ourselves as researchers. This does not, however, make interviews useless, just more complex to negotiate and requiring a more sophisticated theory (Gubrium & Holstein 1995).

Further, Estroff argues that interviews need to be seen as relationships that involve mutual obligations and responsibilities as the interviewer and interviewee attempt to make sense of the experience together. This leads to a number of complex ethical and political questions about the extent to which participants can or should be involved in the research process. Some qualitative researchers have attempted to include participants as co-researchers. Others take a more guarded approach. Estroff concludes:

> I believe that it is possible, however, to reduce exploitation and trespass, to minimize violation of individual rights, ethical principles, and reasonable expectations, and to conduct the work in a way that increases the opportunity for mutual benefit and reduces the chances of harms and wrongs. I do not think it is possible to work in complete collaboration, in actual equality, or in total accord or consensus with our informants (1995, p. 97).

Some qualitative innovators have experimented with other aspects of the research process, exploring new writing styles, and making the research the subject of the research. For example, Ellis (1995; 1998) provides a detailed study of loss and illness through her **autoethnographic** account of her ten-year relationship with her dying partner. An autoethnography is, as the name implies, an **ethnographic** study that focuses on the experience of the researcher. 'Autoethnography blurs distinctions between social science and literature, the personal and the social, the individual and culture, self and other, and researcher and subject' (Ellis 1998, p. 49). Ellis's autoethnography *Final Negotiations* is a story-like account that at times feels like a popular autobiography, but also demonstrates the influence of a careful social science approach to observation, analysis, and recording of experience. Ellis says that the aim of writing about her intimate experiences grew out of her frustration with traditional methodologies and reports that failed to engage with the detail of daily experiences of those living with chronic illness.

Autoethnography, the inclusion of participants as researchers, and various other innovations developed among qualitative researchers are hotly debated. Some argue that autoethnography is literature, not social research. Others point out that there is considerable value in experimenting with a variety of methodologies, analytic procedures, and writing styles in order to better understand social life, and to respond to the epistemological and

autoethnography An ethnography that focuses on the experience of the researcher.

ethnography A research method that is based on direct observation of a particular social group's social life and culture—of what the people actually do.

methodological issues raised by the postmodernists (Richardson 1994). Box 3.1 provides a detailed example.

Box 3.1 A detailed example

In my research on the experience of living with HIV/AIDS in Australia, I have focused on the relationship between religious belief, orientations towards the future, and people's sense of hope or depression (Ezzy 2000a; in press). This study draws on all three types of research described above. It comprises a statistical survey, a qualitative study utilising traditional analytic strategies, and a report that takes a more novel approach by including a poem and some self-reflection.

The survey, involving 914 respondents and conducted in 1997, is a national representative survey of people living with HIV/AIDS in Australia. It includes a number of attitude scales, demographic indicators, and questions about clinical indicators. The survey provided a number of important results; here, however, I focus only on the relationship between religious belief, future planning, and health status. Results from the survey show that religious belief is correlated with how people plan for the future. Surprisingly, people with religious beliefs were more likely to plan for the short term. This seems a strange outcome, given that you might expect religious belief to be associated with hope and therefore with greater confidence about the future. Further analysis demonstrates that this holds irrespective of disease progression. That is to say, it could be argued that as people become more ill they are more likely to both plan for the short term and become religious. However, the survey data demonstrate that this is not the case (Ezzy 2000a). The data pose an interesting problem: why is it that people with HIV/AIDS tend to develop a religious orientation and plan for the short term?

In the qualitative part of the study I demonstrate that there are three types of responses to HIV/AIDS that revolve around different meanings of life, death, and the future (Ezzy 2000a). These types of response are linked to different stories about the future, and different religious orientations. One story is of confidence in a long future that is typically secular, relying on the success of medical science for its optimism. A second story is of despair, anticipating a short life and an early death that is also secular. The third type of story is more complex. It is hopeful, but involves 'living with a philosophy of the present', in which the short term is celebrated. It is this narrative that is typically religious. Only qualitative research can identify the way that stories are constructed, and how these stories shape the way that people respond to illness. In a culture that often devalues the spiritual and religious dimensions of life, this study underlines the importance of spirituality, and particularly non-traditional spirituality, in helping people living with HIV/AIDS to come to terms with their illness.

Finally, in a subsequent paper I wrote a poem about confronting death (Ezzy in press). One of the most confronting aspects of interviewing people living with HIV/AIDS is that I, as the interviewer, had to come to terms with my own sense of mortality. Poetry expresses some of the emotional, symbolic, and spiritual dimensions of experience that are often difficult to put into more traditional prose. While I do not advocate that sociologists should write only poetry, there is considerable value in exploring alternative ways of communicating the experiences of health and illness that we study, even if only as a small part of an overall research project.

Conclusion

Despite some authors' claims and assumptions to the contrary, no research methodology is objective or inherently superior to another. Each type of research method reflects particular philosophical, political, and theoretical interests that can influence the collection of data and their interpretation. This means that the privileging of biomedical research methods tends to benefit the political interests of those involved in biomedical professions and industries. This chapter advocates a more balanced approach and highlights the contributions of epidemiology, and traditional and innovative qualitative methodologies to health research.

Summary of main points

- Health research includes a number of different methodologies. Each methodology has its place and provides important and useful information about different aspects of contemporary experiences of health and illness.
- Some methodologies such as RCTs are considered more important than others, and as a consequence our contemporary understandings of health tend to emphasise biomedical and individualistic responses to health.

- In contrast, epidemiological and qualitative methodologies informed by sociological theory recommend health policy responses that are more focused on social, cultural, and public health factors.
- No research methodology is objective. Each reflects particular political and theoretical interests.
- This chapter advocates a more balanced approach that values the contributions of epidemiology, and traditional and innovative qualitative methodologies, alongside the contributions of bio-medical research.

Discussion questions

1 What are the implications for public health of the privileging of randomised control trials?
2 What is evidence-based medicine (EBM)? What are some of the limitations of EBM?
3 Identify one health issue that can and one that cannot be addressed by epidemiological research.
4 What distinctive contribution do qualitative methods make to health research?
5 Why are qualitative researchers often ignored or undervalued in health research?
6 Why is it important to have alternative ways of studying, interpreting and reporting research findings?

Further investigation

1 Find a recent journal article that reports a randomised control trial for the treatment of HIV/AIDS or tuberculosis. Drawing on sociological or public health research that examines the same disease, provide a critical commentary on the first article, focusing on the role of social and economic factors that shape the distribution of the disease.
2 Why is it important to study meanings and culture in order to understand health in contemporary society? Draw on at least three published qualitative studies of a health issue to illustrate your argument.

Further reading and web resources

Alasuutari, P. 1995, *Researching Culture: Qualitative Method and Cultural Studies*, Sage, London.

Crotty, M. 1998, *The Foundations of Social Research: Meaning and Perspective in the Research Process*, Allen & Unwin, Sydney.

Daly, J., Kellehear, A., & Glicksman, M. 1997, *The Public Health Researcher*, Oxford University Press, Melbourne

Denzin, N. 1997, *Interpretive Ethnography*, Sage, London.

Ezzy, D. 2001, *Qualitative Analysis*, Allen & Unwin, Sydney

Grbich, C. 1999, *Qualitative Research in Health: An Introduction*, Allen & Unwin, Sydney.

Orona, C. 1990, 'Temporality and identity loss due to Alzheimer's disease', *Social Science & Medicine*, vol. 30, no. 11, pp. 1247–56.

Rice, P. & Ezzy, D. 1999, *Qualitative Research Methods: A Health Focus*, Oxford University Press, Melbourne.

Web sites

Resources for Methods in Evaluation and Social Research:
<http://gsociology.icaap.org/methods>

SocioSite – Methodology Section:
<www.pscw.uva.nl/sociosite/topics/ research.html>

Part 1

The Social Production
and Distribution
of Health and Illness

All animals are equal but some animals are more equal than others.

George Orwell 1945, Animal Farm, p. 114

* Why do manual labourers have a lower life expectancy than other people?
* Why do women outlive men but report greater illness during their lives?
* Why is Aboriginal life expectancy 20 years below the Australian average?

   The chapters in part 1 concern the first dimension of the social model of health introduced in chapter 1: the social production and distribution of health. It is generally assumed that health and illness are simply undisputed facts, that medicine is best equipped to deal with health problems, and that illness is a matter of bad luck, fate, or individual responsibility. Health sociology debunks the myth that illnesses are solely the fault or responsibility of the individual. While health problems are experienced by individuals, they also have wider social determinants.

   The chapters in this part address the above questions by examining the evidence and explanations of health inequalities in Australia; and focus on three social criteria: class, gender, and 'race'. The fact that there are significant social patterns in the distribution of health and illness, in which some groups of people suffer much higher rates of illness and premature death than others, implies not only that health inequalities have social origins, but also that the removal of such inequalities requires social action and social reform.

   Part 1 is divided into three chapters:

* Chapter 4 examines the links between class, work, and health inequality.
* Chapter 5 explains how gender is an important determinant of health and illness.
* Chapter 6 explores the reasons for the poor health status of Aboriginal people.

4

Class, Health Inequality, and Social Justice

John Germov

Overview

* What is class and how can it help to explain health inequalities in Australia?
* What does the organisation of work have to do with health?
* What can be done to address class-based health inequalities?

There is a significant amount of research that shows the connection between class and health. Working-class people have higher rates of death and illness as a result of their living and working conditions. This chapter discusses the concept of class, provides up-to-date evidence of class-based health inequality, and examines five main explanations of health inequality: artefact, natural/social selection, cultural/behavioural, materialist/structural, and psychosocial/social capital explanations. Classes arise from the social structure, and therefore class-based health inequality needs to be addressed primarily through structural changes to the economy, the workplace, and the community, guided by public policies based on social justice. The chapter ends with a discussion of a number of ways of tackling health inequality with the aim of achieving an equality of health outcomes.

Key terms

accident-proneness
biomedical model
class
economic rationalism
empirical
epidemiology/social
  epidemiology
gross domestic product (GDP)
life chances

lifestyle factors
occupational welfare
public health
risk factors
ruling class
social cohesion
social capital
social Darwinist
social model of health

social justice
social structure
social support
social wage
structure/agency debate
trickle down
victim-blaming

Introducing class

class (or social class) A position within a system of structured inequality based on the unequal distribution of power, wealth, income, and status. Class membership is determined by three characteristics: ownership and control of scarce economic resources; ownership of marketable skills and qualifications; and wage labour. People who share a social-class position typically share similar life chances.

life chances A term derived from Max Weber that refers to the opportunities available to people in society. People with different social-class locations have different life chances, including different opportunities with regard to education, wealth, and health.

We all have some basic notion of **class**—we see it everyday in the differences between low-priced and expensive cars, take-aways and fine dining restaurants, public and private schools, and over-crowded and exclusive suburbs. In fact, Australian surveys have regularly reported that around four-fifths of the population believe that classes exist and have no trouble placing themselves into a class; only one in ten believe that Australia is classless (Graetz & McAllister 1994). Debates over the importance of class focus on the extent to which being in a particular class determines your **life chances**—that is, your chances of social mobility, of gaining an education, and of getting a certain type of job. While most people acknowledge the existence of class, few recognise that health status is one of the clearest indicators of class inequality in Australia. Despite access to free public health services through Medicare, the most disadvantaged people in Australia still die younger and have the highest rates of illness and disability. As the evidence presented in this chapter will show, class is a significant basis of health inequality in Australia. Yet what exactly is class?

Defining class

Popular notions of class tend to focus on lifestyle differences, particularly fashion, as a social marker of status. While consumption patterns may indicate class membership in a general sense, they shed little light on how class differences are generated in the first place. Sociological analyses of class tend to focus on the underlying factors that actually produce and reproduce class differences. It is important to note that different theoretical perspectives used by sociologists (as discussed in chapter 2) have resulted in continuing debate over appropriate definitions and theories of class, most of which focus on Erik Olin Wright's neo-Marxist and John Goldthorpe's neo-Weberian class models, but these debates are not addressed here (see Wright 1997; Goldthorpe 1996; Crompton 1998; Crompton et al. 2000; Baxter, Emmison, & Western 1991). To help clarify the concept of class, we will consider an admittedly simplified three-class model based on a hybrid of Marxist and Weberian social theories in which class is defined according to three characteristics: ownership and control of scarce economic resources; ownership of marketable skills and qualifications; and wage labour.

The *upper class* refers to those who own and/or manage economic resources (capital), such as raw materials, technology, and workplaces, and employ others to create profit for them. This group includes many directors and senior executives who may not own a company, but nevertheless have access to the company's profit through share ownership, profit-sharing arrangements, and high incomes. This group 'controls' how money is spent and how work is organised and carried out, including the power to hire and fire. The *middle class* represents a diverse group of people who possess some form of qualification and skill, such as health professionals and teachers, that attracts higher wages and better working conditions than unskilled workers. This group can also include small-business owners and the self-employed. The *working class* consists of unskilled manual and non-manual (blue and white collar) workers who gain employment solely by selling their labour power. Based on 1993 data from the Class Structure in Australia Project (see Baxter et al. 1991; Western 2000) we can construct the following three-class model of Australian society:

- upper class: 9 per cent
- middle class: 47 per cent
- working class: 44 per cent.

All class models have 'grey areas'. For example, is a plumber working class or middle class? Can plumbers, teachers, and administrative officers all be middle class? The answers depend on the definitions used in a particular model of class.

While it is relatively easy to fit people into a class model, it is important at this point to avoid any confusion between the terms class and socioeconomic status (SES). These terms are often used interchangeably, but they do not mean the same thing. SES is determined by ranking people according to wealth, education, and occupation levels (among other criteria), and grouping them into corresponding high, medium, and low SES groups. It is a relatively straightforward process to categorise people into SES groups, and this is why most of the **empirical** evidence of class inequality tends to be based on SES; also, it is often where the confusion arises between the two terms (see Connell 1977; 1983 for more discussion of this issue). Measures of SES can only indicate levels of inequality in a society. It is a descriptive classification system and offers little insight in analysing how and why such inequality exists, effectively ignoring such questions by transforming 'the lived reality of class ... to an abstraction for the purpose of statistical treatment' (Connell 1977, p. 33). The 'lived reality' of class refers to people who are class conscious, have class-based values and lifestyles, and mobilise politically as a class on certain issues. As Bob Connell and Terry Irving state, 'class structure exists only in what people do, in particular times and places. Conversely, what people do presupposes the structure that defines the situation they are acting in and the resources they act with' (1992, p. 5). To substitute SES for class ignores the key insight of class analysis—that the unequal distribution of wealth and power is embedded in the **social structure** and thus class is not simply a label or status easily acquired or discarded.

empirical Describes observations or research that is based on evidence drawn from experience. It is therefore distinguished from something based only on theoretical knowledge or on some other kind of abstract thinking process.

social structure The recurring patterns of social interaction through which people are related to each other, such as social institutions and social groups.

Class inequality in Australia

One of the key indicators of class inequality is the distribution of wealth. Andrew Dilnot (1990) provides evidence of significant inequality in terms of Australia's wealth distribution (see also Stilwell 1993; Rees et al. 1993). Figure 4.1 shows that the top 10 per cent of the population own over 55.2 per cent of the nation's wealth; the top 20 per cent own 72 per cent of the wealth; and the top 50 per cent own 98.4 per cent. This means that the other 50 per cent own only 1.6 per cent of all the available wealth in Australia. In terms of the proportion of income acquired by the top 20 per cent, Australia ranks third highest out of nine advanced industrialised countries (Stilwell 1993). Such figures indicate that Australia is among the most unequal of countries and challenges the view that we live in a classless society.

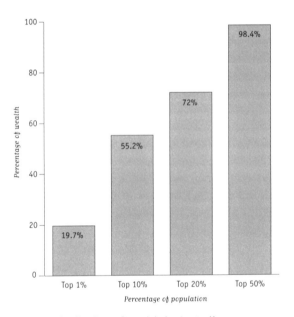

Figure 4.1   Distribution of wealth in Australia

Source: Dilnot 1990

Upper class or ruling class?

Each year, the *Business Review Weekly* (*BRW*) publishes a list of the richest 200 people and families in Australia. The cut-off point for entry to the top 200 has steadily increased over the years, rising from $42 million in 1995 to $80 million in 2001, indicating how well the rich have been doing. Between 1984 and 2001, the aggregate wealth of the richest 200 increased from A$7.3 billion to A$60.4 billion (an eight-fold increase), and the top five—the 'super rich'—have done even better as Table 4.1 shows (*BRW*, 18 May 2001). It is worth noting that these figures are 'guesstimates', based on the officially declared assets and earnings of the wealthy, and as such are likely to significantly underreport the full extent of wealth. The World Wealth Report 2001 found that the combined wealth of individuals around the world was A\$54 trillion in 2000, and that the number of 'high net worth individuals' in Australia (people with investment assets of at least A\$2 million, excluding real estate) was 74 000 (Merrill Lynch et al. 2001). The wealth of the super rich is difficult to fathom, but people such as Kerry Packer make as much money per year as most people earn in a lifetime of paid work.

Table 4.1   The super rich, 2001

Individual or family	Estimated wealth (A$ billion)
Kerry Packer	6.2
Frank Lowy	3.5
Richard Pratt	3.3
Victor Smorgon	1.7
David Hains	1.6

Source: Adapted from *BRW*, 18 May 2001

ruling class This is a hotly debated term used to highlight the point that the upper class in society has political power as a result of its economic wealth. The term is often used interchangeably with 'upper class'.

Debates about the upper class concern not only its wealth but also its influence—on whether it acts as a **ruling class**. While few theorists would argue that the upper class rules in a direct way, there is also little dispute that through their companies, the members of the upper class can affect investment, employment, and the stock market. In this way, their economic power provides them with significant political influence. The upper class may not pull the strings directly but its members share similar interests. For example, they may pressure governments to adopt policies of low taxation and deregulation to aid the pursuit of profit maximisation, which tend to benefit the already well-off. However, such a situation is not beyond change; no natural law of profit and wealth operates here. Class inequality is an outcome of the social structure and as recent history teaches us, the structure of a society can be subject to social change—social policies and taxation rates can work to either consolidate or redistribute wealth.

Research by the National Centre for Social and Economic Modelling (Harding & Greenwell 2001; Kelly 2001) found that throughout the 1990s income and wealth inequality increased in Australia. For example, between 1990 and 1999, the most affluent fifth of the population increased their income by 14 per cent, while the income of the poorest fifth only increased by 1.5 per cent. While the **social wage** and targeted welfare programs ensured the living standards of the poor did not deteriorate during this time, the gap between rich and poor grew markedly.

social wage Government spending on health, social security, education, and housing (often referred to as welfare spending).

economic rationalism or economic liberalism Terms used to describe a political philosophy based on 'small-government' and market-oriented policies, such as deregulation, privatisation, reduced government spending, and lower taxation.

trickle down The theory that everyone benefits by allowing the upper class to prosper relatively unfettered. If wealthy capitalists are allowed and encouraged to maximise their profits, it is believed that this increased wealth will eventually 'trickle down' to the workers.

occupational welfare Welfare provision—such as tax relief for business expenses and super-annuation investment—that benefits higher paid workers.

A decade of policies influenced by **economic rationalism**—during which financial and labour markets were deregulated, government spending was cut, and taxation lowered—has revealed the **trickle down** theory to be without substance. Furthermore, **occupational welfare** has been expanded through tax relief for superannuation and share investment and lower business tax rates compared to personal tax rates, all of which provide greater economic benefit to the highest paid workers. In public debates about economic management and government spending, it is interesting to note that there have been few calls for the restraint of profit levels, executive salaries, or occupational welfare.

Intersecting structures of inequality and the death of class?

Class has been a central feature of sociological analysis, particularly the role class structure plays in shaping individuals' beliefs, behaviour, and access to social rewards such as employment, education, and health (Western 2000). However, some authors argue that 'class is dead' in terms of its influence over individuals' lives and as the basis of the distribution of wealth and power. Instead, it is argued that class has been replaced by social inequalities and power struggles based in gender, 'race', or ethnicity and new social movements, such as gay rights, grey power, and environmental groups (for more on this debate see Pakulski & Waters 1996; Westergaard, 1995; Eder 1993; Beck 1992; Crompton 1998). Ulrich Beck (1992) suggests that a process of 'individualisation' has overtaken class as the dominant marker of social distinction, whereby individual identity is now an outcome of lifestyle choice and consumption patterns (admittedly based on the ability to pay). According to Beck (1992, p. 131) tradition and family ties no longer dominate, so that individuals can construct their identity from a variety of lifestyle choices that are increasingly reflective of and 'dependant upon fashions, social policy, economic cycles and markets'. Therefore, class and occupation are no longer the major determinants of social groups or individual identity. The argument here is not that inequality has decreased, but that the class basis of inequality has declined.

Jan Pakulski and Malcolm Waters (1996, p. 10) identify the following four key features of class analysis, arguing that each has diminished in importance in recent times:

1 *Economism*: class structure is an economic phenomenon based on the unequal ownership of productive capital and marketable skills that allows a minority to accumulate wealth.

2 *Groupness*: classes are real social groupings of people that result from conflict over social and economic rewards.

3 *Behavioural and cultural linkage*: members of a class share 'class consciousness', political preferences, common interests and lifestyles.

4   *Transformational capacity*: classes allow for collective action and can transform the social structure; class conflict is the central dynamic that shapes social life.

Given that the gap between rich and poor has increased over the last decade, it may appear curious that some authors are declaring the death of class. One way to accommodate the insights of the 'death of class' argument is to reinvoke the distinction between objective and subjective notions of class, or, following Karl Marx (1818–83) among others, the difference between a class 'in itself' and a class 'for itself' (Crompton 1998). A class 'in itself' refers to the objective dimension of class as the basis of social inequality. The unequal distribution of socioeconomic resources such as wealth, income, occupation, and education means that the population can be readily categorised into distinct classes. In this sense, there is little dispute that class exists, such as an upper class of company owners and senior managers. However, it is one matter to identify an objectively defined class structure, but another issue altogether as to whether people are aware of their class membership and express characteristics of 'groupness', 'behavioural and cultural linkages', and 'transformational capacities', as noted by Pakulski and Waters above. A class 'for itself' refers to the subjective dimension of the lived reality of class in the form of social groups of people who share class consciousness and collective social identity and may engage in political action to promote social change. As Anthony Giddens (1982, p. 40) states, 'class relations obviously involve the conscious activity of human agents. But this is different from groups of individuals being conscious of being members of the same class, of having common class interests'. While the objective dimension of class remains as stark as ever, evidenced by the increasing gap between rich and poor, the subjective dimension of class as the basis of individual identity is less clear-cut and at the very least intersects with, and may have been overtaken by, group distinctions based on gender, 'race', ethnicity, and other social movements. However, the persistence of class-based patterns of illness and health-related behaviour suggests that both the objective and subjective dimensions of class are central to any analysis of health inequality.

Class and health inequality

If we accept that we should aim to live in a society that has an equality of health outcomes—that is, no health inequalities based on group membership such as class—then by current standards there is considerable room for improvement. Studies of morbidity (illness) and mortality (death) have consistently shown that the poor have the highest rates of illness and the shortest life expectancy. As chapter 1 discussed, health inequality was a key focus of early

public health/public health
infrastructure Public policies
and infrastructure to prevent
the onset and transmission of
disease among the population,
with a particular focus on sanitation and hygiene such as clean
air, water, and food, and immunisation. Public health
infrastructure refers specifically
to the buildings, installations,
and equipment necessary to
ensure healthy living conditions
for communities and populations.

public health efforts in the 1800s, particularly through the work of Friedrich Engels, Edwin Chadwick and Rudolph Virchow (Engels 1958/1845; Porter 1997). Despite these early efforts, it was not until 1980 and the publication of *Inequalities in Health* (DHSS 1980) in the United Kingdom, commonly referred to as the Black Report after its chairman Sir Douglas Black, that interest in health inequality was renewed (see Townsend & Davidson 1982; Whitehead 1987; Townsend, Davidson, & Whitehead 1992; Benzeval, Judge, & Whitehead 1995).

Australian research, despite different data-collection methods, has consistently found that men in lower skilled and lower paid jobs had higher rates of mortality and morbidity (see Taylor et al. 1983; Broom 1984; McMichael 1985; Broadhead 1985; Siskind et al. 1987a,b; NHS 1992; Whitehead et al. 1993). There have been few empirical studies of the relationship between women, class, and health status. The most significant Australian study was based on the Australian Longitudinal Study on Women's Health, which found a distinct relationship between class and morbidity for women aged 45–49 years (Wicks, Bryson, & Mishra 1997; see also Lee 2001). Using an occupational classification system to determine class, the authors found that women in machine operator and manual worker categories were more likely than women in managerial and professional occupations to experience chest pain, breathing difficulties, painful joints, headaches, and migraines.

The most comprehensive evidence of health inequality in Australia is presented in the National Health Strategy (NHS) report, *Enough to Make You Sick: How Income and Environment Affect Health* (1992). The NHS report used the Australian Bureau of Statistics (ABS) Index of Socioeconomic Disadvantage to categorise the population into regions of inequality, divided into quintiles (fifths of the population) against which mortality and morbidity rates were compared. Quintile 1 represents the top 20 per cent of the population living in regions with the lowest level of socioeconomic disadvantage. Quintile 5 represents the bottom 20 per cent of the population, who live in regions with the most socioeconomic disadvantage. The benefit of measuring health inequality by the socioeconomic status of a geographic area is that this method includes everyone living in a region. Although factors such as income and education will vary greatly within regions, thus making it a highly generalised measure, this method has consistently uncovered that regions with significant rates of socioeconomic disadvantage have high mortality and morbidity.

Some of the key findings of the NHS (1992) report are provided in Figure 4.2. The bars on the graphs compare the death rates in quintiles 2–5 with the death rate in quintile 1 (therefore quintile 1 has no bar). For example, the figure for pneumonia/influenza shows that the death rate for men and women in quintile 5 (people living in regions with the highest rate of socioeconomic disadvantage) is 3.65 times greater for men and 4.09 times greater for women than the least disadvantaged

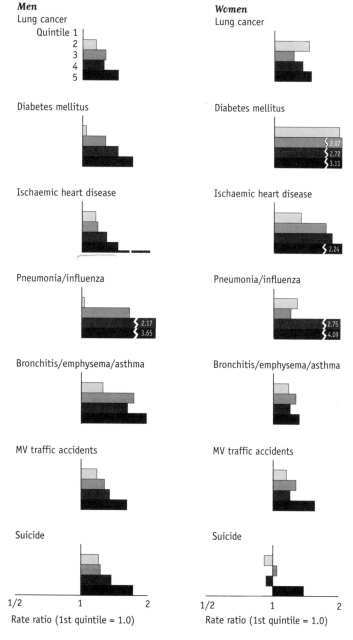

Figure 4.2   Health inequality in Australia by quintile of socio-economic disadvantage

Source: National Health Strategy 1992

area (quintile 1). The NHS report clearly states that 'those of the lowest socioeconomic status have the highest standardised death rates in Australia' (1992, p. 19).

Whereas it generally follows that people living in the most disadvantaged areas have higher morbidity rates, this is not always the case, particularly among women, with conditions such as lung and breast cancer also high among women living in the least disadvantaged areas. The NHS also reported that the lower socioeconomic groups were less likely to use preventative services and dental services. The lack of access to preventative health services reinforces initial health inequalities. As the report states, 'Lack of economic resources may mean that those of low socio-economic status cannot afford to give high priority to use of these services. Consequently, their health may suffer' (NHS 1992, p. 84).

Since the NHS (1992) report, there have been a number of significant Australian and international publications on health inequality (see Box 4.1). In the Australian context, the federal government report, *Better Health Outcomes for Australians* (DHSH 1994) adopted a **social model of health** approach and highlighted the need to address health inequalities. While the report acknowledged the structural basis of health inequality, it remained vague about how these were to be addressed. The availability of data from the *National Health Survey 1995* (ABS 1997) and the 1996 Census have resulted in more recent reports that once again document significant forms of health inequality in Australia, such

social model of health A model of health that focuses on social determinants such as the social production, distribution, and construction of health and illness, and the social organisation of health care. It directs attention to the prevention of illness through community participation and social reforms that address living and working conditions.

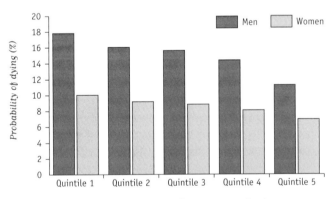

Australian Bureau of Statistics mortality data.
Quintile 1 = most disadvantaged

Figure 4.3 Probability of death between ages 25 and 65 for Australian men and women, by quintile of socioeconomic disadvantage, 1996

Source: Mathers, Vos, & Stevenson, 1999, p. 25, reproduced with permission, © AIHW

as the *Burden of Disease and Injury in Australia* (AIHW 1999) and *A Social Health Atlas of Australia* (Glover et al. 1999). The most recent Australian findings on health inequality, shown in Figure 4.3, are reported by Colin Mathers and colleagues (1999), once again using the Index of Socioeconomic Disadvantage to show that the probability of premature death increases steadily from the least socioeconomic disadvantaged area to the most, in this case represented by quintile 1.

Even though the overall health of the Australian population improved between 1985–87 and 1995–97, 'the extent of socio-economic inequality in mortality has remained fairly stable and, for some conditions, increased' (Turrell & Mathers 2000, p. 435), paralleling similar findings in the United Kingdom (see Acheson 1998; Marmot 2000). Such findings are a reminder that life-expectancy figures oversimplify population health by masking the social patterning of illness, whereby the most disadvantaged groups have far worse health. For example, as Table 4.2 shows, compared to the least disadvantaged areas, mortality rates for certain conditions in the most disadvantaged areas increased significantly over the years for both men and women aged between 25 and 64. For example, mortality from lung disease for men increased from 60 per cent to 98 per cent, and mortality from diabetes for women increased from 204 per cent to 249 per cent.

Table 4.2 Mortality rates for men and women aged 25–64 in most disadvantaged areas, compared with least disadvantaged

	Men			*Women*	
	1985–1987	*1995–1997*		*1985–1987*	*1995–1997*
Heart disease	55% higher	87%	Asthma emphysema	43% higher	194%
Lung cancer	60%	98%	Diabetes	204%	249%

Source: Adapted from Turrell & Mathers 2000, p. 435

The mounting evidence of health inequality even resulted in the federal government releasing a short report, *Health Policy and Inequality* (Hupalo & Herden 1999), a somewhat surprising publication given the conservative nature of the government of the day. However, the report provides a superficial treatment of the topic, and while clearly acknowledging the persistence of health inequality, it relies on vague policy statements such as the need for intersectoral collaboration and more support services to enable general practitioners to deal with the problem, avoiding discussion of policies relating to employment, income support and educational opportunities that may alleviate the long-term socioeconomic determinants of health inequality (Najman & Davey Smith 2000). In *Socioeconomic Determinants of Health,*

Gavin Turrell and colleagues (1999) present a detailed review of existing Australian research on health inequality, including an examination of policies aimed at reducing health inequality, as well as providing some preliminary suggestions for future research and interventions. The authors of the report summarise the available research findings by stating conclusively that:

> persons variously classified as 'low' SES have higher mortality rates for most major causes of death, their morbidity profile indicates that they experience more ill-health, and their use of health care services suggest that they are less likely to act to prevent disease or detect it at an asymptomatic stage. Moreover, socioeconomic differences in health are evident for both females and males at every stage of the life-course (birth, infancy, childhood and adolescence, and adult-hood) and the relationship exists irrespective of how SES and health are measured (Turrell et al. 1999, p. 33).

Following the publication of the reports by Turrell et al. (1999) and Hupalo and Herden (1999), the federal government established the Health Inequalities Research Collaboration (HIRC), which aims to provide a national focus on health inequality research and intervention, with information primarily disseminated from its web site (see <www.hirc.health.gov.au>).

Box 4.1 Major publications on health inequality since 1992

Australian publications

Enough to Make You Sick: How Income and Environment Affect Health (NHS 1992)

Better Health Outcomes for Australians (DHSH 1994)

National Health Survey 1995 (ABS 1997)

For Richer, For Poorer, In Sickness and in Health (Royal Australasian College of Physicians 1999)

Health Policy and Inequality (Hupalo & Herden 1999)

Socioeconomic Determinants of Health: Towards a National Research Program and a Policy and Intervention Agenda (Turrell et al. 1999)

The Burden of Disease and Injury in Australia (Mathers, Vos, & Stevenson 1999)

A Social Health Atlas of Australia (Glover et al. 1999)

International publications

Inequalities in Health: The Black Report and the Health Divide (Townsend, Davidson, & Whitehead 1992)

Tackling Inequalities in Health: An Agenda for Action
(Benzeval, Judge, & Whitehead 1995)
Unhealthy Societies: The Afflictions of Inequality (Wilkinson
1996)
Independent Inquiry into Inequalities in Health (Acheson
1998)
*The Social, Cultural and Economic Determinants of Health in
New Zealand* (National Advisory Committee on
Health and Disability 1998)
The Solid Facts: Social Determinants of Health (Wilkinson
& Marmot 1998)
Social Determinants of Health (Marmot and Wilkinson 1999)
*Taskforce on Equity: Key Issues for the World Health
Organization* (WHO 1998)
Social Inequalities in Health: New Zealand 1999 (Howden-
Chapman & Tobias 2000)
Health for All (HFA) in the 21st Century (WHO 2000)

Explaining health inequality

The most common explanations of health inequality can be grouped
into five main categories:
1   artefact explanations
2   natural/social selection explanations
3   cultural/behavioural explanations
4   materialist/structural explanations
5   psychosocial/social capital explanations.
The first four were initially introduced in the Black Report
(DHSS 1980) in Britain and were also discussed in the Australian
NHS (1992) report *Enough to Make You Sick.* The fifth explanation
is the most recent and has been influenced by the work of
Michael Marmot and Richard Wilkinson (see Wilkinson 1996;
Marmot & Wilkinson 1999).

Artefact explanations
The artefact explanation suggests that links between class and
health are artificial and are the result of statistical anomalies or the
inability to accurately measure social phenomena. This viewpoint
is easily disputed by the vast amount of evidence based on various methods and classificatory schemes that have clearly found
health inequality exists. While the Black Report dismissed the
artefact explanation as without basis, as Sally Macintyre (1997)
suggests, what has been overlooked in the report is that the

authors made the important point that the assumptions under-pinning the way class and health are measured can influence the size of health inequality that is found.

Natural/social selection explanations

social Darwinism The incorrect application of Charles Darwin's theory of animal evolution to explain social inequality by trans-ferring his idea of 'survival of the fittest' among animals to 'explain' human inequality.

The Black Report also briefly discussed **social Darwinist** explana-tions that suggested that social and health inequality were due to biological inferiority. This viewpoint acknowledges the relationship between class and health, but explains it by assuming that inequality is 'natural' and thus inevitable; meaning nothing can or should be done about it. Such a viewpoint has been effectively dismissed by social science research, but Macintyre (1997) suggests there is a 'soft' version (her term) of this explanation that is still commonly ascribed to and has some explanatory power. The soft version suggests that social selection can play a part, whereby poor health early in life results in poor educational performance and occupational achieve-ment. The central idea here is that people's health disadvantage (for example disability) causes social disadvantage such as poverty. Most studies that have examined the social selection explanation have consistently found it can only account for a small percentage of people in groups who suffer health inequality. Furthermore, such an explanation neglects the structural causes of ill health to begin with, such as being born into a family already in poverty, which then leads to ill health and a cycle of disadvantage (such as that found among many Indigenous groups).

Cultural/behavioural explanations

Cultural/behavioural explanations focus on the individual to explain health inequality in the form of risk-taking or illness-related behaviour such as smoking, drug taking, excess alcohol consumption, and poor dietary intake as the cause of ill health. Such accounts have rightly been criticised for their **victim-blaming** and overly simplistic account of inequality. As Wilkinson (1996, p. 21–2), among others, has forcefully argued, such views are unhelpful because

victim-blaming The process whereby social inequality is explained in terms of individuals being solely responsible for what happens to them in relation to the choices they make and their assumed psychological, cultural, and/or biological inferiority.

> the underlying flaw in the system is not put right, it gives rise to a continuous flow, both of people who have suffered as a result, and of demands for special services to meet their needs … even when it comes to tackling the individual risk factors, it may sometimes be more effective to tackle them at a societal level … to tackle the envi-ronment that establishes levels of exposure to risk.

A focus on changing the behaviour of individuals assumes they exist in a social vacuum, ignoring the social context, social relations and social processes that affect their lives. As noted in chapter 1, there are illness-inducing factors that lie outside of an individual's control, such as stressful work environments or the marketing efforts of corporations. Solely concentrating on the individual as the cause and cure of illness (which has often been the focus of much medical, **epidemiological**, and psychological research) also assumes the individual is motivated and has the time and resources for active participation in changing their behaviour and lifestyle.

Macintyre (1997, p. 728) argues that the Black Report did discuss a 'more socially (rather than individually) based model of health-related behaviours'. For example, the report states that behaviour can also be viewed as 'embedded more within social structures; as illustrative of socially distinguishable styles of life, associated with, and reinforced by, class' (Townsend, Davidson, & Whitehead 1999, p. 100). It is indeed true that the working class have higher rates of some health-damaging behaviour such as smoking and use preventative services less. The question remains, 'why are there class differences in health-related behaviour'—an issue that has received scant attention in sociological literature until recently.

Materialist/structural explanations

Materialist/structural explanations concern the role of social, economic, and political factors in determining the social distribution of health and illness. The main thrust of this view has been a focus on how poor living and working conditions, particularly poverty, discrimination, lack of educational and employment opportunities, inadequate nutrition and housing, and the lack of regular income and savings all directly influence illness. Materialist/structural explanations have been particularly addressed by class analysis (see Connell 1988; Waitzkin 1983; 2000) and direct attention away from individualistic and victim-blaming accounts towards the basic class structure of society.

The value of class analysis and a structural approach to explaining health inequality is evident when examining the role played by employment and unemployment in understanding and addressing health inequality. Access to employment and the actual nature of the work that people do can have a significant influence on their health. A growing literature has documented the health consequences of unemployment (see Bartley, Ferrie, & Scott 1999; Mathers & Schofield 1998; Graetz 1993; Smith 1987). Research on the health effects of unemployment is relatively recent and Australian data is incomplete; nonetheless, Mathers and Schofield (1998) provide a significant review of the available Australian and international literature on unemployment and health. Australian findings drawn from the 1989–90 National Health Survey indicate that unemployed women and men aged between 25 and 64 rated their health as poor or fair (compared to good or excellent) at twice the rate of the employed, as well as reporting a 30–40 per

epidemiology/

social epidemiology The statistical study of patterns of disease in the population. Originally focused on epidemics, or infectious diseases, it now covers non-infectious conditions such as stroke and cancer. Social epidemiology is a sub-field aligned with sociology that focuses on the social determinants of illness.

cent greater rate of chronic illness and a 20–30 per cent greater rate of recent health problems (Mathers 1994).

There is continuing debate in this literature over whether unemployment leads to a deterioration of a person's health status or whether poor health status leads to unemployment, echoing the debate over social selection discussed above. Much of the literature on unemployment and health has been influenced by psychological perspectives, which tend to downplay economic insecurity in favour of psychosocial factors such as the impact of unemployment on social isolation, loss of identity, and anxiety, which allegedly increase illness-related behaviour. While these factors are without doubt important, a sociological analysis focuses on the underlying structural basis of unemployment and ill health, whereby low-income groups (Indigenous populations, recent migrants, and unskilled workers) are over-represented among the unemployed and have the poorest health status. According to Mathers and Schofield (1998, p. 181), there is clear evidence from a range of studies to show that the actual experience of unemployment 'has a direct effect on health over and above the effects of socioeconomic status, poverty, risk factors, or prior ill-health.'

Occupational health and safety

For those who are employed, work can also be hazardous to health. For example, those employed in the mining industry have the highest occupational mortality and morbidity rates, followed by agriculture, manufacturing, construction, and transport and communication (Driscoll & Mayhew 1999). Work-related illness is usually divided into two categories:

1 **occupational injuries**: refers to a single incident that results in an immediate, obvious, physically disabling condition (e.g. broken or severely damaged limbs) or death

2 **occupational disease**: refers to ill health that results from prolonged exposure to toxic substances and hazardous work processes, such as radiation, lead, asbestos, and high levels of noise, and which gradually develops over time and does not cause immediately observable damage to a person's health (e.g. asbestos-related cancer, industrial deafness).

Note that these categories avoid the use of the word 'accident' because it tends to imply that work-related health problems are random and unforeseeable events. While accidents no doubt occur, social patterns of injury and disease suggest that many work-related health problems are predictable and preventable.

As Tim Driscoll and Claire Mayhew (1999) report, each year in Australia more than 400 people die from occupational injuries, and a further 2300 die from occupational diseases, with 60 per cent due to cancer (60 per cent of which are lung cancer). More than

700 deaths each year are due to asbestos-related cancer (malignant mesothelioma). It is estimated that by 2010, asbestos-related deaths in Australia will have totalled 18 000, the highest rate in the world (Driscoll & Mayhew 1999). In 1994, the total health costs of work-related death and illness in Australia were estimated at $9 billion per year, a figure likely to have grown substantially since then (Industry Commission 1994).

The workplace has traditionally not been the focus of health policy. This is considered to be due to a number of related factors:

- the profit motive and managerial prerogative
- union attitudes
- state differences
- the dominance of the **biomedical model**, and
- the careless-worker myth.

biomedicine/biomedical model
The conventional approach to medicine in Western societies. It diagnoses and explains illness as a malfunction of one of the body's biological mechanisms. The biomedical approach of most health services focuses on the treating of individuals, and generally ignores social, economic, and environmental factors.

Certain kinds of ill health are effectively created by the social organisation of work. A number of authors have argued that the relationship between work and illness is based on a fundamental conflict of interest between workers' health and profit-maximisation (Quinlan 1993; Quinlan 1988; Willis 1994). Safety is often seen as a cost to be borne by employers, and so precautions are avoided both by employers and by governments who have been unwilling to impose an economic 'burden' on employers. There has also been an unwillingness to encroach upon what has been viewed as managerial prerogative. Managerial prerogative refers to the philosophical belief that views business (at its most extreme) as having little social or individual responsibility. Managers employ workers to do a job, and it is up to employees to accept the risks. A similar view is also considered to have been tacitly held by some unions, which have pursued extra pay ('danger money') without trying to alter dangerous conditions. The representative union body, the Australian Council of Trade Unions (ACTU), only established its OHS Unit in 1981.

OHS is a State government responsibility, but few States monitor work practices or enforce legislation, as they wish to avoid placing extra costs on business, which may result in companies moving to 'friendly' States. David Biggins (1995) notes that little headway has been made in the move towards uniform OHS laws, with significant differences still existing for penalties and compensation payments between States. While there have been some significant reforms—such as the training of thousands of employees as health and safety representatives, and legislation to give employees the right to know about the health implications of their work—there has been no marked decrease in work-related deaths, injuries, and diseases over the last decade. Biggins argues that there is a need for greater democratic representation of workers' interests through unions or through workplace-level employee participation in OHS committees to ensure that substantive progress is made.

Doctors traditionally have had limited training in OHS issues such as toxicology and work practices, with the focus of the medical model being on treating individuals once they are sick or injured, rather than on prevention (see chapters 1 and 10). The individualistic focus of health care has traditionally resulted in victim-blaming (reflecting wider social values), a practice that assumes workers are careless or malingering, despite little evidence to support such a view. For example, repetitive strain injury (RSI) was initially ridiculed by many doctors through the use of derogatory terms such as 'migrant arm', 'kangaroo paw', and 'golden wrist'. Michael Quinlan (1993) argues that such victim-blaming views have a long history, but gained legitimacy from the 1950s onwards through the work of industrial psychologists, who 'explained' workplace illness as the result of '**accident-proneness**'. Despite years of research, no specific personality traits identifying the allegedly 'accident-prone' worker independent of workplace conditions have been substantiated. While human error does occur, it is usually the result of long hours, high noise levels, poor training, or pressure to produce a certain rate of output that leads to errors being made. Industrial psychologists can face a conflict of interest if employers pay their wage, and their training means that the solutions they offer tend to be individualistic—attempting to modify worker behaviour rather than recommending safer equipment or changes in staffing and shift work. Despite the increasing research into the personal, health, and workplace costs of occupational injury and disease, and a number of progressive employers and unions that have begun to address OHS, the continuing high mortality and morbidity rates indicate that there is still much work to be done.

Macintyre (1997, p. 740) notes that in the wider literature since the publication of the Black Report, the four explanations of health inequality discussed above have often been viewed as mutually exclusive, establishing false debates between 'artefact versus real differences', 'selection versus causation', and 'behaviour versus material circumstances'. Such 'either/or' debates have been unhelpful and she makes a clear case that even though the authors of the Black Report favoured the structural explanation, they still acknowledged the minor role of social selection and the role of cultural and behavioural factors. The focus of structural approaches has been class analysis with policy prescriptions based on **social justice** through welfare measures to address poverty, improve workplace safety, and promote health-inducing work and public spaces (such as smoke-free environments). However,

accident-proneness A term invented by industrial psychologists to 'explain' workplace injury and illness. It is based on the false and unproven assumption that workers are careless and malingering, and are therefore solely responsible for accidents.

social justice A belief system that gives high priority to the interests of the least advantaged.

class analysis has been less successful in explaining the continued difference in health-related behaviour among the poor. A more recent explanation has pointed to psychosocial factors and the lack of **social cohesion** or **social capital** as the basis for the persistence of health inequality in developed countries.

social cohesion A term used to refer to the social ties that are the basis for group behaviour and integration.

Psychosocial/social capital explanations

An alternative explanation of health inequality has arisen from the work of social epidemiologists Marmot and Wilkinson (see Wilkinson 1996; Wilkinson & Marmot 1998; Marmot & Wilkinson 1999). While concerned with the social origins of illness, they have turned attention away from class analysis to a narrower focus on income inequality and psychosocial factors. The authors suggest that widening income inequality accompanied by work intensification and rising unemployment has led to increased levels of stress, anxiety, insecurity, anger, and depression among the community, and that these psychosocial factors negatively impact on health not only among the poor, but also on those who experience relative inequality.

social capital A term used to refer to social relations, networks, norms, trust, and reciprocity between individuals that facilitate cooperation for mutual benefit.

Marmot has been the principal researcher in what have become known as the Whitehall studies, which have examined the health of British civil servants since the 1960s and continue today (see Marmot et al. 1978; Marmot et al. 1991; Marmot et al. 1997; Marmot et al. 1999). The first study found a 'social gradient' in the mortality rate, whereby life expectancy increased for each employment level up to the top of the public service hierarchy. Participants in the initial study (all men) were grouped into four employment grades, with those in the bottom two grades found to have a life expectancy 4.4 years shorter than those in the top two grades (Marmot et al. 1978). Furthermore, the social gradient applied to a range conditions such as stroke, cancer and gastrointestinal disease (Marmot 2000).

risk factors Conditions that are thought to increase an individual's susceptibility to illness or disease such as abuse of alcohol or smoking.

There are two sociologically significant aspects to the findings arsing from the Whitehall study. First, the social gradient of health continued along the whole occupational hierarchy, suggesting that health inequality did not only affect those in poverty, but also existed among relatively well-paid, white-collar workers. Second, **lifestyle/risk factors** only accounted for a small percentage of the social gradient. Risk factors such as overweight, smoking, alcohol consumption, and lack of exercise could not explain the health inequality between the occupational grades of the civil servants in the study (see Marmot et al. 1997; Marmot et al. 1999; Marmot 2000). In an attempt to discover what other determinants might be involved, the Whitehall II study (which included women) focused on the impact of stress on employee health, examining the

lifestyle choices/factors The decisions people make that are likely to impact on their health such as diet, exercise, smoking, alcohol, and other drugs. The term implies that people are solely responsible for choosing and changing their lifestyle.

social support The support provided to an individual by being part of a network of kin, friends, or colleagues.

gross domestic product (GDP) The market value of all goods and services that have been sold during a year.

extent of employee control and variety at work, and the role played by **social support**. The Whitehall II study also found a social gradient for morbidity among women as well as men, and its major conclusion was that those with less control over work had higher rates of heart disease, depression and other health problems (see Marmot et al. 1991; Marmot et al. 1997; Marmot et al. 1999; Marmot 2000).

In *Unhealthy Societies*, Richard Wilkinson (1996) presents empirical evidence to support a thesis that societies with lower levels of income inequality have the highest life expectancy. His argument is that once a country reaches a certain amount of wealth determined by **gross domestic product (GDP)** per capita (per head of population) and undergoes the 'epidemiologic transition' from infectious disease to chronic disease as the major cause of mortality, increases in national wealth have little impact on population health. For example, he notes that even though the GDP per head in the USA is almost twice that of Greece, life expectancy in Greece is higher (Wilkinson 1999; see also Wilkinson 1992). Therefore, for developed countries, Wilkinson argues that it is not the total wealth of a society that is important, but rather the distribution of that wealth—the more egalitarian it is, the better the life expectancy and hence the less likelihood of health inequality. As Wilkinson (1996, p. 3) states, there is a 'strong relationship between income distribution and national mortality rates. In the developed world, it is not the richest countries which have the best health, but the most egalitarian.'

Wilkinson's work has spawned a significant literature debating the merits of his study and its conclusions. While a significant number of studies have supported his findings (see Kaplan et al. 1996; Kennedy et al. 1996), others have cast doubt on the accuracy and strength of his claims. For example, in a significant study by Ken Judge and colleagues (1998), statistical associations between income inequality and population health were found not to be great, posing 'a serious challenge to those who believe that the relationship is a very powerful one' (Judge, Mulligan, & Benzenval 1998, p. 578).

The work of Marmot and Wilkinson extends the health-inequality debate beyond a focus on the most socioeconomically disadvantaged groups. Instead, they highlight that a social gradient or continuum of health inequality exists, whereby health gradually worsens as you move down the social hierarchy, so that each social group has worse health than the one above it. For these authors, relative inequality is linked to poorer health, and as Marmot and colleagues found, even for employed white-collar workers, who by definition are not poor or exposed to hazardous work environments. Therefore, it is not only the working class or the poor who experience health inequality, but groups along the whole social hierarchy. Though these findings are yet to be confirmed in Australia, they suggest that materialist/structural explanations offer an incomplete account of health inequality. Subsequently, a range of authors spearheaded by Marmot and Wilkinson has focused on psychosocial factors as the main basis of health inequality.

The psychosocial thesis: the benefits and limits of neo-functionalist approaches

The 'psychosocial thesis' suggests that societies with greater income inequality have less social cohesion or social capital. The idea of social cohesion or social capital is a reworking of Émile Durkheim's (1984/1893; 1951/1897) concept of social solidarity. More recently the concept of social capital has been advanced in the work of Pierre Bourdieu (1986), Jonathon Coleman (1988), and Robert Putnam (1993) and has been popularised in Australia by Eva Cox (1995). Social capital refers to social relations and networks that exist among social groups and communities and that provide access to resources and opportunities for mutual benefit. Social capital depends on a high level of community participation, altruism, trust and an expectation of reciprocity. It has been suggested that the lack of social capital or social cohesion explains why certain social groups adopt health-damaging behaviour. The assumption is that access to social capital will lead to improved health outcomes by lowering stress, providing outlets for social interaction and opportunities for enhancing control over one's life through democratic participation in community life (Winter 2000a,b).

Putnam (1993) and Cox (1995) envisage social capital as a collective property of specific communities or society as a whole, rather than an attribute or trait possessed by individuals. For Cox (1995, p. 46) social capital involves an 'interplay of state and community', and has been a useful concept for counteracting the negative effects of economic rationalism, which she claims has undermined communities by fostering insecurity and anxiety. High levels of social capital are reflected in altruistic activities such as volunteer work that contributes to the welfare of others. Putnam (2000, p. 331) goes so far as to claim that 'if you belong to no groups but decide to join one, you cut your risk of dying over the next year by half.'

Michael Woolcock (1998, p. 195), while supportive of the social capital concept, suggests that it is often used in an uncritical and imprecise way, resulting in a handy catch-all concept that 'risks trying to explain too much with too little'. The vague nature of the concept and its intangible qualities (trust, reciprocity) have allowed it to be used by both progressive and conservative political groups, notably the World Bank, which is a key proponent of the concept (Kawachi & Berkman 2000). Conservative commentators (see Coleman 1988) conceptualise social capital as a property of individuals, whereby social disadvantage is viewed as being overcome by individuals engaging in volunteer work, joining associations and making the most of their own support networks. In this formulation, social capital becomes a code word for mutual obligation and individual responsibility. Therefore, social capital can be used to support economic rationalist policies of cutting expenditure on the social wage and public health by placing an increased emphasis on community and family responsibility and voluntary work. It is interesting to note that working-class examples of social capital, such as collective action through union involvement, tend to be ignored and are not taken into account as evidence of social cohesion and democratic participation in community life (Muntaner & Lynch 1999). Proponents of social capital also downplay the possibility that it can have negative implications, whereby communities and membership of certain clubs and associations can be used for the social exclusion of others such as ethnic minorities. It is even possible to view the close-knit and mutually supportive nature of criminal gangs as exhibiting strong social capital—a particularly unhealthy scenario (Muntaner, Lynch, & Davey Smith 2001).

Social capital resembles community development approaches advocated in the 1970s and fits well with current health promotion efforts that advocate empowering individuals to participate in community activities (Baum et al. 2000). However, these have often met with limited success because they ignored the important role that economic resources and public policies play in facilitating community development and fostering notions of social cohesion or social capital (Winter 2000b; Muntaner, Lynch, & Davey Smith 2001; see also chapter 18). High rates of poverty and unemployment in a community are unlikely to facilitate social cohesion. As Putnam states (1993, p. 42), 'Social capital is not a substitute for effective public policy but rather a prerequisite for it and, in part, a consequence of it.' Public policies that facilitate employment opportunities, social services, and access to social institutions such as education set the conditions for social capital and health-enhancing environments.

Bringing class analysis back in: the structure/agency debate and health behaviour

structure/agency debate A key debate in sociology over the extent to which human behaviour is determined by social structure.

The benefit of the psychosocial/social capital approach is its engagement with the **structure/agency debate** (discussed in

- While class is a major form of social inequality, there are other important intersecting structures of inequality based on gender, 'race', ethnicity, and other social groups, such as youth and the aged. While there is disagreement in the wider literature between objective (class 'in itself') and subjective (class 'for itself') notions of class, with some suggesting class in subjective terms 'is dead', class is still strongly associated with health status.
- Numerous studies using different research methods and forms of measurement have consistently documented that the poor/low SES groups/low income groups/working class have higher rates of mortality and morbidity.
- Recent studies have also exposed a social gradient of health, whereby a continuum of health inequality exists from top to bottom of the occupational and income hierarchy.
- There are five main explanations of health inequality: artefact, natural/social selection, cultural/behavioural, materialist/structural, and psychosocial/social capital explanations.
- Health inequality can only be reduced through social justice strategies that address class inequality through structural change in the economy, the workplace, and the community.

Discussion questions

1 What class are you? Do you believe class has influenced your beliefs, lifestyle, and life chances?
2 In what ways might the upper class in Australia also be considered a ruling class? Think of some real-life examples in your response.
3 In what ways can class analysis shed light on why health inequality exists? What are the limits of class analysis?
4 What are the benefits and limitations of psychosocial/social capital explanations of health inequality?
5 Why do the working class exhibit higher rates of health-damaging behaviour?
6 Given that there are social patterns of health-related behaviour, to what extent are individuals responsible for their health?

Further investigation

1 Examine why the workplace is a major cause of premature death and illness.
2 Why does equal access to health care not lead to equal health outcomes?
3 Compare and contrast the neo-functionalist approach of psychosocial/social capital explanations of health inequality with neo-Marxist and neo-Weberian analyses. Which provides the best fit in explaining health inequality in Australia?

Further reading and web resources

Class and health inequality

Annandale, E. 1998, *The Sociology of Health and Medicine: A Critical Introduction*, Polity Press, Cambridge, Chapter 4, pp. 89–122.

Bartley, M., Blane, D., & Davey-Smith, G. (eds) 1998, *The Sociology of Health Inequalities*, Blackwell, Oxford (also published in *Sociology of Health & Illness*, vol. 20, no. 5).

Benzeval, M., Judge, K., & Whitehead, M. (eds) 1995, *Tackling Inequalities in Health: An Agenda or Action*, King's Fund, London.

Berkman, L. F. & Kawachi, I. (eds) 2000, *Social Epidemiology*, Oxford University Press, New York.

Burdess, N. 1999, 'Class and Health', in C. Grbich (ed.), *Health in Australia*, 2nd edn, Prentice Hall, Sydney, Chapter 8, pp. 149–71.

Coburn, D. 2000, 'Income Inequality, Social Cohesion and the Health Status of Populations: The Role of Neo-liberalism', *Social Science & Medicine*, vol. 51, no. 1, pp. 135–46.

Connell, R.W. 1988, 'Class Inequalities and "Just Health" ', *Community Health Studies*, vol. 12, no. 2, pp. 212–17.

Glover, J., Harris, K., & Tennant, S. 1999, *A Social Health Atlas of Australia*, vol. 1, 2nd edn, Public Health Informational Development Unit, Adelaide.

Graham, H. (ed.) 2000, *Understanding Health Inequalities*, Open University Press, Buckingham.

'Health Inequalities in Modern Societies and Beyond' 1997, *Social Science & Medicine, Special Issue*, vol. 44, no. 6, March.

Macintyre, S. 1997, 'The Black Report and Beyond: What are the Issues?', *Social Science & Medicine*, vol. 44, no. 6, pp. 723–45.

Marmot, M. & Wilkinson, R. G. (eds) 1999, *Social Determinants of Health*, Oxford University Press, Oxford.

National Health Strategy 1992, *Enough to Make You Sick: How Income and Environment Affect Health*, AGPS, Canberra.

Navarro, V. (ed.) 2001, *Political Economy of Social Inequalities: Consequences for Health and Quality of Life*, Baywood, Amityville.

Turrell, G., Oldenburg, B., McGuffog, I., & Dent, R. 1999, *Socioeconomic Determinants of Health: Towards a National Research Program and a Policy and Intervention Agenda*, Queensland University of Technology, School of Public Health, Centre for Public Health Research, Brisbane.

Wilkinson, R. G. 1996, *Unhealthy Societies: The Afflictions of Inequality*, Routledge, London.

Class debates

Baxter, J. H., Emmison, J. M., Western, J. S., & Western, M. C. (eds) 1991, *Class Analysis and Contemporary Australia*, Macmillan, Melbourne.

Connell, R. W. & Irving, T. H. 1992, *Class Structure in Australian History: Poverty and Progress*, 2nd edn, Longman Cheshire, Melbourne.

Crompton, R. 1998, *Class and Stratification: An Introduction to Current Debates*, 2nd edn, Polity Press, Cambridge.

McGregor, C. 1997, *Class in Australia*, Penguin, Melbourne.

Pakulski, J. & Waters, M. 1996, *The Death of Class*, Sage, London.

Western, M. 2000, 'Class in Australia in the 1980s and 1990s', in J. M. Najman & J. S. Western (eds), *A Sociology of Australian Society*, 3rd edn, Macmillan, Melbourne, Chapter 4, pp. 68–88.

Wright, E. O. 1997, *Class Counts: Comparative Studies in Class Analysis*, Cambridge University Press, Cambridge.

Social capital and health

Kawachi, I. & Berkman, L. 2000, 'Social Cohesion, Social Capital, and Health', in L. F. Berkman & I. Kawachi (eds), *Social Epidemiology*, Oxford University Press, New York, pp. 174–90.

Muntaner, C. & Lynch, J. 1999, 'Income Inequality, Social Cohesion, and Class Relations: A Critique of Wilkinson's Neo-Durkheimian Research Program', *International Journal of Health Services*, vol. 29, no. 1, pp. 59–81.

Muntaner, C., Lynch, J., & Davey Smith, G. 2001, 'Social Capital, Disorganized Communities and the Third Way: Understanding the Retreat from Structural Inequalities in Epidemiology and Public Health', *International Journal of Health Services*, vol. 31, no. 2, pp. 213–37.

Winter, I. (ed.) 2000, *Social Capital and Public Policy in Australia*, Australian Institute of Family Studies, Melbourne.

Woolcock, M. 1998, 'Social Capital and Economic Development: Toward a Theoretical Synthesis and Policy Framework', *Theory & Society*, vol. 27, pp. 151–208

Health and work

Daykin, N. & Doyal, L. (eds) 1999, *Health and Work: Critical Perspectives*, Macmillan, London.

Mayhew, C. & Peterson, C. L. (eds) 1999, *Occupational Health and Safety in Australia*, Allen & Unwin, Sydney.

Peterson, C. L. 1999, *Stress at Work: A Sociological Perspective*, Baywood Press, Amityville.

Quinlan, M. 1988, 'Psychological and Sociological Approaches to the Study of Occupational Illness: A Critical Review', *Australia and New Zealand Journal of Sociology*, vol. 24, no. 2, pp. 189–206.

Web sites

Health Inequalities Research Collaboration (HIRC): <www.hirc.health.gov.au>

Health Variations Programme (Social Determinants of Health Inequalities): <www.lancs.ac.uk/users/apsocsci/hvp/intro.htm>

Independent Inquiry into Inequalities in Health—the Acheson Report (UK) <www.doh.gov.uk/ih/main.htm>

Inequality.org: <www.inequality.org>

International Society for Equity in Health: <www.iseqh.org>

National Institutes of Health (USA), Addressing Health Inequalities: <http://healthdisparities.nih.gov>

National Occupational Health and Safety Commission: <www.nohsc.gov.au>

Social Determinants of Health—The Solid Facts: <www.who.dk/
    healthy-cities/determ.htm>
Social Health Atlas of Australia: <www.publichealth.gov.au/atlas.htm>
Social Inequalities in Health (NZ): <www.hfa.govt.nz/moh.nsf/wpgIndex/
    Publications-Online+Publications+Contents>
UK Health Equity Network: <www.ukhen.org.uk>
Whitehall II Study: <www.ucl.ac.uk/epidemiology/white/white.html>
World Bank Social Capital:
    <www.worldbank.org/poverty/scapital/index.htm>
World Wealth Report 2001: <www.ir.ml.com/news/ML051401.pdf>

5

Gender and Health

Dorothy Broom

Overview

* *How is gender important in understanding health and illness?*
* *What have been the main activities of the women's health movement?*
* *Why has a men's health movement arisen?*

Women are more likely to report illness, seek help from a doctor, and use alternative therapies than men are, but they live, on average, five years longer than men do. Women tend to have higher rates of psychological distress, but more men commit suicide. The simplistic conclusion to be drawn from such findings is that 'women get sick and men die'. However, a closer examination shows that the statistics are less contradictory. While there are a number of sex-linked diseases—such as breast cancer for women and prostate cancer for men—women and men are equally likely to be hospitalised (excluding hospitalisation for pregnancy). Differences in mortality and morbidity reflect social differences in male and female behaviour (related to notions of masculinity and femininity) and the nature of the work that men and women perform.

Key terms

class	'race'
ethnicity	risk factors
gender/sex	randomised control trials (RCTs)
gendered health	sexism in medicine
health promotion	sexual division of labour
men's health	women's health movement
norms	

Introduction

gender/sex This term refers to the socially constructed categories of feminine and masculine (the cultural values that dictate how men and women should behave), as opposed to the categories of biological sex (female or male).

sexual division of labour This refers to the nature of work performed as a result of gender roles. The stereotype is that of the male breadwinner and the female home-maker.

norms Expectations about how people ought to act or behave.

Because **gender** is such a significant dimension of social difference in contemporary Western societies, we tend to take it for granted. It is hard to imagine that gender roles could be less socially important or organised differently from the familiar patterns that we see every day. So it can be surprising to learn that, while gender is socially recognised in all known societies, there is wide historical and cultural variation in the way it is expressed. In every society, at least some work is allocated on the basis of gender; this allocation is called the **sexual division of labour**. In some societies, females and males undertake sharply differentiated activities, and may be physically segregated for substantial periods, either as a specific social **norm** or as a consequence of the sexual division of labour. In other societies, children of both sexes are treated in much the same way, but gender difference becomes important in adolescence or young adulthood. In many societies, only a few activities are specific to one sex, and the sexual division of labour is minimal. Men dominate overtly in certain cultures; elsewhere, the lives and powers of the two sexes are largely balanced and complementary. In developed societies, the norms and symbols that govern gender tend to vary according to class, subculture, and ethnicity. And everywhere, gender patterns are dynamic: they change over time. The very terms we use are being contested. In the early 1970s, a distinction was drawn between sex (biological) and gender (psychosocial) (Oakley 1972). However, subsequent theoretical discussions have unsettled that clear dichotomy (Gatens 1991), and whereas the distinction is still often cited, in this chapter the words are used without any intention to communicate a sharp distinction.

In the face of such variation and fluidity, making useful generalisations about gender and health is a challenging task. As with class and ethnicity, the relationship between health and gender is a complex interaction among material circumstances, physical entities, cultural processes, and social organisation. The discussion here concentrates on the interplay between health and gender, both in Australia and in similar contemporary societies.

Gendered health

On the face of it, one might think there is little to explain. Humans have sexually specific organs and processes, and malfunction in those organs and processes *is* the relationship between gender and health. Females can get breast and cervix cancer; males can get testicular and prostate cancer. According to this view, the rest of health is just human, not gendered. A discussion of sexually specific complaints hardly exhausts the topic, however. Many of the conditions that occur in both sexes appear more often in one sex than the other, or they occur at very different ages. For example, stomach cancer is much more common among males than females; cardio-vascular disease is common in both sexes, but tends to occur at later ages among women than among men. These kinds of comparisons suggest that the health of women and men is a product of many elements, and not just differences in reproductive organs. The sexes differ in the types of lives that they typically live, and these differences can influence health. That is, gender is a significant and complex element in the social production of health and illness.

Disease and death: sex comparisons

Except for a very few nations (mostly in South Asia), there are slightly more females in the population than males because female life expectancy is greater than male life expectancy (Kane 1991), and this is true for contemporary Australia. More than half of the Australian population (50.2 per cent) is female, but because female life expectancy exceeds male life expectancy by more than five years (AIHW 2000), there are proportionally more women in the older population (57 per cent of those aged 65 years and over) (ABS 1995a). Life expectancy for the Indigenous population is markedly shorter than for the total Australian population, but sex differences in longevity prevail among Indigenous, as well as non-Indigenous, people. The main causes of death are largely similar for both sexes, and sexually specific diseases contribute only a small proportion of the overall death rate, as is evident in Table 5.1. However, respiratory and infectious or parasitic diseases figure much more significantly in the deaths of Indigenous people than the table would suggest.

Table 5.1   Leading causes of death, 1997 (standardised death rates per 100 000 persons of the population of the same sex)

Cause of death	Females	Males
Ischaemic heart disease	100	183
Stroke	52	59
Breast cancer	24	—
Prostate cancer	—	29
Diseases of respiratory system	47	84
Trachea/bronchus/lung cancer	19	52
Motor vehicle traffic accidents	6	14
Suicide	6	23

Source: OSW 1999, p. 33

Depending on how health is measured, some health surveys find that proportionally more women than men report illness. For example, in the 1995 National Health Survey, 73 per cent of women and 65 per cent of men reported having had some medical condition in the previous two weeks. Many of these health problems were comparatively minor, such as headaches and colds. However, sub-stantial (and similar) proportions—76 per cent of women and 73 per cent of men—experienced a long-term condition. Many of these are minor problems like visual deficiencies that are readily managed, but some are disabling sensory or mobility impairments, or life-threatening diseases, such as cancer (AIHW 1998).

Excluding hospitalisation related to pregnancy, women and men are equally likely to be admitted to hospitals. But women are more likely to go to the doctor, even when pregnancy-related consultations are excluded, and they are also more likely to visit complementary and allied therapists, such as naturopaths and dietitians. For example, in 1995, 60 per cent of women and 50 per cent of men had con-sulted a doctor in the previous three months, and 28 per cent of women and 31 per cent of men had been in hospital during the year (OSW 1999, ABS 1998). Previous surveys also find that more women took medication and were absent from work due to health.

Some analyses of such statistics have identified a paradox: women apparently have higher rates of illness, but men die younger. However, the apparent paradox is at least partly a consequence of oversimplifications—attempts to make sweeping generalisations about the sexes—such as 'women get sick; men die'. On closer examination, the statistics are less contradictory. Men tend to expe-rience comparatively higher rates of several life-threatening conditions and **risk factors**, such as alcohol abuse and dangerous driving. Women, on the other hand, have a relatively high prevalence of painful, unpleasant, but not lethal, conditions, such as migraines and arthritis. For example, according to most measures, psychologi-cal distress appears to be more common among women than among men (AIHW 1996a), but men commit suicide more frequently. Furthermore, over the course of people's lives, there are variations in certain conditions. More men have elevated blood pressure at younger adult ages than do women, but by the age of 65 years, more women are hypertensive. Such variations mean that we must treat contrasts between the sexes with caution, since they can conceal as much as they disclose (Macintyre et al. 1996).

An emphasis on sex differences tends to draw our attention to those conditions for which simple contrasts can be drawn. But in many general respects, the sexes are more alike than different, and variations within gender categories (by age or ethnicity, for example) may be more significant. As we have seen in Table 5.1, cardiovascular disease is the major cause of mortality for all adults. Although there are sex contrasts in the distribution of specific malignancies, cancer is a major threat to the survival and health of adults of both sexes. Everyone falls prey to colds and 'flu', and long-term health problems such as sensory impairment can affect anyone. However, the fact that both sexes can get a condition—even that they get it equally

risk factors Conditions that are thought to increase an individ-ual's susceptibility to illness or disease such as abuse of alcohol or smoking.

frequently—does not mean that gender is irrelevant to that condition. Instead, we must look to more subtle patterns to detect the interplay between health and gender, as gender can shape both exposures to health problems and the experience of illness.

Gendered exposures

While the main causes of many illnesses remain uncertain, others have clearly identified risk factors. For example, smoking is a well-known hazard in relation to a range of serious diseases, and smoking behaviour is sexually differentiated. Among Australians over the age of 18, more men than women smoke—27 per cent compared with 20 per cent—and in the past this sex difference was much more marked (AIHW 2000). Consequently, it is not surprising that more men than women die from lung cancer. Smoking also probably contributes to the higher rates among males of premature morbidity and mortality from cardiovascular diseases. Indeed, some writers have suggested that a substantial portion (perhaps half) of the sex difference in longevity may be attributable to smoking (Waldron 1995). While overall smoking prevalence has gradually declined, the decline began earlier and has been more dramatic among males, and some surveys now find that smoking is more common among adolescent girls than in boys of a similar age. These comparisons illustrate a dynamic interaction between gender and health: specifically a relationship between gender and exposure to a major illness risk factor. Most of the illness effects of current exposure will appear many years hence, when the relationship between smoking (the 'exposure') and gender may have changed yet again. If young women continue to take up smoking, we can expect the sex difference in lung cancer to diminish or even disappear in time.

Certain occupations are significant sources of injury and disease, and the sexual division of labour has tended to concentrate men in the occupations in which such hazards are greatest. Construction work, mining, waterside work, and farming are examples of comparatively hazardous occupations with high proportions of male occupants. Few female-dominated occupations are as dangerous, although the health hazards of women's work (such as office jobs, nursing, and unpaid household work) are often harder to detect and may be underestimated (Broom 1986; Doyal 1995). The hazards may also differ. For example, the low levels of autonomy, pay, and other rewards in many female-dominated jobs may contribute to women's poor mental health.

Exercise is a health-beneficial behaviour with preventative effects on a wide range of significant illnesses, and nearly all children participate in vigorous activity regularly. A persistent sex difference begins to emerge in adolescence. Consequently, many more adult men are exposed to the beneficial health effects of exercise than are women. The exception to this generalisation is that some forms of exercise, particularly contact sports, also expose people to injury. Despite the tendency for women to reduce their involvement in exercise, overweight and obesity are more prevalent among men than among women, and more females are underweight than are males. These differentials suggest that eating patterns are, to some extent, gendered. The prevalence of disordered eating among young women is a well-known example (MacSween 1993).

Males, especially young men and adolescents, are more likely to engage in a range of activities such as risky driving, contact sports, and physical aggression. Consequently, males suffer higher rates of accidental and non-accidental injury. There is considerable debate about gender differences in exposure to violence and its health consequences (Hurst 1996). Males are undoubtedly the main perpetrators of violent acts, but they are not the main victims of all kinds of violence (Fletcher 1995). The most visible kinds of violence—such as mugging, street assault, and fights in public places—usually involve males as both aggressor and victim. But sexual assault and domestic violence are overwhelmingly crimes against women, and they constitute a serious threat to the health of many women. In the USA, 'domestic violence is the leading cause of injury among women of reproductive age' (World Bank 1993, p. 50), and women appear to be at particularly high risk when they are pregnant (Stark & Flincraft 1991). While there is some debate about exact numbers, the overall picture is similar in Australia (as in many developed societies). A woman is in more danger of being attacked (ABS 1996b) or killed (Easteal 1993) by a man she knows—particularly by her husband or for-mer partner—than by a stranger. For example, the Women's Safety Survey found that 338 700 women were victims of physical vio-lence, and 180 400 of these assaults were committed by the women's partners or former partners, whereas strangers committed 67 300 of these assaults (ABS 1996b, p. 19). Two years of coroner's data from Victoria show that, of all deaths from assault, 71 per cent (1991) and 42 per cent (1992) of women's deaths resulted from domestic violence, compared with between 2 per cent and 3 per cent of men's deaths. Ninety per cent of all domestic violence deaths were women (Sherrard et al. 1994, p. 42).

Gendered experiences

The example of violence points directly to a consideration of how gender shapes the experience of health conditions. A particular injury, such as a concussion or laceration, may be physically the same, regardless of how one was injured. But the personal meaning and social consequences will be very different depending on whether the injury was sustained in a car accident, a mugging by a stranger, a pub fight with a drinking companion, or an attack by one's intimate partner. The first three of those sources of injury are likely to be singular or rare events, to be publicly recognised, and to receive immediate assistance. By contrast, 'wife bashing' is apt to be repeated and escalating, shrouded in shame and secrecy, and often concealed from health care workers. Indeed, the source of injury is frequently undetected, even when injuries are so severe that the victim presents at an emergency service (Roberts 1994). And while any injury can leave emotional scars, the psychological impact of being attacked by a loved and trusted partner is particularly devastating and personally debilitating. Because females are typically shorter and lighter than males, and have learned fewer skills of self-defence, women are often poorly equipped to protect themselves if their partner becomes violent. In the rare instance in which a man is attacked by a female partner, other elements of shame and denial may enter the equation because of the implicit insult to masculine power and strength. Thus, the experience of violent assault is highly variable and contains important gender dimensions.

The sex difference in the age at which cardiovascular diseases appear points to another area in which gender shapes the experience of illness. Recent United States, British, and Australian research suggests that cardiovascular symptoms may be investigated less thoroughly and treated less intensively in women than they are in men (Ayanian & Epstein 1991; Steingart et al. 1991). Sometimes the difference may reflect excessive intervention in the treatment of men (Bicknell et al. 1992), or variations in living arrangements and mortality before admission (Sonke et al. 1996), while other research suggests that certain women may miss out on potentially beneficial therapies (Tobin et al. 1987). Although some researchers believe that women's high mortality after heart attack is accounted for by pre-existing risk factors, this does not fully explain the sex discrepancy (Feibach et al. 1990), and there is some evidence of systematic under-diagnosis of women. The failure to pursue symptoms vigorously would be an understandable result of a widespread, though incorrect, belief that women do not get heart disease. Such a belief might make doctors less likely to suspect heart disease in a woman, and hence less likely to investigate it thoroughly or manage it aggressively when it occurs (McKinlay 1996). It may also promote a belief among women and their families that heart disease is not a women's health problem, and therefore that the risk factors or symptoms are not important. An idea prevails that men are prone to ignore symptoms, and that their elevated mortality is a consequence of their reluctance to seek medical care, but systematic research does not confirm that belief

class (or social class) A position within a system of structured inequality based on the unequal distribution of power, wealth, income, and status. Class membership is determined by three characteristics: ownership and control of scarce economic resources; ownership of marketable skills and qualifications; and wage labour. People who share a social-class position typically share similar life chances.

'race' A term without scientific basis that uses skin colour and facial features to describe allegedly biologically distinct groups of humans. It is a social construction that is used to categorise groups of people and usually infers assumed (and unproven) intellectual superiority or inferiority.

ethnicity Sociologically, the term refers to a shared cultural background, which is a characteristic of all groups in society. As a policy term, it is used to identify migrants who share a culture that is markedly different from that of Anglo-Australians. In practice, it often refers only to migrants from non-English-speaking backgrounds (NESB migrants).

(Macintyre 1999). By contrast, an American study found that women who have symptoms of a heart attack are more likely than men to delay calling an ambulance (Meischke et al. 1993).

Even such apparently trivial illnesses as colds and 'flu' may be experienced in ways that are organised and given meaning by gender. For example, because of women's responsibilities for unpaid domestic work (Bittman 1991) and their concentration in casual employment, they may find it particularly difficult to stay in bed when they are ill. Married women's husbands are more likely to be in full-time employment and hence to be unavailable to supply domestic care to ailing family members. However, when those same men get sick, they may have paid sick-leave as well as a supportive wife. These patterns, and the life-long habits and material circumstances to which they contribute, are particularly important health issues with regard to the care of people with severe or chronic illness or frailty. Among older people, women are twice as likely as men to live alone and hence to have no co-resident who can care for them when they are sick or frail. Women are more likely to need care from outside the household at some time during their lives, and so have a different interest in State-funded services (Gibson & Allen 1993; OSW 1999).

Many of the patterns described above are inflected by other social variables such as **class**, **'race'**, and **ethnicity**. For example, in some cultures, the expectation that health care will be supplied by members of the family, usually women, obstructs access to health and community services delivered by agencies or professionals. When family members cannot supply needed support, ill and elderly migrants can be disadvantaged by their reluctance to use the services they need.

Class has been found to correlate with most measures of health; better health is consistently associated with higher status. The relationship between health and socioeconomic status prevails for both sexes, but the relative importance of various elements of social and material circumstances is, to an extent, distinctive for women and men (Arber 1991; Macintyre 1997). It has also been difficult to establish appropriate measures of status for the whole population because of women's interrupted labour-force involvement. All these examples show how the experience of illness may be gendered in subtle and complex ways, even for conditions that are not sexually specific. They also illustrate the way that the relationship between health and gender can be complicated by other dimensions of social difference (see chapters 4, 6, and 7 for further detail).

Responding to gendered health and illness

For many years, it was commonly assumed that the gendered patterning of disease and death was a simple 'fact of nature' about which human beings could do little or nothing. However, culture and medicine routinely modify facts of nature. Many health problems lead to severe illness, injury, or death if they are not treated; we do not allow them to run their course if they can be controlled. But the best approaches to **gendered health** are less obvious than how to treat post-operative infection or catastrophic bleeding. It is one thing to describe the way gender interacts with health and illness; it is quite another to determine when those interactions are creating problems, and to discern how individuals, communities, and societies might respond constructively.

One of the most widely recognised problems has been referred to as **sexism in medicine**. Originally this term pointed to the sexual division of labour in medical care where most doctors are men while nearly all nurses are women. It also focused on the 'sexist' behaviour of some doctors. Far from signalling a constructive sensitivity to the potential relevance of gender, sexism in medicine included a range of ways of treating women that were at best objectionable and at worst harmful. Anecdotal evidence was substantiated by systematic research showing that doctors sometimes did not interact appropriately with their women patients (Broom-Darroch 1978). They failed to hear or accept women's accounts of their symptoms, did not inform women about unwanted effects of drugs and other therapies, and were prone to label women's problems as 'psychosomatic' rather than 'real' (Barrett & Roberts 1978; Woodward et al. 1995). Women have had difficulty getting access to birth-control services (Matthews 1984), especially if the doctors felt that those women (young, unmarried, divorced, or widowed) should not be sexually active. A few doctors have abused their position of trust to exploit clients sexually. Obstetricians and surgeons have often subjected women to unwarranted and even injurious interventions in the management of childbirth (Oakley 1980), the treatment of gynaecological disorders (Frankfort 1972), or care of breast cancer (Batt 1994). But even doctors who strive to give women the best possible care have been handicapped by limited medical research on women and their health problems.

Research

Until recently, men and male animals have been the main, or only, subjects of most studies of disease, diagnostic procedures, management, therapy, and prevention (Melbourne District Health Council 1990). Sometimes, when women were included, the results derived from women were discarded because they did not conform to the pattern based on results from men. One consequence has been the comparative neglect of most women's health concerns, except those that are directly relevant to fertility (Eckerman, 1999), which is arguably the women's health domain

gendered health A term used to acknowledge the different experiences and exposures to health and illness that result from gender.

sexism in medicine Refers to discriminatory and harmful treatment of women by doctors in terms of ignoring women's health concerns in medical research and intervention, not informing women about alternative treatments or the side effects of drugs/therapies, and labelling women's problems as 'psychosomatic' rather than 'real'.

of most interest to men. However, it also means that we often know relatively little about how non-reproductive disorders may manifest themselves differently in women and men, how risk factors may vary, or how the sexes may differ in their response to therapeutic interventions. Such lopsided investigation often arises from an effort to simplify study designs and save money, but it relies on the assumption that findings from males are relevant to everyone. This assumption in turn rests on an implicit conviction that the 'normal' body is not subject to such perturbations as hormonal cycling, pregnancy, lactation, or menopause, and that it is therefore acceptable to exclude the bodies subject to such perturbations from medical research because they 'complicate' the results. An understanding of all bodies—not only female bodies— as sexed suggests that there can be no gender-neutral body, and that menstruation is as much a normal human process as spermatogenesis or the secretion of digestive enzymes.

This history of research exclusion has significant effects for women's health. For example, progress in effective treatment of breast cancer has been remarkably slow, despite an apparent long-term increase in incidence; true prevention of this disease remains a distant hope. Furthermore, a variety of non-lethal but difficult conditions, such as endometriosis, remain poorly understood. Also, concerns that have been identified by women, such as overweight, poverty (Redman et al. 1988), and violence (Jones 1996), have rarely been considered as 'health' issues by researchers and have largely escaped scrutiny.

Recently, the Commonwealth government sought to remedy the neglect of women's health research by funding a major longitudinal study, beginning data-collection in 1996 (Brown et al. 1996). The study has recruited more than 40 000 respondents to investigate such issues as reproductive health problems, access to services, stress, and time-use. One of the most ambitious clinical research programs has been undertaken in the USA by the National Institutes of Health (Finnegan 1996). The Women's Health Initiative consists of several multi-centre studies, including **randomised control trials** of the effects of diet and hormone replacement therapy in preventing breast and colorectal cancer, heart disease, and osteoporosis (for current information see their web site: <http://www.nhlbi.nih.gov/whi/index.html>).

Perhaps a surprising consequence of attempts to refigure health research is that we have become more aware of the neglect of masculinity—as well as femininity—in health and health research. This may seem ironic in light of the male domination of medicine, the focus on males in research, and the privileging of the male body as normal. But it is less surprising when we note that these processes have occurred without being explicitly

randomised control trials (RCTs) A biomedical research procedure used to evaluate the effectiveness of particular medications and therapeutic interventions. 'Random' refers to the equal chance of participants being in the experimental or control group (the group to which nothing is done and is used for comparison), and 'trial' refers to the experimental nature of the method. It is often mistakenly viewed as the best way to demonstrate causal links between factors under investigation, but privileges biomedical over social responses to illness.

health promotion Any combination of education and related
organisational, economic, and
political interventions designed
to promote behavioural and environmental changes conducive to
good health. This promotion may
cover a variety of strategies,
including legislation, health education, community development,
advocacy, and so on. Health promotion has usually, however,
been restricted to interventions
focusing on the behavioural end
of the spectrum.

theorised, and hence there was no conscious or thoughtful attention to masculinity *per se*. While men have featured in medical
research and **health promotion** campaigns, there has, until
recently, been little detectable effort to consider how masculinity
may figure in health and disease. The example of smoking has
already been introduced. While it was mainly a male activity for
several decades, few people except advertisers have paid attention
to its function as a means of confirming and displaying certain
forms of masculinity. More interest in the gender—not to mention class—implications of smoking, and hence of quitting, might
have reduced men's smoking sooner. The effort to promote
dietary change and exercise must also take gender seriously if it is
to be effective. Alcohol consumption and drunkenness have been
socially accepted behaviours for men, and are almost required in
some circles of adolescent and young-adult men. Specific foods
and styles of food preparation are associated with masculinity, and
if men are to eat healthier diets, the symbolic connotations of
food will have to be considered.

If there has been inadequate attention to masculinity and
health, there has been even less interest in specific forms of masculinity or in a sophisticated analysis of their relevance. Instead,
there has been unsubstantiated talk of men's reluctance to seek
medical help 'until it is too late', or generalised allusions to male
risk-taking behaviour, without much serious theorising or research
concerning which males take risks, in what circumstances, how
their masculinity might be implicated in their behaviour, or how
masculinity might be mobilised to diminish risk.

A striking exception to the tendency to ignore or oversimplify masculinity is the activity of homosexual men dealing with
HIV/AIDS. Their efforts have been distinguished by a focus on
the lives of specific groups of men, and they have sought to transform prevention into a positive and pleasurable part of gay
masculinity. Research into how these changes have been insti-
gated may supply valuable directions for the appropriate
incorporation of gender in future research. These examples point
to the need for five major shifts in order to improve research
(including applied research) on health:

1 the inclusion of women in clinical trials
2 the investigation of health issues to which women themselves give priority
3 an understanding that 'women's health' and 'men's health'
   include conditions beyond reproduction
4 the study of women's and men's health in their own right,
   and not simply in comparison with each other
5 the study of how specific forms or aspects of gender are
   distinctively related to health.

The women's health movement

By some accounts, contemporary sensitivity to the relationship between gender and health was initially created by the renascent women's movement, beginning in the late 1960s. Since that time, what might loosely be termed the **women's health movement** has worked to change the face of health services for women, and there is now substantial evidence of such change. Participants in this movement were the first to identify sexism in medicine (discussed above), and many of the movement's activities are efforts to overcome that sexism. Women have advocated innovations such as:

women's health movement
A term used broadly to describe attempts to address sexism in medicine by highlighting the importance of gender in health research and treatment. Achievements include women's health centres and the National Women's Health Policy.

- improvements and expansion in health services
- safer, cheaper, and more accessible contraceptives
- better access to terminations of pregnancy
- enlargement of services provided by Family Planning clinics
- changes in medical education and increases in the number of women in medical practice
- encouragement of multidisciplinary teams in the delivery of health care
- fostering support groups to enable women to help one another.

To some extent, all of these are happening.

In the twenty-first century, perhaps the single most visible transformation is the existence of several dozen more-or-less community-based, more-or-less feminist women's health centres. At the time of writing, these centres are located in every State and Territory, mostly in large urban areas, but some in regional centres, country towns, and smaller cities. They have come into being largely as a result of community-based action that has sought to establish services that would be controlled by women and would be more appropriate to women's needs, as defined by women themselves (Broom 1991). Because they are now such a familiar part of the Australian health care landscape, readers may be surprised to learn that their origins were highly contentious. Despite the fact that most of the activities of women's health centres are different from those supplied by mainstream medicine (Broom 1997), doctors feared that centres would compete for their clientele, or they objected to the employment of 'unqualified' women's health workers. Several women's health centres were opened with minimal funding and relied heavily on volunteer labour and donations of money and materials. A few centres were notorious for their political radicalism, but almost all have sought to influence the mainstream, recognising that most women will obtain most of their health services from conventional sources. Reliance on government funding, a commitment to attracting the most vulnerable clients, and the desire to encourage doctors and hospitals to become more 'woman friendly' are all issues that have confronted women's health centres with dilemmas and challenges: how are they to preserve their feminist independence and still be respectable enough to exert influence? They are now partially legitimised as a strategy of the National Women's Health Policy and have become better established since the first centres opened in 1974. Nevertheless, opposition persists. For example, the Australian Medical Association makes an explicit objection to women's health centres in its otherwise uniform affirmation of the National Women's Health Policy (Australian Medical Association 1993).

Governments respond

Governments—both State and Commonwealth—have responded to women's community-based action by developing women's health strategies, policies, and programs. Most of this activity took place during the 1980s and early 1990s, with particular focus on the National Women's Health Policy (Commonwealth Department of Community Services and Health 1989) and the program for its implementation. Such developments have not been without their critics, however. During the early 1990s, considerable energy was expended defending a complaint against women's health initiatives and services brought by a male doctor (employed by the Commonwealth Department of Health). The complaint used the *Sex Discrimination Act 1984* (Cwlth) to assert that women's health services discriminate against men. It was heard by the President of the Human Rights and Equal Opportunities Commission in 1991 and 1992, and the decision upheld the lawfulness of special women's health activities (Broom 1994). Nevertheless, by the mid-1990s, diminished resources for health, reallocation of previously targeted women's health funding, and an increasingly conservative political climate began to accomplish what the discrimination complaint could not: the gradual winding-back of women's health services.

The Fourth World Congress on Women brought women's health issues to an international forum (Van Wijk et al. 1996). At the international level, a very broad range of common principles in health care (universal access, and gender sensitivity and appropriateness) were identified. The most urgent health needs, however, are nationally and locally specific, with the emphasis in developing countries being on clean water, adequate fuel for cooking and heat, food supplies, and basic maternal and infant health. In developed countries, the emphasis tends to be more on reducing inequalities in access to services, dignity in medical treatment, participation in decision-making, and better care for chronic conditions such as cancer. Clearly there can be overlap on many issues—such as access to safe means of fertility control and real choice about when to employ them—but most priorities tend to be specific rather than universal.

Men's health: progress or threat?

men's health Running parallel
to women's health initiatives,
the men's health movement
recognises that certain elements
of masculine identity and behaviour can be hazardous to health.

Following the women's health movement by about 20 years is an
emerging focus on **men's health** in Australia and other English-
speaking countries (Primary Health Care Group 1996; Sabo &
Gordon 1995). It has benefited from a number of the theoretical
and political developments that have resulted from the women's
health movement, but identifies distinctive issues and strategies
(Fletcher 1995). For example, goals such as reducing drink-driving
and other highly risky behaviours loom large on a men's health
agenda, particularly for young men. Suicide is an urgent priority.
Specific subgroups of men have particular needs, as is evident from
the activities of gay men in relation to HIV/AIDS. In parallel to
women's health initiatives, men's health advocates have identified
the importance of dissecting the role of masculinity in men's health,
recognising that certain elements of masculine identity and behaviour can be hazardous to health. These insights suggest that
improving men's health will entail slow and careful shifts in understandings of what it means to be a man in contemporary society.

Three Commonwealth-sponsored national men's health conferences have been held (1995, 1997 and 1999). Although progress
subsequently halted, an effort to formulate a national men's health
policy (Primary Health Care Group, 1996) was begun in the mid-
1990s at the direction of the then Commonwealth Health
Minister, Carmen Lawrence, and several States are taking initiatives. A variety of school and community-based health training
and education, and health promotion programs have also been
developed to target men's health issues.

Some women's health advocates are nervous about men's
health initiatives. The anxiety is provoked in part by the stark realities of shrinking (in real terms) health budgets, and a perception
that resources for men's health will be taken from hard-won, vulnerable and poorly funded women's health programs. Such fears
are inflamed by episodes such as the discrimination case mentioned above, and by the rhetoric of a small number of individuals
who assert that the accomplishments of women's health services
have been made at the expense of men's health. Some of these
commentators argue that women's health initiatives rely on feminist claims that women are 'victims' and that women are 'sicker'
than men. These critics of women's health go on to assert that it
is not women but men whose health is disadvantaged by sex, and
that attention to women's health is misplaced and should be
shifted to men. As we have seen above, such generalisations
about which sex is 'sicker' are unlikely to be informative.

Most men's health advocates see neither women nor women's
health services as enemies. They are aware that both lay people
and health professionals—both women and men—are now

beginning to explore how various forms of masculinity may enhance or detract from men's health. Mothers and wives who become aware of neglected health problems in their sons and husbands have been among those who have stimulated the increased activity and awareness of diseases such as testicular cancer. Equally important, attention to the relationship between gender and health stands to benefit women and men both.

Future directions: towards a gendered understanding of health

In future we may have to think of gender as a much more complicated concept than the simple dichotomous variable to which most of us are accustomed. Some writers now suggest that it is time to move towards gender-specific approaches that 'provide greater interpretive richness and give full voice to the complexity of the socially constructed meaning of gender' (Kunkel & Atchley 1996, p. 295; Eckerman 1999). We must remember that such dimensions as 'race', ethnicity, and age are all implicated in gender in ways that cannot be reduced to binary thinking. A person is not Black at one moment and male the next: he is always a Black male (among many other things). The implications of such connections present challenges to accurate and constructive research about health and gender, and to the development and delivery of appropriate health care services. More complex models may be awkward and more intellectually demanding than a simple bivariate model, but greater complexity promises more fruitful and practical ways of thinking about contemporary social life and the health patterns with which it is inextricably entangled. A productive analysis of gender involves taking both masculinity and femininity seriously, and understanding that gender is an aspect of every person's individual experience and social life. Femininity and masculinity are complex sources of risks and benefits, simultaneously—but differently—constraining and empowering.

Broad social, political, and economic change, the accomplishments of the women's health movement, and the emergence of activity regarding men's health have all altered the context in which health is created and managed. They have also effected subtle shifts in the meanings of gendered subject positions. For example, from the embattled beginnings of the women's health movement in the early 1970s, women's health has become more 'mainstream' and established, despite its continuing vulnerability, and the identities of all the actors (participants, supporters, and opponents) are modified by these developments (Singleton 1996). Approaches to funding health services and measuring their productivity are also in considerable flux throughout the developed world. All these—and other—changes have altered irrevocably fundamental aspects of the way health and gender are understood, and therefore the way research, services, and advocacy will proceed in the future. While it is too early to know how the next phase will be defined, and by whom, it seems likely that revised assumptions and alliances will be necessary, and that attention to gender—not just to women—will be a feature of developing understandings of health. If that is so, it will not be before time.

Summary of main points

- The typical way of life of each sex differs, and these differences can influence health. The statement that 'women get sick; men die' is an oversimplification. Men experience comparatively higher rates of life-threatening conditions, while women have a relatively high prevalence of some painful, but not lethal, conditions. Gender variations must be treated with caution since they can conceal as much as they disclose.
- A number of studies have shown that sexism in medicine has resulted in objectionable and harmful treatment of women by doctors, such as ignoring women's accounts of their symptoms, not informing women about unwanted effects of drugs and other therapies, and labelling women's problems as 'psychosomatic' rather than 'real'.
- Until recently, men and male animals have been the main subjects of most medical research. Such bias is based on an implicit assumption that the 'normal' body is not subject to such processes as hormonal cycling, pregnancy, lactation, or menopause, and that females can therefore be excluded from research.
- The women's health movement has advocated: safer, cheaper, and more accessible contraceptives; better access to terminations of pregnancy; enlargement of services provided by Family Planning; changes in medical education and increases in the number of women in medical practice; encouragement of multidisciplinary teams in the delivery of health care; women's health centres; and the National Women's Health Policy.
- Most men's health advocates see neither women nor women's health services as enemies. Attention to gender and health stands to benefit both women and men.

Discussion questions

1 Why is gender an important factor in determining the exposure to, and experience of, health and illness?
2 Why is the statement 'women get sick; men die' an oversimplification of the link between gender and health?

3　What are some examples of 'sexism in medicine' and how can it be addressed?
4　What are some of the explanations of why sexual assault and domestic violence are overwhelmingly perpetrated by men against women?
5　Why is the women's health movement necessary?
6　Why is the men's health movement necessary?

Further investigation

1　How successful has the women's health movement and the entry of increasing numbers of women into the medical profession been in addressing 'sexism in medicine'?
2　Examine the ways in which femininity and masculinity result in gendered exposures and gendered experiences of health and illness.

Further reading and web resources

Annandale, E. & Hunt, K., 2000, *Gender Inequalities and Health*, Open University Press, Buckingham.

Broom, D. H. 1991, *Damned if We Do: Contradictions in Women's Health Care*, Allen & Unwin, Sydney.

Doyal, L. 1995, *What Makes Women Sick: Gender and the Political Economy of Health*, Macmillan, London.

Ehrenreich, B. & English, D. 1979, *For Her Own Good: 150 Years of Experts' Advice*, Pluto Press, London.

Fee, E. & Krieger, N. (eds) 1994, *Women's Health, Politics, and Power: Essays on Sex/Gender, Medicine, and Public Health*, Baywood, New York.

Sabo, D. & Gordon, D. F. (eds) 1995, *Men's Health and Illness: Gender, Power and the Body*, Sage, Thousand Oaks, Calif.

World Health Organization 1998, *Gender and Health: Technical Paper*, Geneva, Women's Health and Development.

Web sites

Eating disorders links: <www.uq.net.au/eda/documents/links.html>

Gender & Health Equity (Harvard University):
　　<www.hsph.harvard.edu/grhf/HUpapers/gender/index.html>

Global Reproductive Health Forum (Harvard University):
　　<www.hsph.harvard.edu/Organizations/healthnet/frame1/frame1.html>

Men's Bibliography by Michael Flood: <http://www.xyonline.net/mensbiblio>

National Centre for Epidemiology and Population Health:

Women's Health Australia project: <www.newcastle.edu.au/centre/wha/>

Women's Health Initiative (US): <www.nhlbi.nib.gov/whi/index.html>

6

Indigenous Health

The Perpetuation of Inequality

Dennis Gray and Sherry Saggers

Overview

* *What is the extent of Aboriginal health inequality?*
* *What has been done to address this inequality?*
* *Why do health inequalities persist?*

Everyone in Australia knows that Indigenous people have poor health, and many people believe they know why. This chapter attempts to peel away these common-sense understandings of the causes of Indigenous ill health, by locating explanations within the broader social context of both the past and the present. This type of analysis reveals the historical development of Indigenous inequality through processes of colonisation, dispossession, and marginalisation from the dominant economy, as well as the health implications of these processes. Although Indigenous people have struggled to improve their health status, these efforts have been impeded by the unwillingness of successive governments to significantly address the underlying structural inequalities.

Key terms

alcohol misuse
assimilation
biomedical
colonisation/colonialism
dispossession
ethnocentric

Indigenous community-
    controlled health services
institutionalisation
primary health care (PHC)
public health infrastructure
risk factors

self-determination
sociological imagination
'stolen children'
terra nullius
traditional medical system

Introduction

Mary is 62 years old. She is a battler who has lived a hard life. Under the old **assimilation** policy, she was taken from her Aboriginal mother and put in a 'home'—the memories of which still induce occasional bouts of depression. Her husband Jack, who was four years older than her, died at the age of 46 of smoking-induced lung cancer. However, for a long period before his death—after being evicted from a pastoral station at around the time that 'equal wages' and 'drinking rights' were introduced—he drank heavily. Mary had five children, two of whom are dead—a boy from diarrhoea at the age of 18 months, and another boy who died in a car accident when he was 22 years old. She loves them all, but of the three children who are living, she is most proud of Ron, who is an artist living in Sydney.

Mary moved to the city about 15 years ago, where she now lives in a three-bedroom government house in an outer suburb. The house is also occupied by her daughters Joan and Margaret, Joan's 'man' Ken, and Joan's and Margaret's six children. Given the length of waiting lists for government housing and the high cost of private rental, Mary's family has no choice but to all 'bunk-in' together. The house was not designed for this many people, and the overcrowding creates various problems. Although Mary and her daughters do their best, it is almost impossible to keep the place clean. And, with all the wear-and-tear, fittings such as fly screens are broken and the septic tank often overflows.

Mary has moved into the smallest of the bedrooms, which she shares with Shantelle, Margaret's 18-year-old daughter. Margaret sleeps on a couch in the 'lounge' room, and her 12-year-old and 10-year-old daughters share the largest bedroom with Joan's 7-year-old daughter and 5-year-old son. Joan and Ken sleep in the other bedroom with their 11-month-old son. With so many children together on mattresses on the floor in one room, they often transmit infections and parasites to each other—such as 'colds', 'flu', and sometimes lice—that they have picked up at school.

Ken counts himself as 'one of the lucky ones'. Unlike many of the Aboriginal men in the neighbourhood, he has a job—as a storeman at a freight terminal. 'It don't pay much,' he says, 'but it stops me from goin' nuts an' keeps me off the piss.' With the money Ken earns, along with Mary's pension and Margaret's supporting mother's benefit, none of the family goes hungry. However, because it is difficult to cook for so many at once, or for everyone to be in the kitchen, they eat a lot of fast food, such as 'KFC' and chips, which the kids love. Mary knows that this food is not good for them, particularly in such quantities and without vegetables. She tries to supplement the fast food with fruit—which the kids all like—but on their income it is so expensive.

For a long time now, Mary has been considerably overweight; she has diabetes, and she finds it difficult to get around. Nevertheless, as well as keeping her own family together, Mary is still active on the committee of the local Aboriginal child-care centre that she helped to establish. 'It's important to do things for the young people,' she says, 'We had nothin'. No decent education. No good jobs. Always poor. Always battlin'. Same for my kids— 'cept maybe for Ronnie. But we gotta keep tryin'. Do things ourselves. Make it better for the grannies.'

Mary is not simply a statistic. Her story represents the life experiences of many Indigenous people in this country, and it helps to explain why too many of them are sick and die early. In this chapter we attempt to reveal the 'public issues' behind these intensely 'personal troubles' (Mills 1959, p. 14).

Evidence of health inequality

Despite calls going back almost three decades, there is still no comprehensive national system for the collection of data on the health of Indigenous Australians. Nevertheless, the data that is available provides dramatic evidence of the health inequalities faced by Indigenous people. Life expectancy is one valuable indicator of the health status of a population. The measure 'represents the average number of years a newborn baby could expect to live if the mortality rates of today were to continue throughout that baby's life' (McLennan & Madden 1999, p. 134). As the case study of Mary shows, Indigenous people have become accustomed to illness and early death. Based on data for the period 1991–96, life expectancy at birth for all Australian males and females was estimated to be approximately 75 and 81 years respectively. However, based on data for the same period from Western Australia, South Australia and the Northern Territory, for Indigenous Australian males and females the expectancies were approximately 18 and 19 years less (McLennan & Madden 1999).

The main causes of mortality (death) among Indigenous and non-Indigenous Australians are similar—cardiovascular diseases; external causes such as accidents, poisoning, and violence; respiratory disorders; various forms of cancer; and diseases of the digestive system. However, Indigenous people die from these causes at between 1.4 and 6.0 times the rates among non-Indigenous people. In addition, the mortality rate for endocrine, nutritional, and metabolic diseases (especially diabetes) is six times greater among Indigenous men and 11 times greater among Indigenous women (McLennan & Madden 1999).

Hospital separation data (for example discharges, transfers, or deaths) are a key indicator of morbidity (sickness). In the case of

Indigenous people these data are likely to be an under-estimate. Nevertheless, they again provide clear evidence of the health inequalities faced by Indigenous Australians. In 1996–97, the rates of hospital separations among Indigenous males and females were 1.8 and 1.9 times the rates among their non-Indigenous counterparts. In this period, the most common reasons for hospitalisation of Indigenous males and females were injury, respiratory disease, digestive disease, and renal disease (primarily kidney dialysis), and for women complications of pregnancy and childbirth. However, Indigenous people were also twice as likely as non-Indigenous people to be hospitalised for infectious and parasitic diseases and diseases of the skin and subcutaneous tissue. Like mortality data, hospital morbidity data are only indicators of ill health. They do not include the heavy burden of illness that is either treated by medical and other health-care practitioners or that goes untreated. As well as particular illnesses *per se*, there are several key health issues that both health professionals and Indigenous people identify as serious. These include alcohol misuse, smoking, violence and self-harm, and mental health concerns. Understanding the higher prevalence of these health problems requires a sociological imagination (Mills 1959), in addition to mere medical awareness.

risk factors Conditions that are thought to increase an individual's susceptibility to illness or disease such as abuse of alcohol or smoking.

Among all Australians, excessive alcohol use represents a major health **risk factor** and has been linked to health problems such as traffic accidents, cirrhosis of the liver, suicide, and stroke (Unwin et al. 1994). Indigenous people are less likely to be current regular drinkers than the general population (33 per cent versus 45 per cent), and are more likely to no longer drink alcohol (22 per cent versus 9 per cent) or to have been lifetime abstainers (19 per cent of males and 34 per cent of females). These facts are now more widely known (McLennan & Madden 1999), but they still cause surprise among many people. In part this can be explained by the impact of higher levels of consumption among those Indigenous people who drink; with 21 per cent of male and 9 per cent of female drinkers consuming alcohol at high risk levels, compared with 8 and 3 per cent, respectively, of non-Indigenous males and females (McLennan & Madden 1999).

Again, national figures on alcohol-related mortality and morbidity are not available. However, a study from Western Australia showed that Indigenous males were 5.2 times, and Indigenous females 3.7 times, more likely to die and were 9.3 and 12.8 times more likely to be hospitalised for alcohol-related conditions than non-Indigenous males and females (Unwin et al. 1994)

The personal and social costs of alcohol-related deaths in Indigenous communities cannot be exaggerated. Pam Lyon (1990, p. 41) described the toll for one person in Central Australia:

Funerals have become a feature of daily camp life. The alcohol-related death toll within Tyapewe Rice's family alone is horrendous: his father's four sisters, two of his mother's three brothers, two of his own brothers, not to mention cousins and friends. He has had two friends die in his arms from alcohol-related disease or injury. 'A lot of people are dying from grog,' he said. 'Too many people are dying.'

Just as important, from the perspective of many Indigenous people, are the harmful social effects with which misuse of alcohol is associated. Alcohol contributes to accidents and violence, sexual assaults, neglect of children, crime and social unrest, and threats to culture and tradition (Langton 1992). This is why alcohol, among many other risk factors to health, is regarded by many Indigenous people as the greatest threat to their health and well-being (Madden 1995).

alcohol misuse Excessive consumption of alcohol leading to health and/or social problems.

Tobacco smoking is not regarded as seriously as **alcohol misuse** by many Indigenous people because it does not have the same acute social consequences. In the Australian population as a whole, it has been estimated that almost 10 per cent of the total burden of disease is attributable to tobacco smoking (Higgins et al. 2000). In the Indigenous population—where the prevalence of smoking is double that among the non-Indigenous population—its impact is even greater. It underlies the higher rates of stroke, heart disease, lung cancer, and respiratory diseases such as emphysema and chronic bronchitis and is the single most preventable cause of mortality and morbidity.

Indigenous people are much more exposed to violence than people in the general population. Much of this violence is under-reported for a variety of reasons, but one measure of this is hospitalisation for related injuries. In 1991–92 the rate of interpersonal violence resulting in hospitalisation was seventeen times higher among the Indigenous population in Australia (excluding the Northern Territory). Self-harm—including suicide and attempted suicide, poisoning, hanging, cutting or piercing, or injuries associated with firearms—occurs more frequently among Indigenous people. To take suicide alone, Indigenous males in South Australia, Western Australia, and the Northern Territory in 1992–94 were twice as likely as the non-Indigenous population to take their own lives (Anderson et al. 1996).

'stolen children' Children who were forcibly removed from their families during the nineteenth and twentieth centuries by the agents of government in order to assimilate them into mainstream Australia.

Linked to issues of self-harm are broader questions to do with mental health. Given the history of interaction between Black and White Australians in this country, resulting in both physical illness and traumatic social upheaval—including the **'stolen children'**—it comes as no surprise to learn of the increasing concern about levels of mental illness in the Indigenous population. In 1997 the report of the National Inquiry into the Separation of

Aboriginal and Torres Strait Islander Children and their Families estimated that, in the years 1910–70, between one in three and one in ten children were forcibly removed from their families (Human Rights and Equal Opportunity Commission 1997). Many of these people and their descendants have suffered and continue to suffer a wide range of health and social conditions that they relate to these experiences. In confidential evidence to the inquiry, one informant said:

> I look at my son today who had to be taken away because he was going to commit suicide because he just can't handle it; he just can't take any more of the anxiety attacks that he and Karen have. Have I passed that on to my kids because I haven't dealt with it? How do you sit down and go through all those years of abuse? Somehow I'm passing down negativity to my kids (Human Rights and Equal Opportunity Commission 1997, p. 222).

Although mental health data are inadequate, a national study found that Indigenous people 'suffer mental health problems such as depression at a very high rate, compared to non-Indigenous people, that rates of self-harm and suicide are higher and that substance abuse, domestic violence, child abuse and disadvantage are continuing additional risk factors. Trauma and grief were seen as overwhelming problems' (Swan & Raphael 1995, p. 1). However, rather than focusing narrowly on mental illness, the authors of the same study argued that key principles to be incorporated include the notion of holistic health; the place of history in trauma and loss; the right of peoples to self-determination; and the importance of kinship to Indigenous well-being (Swan & Raphael 1995).

All of the above demonstrate vividly the extent to which health inequalities are experienced by Indigenous people in Australia. Most people have an opinion about why these inequalities persist, despite increasing allocations of funds to health care. As sociologists, we need to examine how ill health is socially produced and maintained.

biomedicine/biomedical model The conventional approach to medicine in Western societies. It diagnoses and explains illness as a malfunction of one of the body's biological mechanisms. The biomedical approach of most health services focuses on the treating of individuals, and generally ignores social, economic, and environmental factors.

Social production of Aboriginal ill health

Sociological, as opposed to **biomedical**, explanations of ill health attempt to throw light on why people are not randomly afflicted by disease and illness. Indeed, many studies have revealed the relationship between health status and social indicators such as class, ethnicity, and gender. The most dramatic illustration of this is the link between low socioeconomic status and poor health (Saunders 1996; Marmot & Wilkinson 1999). In the so-called 'Whitehall' study of civil servants in the United Kingdom, men in the lowest employment category had a mortality rate that was four times higher than that for those in the highest administrative category, and there was a clear social gradient affecting total mortality and all major causes of death (Marmot 1999, pp. 10–12). Similar inequalities based on socioeconomic disadvantage have been demonstrated in Australia. Mortality rates for men and women in the most disadvantaged group were 23 per cent higher than those in the least disadvantaged group (Glover & Woollacott 1992; see also chapter 4).

Harmful risk factors, such as smoking, are also associated with class, or socioeconomic disadvantage (Jarvis & Wardle 2000). In Australia, men and women in the most disadvantaged group were 34 per cent and 44 per cent, respectively, more likely to be smokers than men and women in the least disadvantaged group (Glover & Woollacott 1992). Given the overwhelming concentration of Indigenous people in the most poverty-stricken groups, and given that Indigenous people tend to have less education and training than the general population (see Table 6.1), poor Indigenous health should come as no surprise (Cunningham et al. 1997).

Table 6.1   Median weekly individual income and highest post-school educational qualification for Indigenous and non-Indigenous Australians 1996

Median weekly individual income	Indigenous	Non-Indigenous
Male ≥15 years	$189	$415
Female ≥15 years	$190	$224
Highest post-school educational qualification	% of Indigenous population	% of non Indigenous population
Degree or higher	2.0	10.9
Diploma level	2.2	6.3
Skilled vocation	4.5	11.0
Basic vocation	1.9	3.0
No post-school qualifications	76.3	59.1
Not stated or inadequately described	13.0	9.7

Source: Adapted from McLennan & Madden 1999: pp. 19, 22

Studies such as those cited above illustrate the need to go beyond individualistic explanations for poor Indigenous health. Much health sociology tries to do just that by locating the sources of ill health in the material and social domains. This is not to say that the behaviour of individuals does not influence their health. Increasingly, however, in both the public domain and among health and medical professionals, discourses about health are becoming dominated by theories attributing most ill health to the risky behaviour of individuals (O'Malley 1996, pp. 199–200). One prominent journalist has recently described much Aboriginal ill health as 'self-inflicted', and claimed that the so-called 'cycle of poverty', which exacerbates poor health, 'can only be broken by their own efforts' (McGuinness 1996, p. 17). Here Paddy McGuinness is simply reflecting the dominant racist views that Indigenous people are lazy and that they all drink excessively and are irresponsible parents and citizens. The trouble with this type of analysis is that it ignores the demonstrated links between health and socioeconomic status and blames those least able to take control of their lives and institute healthy practices (Marmot & Wilkinson 1999; McLennan & Madden 1999, p.55).

One illustration of the social, as opposed to individual, causes of ill health are comparative Indigenous health data from Canada and New Zealand. Like Australia, both these countries have colonial histories involving the **dispossession** and subsequent marginalisation of Indigenous peoples. The health consequences of those colonial histories are distressingly familiar. A recent profile of native Canadians, for example, reveals an average life expectancy almost 10 years less than that of other Canadians, only marginal improvements in health and education over the past 25 years, incarceration rates that are much higher than those for the general population, and frightening records of violence and self-harm. According to this source, 'Aboriginal people destroy themselves at a phenomenal rate through violence, accidents and suicide … As one Western newspaper columnist noted in the late 1980s, in a story about a young native boy's suicide, "We used to hang them. Now they hang themselves" ' (Comeau & Santin 1995, p. ix).

dispossession The removal of people from land they regard as their own.

colonisation/colonialism
A process by which one nation imposes itself economically, politically, and socially upon another.

Colonialism and dispossession

The invasion and subsequent settlement of Australia by the British was based on the legal fiction of *terra nullius*, a concept concerning supposedly vacant or unoccupied territory. The term reveals the **ethnocentric** belief that the original inhabitants of the continent had no equivalent claim to the land, because of their very different economies and societies. With a population estimated at around 750 000, and consisting of groups with hundreds of distinct languages and cultures, Indigenous peoples maintained a hunter-gatherer existence in highly diverse environments—from the deserts of central and western Australia, to the wet tropics of north-eastern Australia and the cold climate of Tasmania (White & Mulvaney 1987). Their antiquity in Australia is conservatively established at 50 000 years (Flood 1999). Unlike sedentary agriculturalists, Indigenous Australians depended upon large tracts of land for their foraging, and their relationship to that land was cemented in the complex network of myths and rituals binding people to country.

terra nullius A Latin term used by the British to legally define Australia as an unoccupied land belonging to no one and therefore open to colonisation.

ethnocentric Viewing others from one's own cultural perspective. Implied is a sense of cultural superiority based on an inability to understand or accept the practices and beliefs of other cultures.

Citing evidence from early historical accounts, and from comparative studies among extant hunter-gatherers, the health of the original Australians at the time of the European invasion has been described as 'physically, socially and emotionally healthier than most Europeans of that time' (Thomson 1984, p. 939). This does not mean, however, that they were free from disease. Parasitic and infectious diseases were present, although experienced far less frequently than in settled populations. Diseases and conditions included diarrhoea, lice and hookworm, various respiratory diseases, skin complaints, joint disease, and injuries from accidents (Moodie 1973). An extensive pharmacopoeia of herbal remedies, mineral treatments, and animal substances were used to treat illnesses that were believed to have natural causes. In addition, Indigenous people had access to specialist healers whose expertise was religious in origin. These 'men of high degree' (Elkin 1977) diagnosed and treated illness that people believed to be supernaturally caused.

traditional medical system
Indigenous beliefs and practices about health and illness.

This **traditional medical system** was not equipped, however, to deal with the health consequences of the colonial invasion. Within a few years of European settlement, the basics of good health—adequate shelter, suitable nutrition, companionship, income, and a healthy environment (Better Health Commission 1986)—were no longer available to many Indigenous people. Understanding the historical context in which dispossession, depopulation, and the disintegration of traditional societies occurred is fundamental to an understanding of the current health status of Indigenous people in this country.

The new colony had the twin aims of providing a dumping ground for convicts and thwarting French colonial intentions. It was expected that the colony would become economically self-supporting as soon as was possible. The availability of convict labour meant that Indigenous labour was largely superfluous to colonial requirements. However, the colonists were instructed by the British government to live at peace with the Aboriginal people. Initial dispossession occurred around town sites and nearby rural areas, and it was in those locations that the disastrous effects of introduced diseases such as smallpox and chickenpox were soon described. Pastoral expansion in the early nineteenth century led to intense struggles between the Europeans and Indigenous people, as the latter realised that the newcomers were there to stay. It is only relatively recently that the Aboriginal resistance to the invading forces has received serious historical attention (Reynolds 1995).

Although the estimates of Indigenous depopulation are contentious, it is clear that within 150 years of European settlement the Indigenous population was decimated as a result of direct frontier violence and the effects of introduced diseases. Indigenous social organisation and religious life also suffered, dependent as they were upon an abundant hunter-gatherer economy in which all able-bodied adults were autonomous and self-sufficient (Saggers & Gray 1991a).

Australian economic development is largely based upon the exploitation of natural resources appropriated from Indigenous peoples. The private sector has been primarily concerned to remove Indigenous people from their land in order to facilitate that development and maximise returns on its capital investment. Except in the pastoral industry—and, to a lesser extent, the pearling and sealing industries—where their labour was required, Indigenous people have been marginal to this economic development. On one hand, government policy has been to appropriate, or sanction the appropriation of, land and to curb any resistance to it. On the other hand, it has been to implement policies and practices to ameliorate the effects of this.

Institutionalisation and beyond

During the nineteenth century, government reserves and Christian missions were established throughout Australia on Crown lands. Their purpose was to protect Aboriginal people from the violence of Europeans and to provide a civilising environment in which children, in particular, could be introduced to European ways of life (Brock 1993; Rowse 1998). Indigenous people today have many conflicting memories of these places. For some, they are searing memories of being 'stolen' from their families and communities, of enduring life-long **institutionalisation** in every aspect of their life—from the meagre rations supplied to the demeaning regulation of their employment and personal lives (Haebich 2000). Others have less harsh memories, particularly in those areas where people were able to maintain aspects of their hunting and gathering way of life, as well as elements of their social and religious institutions (Rowley 1978).

institutionalisation A process by which the lives of individuals are regulated in every way, and which creates dependent relationships between the institutionalised person and authority figures.

The economic precariousness of most Christian missions led them to become agents for government welfare, and hence the controllers of individual welfare entitlements. This set in place relations of dependence in which the missionaries were depicted as benevolent fathers tending to the needs of their charges, who in turn were seen as wilful children, requiring constant supervision and moral guidance. These unhealthy relationships would remain in place until the 1950s, when the gradual implementation of policies of assimilation saw the revocation of these settlements and missions. Under assimilation policies, initially introduced in 1939, Indigenous people were expected to become indistinguishable from mainstream Australia, with the same rights and responsibilities as other citizens. However, until after the 1967 referendum, unless Aborigines renounced any association with Indigenous relatives and friends, they were unable to become citizens. At the heart of assimilation policies was the assumption that harmonious relationships between Black and White Australians could only be achieved by breeding out Aboriginality (Brock 1993, pp. 14–19; Rowley 1970, p. 343). Only in the past three decades have these racist policies been replaced by policies, first, of integration, then **self-determination**, and self-management, which allow for the expression of cultural difference and for the rights of Indigenous people to have some control over their destiny. Contemporary political debate ranges from simplistic calls by members of various conservative parties to abolish all affirmative action for Indigenous people, to sophisticated, but contentious contributions from Indigenous people like Noel Pearson, who advocates a more critical assessment of the impact of welfare policies on Indigenous people (Pearson 1999). It is within these broader political and economic debates that the struggle for Indigenous health must be carried on.

self-determination A government policy designed to ensure that Indigenous communities decide the pace and nature of their future development.

History and political economy of alcohol and Indigenous Australia

The drinking patterns observed among Indigenous Australians are the consequence of both supply and demand, and the complex interplay of political, economic, and sociocultural factors. These patterns illustrate the way in which illness, such as that described previously, is socially produced.

The early British colonists, who themselves consumed large amounts of alcohol (Lewis 1992), introduced commercial quantities of alcohol to Indigenous Australians. While initially cautious towards it, some Indigenous Australians soon developed a taste for alcohol and colonists used it 'unconsciously or consciously as a device for seducing Indigenous people to engage economically, politically and socially with the colony' (Langton 1993, p. 201). For many Indigenous Australians, as for other people, intoxication was a pleasurable experience. However, as they were dispossessed of their lands, as their cultures were undermined, and as they were relegated to increasingly marginalised positions in the wider political economy, some turned to excessive alcohol consumption both as a way of dealing with the consequent psychological trauma and as one of the few pleasures available to them.

The relationship between high levels of alcohol misuse and socioeconomic deprivation observed in the broader society are reproduced within the Indigenous population. A national study of Indigenous people found that the unemployed and those on low incomes were more likely to be high-risk drinkers (McLennan &

Madden 1999, p. 55); and a local study of Indigenous young people found that those who were unemployed were 13 times more likely to be frequent users of alcohol and other drugs than those who were still at school or in training, or who had a job (Gray et al. 1996).

For some Indigenous people, drinking is about not accepting such inequalities. For much of the nineteenth and twentieth centuries, consumption of alcohol by or the sale of alcohol to Indigenous people was illegal; though some employers obtained exemptions to these laws and other Europeans profited from the illicit sale of alcohol to Indigenous people. Exemptions to these laws were granted to Indigenous people who became citizens. This latter association—and approximate coincidence of the repeal of prohibitionary legislation with the granting of citizenship to all Indigenous people in the 1960s—meant that for at least some Indigenous people to be intoxicated without legal sanction became a strong expression of equality (Sansom 1980). For some also, public intoxication became a form of protest against the imposition of non-Indigenous laws and social norms (Sackett 1988).

The pattern of drinking among Indigenous Australians is similar to that observed in countries such as New Zealand and Canada among people who are both ethnically and culturally diverse. What accounts for the pattern is their similar history of colonialism, dispossession, and marginalisation. The demand for alcohol growing out of this history is further fuelled by global and local factors that ensure that alcohol is relatively cheap and easily available (Saggers & Gray 1998a; Saggers & Gray 1998b).

Indigenous communities acknowledge the harm that excessive alcohol use causes, and many have developed programs to tackle the issues of both demand and supply. Across Australia, more than 340 programs conducted by Indigenous community organisations provide a wide range of services designed to reduce the harm caused by alcohol and other drug misuse (National Drug Research Institute 2000). Indigenous people are also insisting that government agencies, such as liquor licensing authorities, pay more attention to their demands that alcohol be restricted. These actions demonstrate that Indigenous people are not hapless victims of broader political and economic forces, but their relative powerlessness must nevertheless be acknowledged (Saggers & Gray 1998b).

Addressing Indigenous ill health: rhetoric and reality

Interventions aimed at reducing Indigenous health inequalities have been undertaken by Indigenous people themselves and by governments. To understand these interventions and their impact, it is necessary to know something about the structure of the Australian health care system and the way in which it is financed.

Except in some rural and remote areas, where it is unprofitable, most primary medical care in Australia is provided by medical practitioners in the private sector. This care is funded privately through private medical insurance and direct payment to providers; and publicly through rebates from the national health insurance scheme, Medicare (see chapter 13), and the subsidisation of medications through the Pharmaceutical Benefits Scheme (PBS). Recent work has shown that—largely because of the inaccessibility or inappropriateness of services—the level of Medicare and PBS funding accessed by Indigenous people is incommensurate with the greater burden of morbidity they face (Deeble et al. 1998). Hospital care is provided both by private organisations and, generally, by State or Territory health departments—although, outside urban areas there are few private hospitals. In some rural and remote areas, public hospitals also provide the primary medical care that is not available from private practitioners, and Indigenous patients frequently use such services. Like primary medical care, hospital care is both privately and publicly funded. Public funding of State hospitals is largely through funds provided by the federal government under Medicare agreements and from the financial resources of the States themselves.

primary health care Both the point of first contact with the health care system and a philosophy for delivery of that care.

In contrast—with the exception of some occupational health and safety programs—public health (including some aspects of **primary health care** (PHC), such as health promotion and community health services) is almost exclusively provided by State and Territory governments. Again this is funded from State or Territory financial resources and by Commonwealth government grants to the States and Territories.

public health/public health infrastructure Public policies and infrastructure to prevent the onset and transmission of disease among the population, with a particular focus on sanitation and hygiene such as clean air, water, and food, and immunisation. Public health infrastructure refers specifically to the buildings, installations, and equipment necessary to ensure healthy living conditions for communities and populations.

Public health infrastructure has the greatest impact on health status. Housing, which is particularly important in this regard, is provided by both the private and public sectors. Other aspects, such as water and electricity supply, and waste disposal services, are provided by State and local governments, with financial grants from the Commonwealth, and with a 'user-pays' component for some services. Indigenous people generally have less access to such infrastructure—as a result of poverty and location—than do non-Indigenous people, and this contributes significantly to their poor health status.

In recent years both Liberal–National and Labor federal governments have sought to shift the burden of financing the health care system—particularly for primary medical and hospital care—from the public sector to private individuals. However, despite their efforts, the cost of private health insurance remains beyond the means of many Australians—including most Indigenous people. In addition, various governments have sought to reduce expenditure on health services either by reducing them or by not increasing them to match growth in demand or costs. They have also sought to increase the 'user pays' component of utility services. This cost-shifting further restricts the access of Indigenous people to health services and infrastructure. The World Health Organization's (WHO) Alma Ata Declaration (1978) stated that to be effective, primary health care (and other levels of care) should be affordable, accessible, appropriate, and acceptable. To varying degrees—and despite attempts to address them—most private and mainstream medical and health services fail to meet these criteria with regard to Indigenous people.

Indigenous people themselves have taken a significant initiative to address the short-comings of mainstream private and public health services. In 1972, the first Aboriginal medical service was established in the inner Sydney suburb of Redfern. The service began on a shoestring budget, with nursing and medical staff donating their time, and it was only after it had been operating for a period of twelve months that it was able to attract government funding.

Indigenous community-controlled health services
Independent local organisations, controlled and managed by indigenous people, that provide a range of services to meet the needs of their particular communities.

Currently, there are about 60 fully-fledged **Indigenous community-controlled health services** throughout the country—although this number does not nearly meet the demand for such services. As well as providing primary medical care, they conduct a varying range of health promotion and public health activities. In addition, there are about 20 small community-controlled services, which provide limited levels of care. These organisations are represented nationally by the National Aboriginal Community Controlled Health Organisation (NACCHO), which has played a leading role in representing their interests to State and Territory and Commonwealth governments and developing health policy and standards of care.

In addition to health services, there are another 90 Indigenous-controlled organisations that provide services aimed at preventing and/or treating the misuse of alcohol and other drugs and the associated harms. These services include night patrols, sobering-up shelters, counselling programs, residential treatment centres, education programs, and after-care.

Funding for these organisations comes from a variety of sources. These include grants from various State and Territory and Commonwealth government agencies, from Medicare rebates (in the case of medical services), and from State lotteries commissions for some capital items. Most importantly, it also includes significant amounts of time provided voluntarily by community members, without which most organisations could not survive.

It is often claimed by those seeking to reduce government expenditures that community-controlled services duplicate services provided by the private sector and by mainstream government agencies. This argument is fallacious on two grounds. First, such services are often located where no other services exist; and, second, they provide services that others have either failed to provide, or have inadequately provided in terms of the WHO criteria cited previously.

The other claim of critics is that community-controlled organisations do not deliver adequate levels of service. The development of appropriate criteria for the evaluation of such services is fraught with difficulty (Gray et al. 1995). However, when judged by the criteria of the people who have established and continue to support them, such services are clearly addressing community needs. Where difficulties arise, they have less to do with the objectives than inadequate levels of resources. In this regard, NACCHO has stressed the reciprocal obligations that should exist between funding agencies and community-controlled organisations. That is, it argues that funding agencies, while recognising that community organisations have an obligation to account for the funds provided, should also recognise that in return they have an obligation to provide adequate levels of resources and training to community organisations.

Major government initiatives aimed at alleviating Indigenous ill health are a relatively new phenomenon. It was not until the late 1960s and early 1970s that State and Territory governments began to introduce special Aboriginal health programs. The focus of these was upon health education and promotion campaigns and making mainstream health services more accessible and acceptable to Indigenous people. The latter included the training of health workers to provide the first line of contact between services and Indigenous people. In those remote and rural areas where governments provided medical care, these initiatives also included attempts to make such care more available. At the same time, the Commonwealth began to provide funds to the States and Territories to support those initiatives. Through the newly formed Department of Aboriginal Affairs (later to become the Aboriginal and Torres Strait Islander Commission, or ATSIC), the Commonwealth also began to fund the newly emerging Indigenous community-controlled health services, and housing and community infrastructure projects including sewage and waste disposal. Importantly, these funds were intended to supplement the services that the States were obligated to provide.

In 1973, the Commonwealth Department of Health and the Department of Aboriginal Affairs developed a rudimentary Ten Year Plan for Aboriginal Health. However, in the absence of firm agreements with the States, the Plan was never implemented, and health care for Indigenous people continued to be addressed in a piecemeal fashion by State and Territory governments with financial assistance from the Commonwealth (Saggers & Gray 1991b; Australian Indigenous HealthInfonet 1999).

The initiatives of the late 1960s and 1970s did have some impact. However, the 1979 report on Aboriginal Health by the House of Representative Standing Committee on Aboriginal Affairs highlighted the continuing poor health status of Indigenous people. The report attributed this to unsatisfactory environmental and housing conditions, socioeconomic factors, and the provision of inappropriate health services. It also questioned the commitment of some State governments to improving Indigenous health. Recommendations by the Committee focused upon improvements to the physical environment and the provision of essential services; and the upgrading of health services, including a greater role for Indigenous community-controlled services. While the Committee identified the importance of underlying socioeconomic factors, it made no recommendations to address them (Saggers & Gray 1991b; Australian Indigenous HealthInfonet 1999).

Over the next decade, gains in Indigenous health status remained modest. To address this, a National Aboriginal Health Strategy (NAHS) Working Party was established. In essence, its recommendations both reflected and extended those made ten years earlier in the Aboriginal Health report (National Aboriginal Health Strategy Working Party 1989). In 1990, with some modification, the recommendations were endorsed by a Council of Commonwealth and State Ministers for Health and Aboriginal Affairs; and the Commonwealth announced that, over the following five years through ATSIC, it would provide an additional $232 million to implement the strategy. Some of that money was to be allocated to Indigenous community-controlled health services, but the bulk was to be allocated for essential services infrastructure, contingent upon matching new allocations by the State and Territory governments (Gray & Saggers 1994; Australian Indigenous HealthInfonet 1999).

An evaluation of the NAHS was conducted by ATSIC in 1994. It found that the National Council of Aboriginal Health, which was established to oversee implementation of the NAHS, lacked political support from Commonwealth and State and Territory ministers, that all governments had grossly under-funded the NAHS, that the NAHS had never been adequately implemented, and as a result there had been 'minimal gains in the appalling state of Aboriginal health' (ATSIC 1994, pp. 2–3). The evaluation team also reported that the Commonwealth Department of Finance estimated that 'at least a quarter of Commonwealth Aboriginal specific expenditures appear to substitute for expenditures which otherwise would occur within mainstream services' (1994, p. 84).

In the early 1990s there were increasing concerns that ATSIC did not have the expertise to administer Indigenous health and substance abuse programs and that, in the face of competing priorities, the level of funding for them could not be maintained. As a consequence, in 1995, responsibility for the administration of those funds was transferred to a new Office of Aboriginal and Torres Strait Islander Health Services (now the Office of Aboriginal and Torres Strait Islander Health or OATSIH) within what is now the Department of Health and Aged Care (DHAC).

One of the most important initiatives undertaken by OATSIH has been the attempt to put in place 'framework agreements' between Commonwealth and State and Territory governments and NACCHO (Department of Health and Aged Care 2000). The aim of the agreements is to transfer Medicare and PBS funds to the provision of improved health services for Indigenous people, within the context of agreed-upon Indigenous health plans. However, while supporting the framework agreements in principle, NACCHO has been critical of delays in their adoption. NACCHO has also been critical of the fact that despite the increase in funding for Indigenous health, this expenditure remains at less than one per cent of DHAC's total budget and remains insufficient to adequately address the magnitude of the Indigenous health problem (NACCHO 1999).

The focus of this section of the chapter has been upon those policies and practices developed and implemented by the public sector and Indigenous people themselves to alleviate Indigenous ill health. These initiatives have had some impact. However, this impact has slowed in recent years and the gap in the health status of Indigenous and non-Indigenous people remains wide.

Conclusion

The inequalities in Indigenous health status are a consequence of, and reflect, more fundamental structural inequalities related to the dispossession of Indigenous people and their continued economic and political marginalisation. The 'common-sense' ideology of liberalism that dominates Australian thought obscures those structural inequalities by proclaiming that individuals are responsible for their 'successes' and 'failures'. In also proclaiming that all should be treated equally, it mitigates against solutions, for nothing more assures the perpetuation of inequality than the equal treatment of unequal individuals.

The inadequacy of funding for Indigenous health programs reflects what has occurred in other areas of Indigenous affairs. Australian governments of all persuasions have loudly avowed their commitment to reducing Indigenous inequalities and proudly announced increasing levels of funding. However, such claims are to some extent illusory. On the one hand, they have simply shifted funds from mainstream programs and claimed them as new Indigenous allocations—as did the Commonwealth when it transferred unemployment benefits (now Newstart) from the Social Security budget to the Community Development Employment Projects (CDEP) scheme, enabling it to claim an increase of more than 30% in the Indigenous affairs budget for no further expenditure! On the other hand, governments have allowed Indigenous programs aimed at supplementing existing programs to substitute for them—as State governments have done in cutting back their own spending on infrastructure programs as the Commonwealth has increased its spending.

These claims and accounting sleights-of-hand have created the false perception in the broader community that, on a per capita basis, Indigenous people receive far more in government assistance than do other Australians. In turn, this has allowed some casual observers to conclude erroneously that many Indigenous programs have not achieved their objectives because funds are 'wasted', rather than because they are under-resourced. These illusions and false perceptions fuel support for right-wing, extremist political parties such as One Nation, but cannot be adequately countered by mainstream parties without exposing their own duplicity.

The rhetoric of both Liberal–National Party and Labor Party governments over the past quarter of a century has been that they have taken significant measures to reduce the health inequalities faced by Indigenous Australians. The reality is that—although there have been real improvements—these have been circum-scribed by past and present policy and practice in other areas, which have had far greater impact in creating and maintaining Indigenous ill health.

Summary of main points

- While the causes of illness and death among Indigenous and non-Indigenous Australians are similar, Indigenous people are between two and five times more likely to be hospitalised and to die from these causes.
- People are not randomly afflicted by disease. The patterns of health and illness in any population reflect social inequalities such as ethnicity, social class, and gender.
- Attempts to explain poor Indigenous health in terms of lifestyle and risk factors focus on individual attributes, rather than broader struc-tural factors that inhibit people's abilities to lead healthy lives.
- The contemporary ill health of Indigenous people must be located in the historical context of colonialism and existing inequalities.

- Public health infrastructure, such as housing, water, electricity, and waste disposal, has the greatest impact on health status.
- Indigenous community-controlled health services are an important part of a total health service that should be accessible, appropriate, affordable, and acceptable to Indigenous people.
- For more than two decades there has been a gap between the rhetoric and reality of Indigenous health policy, with insufficient attention and resources directed to the fundamental inequalities experienced by Indigenous people.

Discussion questions

1 How is health inequality measured, and what evidence is there of inequalities between Indigenous and non-Indigenous Australians?
2 Discuss the historical context of the social production of contemporary Indigenous health, including some assessment of the traditional Indigenous health system.
3 Describe the past and present impact of the reserve and mission system on the health of Indigenous people.
4 How is the Australian health care system organised and how well equipped is it to deal with the health problems of Indigenous people?
5 Why has the money going into Indigenous health not resulted in significant improvements in Indigenous health status?
6 What have been some of the key policies designed to improve Indigenous health over the past 25 years?
7 What are some of the major differences between mainstream health services and those that are community controlled?

Further investigation

1 Discuss the demand for and supply of alcohol to Indigenous people in an historical context, and the efforts by Indigenous communities to address substance misuse.
2 What do contemporary political debates about the 'stolen generation' and reconciliation have to do with the status of Indigenous health in the past and present?

Further reading and web resources

Hunter, E. 1993, *Aboriginal Health and History*, Cambridge University Press, Melbourne

Langton, M. 1993, 'Rum, Seduction and Death: "Aboriginality" and Alcohol', *Oceania*, vol. 63, no. 3, pp.195–206.

Reid, J. & Trompf, P. (eds) 1991, *The Health of Aboriginal Australia*, Harcourt Brace Jovanovich, Sydney.

Saggers, S. & Gray, D. 1991a, *Aboriginal Health and Society: The Traditional and Contemporary Struggle for Better Health*, Allen & Unwin, Sydney.

—— 1991b, 'Policy and Practice in Aboriginal Health', in J. Reid & P. Trompf (eds), *The Health of Aboriginal Australia*, Harcourt Brace Jovanovich, Sydney.

—— 1998, *Dealing with Alcohol: Indigenous Usage in Australia, Canada and New Zealand*, Cambridge University Press, Melbourne.

Web sites

Australian Indigenous HealthInfoNet, Edith Cowan University, Perth— provides access to published, unpublished, and specially developed material on Indigenous health. Services include a noticeboard; details of conferences; a listserve; sections on media, media releases and speeches; and courses for Indigenous health workers and those concerned about Indigenous health: <www.healthinfonet.ecu.edu.au>

Danila Dilba Health Service—a community-controlled Indigenous health service based in Darwin: <www.daniladilba.org.au>

IndigiNet Multimedia and InterNet Services—designed to meet the needs of communities and community organisations and individuals. Includes details on the Congress of Aboriginal and Torres Strait Islander Nurses (CATSIN): <www.indiginet.com.au>

National Aboriginal Community Controlled Health Organisation (NAC-CHO)—the umbrella organisation for the Indigenous community-controlled health services, and a national peak body on Australian Indigenous health: <www.cowan.edu.au/chs/nh/clearing-house/naccho/>

National Drug Research Institute: Indigenous Australian Alcohol and Other Drugs Databases, Curtin University of Technology, Perth—includes databases with references and information on Indigenous Australian use of alcohol and other drugs, including intervention projects: <www.db.ndri.curtin.edu.au>

Office for Aboriginal and Torres Strait Islander Health—within the Commonwealth Department of Health and Aged Care: <www.health.gov.au/oatsih/cont.htm>

Part 2

The Social Construction of Health and Illness

I enjoy convalescence. It is the part that makes illness worth while.

George Bernard Shaw 1930, Back to Methuselah

The second dimension of the social model of health, and the theme of this part, is the social construction of health and illness. Social construction refers to the socially created characteristics of human life—the way people actively *make* the societies and communities in which they live, work, and play. The sheer differences in values, traditions, religions, and general ways of life across the globe are manifestations of the social construction of reality. In other words, human life and the way we interact with one another is neither 'natural' nor inevitable, but varies between cultures and over time. In the same way, social construction can be applied to how we view health and illness, revealing that assumptions about normality/abnormality, right/wrong, and healthy/unhealthy reflect the culture of a particular society at a given point in time.

Part 2 consists of six chapters that demonstrate how culture, morality, politics, and economics play a part in socially constructing notions of health and illness in the following ways:

* Chapter 7 deals with the issues of ethnicity, cultural difference and multiculturalism, highlighting the discriminatory practices and stereotyped views that some migrants experience in the health system.
* Chapter 8 examines the medical treatment of deviant behaviour, showing how medical definitions of normality and abnormality can lead to the abuse of patient rights and reinforce prejudice and discrimination against certain social groups.
* Chapter 9 explores how medicine and public health have subjected the body to surveillance and regulation in terms of appearance, sexuality, health and the illness experience.
* Chapter 10 discusses health promotion and highlights the limitations of approaches preoccupied with behaviour change, highlighting the need to address wider living and working conditions.
* Chapter 11 examines the social implications of the search for genetic explanations and cures of disease and behavioural problems.
* Chapter 12 concludes this part by exploring the social construction of ageing, death, and dying. While ageing and death are biological realities, how we experience ageing, dying, and death are distinctly social processes as the continuing debate over euthanasia shows.

7

Ethnicity, Health, and Multiculturalism

Roberta Julian

Overview

* *What does the research evidence tell us about the health of Australia's ethnically diverse population?*
* *How important is ethnicity (or culture) in determining health outcomes for Australia's ethnically diverse population?*
* *Are class and gender more powerful determinants of health than ethnicity, or is it the migration and settlement experience that distinguishes the health profiles of immigrants, rather than ethnicity per se?*

This chapter traces the introduction of mass immigration in Australia, the ethnic composition of Australia, how ethnicity relates to health and illness, and the implications of multiculturalism for the health system. The salience of cultural or 'ethnic' factors as causal factors in differential health outcomes is questioned, and the relevance of class, gender, and immigrant status is highlighted. Thus ethnicity is examined in terms of its implications for social location rather than as a purely 'cultural' phenomenon. Research evidence is utilised to support the argument that structural factors are of greater significance than (cultural) ethnicity *per se*. A critique of the policy of multiculturalism in Australia is offered. This critique argues that the policy focuses on cultural tolerance rather than structural change. The capacity of such a policy to address issues of social inequality in the area of health is thus problematic. It is argued that the provision of health care in a culturally diverse society requires structural changes, especially changes in the structure of health care services.

Key terms

accident-proneness	ethnic group	materialist analysis
assimilation/assimilationism	ethnic minorities	multiculturalism
biomedicine	ethnicity	norms
citizenship	ethnocentric	pluralism
class	ethnospecific services	postmodernity
cultural diversity	gender	'race'
cultural stereotypes	immigrants	racism
discourse	life chances	risk
epidemiology	lifestyle	social construction
ethnic communities	mainstreaming	social justice

Introduction

immigrants The overseas-born population in a society. The term is sometimes extended to refer to the descendants of immigrants through the terms 'second-generation' and 'third-generation immigrants'. However, this usage tends to confuse the term, as it obscures the important fact that those born overseas have a set of immigrant experiences that their descendants do not.

As two-fifths of the Australian population are **immigrants** or the children of immigrants, it is not surprising that there has been a growing interest in issues relating to the health and illness of Australia's **ethnic minorities** (Reid & Trompf 1990; Manderson & Reid 1994). This interest has arisen as service providers have had to address the needs of Australians whose understandings of health and illness are 'different' from those of the Anglo-Australian majority. Within this context, migrants are often viewed as 'people with problems' because they do not fit neatly into the culture and structure of the Anglo-Australian health care system. This pragmatic interest has led policy developers and service providers to examine the work of sociologists and anthropologists, who have long had an interest in the social and cultural factors influencing health (see, for example, Kleinman 1980; 1988).

ethnic minorities Ethnic groups that are not the dominant ethnic group in a society. Unlike the term 'ethnic group', it highlights the power differences between different ethnic groups in society.

This chapter adopts a sociological perspective to explore issues relating to the health of Australia's ethnically diverse population. It discusses the **social construction** of health, illness, and ethnicity, and examines the relationship between ethnicity, class, and health. Importantly, this discussion is located within the socio-historical context of Australia's postwar immigration program, which profoundly affected patterns of structural inequality and cultural difference in Australian society. The chapter concludes with a critical discussion of Australia's health care system in the context of multiculturalism.

The social and cultural construction of health and illness

social construction/ constructionism Refers to the socially created characteristics of human life based on the idea that people act-ively construct reality, meaning it is neither 'natural' nor inevitable. Therefore, notions of normality/abnormality, right/ wrong, and health/illness are subjective human creations that should not be taken for granted.

'Health' and 'illness' are terms that we typically take for granted. We know what it means to be healthy, and we know when someone is ill. We tend to assume that these are objective facts: states of the body and the mind that can be measured against what is 'normal'. Sociologists and anthropologists, however, have shown us that health and illness are social constructions; they are not objectively defined. Thus, definitions of 'health' and 'illness', and understandings of appropriate health care vary over time and across cultures. For example, in Australia during the 1950s and 1960s, many childhood diseases, such as measles, were defined as 'normal'. Thus children were encouraged to interact with others who had the virus so that they would be exposed and 'get the measles'. However, since the development of new medical knowledge—in this case a vaccine— measles are defined as a serious illness and children are encouraged to avoid exposure to the virus (Manderson & Reid 1994).

Furthermore, in any society, some members have more power than others to define health and illness. Some people are the custodians of 'legitimate' medical knowledge, while other members of society, who do not have specialist knowledge, are encouraged to define health and illness in the same ways as the 'experts'. In Australian society, the dominant cultural model of health and illness is that of **biomedicine**, and the 'experts' are health professionals such as doctors. The structure of the health care system (for example, hospitals and general practice) reflects the dominance of this model; it locates these medical 'experts' in positions of power. In other societies, however, there may be a different model of health and illness. Among the Hmong in Laos, for example, health and illness are believed to have organic and/or inorganic causes. The medical 'experts' are the shamans. They have the power to interact with the spirits, and their involvement is crucial in the ritual management of illness (Julian & Easthope 1996; Adler 1996; Rice 1994; Rice 2000; Fadiman 1997).

Health and illness are thus social constructions. Different cultures have different understandings of health and illness, and people within societies are differentially located with respect to access to 'expert' knowledge in this area. Cultural understandings and the structure of health care both play important parts in determining health and illness.

biomedicine/biomedical model The conventional approach to medicine in Western societies. It diagnoses and explains illness as a malfunction of one of the body's biological mechanisms. The biomedical approach of most health services focuses on the treating of individuals, and generally ignores social, economic, and environmental factors.

Ethnic groups in Australia

It is relatively easy to comprehend that there are significant cultural differences between different societies, but it is also important to recognise the existence of cultural diversity within a single society. Diversity can arise from a range of factors such as class, gender, 'race', and ethnicity (see chapters 4, 5, and 6).

Studies of ethnic groups in Australia have demonstrated that differences exist with respect to cultural understandings of health and illness. For example, the Hmong, whose beliefs and practices are outlined above, are an **ethnic group** in Australia. The Vietnamese believe that physical and emotional illness is caused by an imbalance in the forces of *am* and *duong* (similar to the Chinese *yin* and *yang*). One cause of mental illness is believed to be possession by ancestral spirits who have been offended and have become angry (Lien 1992). Among Latin Americans, the word *susto* refers to illnesses associated with unexpected experiences of fright that produce symptoms such as loss of appetite, nervousness, and depression. According to folklore, it is caused by 'the separation of the spiritual element from the physiological element of the person' (Holloway 1994).

ethnic group A group of people who not only share an ethnic background but also interact with each other on the basis of their shared ethnicity.

Different ethnic groups may also have different expectations of what constitutes appropriate treatment. These will, in part, reflect different cultural understandings of the causes of health and illness. For example, in the post-partum period, a Vietnamese mother must not leave the house for 30–40 days, must not speak loudly, must not clean her teeth with a toothbrush, must not read or strain her eyes, and must not wash her hair or have a bath for at least a week, and in some cases a month (Tran 1994). However, even among ethnic groups for whom a biomedical model is taken for granted, there may be cultural differences in expectations of appropriate medical or health care, and in appropriate ways of articulating and managing pain. El Salvadorans, for example, are used to general practitioners treating a wide range of illnesses with injections and are therefore often dissatisfied with the oral treatment that predominates in the Australian health system (Macintyre 1994). Greek and Italian mothers vocalise pain during childbirth more than do mothers from Vietnamese cultural backgrounds—a fact that, in the past, often led nursing staff to assume (incorrectly) that the former were exaggerating their pain, while the latter 'don't feel pain like we do' (Manderson & Reid 1994).

Clearly, an adequate understanding of the ethnic patterning of health and illness must take into account the cultural factors influencing the ways in which different ethnic groups understand, experience, and manage illness. However, in the quest to demonstrate the significance of 'culture' among ethnic groups, a number of problems have arisen that have confounded rather than contributed to our understanding of the cultural influences on health and illness. First, culture has been equated with ethnicity. In other words, it has been assumed that 'culture' has an impact on health for ethnic minorities, but Anglo–Australian views of health and illness are viewed as 'scientifically based' and therefore not influenced by culture. Such a view is **ethnocentric**. Second, 'culture' and 'ethnicity' have been reified in explanations of immigrant health (Manderson & Reid 1994). In other words, 'ethnic' culture is invoked as the major (if not the only) factor affecting differential patterns of health and illness among different ethnic groups. Such 'culturalist' explanations fail to examine the significance of alternative factors, such as class, gender, and age, which may be more important variables than 'culture' or 'ethnicity' in the incidence, diagnosis, and treatment of some illnesses.

In order to overcome these problems, cultural analyses of health and illness need to be balanced with structural analyses. Ethnic groups differ not only in terms of culture but also, and perhaps more importantly, in terms of their social location—that is, in terms of their location in the structure of social inequality. It is possible to identify a hierarchy of ethnic groups on the basis of indicators such as income, occupation, education, and access to goods and services such as health. Clearly, ethnicity and class are interrelated.

One of the major debates in research on the ethnic patterning of health and illness has focused on the relative significance of

ethnocentric Viewing others from one's own cultural perspective. Implied is a sense of cultural superiority based on an inability to understand or accept the practices and beliefs of other cultures.

ethnicity in relation to class. Such debates are often represented as 'culturalist' versus 'structuralist' (or 'materialist'). More recently, however, researchers (for example, Smaje 1996; Manderson & Reid 1994) have pointed to the futility of such debates. Both class and ethnicity are significant structural dimensions of Australian society. As such, it is important to examine the ways in which class and ethnicity are interrelated and thus *interact* to produce differential health outcomes, rather than addressing each as separable from the other and attempting to determine which is more important. Such analyses are significant in that they open up the opportunity to examine the interaction of other structural variables, particularly gender and age, both of which have a significant impact on health (see chapters 5 and 12).

The socio-historical context

cultural diversity A term used to refer to the existence of a range of different cultures in a single society. In popular usage, it typically refers to ethnic diversity, but sociologically the term can equally refer to differences based on gender, social class, age, disability, and so on.

The structure of ethnic relations in contemporary Australia, and thus the ethnic patterning of health and illness, is the outcome of a series of socio-historical processes. One of the most significant events in Australian history in terms of its impact on Australian society has been the postwar immigration program (Jamrozik et al. 1995; Jupp 1999). The outcome of this program is a 'multicultural' society, characterised by **cultural diversity** as well as structural inequality between different ethnic groups (Vasta & Castles 1996; Castles et al. 1998).

Australia's postwar immigration program

In the aftermath of World World II, the Australian government embarked on a mass immigration program with the catch-cry 'populate or perish'. The first Minister for Immigration, Arthur Calwell, was committed to the goal of racial purity and promised to accept ten British immigrants for every 'foreigner' (Collins 1991). As this goal proved difficult to achieve, migrants were accepted from other sources but were selected on the basis of an ethnic preference hierarchy. Since 1945, Australia has accepted over five million people from over 100 countries (Collins 1991; Castles 1992). With the dismantling of the White Australia Policy in the 1970s, the proportion who were of European descent declined; since 1976, 35% to 40% have come from Asian countries (Jupp 1999, p. 120)

There was a twofold rationale for the postwar immigration program. A larger population was needed, first, for the purposes of defence and, second, in order to provide workers for the postwar industrialisation program. These goals had an important impact on the types of migrants initially recruited: they were male, single, and predominantly unskilled. Many were 'displaced persons' or refugees who, along with those who had received assistance with their passages, could be sent by the government to work on projects that were being established and that required a large unskilled labour force. Such projects included the Snowy Mountains Scheme in New South Wales, the La Trobe Valley in Victoria, and the hydroelectric development schemes in Tasmania. The types of immigrants entering Australia have varied over the years, with a recent emphasis on skilled and business immigration (Collins 1996, p. 84), along with a growth in the humanitarian program since the 1970s (Williams & McKenzie 1996).

The conditions under which immigrants arrived and settled in Australia, as well as the characteristics of the immigrants themselves, have led to the pattern of cultural diversity and social inequality that exists in Australia today. A number of aspects are important to note.

ethnic communities Those ethnic groups that have established a large number of ethnic organisations, thus providing a shared context for interaction between members. Only some ethnic groups develop the institutional structure that enables them to become ethnic communities.

First, not all immigrants established visible **ethnic communities** in Australia, and none are totally segregated from mainstream Australian society. Ethnic ghettoes have not been characteristic of immigrant settlement in Australia. Ethnic communities are most likely to result from a pattern of chain migration; immigrants who arrive as individuals or single family units thus may not have access to established ethnic communities. Furthermore, the assumption that an ethnic community exists on the basis of a shared aspect of 'ethnic culture' such as language or citizenship (for example, a Salvadoran community) is erroneous. It assumes homogeneity where it may not exist by denying differences based on class, gender, and politics within the social category (Langer 1998). This is an important fact to keep in mind when examining support structures for those suffering ill health. In addition, a number of studies have shown the significance of class, rather than ethnicity *per se*, in the spatial settlement patterns of immigrants in Australia (Collins 1991; Viviani 1996).

Second, while immigrants are spread throughout the class structure in Australia, the labour force is segmented along lines of ethnicity and gender. According to Jock Collins (1991, 1996), the (non-Aboriginal) Australian labour market is divided into four distinct segments. The 'labour aristocrats' in the first segment (the 'primary' labour market) are Australian-born and Anglophone male migrants who work in white-collar jobs or in skilled jobs in the manufacturing sector. In the second segment are non-Anglophone male migrants who work in hard, dirty jobs that are semi-skilled or unskilled. The third segment comprises Australian-born and Anglophone female migrants who tend to work in 'women's jobs' in the tertiary sector. Finally, at the 'bottom of the heap' are non-Anglophone migrant women who are concentrated in shrinking jobs in the manufacturing sector, such as in the clothing, footwear, and textile industries. The labour of Aboriginal men and women is patterned differently, suggesting an additional and completely different segment (Collins 1996). Over the last fifteen years, however, this pattern of labour market segmentation has altered as a consequence of economic restructuring and changes in the immigration program. Many Asian immigrants arriving since the 1990s have been highly skilled and qualified managers and professionals who have been employed in 'primary' sector jobs (Collins 1996, p. 84). The immigrant workforce is thus becoming increasingly bipolar with clustering at the upper and lower levels of the labour market (Castles & Miller 1998).

Third, refugees have very high rates of unemployment and welfare dependency compared with those born in Australia and with other immigrants (Viviani et al. 1993; Healey 1996). This is largely a result of the fact that they arrive in Australia with few, if any, economic resources, are not likely to have the paperwork required to have their qualifications accepted, and are often suffering the effects of post-traumatic stress disorder as a result of experiences in their home country.

Finally, demographic factors affect the experiences of immigrants. The early postwar immigrants now constitute an ageing population and there is a growing number of second- and third-generation 'immigrants'. While there is evidence to suggest that non-English-speaking background (NESB), second-generation immigrants have achieved upward social mobility, such observations must be treated with caution. It is important to recognise the wide variation in rates of mobility between different ethnic groups and the higher-than-average unemployment rates among migrant youth (Collins 1991).

Clearly, when exploring the relationship between ethnicity and health, it is important to examine ethnicity not only as a cultural phenomenon associated with lifestyle and identity, but also as it impacts on social location and thus on life chances. In other words, ethnicity is both a cultural and a structural dimension of society. It is the nexus between the two that determines the health of the Australian population.

The health of Australia's ethnically diverse population

What does the research evidence tell us about the health of Australia's ethnically diverse population? As the following review of research shows, the effects of ethnicity cannot be separated from the effects of immigrant status, class, gender, and age; rather, ethnicity interacts with each of these factors, rendering their effect somewhat differently for members of different ethnic groups.

Mortality and morbidity

Most research on the ethnic patterning of health begins by noting that the on-arrival health status of immigrants is generally better than that of the Australian-born population. In general, levels of mortality and morbidity for immigrants tend to be lower than those for the Australian-born population (Wooden et al. 1994; Australian Institute of Health and Welfare 1994).

There are a number of explanations given for this. First, migrants are positively selected on the basis of their health. A 'healthy worker effect' may occur as a result of the emphasis on labour migration in the postwar era. While this phenomenon cannot be proven, it is likely that the population of migrants seeking work in another country would be healthier than the general population, which also includes those not in the labour market (Smaje 1996; Wooden et al. 1994). More specifically, in the case of Australia, the superior health outcomes of migrants are the direct effect of a selection process that involves stringent health tests (Wooden et al. 1994). Importantly, the generally lower mortality rates among immigrants declines with length of residence in Australia.

One hypothesised explanation—both of differential mortality rates between immigrants and the Australian-born population, and of the increase in mortality rates with length of residence among immigrants—focuses on the effect of different lifestyles, particularly in relation to diet. Research has shown that southern European immigrants consume less animal fat and protein than the Australian-born population and that diets begin to look more like the Australian norm with length of residence. However, recent research has shown that, for some birthplace categories, mortality rates do not converge on the rate for the Australian-born population: differential rates are sometimes maintained, even after 15 years of residence in Australia (Young 1989, cited in Wooden et al. 1994, p. 74).

Mental health

epidemiology/

social epidemiology The statistical study of patterns of disease in the population. Originally focused on epidemics, or infectious diseases, it now covers non-infectious conditions such as stroke and cancer. Social epidemiology is a sub-field aligned with sociology that focuses on the social determinants of illness.

Epidemiological studies in the postwar period demonstrated a high level of psychiatric disorder, such as depression and schizophrenia, among immigrants (Wooden et al. 1994). However, more recent discussions of the relationship between ethnicity and mental illness note the problematic nature of Western psychiatry's criteria for, and diagnosis and treatment of, mental illness in the context of higher rates of Asian immigration (Jayasuriya et al. 1992). This suggests that the conclusions of earlier studies should be treated with some caution.

Research has identified a number of high-risk categories within the immigrant population: refugees, women, children and adolescents, and the aged (Easthope & Julian 1996). A longitudinal study of Indochinese refugees found a high level of psychiatric morbidity (Krupinski & Burrows 1986). This study stressed the transitional nature of psychiatric disorders among refugees, while other research indicates the long-lasting effects of post-traumatic stress disorder (Silove et al. 1991). Psychiatric illness among immigrant women is often attributed to high levels of isolation from the receiving society (Cox 1989). A review of the literature on youth states that 'There are no conclusive results suggesting that young people of NESB have higher or lower rates of mental health morbidity than other young people' (Bevan 2000, p. 50). Nevertheless, there is universal agreement that refugee children and adolescents 'constitute a high risk for the development of mental health problems' as a consequence of both settlement factors and traumatic pre-migration experiences (Klimidis & Minas 1995). The ethnic aged are vulnerable to psychological distress and depression (Ames 1991), and the tendency among those from a non-English-speaking background to revert to their first language has been attributed to age-related psychosis (Rowland 1991).

Settlement experiences have been found to contribute to mental illness. These include employment and accommodation difficulties, downward social mobility, separation from family and social networks, and communication problems as a result of language difficulties (NHS 1993b), as well as **racism** and discrimination (Jayasuriya et al. 1992). Importantly, research has consistently found that socioeconomically disadvantaged ethnic groups have higher rates of mental disorders than socioeconomically advantaged ethnic groups (Minas 1990). The interactive effects of socioeconomic status, gender, and migration are evident in a study by Taylor et al. (1998) of suicides in New South Wales. They found that among Asians, immigrants from English-speaking countries, and Australian-born males, suicide rates are higher for those with lower socioeconomic status. However, this did not apply to males or females from non-English-speaking European countries.

racism Beliefs and actions used to discriminate against a group of people because of their physical and cultural characteristics.

Occupational health

Work-related injuries are more common among migrant men and women than among the Australian-born population. This is largely because immigrants have been over-represented in dangerous industries (Lin & Pearse 1990). However, while more than 50 per cent of accident victims are migrants, they make up only 5 per cent of those rehabilitated (Holloway 1994). Furthermore, while NESB women make more workers' compensation claims than women from English-speaking backgrounds, these 'last longer and result in a less successful return to work experience' ('Work' 1993, p. 12). As one NESB woman states,

We only get one 10-minute teabreak per day. There is no first-aid or rest room. Workers who injure their hands are forced to keep working. The bosses give them first aid and then send them back to the machines … One worker injured her hand by machining over her fingers. She returned 3 days later. They transferred her from an automatic to a manual machine. This is just one of the ways they punish us. (Savcigil 1982 p. 32)

High rates of work-related illness, injury, and disability among immigrants are often interpreted as a consequence of cultural predispositions. This has contributed to the myth of the 'lazy, **accident-prone** and malingering immigrant worker'. The research reported here, however, supports a more adequate explanation, which is that location in the labour market is primarily responsible (see chapter 4).

accident-proneness A term invented by industrial psychologists to 'explain' workplace injury and illness. It is based on the false and unproven assumption that workers are careless and malingering, and are therefore solely responsible for accidents.

Migrant and refugee women

The health status of many NESB women has been shown to deteriorate as a result of living and working in Australia (Alcorso & Schofield 1991). Immigrant women experience high rates of isolation, loneliness, mental stress, depression (NHS 1993b), and emotional stress (Fitzgerald et al. 1999, p. 123), while the effects of trauma on the health of refugee women have also been noted (Pittaway 1999). Work-related disability in the form of diseases of the musculo-skeletal system and connective tissues (including back pain disorders, arthritis, rheumatism, absence of limbs or parts of limbs, and over-use injuries) account for '40.3% of all disabling conditions experienced by NESB women compared with 29.2% of Australian-born women and 36.2% of women from English-speaking countries' (Alcorso & Schofield 1991, p. 50). High rates of suicide have also been reported among females from Austria, Poland, Czechoslovakia and Greece (McDonald & Steel 1997).

With respect to obstetric indices, NESB immigrant women do not appear to be generally disadvantaged. However, there are some specific areas of concern. These relate to access to antenatal care, high rates of Caesarean section, and high rates of infant mortality (Wooden et al. 1994). NESB women are less likely to be admitted to an *in vitro* fertilisation (IVF) program than those who speak English (NHS 1993b) and, with respect to refugee women, research indicates that 'Cambodian women giving birth are at high risk for acute and, perhaps, chronic postnatal depression' (Fitzgerald et al. 1998 p. 124).

The prevalence of domestic violence among the overseas-born is difficult to determine. Some research suggests that the incidence of domestic violence is no higher among immigrants than it is among the Australian-born population (Morrissey et al.

1991). Nevertheless, there is a belief that domestic violence is more common among some ethnic groups than among others. The stress of exile, migration, and settlement is sometimes used as an 'explanation' of high rates among refugee groups. Pittaway (1999, p. 10) also notes the '[i]ncreasing and disturbing evidence [that] shows that refugee men who have both witnessed and experienced torture are more likely to resort to domestic violence'. On the other hand, concern is sometimes expressed that such beliefs stem from racism in the Australian community in that they 'reinforce stereotypes about the submissiveness of overseas-born women and the violence of males from other cultures' (Easteal 1996, p. 2). While acknowledging that her study of marital violence against overseas-born women in Australia does not provide 'an unambiguous answer to the question of prevalence' (1996, p. 11), Easteal argues that her findings 'suggest that spouse abuse is at least under-reported and under-counted in NESB communities; at the most it may occur more often' (1996, p. 2). There are great difficulties in determining the incidence of domestic violence in both migrant and Australian-born households because it takes place in the private sphere. Easteal concludes that the level of invisibility is likely to remain higher among the overseas-born (1996, p. 10).

Age

Age is a key factor influencing the health of Australia's overseas-born population. Early postwar arrivals, the majority of whom are from European countries, are now in age categories in which chronic diseases such as coronary heart disease and cancer are more common (Wooden et al. 1994). It should also be noted, however, that the ethnic aged do not comprise a homogeneous category: class, ethnicity, and gender are important bases for differentiation and are reflected in the diversity of health problems. For example, McDonald and Steel (1997) found particularly high rates of suicide among elderly immigrants from Eastern Europe, Southern Europe, Middle East/Egypt and Northeast Asia. Furthermore, the health of the ethnic elderly varies according to whether they arrived as young men and women in the immediate postwar years or more recently as elderly parents under the family-reunion scheme.

Myths and stereotypes abound in relation to the ethnic aged. Not all immigrants are members of large, cohesive ethnic communities. This is particularly true for a large proportion of the ethnic aged, many of whom suffer problems of isolation. The view that low levels of institutional care among the ethnic aged result from the fact that they are typically cared for by kin and community is thus misleading (Rowland 1991). Low levels of institutional care may have more to do with limited access caused by financial barriers and cultural inappropriateness.

Most research on ethnicity and health in Australia has focused on first-generation immigrants (the overseas-born). Recent data suggest that children of NESB migrants are less likely to receive preventative health care than the children of English-speaking-background migrants and the Australian-born (Wooden et al. 1994). This would suggest the possibility of differential health outcomes among the younger generation. However, there is a paucity of research on the impact of culture and ethnicity on young people's health. As Bevan (2000, pp. 49–50) notes: 'The lack of a cross-cultural perspective on adolescent development and life-stage transitions is particularly problematic because these concepts are so central in almost all research and literature on young people's health.'

Treatment and health services

Immigrants are generally underserviced when compared with the Australian-born population (Wooden et al. 1994; NHS 1993b). Research shows that people from non-English-speaking backgrounds 'are less likely to go to hospital, visit dentists, live in nursing homes, make use of community-based services, and use preventive services (immunisations, Pap smears and breast screening)' (NHS 1993b, p. 64). Hospitals have been slow to respond to Australia's changing population. Problems of cultural inappropriateness in health care are often ignored, and people from non-English-speaking backgrounds experience intolerance because of their cultural beliefs and practices, which, as noted earlier, are vital to the healing process (NHS 1993b). In the area of mental health, numerous studies have demonstrated that people from non-English-speaking backgrounds receive poorer quality services and their treatment outcomes are worse than those for people from English-speaking backgrounds (NHS 1993b; Minas et al. 1996). For example, research has shown that NESB migrants with schizophrenia or depression have been more likely than their Australian-born counterparts to be treated with electro-convulsive therapy (Minas 1990).

Immigrant women are often unaware of the services available. Furthermore, services that are available are often culturally inappropriate (NHS 1993b) and thus not accessed by immigrant women. Antenatal care, for example, is accessed less by NESB women than by women of English-speaking backgrounds and by Australian-born women (Wooden et al. 1994). Research has shown that this is particularly the case for Arabic women. They tend to have a strong cultural preference for antenatal care provided by women, but this is often unavailable (Bennett & Shearman 1989). Research has highlighted the need for hospitals to take account of different cultural practices in relation to child-birth and post-partum confinement (Manderson & Mathews 1981; 1985; Rice 1994; Rice et al. 1994).

Clear communication between patient and health care worker is crucial in the delivery of quality health care. Interpreters are necessary in order to make appropriate diagnoses and to comply with treatment regimes. For this to occur, however, it is necessary to employ professionally trained interpreters who 'have a good grasp of medical technology' (NHS 1993b, p. 82). A number of studies have found that people from non-English-speaking back-grounds prefer bilingual health care workers (NHS 1993b); in particular, they prefer to visit general practitioners who speak their own language. However, given the small proportion of general practitioners (7.4 per cent) who are from non-English-speaking backgrounds, this is more an ideal than a reality. In addition, the attitudes of those who work with refugees affects mental health outcomes. For example, research has shown that 'workers who regard PTSD as a normal reaction to repetitive trauma are more likely to seek innovative and culturally appropriate responses for their client group' (Pittaway 1999, p. 7).

Theoretical explanations

How important is ethnicity (or culture) in determining health outcomes for Australia's ethnically diverse population? Are class or gender more powerful determinants of health than ethnicity? Is it the experiences of migration and settlement—rather than ethnicity *per se*—that distinguish the health profiles of immigrants from those of the Australian-born population? The answers to these questions have direct implications for appropriate health care policies based on principles of equality and **social justice**.

social justice A belief system that gives high priority to the interests of the least advantaged.

A number of arguments have been presented to explain the research findings discussed above. Culturalist explanations, which emphasise the significance of ethnicity as the major cause of health outcomes, predominate within the Australian **discourse**. These types of explanations take two basic forms. First, there are 'explanations' based on simplistic accounts of cultural difference. These so-called 'explanations' do not examine the complex ways in which culture influences health; rather, they tend to assume that people with particular ethnic backgrounds are more likely to exhibit certain illnesses simply as a function of their 'ethnicity'. This view is evident, for example, in references to the 'Mediterranean back' or in the belief that Southern European women experience more pain during childbirth than women from Asian countries. Such views, in addition to taking an overly simplistic view of ethnicity and/or culture, homogenise people of

discourse A domain of language-use that is characterised by common ways of talking and thinking about an issue (for example, the discourses of medicine, madness, or sexuality).

a similar ethnic background and reify culture, thereby contributing to the perpetuation of racist stereotypes. They are of little value in addressing the health care needs of Australia's ethnically diverse population.

Second, there are more sophisticated culturalist explanations of health outcomes, and these focus on the processes of interaction between patient and health care provider. In other words, they recognise the importance of cultural differences in the meaning of health and illness among people of different ethnic backgrounds, as well as the effects of these in diagnosis and treatment. Such explanations often incorporate a critique of the biomedical model that is taken for granted in the Anglo-Australian health system. More specifically, such explanations emphasise the problems that arise through cultural misunderstandings and poor communication. These have been noted above, for example, in the area of mental health.

structural explanations

Explanations that locate causality outside of the individual. For instance, these may include one's social class position, age, or gender.

In contrast to culturalist explanations, **structuralist** (or materialist) **explanations** stress the significance of social location as the major causal factor in health outcomes. Such explanations emphasise the role of one or more of the following aspects of social location: social class, gender, age, or immigrant status. Once again, there are two main types of structuralist accounts. The first tends to dismiss the significance of ethnicity as a causal factor altogether. Such explanations typically view health outcomes as a function of social-class position. If the influence of other factors is acknowledged at all, these are viewed as secondary. For example, according to this type of account, the high incidence of work-related injuries among immigrants would be explained in terms of the over-representation of immigrants in dangerous working-class occupations.

The second type of structuralist account views social location as a function of the intersection of a range of factors such as class, ethnicity, gender, age, and immigrant status. These explanations acknowledge the influence of both class and ethnicity, and attempt to examine the complex interrelationships between these variables, as well as how the relationship differs among various subgroups or individuals (for example, migrant women, the ethnic aged, second-generation youth, or refugees). Importantly these explanations examine each of these factors as both a cultural and structural phenomenon. For example, they recognise that class, ethnicity, and gender determine both social location (and thus access to health and health care services) and cultural orientation (and thus the meaning of health and illness, as well as views of culturally appropriate health care). These more sophisticated structuralist accounts thereby incorporate the influence of culture; however, they do not reify culture, and they acknowledge difference within ethnic categories. They therefore avoid the problems of stereotyping inherent in most culturalist explanations.

Current policies

multiculturalism A policy term referring to the expectation that all members of society have the right to equal access to services, regardless of 'race', ethnicity, culture, or religion. It is based on the recognition that all people have the right to maintain their cultural beliefs and identity while adhering to the laws of the nation state.

Multiculturalism is a policy that emerged in the 1970s as the government began to recognise the failure of **assimilationism**. The assimilationist policy, according to which immigrants were expected to become indistinguishable from the Anglo–Australian majority (Castles 1992; Jupp 1999), regarded immigrants as having no special needs. One consequence was that the needs of a large number of people were not being met. Demands on service providers led to the perception that migrants were 'people with problems', many of which were health related (Martin 1978).

Multiculturalism was introduced in an effort to redress many of the problems brought about by expectations of rapid assimilation. It was based on the recognition that some ethnic groups had distinct cultures and special needs. However, since multiculturalism began, along with changes in its meaning, there have been significant changes in its institutional structure. In the 1970s the emphasis was on the value of cultural diversity and on the view that migrant welfare was predominantly the responsibility of ethnic groups: 'The ethnic group model was based on the notion that the main determinant of social relations and identity was culture, defined in static terms as the language, customs, traditions and behavioural practices which migrants brought with them as "cultural baggage" '(Castles 1992, pp. 195–6).

assimilation/assimilationism A policy term referring to the expectation that indigenous people and migrants will 'shed' their culture and become indistinguishable from the Anglo-Australian majority.

Much criticism was aimed at this version of multiculturalism. In particular, it was argued that it did little, if anything, to address issues of structural inequality in Australian society or, more particularly, the disadvantages experienced by immigrants and ethnic minorities. As Laksiri Jayasuriya (1992) argues, the policy focused on issues to do with lifestyle rather than life chances. It emphasised the need for cultural tolerance while deflecting attention from issues of social inequality. At the same time, however, its static and unsophisticated view of culture tended to trivialise cultural difference by equating it with food and dance. In this way it contributed to the maintenance of **cultural stereotypes**, which often served to increase, rather than decrease, the level of disadvantage experienced by ethnic minorities.

cultural stereotypes Shared images of the members of an ethnic group that are often negative and are based on a simplistic, overgeneralised, and homogenous view of an 'ethnic' culture.

During the 1980s and 1990s the meaning of multiculturalism changed. The *National Agenda for Multicultural Australia* (1989) placed emphasis on 'removing structural barriers (defined … as those based on race, ethnicity, culture, religion, language, gender or place of birth) to participation in Australian society' (Castles 1992, p. 196). This was recognised as a key component of meeting equity goals. Since 1996, however, there is evidence of a shift away from support for multicultural policies (Castles & Davidson 1998, p. 165), which reflects an ambivalent attitude towards 'multiculturalism' at the Commonwealth level (Jupp 1999, p. 139). Despite the experience of three decades of multiculturalism, the major institutions in Australian society, including health institutions, are still based on a British model: 'This suggests that the political task of changing central institutions to truly reflect a multicultural society has yet to be undertaken' (Castles 1992, p. 198). Nowhere is this more true than in Australia's health care system.

The health care system

Discussions about appropriate health care services have traditionally been couched in terms of the debate between **ethnospecific services** and **mainstreaming**. Support for ethnospecific programs is based on the fact that linguistic and cultural barriers significantly affect access to health care for Australia's ethnic minorities. However, such services are often viewed as temporary measures. Today, governments typically support mainstreaming for reasons of cost–effectiveness.

Critics of mainstreaming argue that its attraction 'seems to lie with the short–term cost savings rather than any long–term policy focusing on the best interest of migrants' (Collins 1991, p. 243). Such a view led Stephen Castles and others (1986, p. 10) to argue that mainstreaming may be the beginning of the end of multiculturalism: 'Although mainstreaming aims to strengthen multiculturalism—and, if sensitively handled, would have that effect—it could become a pretext for dismantling the capacity of services and programs to meet special needs'. For example, while acknowledging the introduction of a new range of services for refugees in the last decade, Pittaway stresses that 'It is essential that these new services are examined from a gender perspective, to ensure that once again, the special needs of refugee women are not subsumed and ignored in the name of mainstreaming' (1999, p. 19). Herein lies the challenge for the future. As Castles notes, 'There is a very real problem here: basing service delivery on ethnicity tends to segregate and marginalise migrants, but ignoring ethnicity and catering for migrants only within general services can mean neglecting special needs and perpetuating structural discrimination' (1992, p. 197).

To address this challenge, we must move beyond the narrow confines of the debate as it has been couched in the past. The need for more radical structural changes in the provision of health care services has become increasingly recognised in recent years. This has occurred in response to two major changes. First, there has been increased recognition of diversity and 'difference' within the

ethnospecific services
Services established to meet the needs of specific ethnic groups or a number of ethnic groups. Members of the ethnic group(s) are the targeted clientele, so that these services are distinct from, and often run parallel with, mainstream services.

mainstreaming A policy term that refers to the provision of services to all members of the community through the same institutional structure. In Australia, it refers to a structure of service provision that is contrasted with that of ethnospecific services.

Australian community. Importantly, this relates not only to difference based on ethnicity, but also to difference based on factors such as gender, age, and disability. Second, critiques of biomedicine have been associated with critiques of the structural organisation of hospitals and other health care services. Alternative modes of service delivery for the provision of health care to all Australians are thus being suggested. As Cherry Russell and Toni Schofield (1986, p. 205) argue with respect to the Australian community as a whole, 'the interests of both sick people and health care workers would appear to be optimised by a situation in which the management of illness occurs in an atmosphere of participation—of activity and interaction—rather than of patient passivity and "expert" control'. By encouraging the participation and involvement of patients in the management of illness, these views also have the potential to lead to the provision of quality care to people of differing ethnic backgrounds.

Future directions

The review of research on the ethnic patterning of health in Australia indicates the need to move beyond 'either/or' debates about the relative significance of class and ethnicity and to address the 'key analytical question, namely the nature of the relationship between ethnicity, socioeconomic status and health' (Smaje 1996, p. 158). Such research should focus not just on immigrants and minority ethnic groups, but should recognise ethnicity as a significant factor in the lives of all Australians.

The same logic can be applied to a discussion of future directions for the Australian health care system. Multiculturalism, as a social policy informing the structure of health care, needs to move forward to correspond with emerging views of **citizenship** in the context of **postmodernity**. As Castles explains, in this sense 'multiculturalism is essentially seen as a system of rights and freedoms … Multiculturalism is not defined in terms of cultural **pluralism** or minority rights, but in terms of the cultural, social and economic rights of all citizens in a democratic state' (Castles 1992, pp. 190, 196). It is this conceptualisation of multicultural citizenship that is needed to effect the necessary structural changes in Australia's predominantly Anglo institutions. This version of multiculturalism recognises difference within the Australian population and ethnicity as an identity option available to all Australians. From this perspective, it is clear that our current health care system is structured to meet the 'ethnic' needs of its Anglo-Australian population but creates barriers for those whose appearance, speech, behaviours, or values reflect cultural difference. Efforts to encourage cultural tolerance, while beneficial in

citizenship A collection of social rights and obligations that determine legal identity and membership of a nation state, and function to control access to scarce resources.

postmodernity A hotly debated term in sociology that broadly refers to a social condition following modernity, in which society becomes fragmented as a result of a high level of social differentiation and cultural diversity.

pluralism A theory whereby state power is shared with a large number of pressure or interest groups.

their own right, will do little to achieve a socially just health system. Structural change in the health care system is the key, and this should not be limited to addressing cultural difference among Australia's ethnic minorities. More pervasive structural changes are required. These will be based more broadly on the recognition of structural and cultural diversity within the Australian community as a whole. Only then will we begin to see the emergence of a truly multicultural society and a health care system that can adequately begin to address the health needs of all Australians.

Summary of main points

- Health and illness are social constructions. Definitions of health and illness, and understandings of appropriate health care, vary over time and between cultures.
- Ethnic groups in Australia (both the dominant Anglo-Australian group and ethnic minorities) have different cultural understandings of health and illness, and different expectations of appropriate treatment.
- Ethnic groups are differentially located in the structure of social inequality in Australia. Thus, ethnicity and class are interrelated.
- Rather than arguing about the relative significance of ethnicity in relation to class in producing differential health outcomes, it is more fruitful to examine the ways in which class and ethnicity are interrelated.
- The ethnic patterning of health and illness in Australia is the outcome of a series of socio-historical processes. The postwar immigration program is one of the most significant. This determined the social and cultural characteristics of Australia's immigrant population.
- In general, levels of mortality and morbidity for immigrants tend to be lower than those for the Australian-born population. With length of residence, these tend to converge on the Australian rates.
- Research has identified a number of areas of concern with respect to the health of Australia's immigrants. These are mental health, occupational health, the health of migrant women and the ethnic aged, and the need for culturally appropriate health care services.
- There are two broad types of explanation for the ethnic patterning of health: culturalist and structuralist (materialist). Culturalist explanations emphasise the problems that arise from cultural misunderstandings and poor communication; however, they tend to reify culture. Structuralist explanations stress the significance of social location and view health as a product of the intersection of a range of factors, such as class, ethnicity, gender, age, and immigrant status.

- Multiculturalism was introduced to redress many of the problems brought about by assimilationism. Early versions of multicultural-ism were criticised for focusing on cultural tolerance and deflecting attention from issues of social inequality.
- The equitable provision of health care in a culturally diverse society requires structural changes that go beyond the debate over ethno-specific versus mainstream services. A diversity of structures is required to meet the needs of Australia's diverse population.

Discussion questions

1 Discuss either immigrant women, the ethnic aged, or refugees. In what ways would their health concerns be similar to and/or different from those of the Australian-born population?

2 Discuss the ways in which class, ethnicity, and gender might affect the health of the following categories: migrant women, the ethnic aged, second-generation ethnic youth, and refugees.

3 What does 'multiculturalism' mean to you? Compare your views with those of one or more class members.

4 In what ways has multiculturalism as a social policy had an impact on health services in contemporary Australia?

5 Stephen Castles (1992) states that contemporary multiculturalism 'is about equality of access to government services, rather than about the quality of the services offered'. With respect to health care, do you agree or disagree with this statement?

6 Debate the 'pros' and 'cons' of providing ethnospecific health care services. How would you move beyond the 'either/or' debate with respect to ethnospecific services and mainstreaming?

Further investigation

1 Critically assess the relative significance of pre-migration and post-migration factors on the health of immigrants in Australia. What patterns (if any) are apparent?

2 *The Spirit Catches You and You Fall Down* (Fadiman 1997) is a fascinating account of the difficulties that arise when the mem-bers of an ethnic minority with a non-Western view of health and illness (in this case the Hmong in the USA) interact with the Western health care system and its experts. Read this book and (a) identify the key factors contributing to the 'problems' that arose, and (b) suggest possible changes to the Australian health care system that would increase the likelihood of positive health outcomes. (Note: You will need to consider who is defining the 'problem' and who is defining 'positive health outcomes'.)

3 Find out the ethnic composition of the population in your area (if possible, you might also get an age and gender breakdown).

What changes would you make to current services in your area in order to meet the needs of the whole community?

Further reading and web resources

Castles, S., Foster, W., Iredale, R., & Withers, G. 1998, *Immigration and Australia: Myths and Realities*, Allen & Unwin, Sydney.

Donovan, J., d'Espaignet, E., Merton, C., & van Ommeren, M. (eds) 1992, *Immigrants in Australia: A Health Profile*, Ethnic Health Series, no. 1, Australian Institute of Health and Welfare & AGPS, Canberra.

Fadiman, A. 1997, *The Spirit Catches You and You Fall Down*, Farrar, Straus and Giroux, New York.

Ferguson, B. & Pittaway, E. (eds) 1999, *Nobody Wants to Talk About It: Refugee Women's Mental Health*, Transcultural Mental Health Centre, Sydney.

Jayasuriya, L., Sang, D., & Fielding, A. 1992, *Ethnicity, Immigration and Mental Illness: A Critical Review of Australian Research*, AGPS, Canberra.

Jupp, J. 1999, *Immigration*, 2nd edn, Oxford University Press, Melbourne.

Klimidis, S. & Minas, I. H. 1995, 'Migration, culture and mental health in children and adolescents', in C. Guerra & R. White (eds), *Minority Youth in Australia*, National Clearing House for Youth Studies, Hobart, pp. 85–99.

National Health Strategy 1993, *Removing Cultural and Language Barriers to Health*, Issues Paper no. 6, AGPS, Canberra.

Reid, J. & Trompf, P. (eds) 1990, *The Health of Immigrant Australia: A Social Perspective*, Harcourt Brace Jovanovich, Sydney.

Rowland, D. T. 1991, *Pioneers Again: Immigrants and Ageing in Australia*, Bureau of Immigration Research & AGPS, Canberra.

Web sites

Center for Cross-cultural Health (USA): <www.ceh.org.au>

Centre for Culture, Ethnicity and Health: <www.ceh.org.au>

Culturally sensitive health care guides (developed by Queensland Health): <www.health.qld.gov.au/hssb/cultdiv/home.htm>

Ethnic Health: <www.australiahealth.com/Community%20Health/ethnic.htm>

Refugee Council of Australia: <www.refugeecouncil.org.au>

WWW VL Public Health: Selected Topics—Ethnic Health: <www.ldb.org/vl/top/top-ethn.htm>

8

The Medicalisation of Deviance

Sharyn L. Roach Anleu

Overview

* *What causes or motivates someone to deviate from social expectations?*
* *Who defines what those expectations are?*
* *When a person is identified as deviating from social norms, to what extent is that person viewed as sick (and thus as requiring a therapeutic response) or as a criminal (requiring a legal response)?*

Throughout the history of psychiatry, attempts have been made to designate various forms of behaviour as evidence of mental illness requiring therapeutic intervention. These forms of behaviour have been defined as deviant by some segments of society. Psychiatry has developed notions of normal (and deviant) behaviour in such areas as sexual behaviour and identity, mental health, gambling, alcohol and drug use, criminal behaviour, eating, reproduction, and child development. Psychiatry has been engaged in the process of normalisation or social control through its relationship with patients (or consumers) and through its role in mental institutions. Nevertheless, psychiatry has never been completely successful, and other disciplines and segments of medicine contest psychiatry's capacity to identify, diagnose, and treat mental illness. This chapter examines psychiatry's attempt to establish jurisdiction over several kinds of deviance, and explores its successes and failures. It looks at the processes of medicalisation and demedicalisation rather than arguing that the influence of psychiatry is always supreme and unidirectional.

Key terms

deinstitutionalisation	medical dominance
deviance	medicalisation
discourse	norms
empirical	risk
epidemiology	risk factors
ethnicity	sick role
gender	social control
individualism	social constructionism
labelling	

Introduction

norms Expectations about how people ought to act or behave.

medicalisation The process by which non-medical problems become defined and treated as medical issues, usually in terms of illnesses, disorders, or syndromes.

This chapter examines the ways in which deviation from some social **norms** and expectations becomes defined and treated as illness, or as a medical phenomenon, requiring intervention and treatment by medical personnel. The **medicalisation** of deviance is a historical and social process, and is the outcome of professional and social-movement activity. The dominance of the medical model in explaining certain types of behaviour or conditions means that the emphasis is on the individual, who must be treated in some way in order to restore conformity or health. The discussion in this chapter first outlines the concepts of deviance and social control, and then examines the relationship between medicalisation and social control. It focuses on the role of psychiatry in identifying and regulating deviance in relation to women and mental illness, criminal deviance, and current debates about sexuality and AIDS.

Deviance and social control

deviance Behaviour or activities that violate social expectations about what is normal.

labelling Labelling theory focuses on the effect that social institutions (such as the police, the courts, and psychiatry) have in labelling (or defining) what is deviant.

social control Mechanisms that aim to induce conformity, or at least to manage or minimise deviant behaviour.

Deviance is behaviour that violates social norms. The emergence of social norms is shaped by political and historical factors, and by specific social structures and situations (Meier 1982, p. 43; Parsons 1951b, pp. 297–8). **Labelling** theorists shift attention away from the person who deviates from social norms to the social audience that reacts to, defines, labels, and punishes behaviour and individuals as deviant. Social movements, interest groups, and individuals affect the shape and application of social norms. Becker terms those engaged in the creation and application of social rules 'moral entrepreneurs'—that is, actors who seek general acceptance of their particular values and perspectives, and who often adopt a self-righteous or crusading stance (Becker 1963, p. 147–63).

Several kinds of questions can be asked regarding the concept of deviance: What causes or motivates someone to deviate from social expectations? Who defines what those expectations are? Does deviance necessarily invoke sanctions? What kinds of sanctions are invoked and under what conditions? What is the relationship between various forms of **social control** (for example, between legal regulation and medical intervention)? To what extent does the type of deviance or societal reaction depend on gender, age, socioeconomic status, ethnicity, sexual identity, or other social attributes and structural inequalities? Medicine is one kind of social audience; it is concerned with identifying various conditions as deviations from a model of health and well-being that makes assumptions and values about normality (Edwards 1988, pp. 143–87).

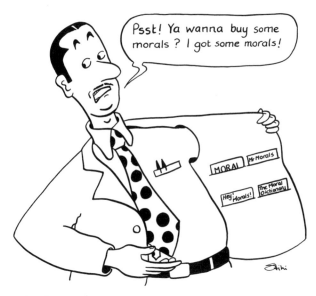

The moral entrepreneur

Medicalisation and social control

Medicalisation describes the process whereby non-medical problems or phenomena become defined and treated as medical issues, usually in terms of illnesses, disorders, or syndromes (Conrad 1992, p. 209). Successful medicalisation means that the dominant form of social control is therapeutic, and that individuals diagnosed as deviating from a model of health confront a new set of normative expectations stemming from the sick role. Talcott Parsons (1951a; 1951b, pp. 455–6) first specified the connections between deviance and illness in his conception of the **sick role**. In addition to the constraints of physiological conditions, the sick role itself exempts people from fulfilling their normal social duties; it does not hold individuals responsible for their conditions (at least to some extent) and obliges them to seek medical assistance. By entering into a relationship with medical personnel, the sick person becomes a patient with attendant expectations and requirements.

sick role A concept used by Talcott Parsons to describe the social expectations of how sick people are expected to act and of how they are meant to be treated.

While the sick role legitimates some kinds of deviance and imposes a new set of social norms (and social control), access to this status is not automatic. The manifestation of certain physiological conditions is not the only, or indeed a necessary, prerequisite for contact with institutionalised medicine. For example, individuals identified as potential deviants from medical (and social) norms may be viewed as being 'at risk' of some types of illness or deviance and may be subject to medical surveillance in the name of preventing or reducing the '**risk**' behaviour. Public health programs may target Aboriginal people, female-headed

risk or risk discourse 'Risk' refers to 'danger'. Risk discourse is often used in health promotion messages warning people that the lives they lead involve significant risks to their health.

households, gay men, or young people for early intervention or education in order to prevent such illnesses or conditions as drug addiction, AIDS, child abuse, and suicide.

The medicalisation thesis posits that physical conditions do not, by their nature, constitute illness; rather, they require identification and classification, which entail subjective and value-laden considerations—that is, they are socially constructed. **Social constructionism** counters medicine's claims to be scientific, objective, and disinterested. Eliot Freidson (1988) argues that medicine actively and exclusively constructs illness, and therefore determines how people must act in order to be treated. Rather than disinterestedly detecting symptoms and physiological causes, and administering scientifically validated therapeutic techniques, medical practice involves interpretation and judgments about what is normal and abnormal—about which circumstances are suitable for medical intervention and which are not. The symptoms do not speak for themselves; their interpretation and categorisation are informed by social values and assumptions about what constitutes health (normal) and illness (deviant). Illness and disease are human constructions: they do not exist without someone proposing, describing, and recognising them; they are neither self-evident nor naturally occurring. The central question becomes: how it is that certain areas of human life come to be defined, or not, as medical issues under certain conditions (Freidson 1988, pp. 30–1)? The success of the medical profession in monopolising definitions of health and illness provides it with considerable authority and scope for social control.

Within this context, **empirical** research identifies the social conditions under which certain illnesses emerge, and it analyses the effect of medical practitioners' claims on the development of conceptions of illness. The medicalisation of infertility is a recent example. Traditionally, involuntary childlessness was considered a personal and private issue, but now it is viewed as a condition warranting medical attention and intervention. The experience of infertility also causes many people, especially women, to feel as though they are deviating from gender norms, which specify motherhood as essential to womanhood, even when their male partners are infertile but they are not. Participants in *in vitro* fertilisation (IVF) programs are subject to complicated medical procedures and expectations, and in some States, legal regimes demand that they comply with marriage and counselling requirements. Nonetheless, conceptive technologies, especially IVF, do not cure infertility but rather circumvent it by attempting to achieve a pregnancy and live birth (Roach Anleu 1993).

Discussions of medicalisation often refer to psychiatry as the primary example or prototype of medical social control. Such discussions tend to emphasise the negative and coercive aspects of

---

social construction/ constructionism Refers to the socially created characteristics of human life based on the idea that people act-ively construct reality, meaning it is neither 'natural' nor inevitable. Therefore, notions of normality/abnormality, right/ wrong, and health/illness are subjective human creations that should not be taken for granted.

empirical Describes observations or research that is based on evidence drawn from experience. It is therefore distinguished from something based only on theor-etical knowledge or on some other kind of abstract thinking process.

discourse A domain of language-use that is characterised by common ways of talking and thinking about an issue (for example, the discourses of medicine, madness, or sexuality).

social control, in contrast to medical **discourses** that focus on medical intervention as positive and necessary for health and well-being. The concept of medicalisation—and of social constructionism in general—has been subject to considerable critique regarding the relativity of its proponents' own position (Bury 1986). Critics point out that these theorists tend to view medicalisation as wholly negative and coercive—as something bad that should be averted. They also suggest that arguments about medical imperialism—and about medicine's displacement of religion and law as a source of social control—are exaggerated, rhetorical, and not borne out in practice (Strong 1979, pp. 199–200). However, the extent to which medicalisation has detrimental consequences is an empirical, not a definitional, question. Historical analyses and case studies identify the ways in which various phenomena come to be defined in medical terms and to be viewed as warranting medical intervention. Medicalisation occurs on several levels:

- *the conceptual level*, at which medical vocabulary is used to describe or define an issue or problem but medical professionals and treatments may not be involved. For example, alcohol abuse, interpersonal problems, and some criminal activities may be defined as pathological or as evidence of sickness or mental impairment, but their management—although it may be viewed as therapeutic—does not necessarily entail intervention by medical personnel.
- *the institutional level*, at which organisations may adopt a medical approach to particular problems, and medical personnel may be gatekeepers for the organisation, but the everyday routine work is performed by non-medical personnel. Access to some workers' compensation schemes requires a referral from a medical practitioner, even when human services personnel such as psychologists, counsellors, or social workers implement the rehabilitation program.
- *the interactional level*, at which medicalisation occurs as part of doctor–patient interaction, with the former medically defining and/or treating the latter's problem. The doctor provides a medical diagnosis and prescribes a medical treatment (Conrad 1992, p. 211).

Psychiatry has always been involved in the identification and regulation of deviance. Both as an emergent occupation and as a segment of the medical profession, psychiatry has developed notions of normal behaviour in areas such as sexual behaviour and identity, mental health, gambling, alcohol and drug use, eating, reproduction, and child development. Psychiatry seeks to locate a pathological basis within the individual for such 'deviance' and views certain types of behaviour as evidence of addiction, syn-

dromes, conditions, personality disorders, or other mental illnesses.
It attempts to attribute causes to—or perhaps, more accurately, to
identify sites of intervention on the basis of—individual rather
than to social or definitional factors. Conditions that psychiatrists
view as warranting their intervention include deviations from
moral or religious norms (for example, gambling or alcohol use,
which may be 'diagnosed' as evidence of addictive behaviour,
personality disorder, or depression), or from legal norms (for
example, child abuse, juvenile delinquency, rape, or homicide).
Multiple crimes or crimes that are especially unusual or particularly violent or cruel are often identified by psychiatrists as being
both caused by, and evidence of, psychoses. The mass media and
members of the public also tend to equate 'abnormal' crimes with
mental illness on the part of the perpetrator.

Case studies of psychiatric hospitals illustrate the power of psychiatric diagnosis, the pervasiveness of psychiatric discourse, and
the high status of psychiatrists (Goffman 1961). A stark example is
provided in D. L. Rosenhan's article 'Being Sane in Insane Places'.
He describes an experiment in which eight sane people gained
secret admission to psychiatric institutions (Rosenhan 1973). The
pseudo-patients claimed that they had been hearing voices but,
upon admission to the hospital ward, ceased simulating any symptoms of abnormality. The only people who detected that they were
not suffering from a psychiatric condition were the other patients,
not the medical staff. Indeed, the label 'schizophrenic'—that is, the
diagnosis—determined psychiatrists' and nurses' perceptions and
interpretations of the pseudo-patients' behaviour, even when it was
completely 'normal' (Rosenhan 1973, p. 253).

Despite the influence of psychiatry, not all attempts to med-
icalise a field of behaviour are necessarily successful. Different
medical specialties may compete with one another for jurisdiction over a problem, or aspects of it, and medical personnel are
not the only ones to advocate the process of medicalisation. Other
occupational groups may adopt a medical frame of reference, and
individuals who experience a condition may seek to have it legitimated medically. The history of psychiatry, its interrelationships
with allied occupations and other segments of the medical profession, and the influence of wider social changes all illustrate
unevenness in the process of medicalisation and great shifts in
psychiatric knowledge and treatments.

The rise of psychiatry

The emergence and dominance of a medical approach to madness
(later to be redefined as mental illness) began in the late eighteenth
century. The asylum emerged during the nineteenth century as the

state's solution to the increasing numbers of people identified as insane, and the history of psychiatry and its authority is inextricably intertwined with this development. In the seventeenth century, enormous houses of confinement had been opened to accommodate diverse populations of 'deviants', including 'mad' people, criminals, libertines, beggars, vagabonds, prostitutes, the unemployed, and the poor—that is, people deemed to be economically (and politically) marginal. These institutions of confinement had arisen in order to accommodate increasing poverty—with growing numbers of people unable to engage in productive work—and as a way of managing or segregating all forms of behaviour defined as immoral (Ingleby 1985, p. 147). The Hôpital Général in Paris, for example, combined the characteristics of an asylum, a workhouse, and a prison, but no medical treatment was administered (Foucault 1988, pp. 38–84).

The next stage was the development of separate institutions to deal with more homogenous subgroups: the almshouse, the workhouse, the insane asylum, and the prison. These institutions remained the dominant way of managing these people until the 1950s. The rationale for separating the insane was not medical but social and economic. Despite the lack of cures or explanatory theories of madness, physicians assumed a small but central role as gatekeepers of the asylums: from 1774, a physician's certificate was required for commitment to a British asylum. As Michel Foucault observes:

> The physician ... played no part in the life of confinement. Now he becomes the essential figure of the asylum. He is in charge of entry ... the doctor's intervention is not made by virtue of a medical skill or power that he possesses in himself and that would be justified by a body of objective knowledge. It is not as a scientist that *homo medicus* has authority in the asylum, but as wise man (Foucault 1988, p. 270).

Nevertheless, there was considerable optimism, and it was hoped that new scientific advances in medicine would be able to solve problems associated with mental illness (Conrad & Schneider 1992, pp. 44–6). By the end of the eighteenth century, reformers sought to eliminate the physically punitive aspects of life in the insane asylum and to reinforce the benefits of moral treatment. They emphasised training, obedience, work, and the value of property. Dr Phillippe Pinel in France developed one of the first typologies of madness by distinguishing between melancholia, mania, dementia, and idiocy. Physicians argued that, as both moral and medical responses were appropriate, they should have a monopoly on dispensing both. Their successful bid to provide moral assistance was especially important since they were unable to show the physiological causes of mental illness and had not demonstrated any cures. The decline of the Church, the scientific discoveries of the Enlightenment, and the humanitarianism of the Renaissance all aided physicians' 'professional dominance' in this area and fostered a unitary conception of mental illness—that is, a single illness category to encompass diverse conditions and symptoms. The Enlightenment, an eighteenth-century philosophical movement, questioned traditional, especially religious, values and doctrines; it emphasised **individualism**, rational thought, and the empirical method in science, and was oriented to human progress. Similarly, the Renaissance, which occurred between the fourteenth and seventeenth centuries, heralded the transition from medieval to modern society, the latter being distinguished by the power and influence of rational science, which displaced some of the authority of religious expertise and its concern for the sacred. At the close of the eighteenth century, the notion of mental illness as a disease and as a topic of medical and scientific intervention was becoming the dominant conception of madness, and the influence of religious or supernatural explanations was waning (Conrad & Schneider 1992, pp. 47–8).

individualism/individualisation

A belief or process supporting the primacy of individual choice, freedom, and self-responsibility.

The separation of deviants was an essential precondition for the development of a medical specialty (the forerunner of psychiatry) that claimed to possess specific expertise in dealing with madness. This, in turn, further legitimised the concept of mental illness as a distinguishable phenomenon (reflecting and caused by an underlying pathology), rather than the amorphous cultural view of insanity that had 'previously prevailed and which had emphasised demonological and non-human influences (Scull 1975, 241–5; 1977, p. 344). During the nineteenth century, psychiatrists identified ill health, religious anxiety, disappointed love, pecuniary embarrassment, acid inhalation, suppressed menstruation, and general poor health as causes of mental illness. Their interventions included physical restraints, cold baths, tooth extractions, and surgery of the brain and reproductive systems. J. R. Sutton describes these classificatory schemes as 'crude nosologies, eclectic arrays of behavioural symptoms loosely organised in terms of prevailing moral judgements [, and] too often[,] prevailing "moral" therapies practised in asylums consisted only of the work and disciplinary routines that contributed to administrative efficiency' (1991, p. 668).

By the close of the nineteenth century, a whole range of new personal problems paralleled enormous social changes, especially in the USA. Everyday problems became defined as nervous diseases, providing a focus for new professional groups. One of the forebears of psychiatry—neurology—dealt with an ill-defined and heterogenous range of residual conditions that conventional medicine was unable to cure or manage. Up to a third of the neurologists' patients in the USA were diagnosed as suffering from 'general nervousness' and complained of conditions that would now be described as depression, anxiety, and insomnia. Discussions about general nervousness included complex theories of psychic and organic aetiology, with treatments ranging from rest cure to electrotherapy and psychotherapy (Abbott 1988, pp. 285–90).

The growth of asylums consolidated the professional development of psychiatrists. However, psychiatry was not approved as a medical specialty until 1934 (Neff et al. 1987, p. 45). The number of patients in mental hospitals increased more than sixfold between 1880 and the mid-1920s, making them the largest of all custodial institutions in the USA. Similar patterns existed in the United Kingdom and France (Ingleby 1985). Psychiatrists had successfully monopolised the treatment of insanity by officially defining it as a medical condition with identifiable causes, but moral judgments and lay concerns still influenced diagnosis. Insanity was an elastic concept—a category of residual deviance—which could be applied to a variety of individuals whose deviance stemmed from poverty, homelessness, or physical disability. Unlike confinement in other custodial institutions, commitment to an insane asylum entailed neither a trial, a fixed term of internment, nor the legal protection associated with criminal proceedings (Sutton 1991, p. 667).

Close links exist between mental hospitalisation and social control. Erving Goffman's classic study of a state mental hospital shows that very few of the everyday activities of the institution are devoted to therapy or treatment; most activities are oriented to maintaining the organisation, performing routine tasks, and maintaining social control among the patients. The psychiatrist's presence is brief and the input non-specific (Goffman 1961). Mental institutions also play a role in wider social policy and in the regulation of sub-populations that are identified as problematic. The increasing numbers of people confined to mental hospitals in the USA between 1880 and the 1920s did not indicate an epidemic of mental illness. Rather, the pattern stemmed from the government's incapacity to systematically address and solve poverty, especially among the aged; from the closure of the almshouses, combined with flexibility in the medical concept of insanity; and from the relatively simple commitment procedures (Sutton 1991, pp. 667–8, 675–6).

Other significant developments in the history of psychiatry include the rise of psychoanalysis, which enabled psychiatrists to help people who were anxious and depressed, and who experienced problems with everyday life, as well as to treat the insane. Sigmund Freud, a physician and a neurologist, provided a new approach to understanding personal problems. He replaced a biological model with a psychogenic explanation and intervention that was based on free discussion (by the patient) in the context of a relationship with the therapist (Conrad & Schneider 1992, pp. 53–4). Parallels between this therapeutic relationship and the Christian confessional are obvious: the penitent/patient confesses his or her sins/deviance to a priest/psychiatrist, who has the power to specify and require remedial action. The one who receives confessions is able to exert social control—that is, instruct penitents/patients how to expiate their sins or manage their deviance in order to become conforming, normal people (Hepworth & Turner 1982, pp. 8–10, 14, 85–107). The popularity of psychoanalysis also provided psychiatry with competition from psychology, which led to a re-biologising of personal problems in the late 1970s (Abbott 1988, pp. 300–3).

A second important development in the 1950s was the availability of new psychotropic (mood-altering) drugs, which were used in mental hospitals as well as to enable more people to be discharged but raised questions of compliance and self-medication. While drug treatment reinforced the medical model of mental illness, the curative effect is contested, and critics argue that the drugs merely sedate, and thereby regulate, the behaviour of people identified as mentally ill. In the 1960s, criticisms of psychiatry, of the unitary conception of mental illness, and of the social control functions of mental hospitals and the 'therapeutic' relationship became more evident. Proponents of the labelling perspective doubted that diverse symptoms, behaviours, and conditions constituted a single classification of mental illness. Thomas Scheff, for example, argues that mental illness became almost a label of convenience for a range of norm-breaking behaviour that could not be accommodated within other types of deviance (what he termed 'residual deviance'), including crime, alcoholism, and illness (Scheff 1966, pp. 31–54). Commentators identified enforced drug therapy—which violated patients' rights by denying them informed consent and due process—as an unacceptable outcome of the influence of psychiatry in the mental health and criminal-justice systems (Kittrie 1971). One of the strongest proponents of the anti-psychiatry movement, Thomas Szasz, maintains that the replacement of the Church by medicine as the institution of social control merely redefines and relabels deviance with medical terminology (1961, pp. 204–20; 1973, 69–78). He argues that the term 'mental illness' is widely used to describe something that is very different from a disease of the brain, and suggests that problems in living derive from the stresses and strains inherent in social interaction between complex human personalities in modern societies (1960, p. 113). The concept of mental illness serves the same social control function in the contemporary world as witchcraft did in the late Middle Ages. Both are imprecise and all-encompassing concepts, adaptable to whatever the priest or physician wishes. The therapeutic model was being applied to all kinds of 'deviance': alcoholism, drug addiction, economic disadvantage, mental disorders, interpersonal problems, and juvenile delinquency.

A contemporary example of a controversial psychiatric classification, and associated diagnosis and treatment, is that of personality disorder. The past 20 years has seen a rapid elaboration of this category in the Diagnostic and Statistical Manual of Mental Disorders (DSM). Nonetheless, personality disorders do not include obvious organic or psychological impairment but are identified through their interpersonal effects, including chaotic and distressing relationships, instability of identity, or criminal records incurred (Manning 2000, pp. 622–3). The DSM distinguishes personality disorders according to such descriptive terms as 'odd and eccentric' and 'anxious and fearful' (Nuckolls 1997, p. 52), thus attesting to the classification's broad scope.

Deinstitutionalisation

Widespread criticism and research demonstrates the coercive dimensions of state mental hospitals and their failure to cure or treat mental illness. This, along with a renewed community interest in the management of all kinds of social problems, legitimates the process of **deinstitutionalisation**: the emptying of publicly funded mental hospitals, the closure of many facilities, and a trend whereby individuals may be admitted for short periods of time (often on many occasions) rather than undergo lifetime hospitalisation. Combined with the continual winding back of the welfare state, which began in most Western industrial nations in the 1970s, such criticisms have been used to justify the closure of state-run mental hospitals and have led to massive changes in mental health policy. There has also been a parallel expansion in the numbers of private psychiatric hospitals and psychiatrists practising privately (DHAC 1998, pp. 105–14).

The National Mental Health Policy, established by the health ministers of the Commonwealth, States, and Territories of Australia in 1992, advocates a shift away from reliance on separate psychiatric hospitals, an increased emphasis on community-based care, and the integration of mental health care with other types of health and community care. It advocates a mix of general hospital, residential, community treatment, and community support services, as well as support from other services such as housing and accommodation, community and domiciliary care, and employment and training opportunities (Australian Health Ministers 1995, pp. 3–4). The policy intends to reduce the stigma associated with mental illness and hospitalisation in a psychiatric institution, and to 'normalise' mental health sufferers. Such an approach emphasises that psychiatrists and separate psychiatric

deinstitutionalisation A trend in mental health treatment whereby individuals are admitted for short periods of time, rather than undergoing lifetime hospitalisation. In theory, such policies are meant to be supported by extensive community resources, to 'break down the barriers' and integrate the mentally ill into the community. However, in practice, this has not occurred on a wide scale because of the lack of funding of community services.

institutions do not have a monopoly on the management of mental illness, and the strategy reallocates resources accordingly. Since the commencement of the strategy, the number of public-sector psychiatric beds and the use of in-patient services nationally have decreased by 20 per cent (DHAC 1998, pp. 27–30). The policy reflects the historical concern with classifying sub-populations and types of mental disorder, but it represents a shift away from public funding and provision of mental health services. The Second National Mental Health Plan (from 1 July 1998 to 30 June 2003) seeks to maintain a national minimum data set and to predict, as accurately as possible, the mental health needs of members of the community. It will closely monitor the demographic and clinical characteristics of consumers, the detail of mental health programs, the attributes of the mental health workforce, program expenditures, and client/consumer outcome data (ABS 1998; DHAC 1999, pp. 5–14).

A new and more legal concern relates to the rights and civil liberties of people with mental health problems. It identifies the importance of consistent mental health legislation to define and protect the rights of individuals with a mental disorders. Indeed, Mulvany suggests that the social approach to disability provides an appropriate framework to analyse the situation of people with psychiatric disabilities or impairment and to formulate social policy (2000, pp. 584–5). It shifts attention from an individual's mental impairment to the social processes of oppression, discrimination, and exclusion that restrict the life opportunities, including access to treatment, of those suffering from an impairment, and focuses on the rights of people with disabilities. In Australia, State and Territory governments have amended their mental health legislation to conform with the United Nations Resolution on the Protection of Persons with Mental Illness and the Improvement of Mental Health Care. The associated Mental Health Statement of Rights and Responsibilities formalises the rights of people with mental illness problems and mental disorders, specifies the rights and responsibilities of the consumer of mental health services as well as those of carers, advocates, service providers, and the community (DHSH 1995). Despite this new discourse around the rights of people with mental illness and the establishment of legal remedies, factors other than discrimination—especially individuals' or advocates' assessment of the personal, social, or financial costs involved in initiating an official complaint—will help to determine whether any legal procedures are activated (Bumiller 1987).

The national mental health strategy does not necessarily refute the underlying medical model of mental illness and includes more types of deviance (for example, child abuse and neglect, behavioural problems, especially among children and young people, health-compromising behaviours, including homelessness and substance abuse, and suicide prevention) (DHAC 1998, pp. 127–34). Community mental health centres retain the medical model by emphasising individual intervention, and they deal with a range of contemporary issues including alcoholism, drug addiction, children's behavioural problems, pre-delinquency, marriage conflicts, job losses, and ageing, as well as the more traditional mental health problems (Roach Anleu 1999, p. 220). The policy also recognises that 'a small number of people, whose disorder is severe, unremitting and disabling, will continue to require care in separate inpatient psychiatric facilities' (Australian Health Ministers 1995, p. 3).

The scope of psychiatric influence

As a profession, psychiatry has never been completely successful: as its authority stems in large part from its institutional base within mental hospitals, governmental policy directly affects psychiatrists' access to patients and resources. Moreover, psychiatrists' ability to identify, diagnose, and treat mental illness is contested by other disciplines that are concerned with human relations or personal problems, such as psychology, social work, and counselling, as well as by other medical specialties and kinds of knowledge. Its claims to provide precise and exact explanations are questioned, and its ability to demonstrate aetiology is difficult, making psychiatry particularly vulnerable to the criticism that its knowledge base is socially constructed and historical. Indeed, psychiatry continues to be one of the most contested areas of medicine. Discussion about the causes of mental illness—genetic, physiological, psychological, and social—is far from conclusive, and psychiatrists' ability to predict the potential for mental illness in patients is highly questionable (Cocozza & Steadman 1978, p. 265). Arguably, then, psychiatry's jurisdiction over certain conditions and patients stems from its own self-interested quest to achieve and maintain professional status. The failure to provide an uncontested scientific rationale for mental illness has led psychiatry to develop a greater interest in prevention, thereby widening its potential for intervention (Abbott 1988, pp. 296–8). Current research—as part of the human genome project to map the genes that (allegedly) determine mental illness, alcoholism, Alzheimer's Disease, and even depression—will renew psychiatrists' claims that they offer scientific explanations, diagnoses, and treatments that are not socially constructed (see chapter 11). Nonetheless, psychiatry remains a dominant and institutionally recognised profession, with psychiatric treatment being covered by national health schemes (for example, Medicare), unlike the services of other human relations personnel.

Psychiatry is not the only medical specialty or type of medical knowledge engaged in designating and normalising deviance. Other segments of medicine (as well as other social movements, occupational groups, and individuals) are involved in normative work—that is, identifying problematic behaviour and proposing medical, including psychiatric, intervention to achieve normality. In other words, psychiatry may dominate current discourses and approaches to problems or issues, even though psychiatrists do not. For example, Alcoholics Anonymous (AA) is a hybrid organisation that combines elements of the disease model of alcoholism with a spiritual program emphasising individual change and recovery and the achievement of inner peace (Valverde & White-Mair 1999). Another example, the National Alliance for the Mentally Ill (NAMI), one of the most influential mental health organisations in the USA, grew from the concern that the families of the mentally ill had insufficient input into the management of their afflicted relatives. NAMI adopts the medical model, viewing schizophrenia and manic depression as diseases caused by chemical imbalances in the brain. This organisation focuses on the mental patient's inability to hold and exercise rights, and criticises the legal extension of rights to individuals involuntarily committed to mental institutions. It maintains that psychotherapeutic approaches—which may view family dynamics, rather than a chemical imbalance, as responsible for the disease—stigmatise care-givers, and that the patient's legal right to refuse medication establishes an inappropriate adversarial relationship between patients and their families (Milner 1989, pp. 653–5).

Other research shows that family members have been particularly influential in the construction of hyperactivity in children as evidence of a psychiatric disorder, namely Attention Deficit (Hyperactivity) Disorder (AD[H]D) (Lloyd & Norris 1999, pp. 505–8). In Britain, as elsewhere, active parents' organisations articulated their 'rights' and the right of their children to be classified as having a medically defined disorder requiring prescribed medication, thus rejecting a more social model of the deviantisation of certain childhood behaviours. Parents' claims for medicalisation have been met by resistance and disagreement from segments of the medical profession.

Additionally, some women have been active participants in the construction of premenstrual syndrome (PMS) as a disorder, and seek its inclusion in the American Psychiatric Association's *Diagnostic and Statistical Manual of Mental Disorders* (*DSM*). It is significant that the original term was 'premenstrual tension'; the use of the term 'syndrome' indicates increased medicalisation. *DSM-IV*—the most recent edition, published in 1994—proposes premenstrual dysphoric disorder (PDD) as an official category for possible inclusion in later editions following further research. The discussion of PDD in the appendix of *DSM-IV* refers to criteria for research on the disorder rather than diagnostic criteria. It identifies symptoms such as markedly depressed mood, feelings of hopelessness or self-deprecating thoughts, marked anxiety, affective lability interspersed with frequent tearfulness, and decreased interest in usual activities as the essential features of the disorder (American Psychiatric Association 1994, pp. 703, 715–18). *DSM-IV* distinguishes PMS (which it specifies as far more common) from PDD in terms of the symptoms' severity and distinctiveness, and resulting impairment. It notes that 'the transient mood changes that many females experience around the time of their period should not be considered a mental disorder' (American Psychiatric Association 1994, p. 716).

Both medical and everyday literatures tend to emphasise the negative, debilitating symptoms of PMS. An analysis of popular magazines and self-help books shows that PMS is portrayed in a generally negative tone, which effectively defines how a normal woman should feel or behave in contrast to an 'abnormal' woman who experiences PMS. Popular discourse identifies the causes as physiological and focuses on women's hormones as the source of the problems. Intervention and alleviation of the symptoms identified—ranging from dizziness, backache, and lack of concentration to decreased school or work performance, mood swings, and irritability—include drug therapy and management of individual lifestyles, through diet, exercise, and rest, rather than considering the relevance of social, structural, or cultural factors (Markens 1996, pp. 46–8; Martin 1987, pp. 113–14).

The medicalisation of PMS presents a dilemma for women: on the one hand, it legitimises the experiences of premenstrual symptoms as real and worthy of medical and public attention, but on the other, it reasserts the pathology of women's bodies, especially their reproductive systems, and views women's actions and thoughts as being determined by biology (in this case, their hormones). Opponents worry that medicalisation could lead to stigmatisation and result in sex discrimination. This is an example of a situation in which some medicalisation—but not necessarily psychiatrisation— may be helpful in order to have complaints taken seriously by medical practitioners, and for strategies to be adopted for the alleviation or management of symptoms. Research on chronic fatigue syndrome finds that diagnosis—that is, medicalising a condition during consultation—can enable patients to explain their symptoms and to feel more in control of their situations; they are not dismissed as having imagined their symptoms or as malingerers. On the other hand, medicalisation that reflects **medical dominance** and preconceived notions about gender-specific behaviour—for

medical dominance A general term used to describe the power of the medical profession in terms of its control over its own work, over the work of other health workers, and over health resource allocation, health policy, and the way that hospitals are run.

example, that women are naturally emotional, hysterical, or prone to depression or hypochondria—is unhelpful (Broom & Woodward 1996, pp. 370–3).

Gender and mental illness

gender/sex This term refers to the socially constructed categories of feminine and masculine (the cultural values that dictate how men and women should behave), as opposed to the categories of biological sex (female or male).

Current debates about the utility of psychiatric categories to explain women's behaviour—especially that which deviates from **gender** norms—have historical parallels. In the nineteenth century, dominant medical theories linked a woman's uterus and ovaries to irrationality, emotional disorder, and mental disease. Indeed, the term 'hysteria' derives from the Greek word for uterus and refers to what was regarded as a quintessential female condition, indicated by weeping, fainting, screaming, tantrums, and moodiness (Turner 1987, p. 89). A scientific explanation of the 'disease' was that it was localised in the nervous system, but its diagnosis reflected expectations and attitudes regarding appropriate female behaviour and demeanour. Attributes thought to be natural and normal for women—affection, emotion, nurturance, preference for the domestic sphere, and moral sensibility—were also viewed as precursors of mental instability. Hysteria was linked to cultural definitions of femininity via its range of physical and emotional symptoms, including sobbing, fainting, fits, laughter, and general malaise (Seale & Pattison 1994, pp. 86–8). The diagnosis of hysteria became a general label for 'abnormal' or nonconforming behaviour on the part of women, and medical intervention became a form of social control.

Medical practitioners were impressed by the preponderance of women in the nervous population, while at least some attributed male nervousness to misdiagnosis (Abbott 1988, pp. 290–1). Theories to explain women's mental illnesses were sex-specific, as were treatments. Gynaecologists (not psychiatrists) performed surgery, including removal of women's sexual and reproductive organs, to alleviate mental illness (Scull & Favreau 1986, pp. 7–18). Such intervention fell into disrepute with the rise of endocrinology and its attention to hormones, and because of its failure to link nervous disease among men to male reproductive organs (Abbott 1988, pp. 291–2; Scull & Favreau 1986, p. 27). Currently, the diagnosis of hysteria is very rare (it is not included in the *DSM*), and it refers to an entirely psychological condition with no specific physical correlates. In addition to reflecting changes in medical knowledge, the decline of hysteria as a flexible diagnostic category indicates changes in gender norms and the activism of women in resisting medicalisation (Seale & Pattison 1994, pp. 78, 93). Nevertheless, the 'hysterical woman' stereotype remains pervasive, and behaviour that, in the past, may have resulted in a diagnosis of hysteria may today be diagnosed as schizophrenia, as a personality disorder, or as PMS.

In professional medical, psychiatric, and psychological journal articles on homosexuality between 1900 and 1950, most of the early discussion of homosexuality among women argued that lesbianism led to masturbation, nymphomania, feeling superior to men, or being a suffragist, thereby contravening both sexual and gender norms. Later, the dominant medical concern was to develop tests and scales to enable classification and 'diagnosis' of homosexuality (Martin 1993, p. 248). Nevertheless, female homosexuality, unlike male homosexuality, has never been the subject of vast medical and psychiatric attention, and has not evoked the same public reaction.

Through history, male homosexuality has been defined as a sin, as a crime, and during most of the twentieth century, as a medical or psychiatric condition. Some of the medical interventions for homosexuality have included hormone therapy, drugs, 'therapeutic' castration, and aversive conditioning using electric shock, while Freudian approaches have emphasised psychoanalysis. The first edition of *DSM* in 1952 included the diagnostic label 'homosexuality' as one of several types of 'sexual deviation' within the more general classification of 'sociopathic personality disturbance' (Conrad & Schneider 1992, pp. 187–93). During the 1970s the gay liberation movement, which was oriented to the rights of gay men, was successful, along with key psychiatrists, in having the category of homosexuality removed from the *DSM*. Despite changing official definitions, there remain people who view homosexuality as sinful, and some laws criminalise same-sex conduct between consenting adults.

Sex differences in the identification of mental illness still persist. Women are more likely than men to consult with a doctor about a mental disorder. They are also more likely than men to report experiencing emotional problems, nerves, and depression, whereas men are slightly more likely to experience psychoses and other mental disorders (Australian Bureau of Statistics 1997, table 14). Such differences may result from the greater likelihood that women will report illness: it is more culturally acceptable for women to be ill and more appropriate for them to express their psychological problems and symptoms, whereas men (or at least those conforming to some forms of masculinity) are more reluctant to admit certain unpleasant feelings and sensations (Phillips & Segal 1969, pp. 69–71). Alternatively, women may actually experience more mental illness than men as a result of their social status (rather than their biology); the stresses and tensions that many women experience in the context of their families and workplaces, and the connections between these areas of their lives, may lead to depression, neurosis, and other mental health problems

epidemiology/

social epidemiology The statistical study of patterns of disease
in the population. Originally
focused on epidemics, or infectious diseases, it now covers
non-infectious conditions such as
stroke and cancer. Social epidemiology is a sub-field aligned
with sociology that focuses on
the social determinants of illness.

(Busfield 1989, pp. 344–6). Some **epidemiological** surveys indicate that depressive and some anxiety disorders are more frequent
among women, while antisocial personalities, and alcohol and
drug abuse or dependence are more common among men
(Aneshensel et al. 1991, pp. 171–2). Some mental illnesses may not
be independent of gender, as they relate to perceptions of 'normal'
male and female behaviour (Busfield 1988, p. 534). Women's deviation from criminal laws has also been interpreted in terms of
mental instability or illness, rather than as a result of rational action,
or environmental or social structural forces. For example, klepto-
mania became an explanation for shop-stealing, with the 'normal'
kleptomaniac being female (Smart 1976, pp. 109–11).

Psychiatry and law

Psychiatry has greater input into the criminal justice system when
the criminal law and sentencing policy move away from emphasising punishment for past illegal activities and towards examining
the causes of the behaviour, the offender's motivations, and ways
of preventing future criminal activity. Violators of the criminal law
may be defined as requiring treatment or rehabilitation, which
implies that they are sick, that they are not entirely responsible for
their actions, and that they require psychiatric intervention. This
type of definition is especially common in the area of juvenile
delinquency, where there is a particular concern to prevent subsequent offending and the perceived risk of developing criminal
careers (Abbott 1988, pp. 297–8).

In Western legal systems the central example of psychiatry's
legal role is the 'insanity defence' for murder, formulated in the
nineteenth century and still used, albeit rarely, in contemporary
criminal trials. To establish a defence on the ground of insanity,
the legal test requires that 'it must be clearly proved that, at the
time of the committing of the act, the party accused was labour-
ing under such a defect of reason, from disease of the mind, as not
to know the nature and quality of the act he [sic] was doing; or,
if he did know it, that he did not know he was doing what was
wrong' (as quoted in Waller & Williams 1993, p. 762).

With the defence of insanity, the court relies on psychiatric
opinion to determine whether or not the accused person was
insane at the time of the alleged offence. The psychiatrist does not
assess whether or not the defendant's actions violated the law;
indeed, if the defence succeeds, that issue disappears altogether:
the defendant is acquitted of murder and is usually hospitalised for
a period of time. As Foucault notes, 'the gravity of the act was not
altered by the fact that its author was insane, nor the punishment
reduced as a consequence; the crime itself disappeared. It was

impossible, therefore, to declare that someone was both guilty and mad' (1978, pp. 17–18). Evaluation of cases is not on the legal status of the alleged offences but on the defendants' personalities, and on the nature or level of danger (as determined by psychiatrists) that they pose to society at large or to themselves. Attention shifts from the criminal offences to an individual's criminality, as assessed by non-legal personnel—a shift that alters the nature of the social control. Again, Foucault writes, 'The purpose of the sanction will therefore not be to punish a legal subject who has voluntarily broken the law; its role will be to reduce as much as possible—either by elimination, or by exclusion or by various restrictions, or by therapeutic measures—the risk of criminality represented by the individual in question' (1978, p. 16).

The therapeutic approach to crime and its control reached its zenith during the 1950s. Various personality tests were developed to identify the differences of emotionality, temperament, and character between criminals and non-criminals, and as a basis for early intervention to prevent criminal behaviour. However, the inaccuracy of such tests, their inability to directly link personality with criminality, and the fact that they were usually performed on prison populations undermined their validity (Schuessler & Cressey 1950, pp. 483–4).

Some penalties within the criminal justice system, particularly parole and probation, adopted a clinical or therapeutic approach to crime management during the 1950s—an approach that dominated until the late 1970s. While psychiatrists developed theory, undertook research, and provided expert testimony to the sentencing court, the role of probation or parole officers (often, but not necessarily, trained in social work, with an emphasis on casework) is to counsel their clients and help them to adjust to the demands of everyday life. Psychiatrists viewed many people who were convicted of crime as experiencing 'adjustment' problems, and the ongoing relationship with the probation or parole officer was believed to have therapeutic effects (Simon 1993, pp. 72–84). Central to this approach was a system of indeterminate sentencing: the court would establish a maximum sentence, but the actual release date was determined by a parole board when the prisoner showed signs of some rehabilitation. This rehabilitative model of corrections fell into disrepute because of its failure to reduce either recidivism or crime levels. It also produced sentencing disparity, because sentences were not entirely based on the offence committed; they were also based on the kind of offender and on assessments of his or her rehabilitation needs.

Increasing reliance on medical conditions or syndromes in defending criminal charges expands the scope for psychiatrists and other human relations professionals to provide expert evidence to the courts. Current examples include the battered woman syndrome and premenstrual syndrome, both of which have been used as defences to homicide charges. A clinical psychologist, Lenore Walker, developed the conceptualisation of the battered woman syndrome, according to which a woman who has suffered repeated violence experiences a psychological condition in which she believes that the only way to change her situation is to kill her batterer (Sheehy et al. 1992, pp. 370–80). The courts' acceptance of this argument places women's criminal deviance in a psychological or medical paradigm: psychological disturbance prevented the woman from thinking and acting rationally (that is, from not killing her abuser), which resulted in her crime.

Another aspect of the criminal justice process into which psychiatry may have further input involves serious crimes and dangerous offenders, which may prompt governments to legislate for protective sentences. Sentencing for 'dangerous' offenders is, in part, based on the probability or risk of a dangerous act being committed in the future, and it is on this probability that psychiatrists provide evidence. Perceptions of dangerousness are often conflated with the seriousness of the offence committed and the perceived need for protection of the public. In England and Wales, the *Criminal Justice Act 1991* makes a form of protective sentence possible and allows for psychiatrists to identify whether or not a person is dangerous (Nash 1992, pp. 337–40). In Australia, a very controversial example of preventative detention legislation is the Victorian government's *Community Protection Act 1990*, which was passed specifically to enable the detention of Gary David, who was deemed to be dangerous to both himself and others. This law sparked controversy because—by targeting a single person—it undermined the 'rule of law' principle, which requires that laws be applied universally, and because it contradicted the traditional legal view of punishment as essentially retributive (that is, as a penalty for past criminal offences). Moreover, psychiatric evidence suggested that David was not mentally ill but, rather, had a personality disorder (Waller & Williams 1993, pp. 793–9). Predictions of dangerousness can be extremely unreliable; definitions of what or who is dangerous are imprecise and make assumptions about the future that can be impossible to verify. This development exemplifies the movement towards prevention and risk-analysis in criminal justice policy (Castel 1991, p. 288). Even so, the structure of psychiatric influence is not unidirectional, and its jurisdiction is not always increasing.

Future directions: towards demedicalisation?

Just as segments of the medical profession gain exclusive or partial jurisdiction over managing certain behaviour or individuals whom they define as pathological and sick, they also lose jurisdiction.

The term 'demedicalisation', the reverse of medicalisation, denotes that an issue is no longer defined in medical terms and that medical intervention is no longer thought to be appropriate. Demedicalisation does not necessarily indicate that the behaviour in question ceases to be subject to normative evaluation and social control. An example is homosexuality, which arguably has been demedicalised. In 1973, as a result of social activism and the work of individual psychiatrists, the American Psychiatric Association agreed that homosexuality was not an illness and voted to exclude it from the *DSM* (Conrad & Schneider 1992, pp. 206–9). This change did not mean that gay men were no longer subject to discrimination or were no longer viewed as 'deviant'. The alacrity with which many people have associated gay men and AIDS in Western societies attests to their lack of integration and acceptance. Because of the increasing prevalence of the human immunodeficiency virus (HIV), gay men (as well as intravenous drug users, prostitutes, and others) are subject to increasing medical scrutiny, albeit in a different form.

risk factors Conditions that are thought to increase an individual's susceptibility to illness or disease such as abuse of alcohol or smoking.

The rise of epidemiology has been central in identifying **risk factors** for a range of illnesses, which in turn has resulted in greater public concern and surveillance in relation to various activities, behaviours, and lifestyles (Petersen 1996, pp. 49–51). Epidemiological knowledge about the incidence and distribution of disease in a population has been central to the identification of the AIDS epidemic with gay men, and in coupling sexual behaviour with sexual identity (Waldby et al. 1995, p. 7). Epidemiology identifies particular correlates with the concentration of diseases in sub-populations in order to provide a basis for clinical and public health intervention and prevention. This area of knowledge and practice makes an important contribution to the health-promotion task of identifying, reducing exposure to, and eliminating 'risk'. In general, the risk-analysis used in recent national health-services provision and health-promotion activities identifies a large range of preventable conditions in relation to various sub-populations, as defined by age, gender, socioeconomic status, occupation, geographic region, Aboriginality, and ethnicity, as well as by lifestyle and sexual practices. Thus, as well as incorporating structural factors, epidemiological research increasingly identifies a range of risk factors that are subject to individual choice: tobacco and alcohol use, sexual practices, exercise, and diet.

The identification of risk factors raises questions of responsibility: individuals who choose to engage in behaviour correlated with disease are, to some extent, responsible for the outcomes of that behaviour. Conversely, individuals are under some social or moral obligation to reduce their chances of contracting particular illnesses, including heart disease, lung cancer, and AIDS; they should minimise their exposure to hazards such as alcohol, tobacco, bad eating habits, and 'unsafe' sexual practices (Castel 1991, p. 289; Petersen 1996, pp. 50–1). Along with helping to track risk populations, epidemiological knowledge provides a base for educating all populations; having received this education, the onus falls on the individual to prevent health risks. Moreover, the proliferation of risk populations effectively narrows the definition of who or what is considered to be normal. For example, one Australian government report lists bisexual and homosexual men, women, needle-sharing drug users, Aboriginal people, prostitutes, and recipients of blood transfusions as specific targets for AIDS-prevention and education programs. Effectively, the only sub-population not included is that of healthy, law–abiding, heterosexual, White men (Roach Anleu 1999, p. 79).

Epidemiological studies of AIDS usually associate the trans-mission of HIV with risk groups, exposure categories, or people defined as engaging in risk behaviour. It is assumed that some sex-ual practices and types of relationships are the exclusive domain of homosexuality, thereby rendering gay men a risk group. This implicitly affirms an ideology of heterosexual marriage as the location of 'normal' sexual relationships with a low risk, or no risk, of HIV transmission. From this frame of reference, it is assumed that anal intercourse and promiscuity are prevalent among homosexual relationships but rare within marriage (Waldby et al. 1995, pp. 5–8, 10–11).

Medical intervention and surveillance aimed at preventing the spread of AIDS do not necessarily confer the sick role. Often the language of law, rather than medicine, is invoked: gay men are viewed as responsible for and therefore 'guilty' of HIV trans-mission; some view the contraction of AIDS as just deserts for engaging in risk behaviour or for deviating from moral precepts. As Josh Gamson observes, 'promiscuity is medically unsafe while monogamy is safe; being a member of certain social groups is dan-gerous to one's health while being a member of the "general population" is dangerous only when the un-general contaminate it' (1989, p.359). Fear of AIDS easily translates into fear of homo-sexuals and homosexuality. This contrasts with the sympathy frequently evoked for those who are viewed as innocent victims of AIDS, albeit victims who are still subject to stigmatisation: chil-dren who contract the virus *in utero*, hospital or sanitation workers who become infected after a needle-stick injury, and blood-trans-fusion recipients, for example. The public discourse surrounding AIDS is intertwined with moral evaluation, which can be shrouded by medical statements that are presented as scientific facts. Biomedical knowledge can be used to legitimate discrimi-natory practices, such as requiring some categories of people to undergo HIV testing before providing or denying medical insurance, or determining the premium. One study of gay men's motivations for taking or not taking the HIV antibody test found that those who avoided taking the test feared social discrimination, repressive governmental actions, and the adverse psychological effect of a positive result. On the other side, those taking the test indicated the importance of monitoring their health status and planning medical intervention (Siegel et al. 1989, p. 381).

Conclusion

This chapter demonstrates how, over the past century, psychiatry has been engaged in the regulation of deviance. Psychiatrists seek to locate the source of deviation—from moral or sexual norms, or from legal norms, for example—within the individual. According to the therapeutic model, the deviant individual suffers from a syndrome, illness, or personality disorder, or experiences 'adjustment' problems, thus requiring psychiatric intervention. There is little attention to social factors, cultural differences, or disagreements about what constitutes deviance and normality. The influence of psychiatry is diffuse: the therapeutic model has been applied to manage or regulate such heterogenous activities, behaviours, and conditions as gambling, sexuality, drug and alcohol use, criminal offending (especially with young and female offenders, and those convicted of serious and violent crimes), mental disorders, premenstrual tension, and child development.

Despite its power and influence, psychiatry has never achieved complete jurisdiction over certain patients, conditions, or resources. This is one medical specialty that has been particularly dependent on government practices and mental health policies, which currently emphasise deinstitutionalisation. Psychiatry's authority has historically been derived from its central role as a gatekeeper for publicly funded mental hospitals, which are currently being closed or reduced in size. The movement towards community-based mental health facilities also highlights the competition that psychiatrists are facing from other human-services personnel, who themselves may adopt a medical model of deviance. The role and influence of psychiatry in the criminal justice system is also changing: there is widespread discontent with the therapeutic and rehabilitative approach to corrections, and renewed emphasis on punishment of offences rather than the treatment of offenders. Nonetheless, the criminal law remains interested in the defendant's motivations or intentions in committing the alleged crime. It often seeks expert evidence from psychiatrists to provide information on various syndromes that might support a related defence.

Summary of main points

- The medicalisation of deviance is a historical and social process, and the outcome of professional and social-movement activity.
- Deviance can be defined as behaviour or activities that violate social expectations about what is normal.
- The term 'social control' refers to the mechanisms that aim to induce conformity, or at least to manage or minimise deviant behaviour and to reaffirm norms.
- Medicalisation is the process whereby non-medical problems or phenomena become defined and treated as illnesses, disorders, syndromes, or problems of adjustment.
- Successful medicalisation means that 'therapy' becomes the dominant form of social control and that individuals diagnosed as deviating from a model of health must confront normative expectations stemming from the sick role.
- Medicalisation can occur on at least three levels: the conceptual, the institutional, and the interactional.
- Psychiatry has always been involved in the identification and regulation of deviance.
- The late eighteenth century was the beginning of the critical period for the emergence and dominance of a medical approach to madness, which was redefined as mental illness.
- Historically, women's reproductive organs were assumed to cause women's mental illness.
- Psychiatrists' involvement in the criminal justice system includes providing expert testimony regarding defences to criminal charges.
- Demedicalisation, the reverse of medicalisation, is the process whereby an issue is no longer defined in medical terms and medical intervention is no longer thought to be appropriate.
- The rise of epidemiology has been central to identifying 'risk' factors for a range of illnesses, including mental illnesses.

Discussion questions

1   What is the role of psychiatry in the medicalisation of deviance?
2   What are the implications of deinstitutionalisation for the professional status and autonomy of psychiatry?
3   Outline the relationship between law and psychiatry as institutions of social control.
4   Has deinstitutionalisation brought about the demedicalisation of various problems? Explain.
5   Discuss the existence of gender differences in relation to mental illness and deviance.
6   Critically assess the assumptions and directions of the National Mental Health Strategy in Australia.

Further investigation

1 Critically analyse the proposition that psychiatry is one of the most powerful institutions of social control in contemporary societies.

2 Discuss the relationship between a number of social problems— for example, crime, juvenile delinquency, homelessness, drug use, poverty—and mental health. To what extent do policy makers and others view social problems as caused by mental illness or individual deficiency?

3 The decline of the welfare state runs parallel with an increasing emphasis on the individual to take responsibility for their own well-being. What role, if any, does psychiatry play in contemporary cultures that increasingly emphasise the individual?

Further reading

Abbott, A. 1988, *The System of Professions: An Essay on the Division of Expert Labor*, University of Chicago Press, Chicago, ch. 10.

Busfield, J. (ed.) 2000, *Sociology of Health & Illness: Special Issue, Rethinking the Sociology of Mental Health*, vol. 22, pp. 543–719.

Conrad, P. 1992, 'Medicalization and Social Control', *Annual Review of Sociology*, vol. 18, pp. 209–32.

Conrad, P. & Schneider, J. 1992, *Deviance and Medicalization: From Badness to Sickness*, 2nd edn, Temple University Press, Philadelphia.

Department of Health and Aged Care 1998, *National Mental Health Report 1997*, AGPS, Canberra.

Foucault, M. 1978, 'About the Concept of the "Dangerous Individual" in 19th Century Legal Psychiatry', trans. A. Baudot & J. Couchman, *International Journal of Law and Psychiatry*, vol. 1, pp. 1–18.

—— 1988, *Madness and Civilization: A History of Insanity in the Age of Reason*, trans. R. Howard, Vintage Books, New York.

Roach Anleu, S. L. 1999, *Deviance, Conformity and Control*, 3rd edn, Longman, Melbourne.

Sutton, J. R. 1991, 'The Political Economy of Madness: The Expansion of the Asylum in Progressive America', *American Sociological Review*, vol. 56, pp. 665–78.

Waldby, C., Kippax, S., & Crawford, J. 1995, 'Epidemiological Knowledge and Discriminatory Practice: AIDS and the Social Relations of Biomedicine', *Australian and New Zealand Journal of Sociology*, vol. 31, pp. 1–14.

9

The Body, Medicine, and Society

Deborah Lupton

Overview

* *Why is more attention paid to women's bodies than to men's bodies?*
* *How does medicine's power to define the body affect treatment?*
* *How has medicine contributed to reproducing unequal social bodies?*

This chapter discusses ways of viewing the human body as a sociocultural, rather than as simply a biological, phenomenon. The chapter draws upon contemporary sociological, anthropological, and historical research as well as theoretical perspectives to explore how medicine and public health define and reproduce understandings, beliefs, and experiences in relation to embodiment. There is an emphasis on the dynamic nature of concepts and experiences of the body, including changes through history, and differences between social and cultural contexts. The chapter also discusses how medical and public health knowledges and practices have reproduced—and in some cases contributed to—the drawing of distinctions between social groups.

Key terms

agency
clinical gaze
commodity culture
discourse
embodiment
men's health
norms
public health

Introduction

The human body is generally understood to be, above all, a biological and 'natural' phenomenon, and this is the view of the body that predominates in medicine and the allied health sciences. From this perspective, there is little that could be regarded as 'social' or 'cultural' about the human body, except perhaps such superficial aspects as the type of clothing that is worn, hairstyles, and body shapes. However, sociologists of the body regard the human body as a sociocultural construction; that is, the ways in which we understand and experience the body are mediated through social, cultural, and political processes. Certain aspects of the human body are, of course, given and immutable—for example, all humans are born and must die, and all humans experience pain and illness. However, the beliefs, understandings, and experiences of different groups in relation to phenomena such as birth, death, pain, and illness vary, in some cases dramatically. Sociologists argue that, in many cases, the reasons for these differences are not simply anatomical but are also social and cultural. Central to understanding the sociological approach to the body is the notion that we both *are* and *have* a body. One's body, therefore, is central to one's self identity; it is the thing or container in which we present ourselves to others, and through which we experience the world.

Social theorists who are interested in the body and medicine deny that medical knowledge, or indeed any other type of knowledge, can be regarded as neutral, scientific, or politically disinterested (see, for example, Foucault 1975; Armstrong 1983; Turner 1992; Turner & Samson 1995). Rather, like the body or any other phenomenon, medicine is socially constructed, is mediated through social understandings, and has political effects. For instance, while we may think that the version of the human body presented in a medical textbook is 'scientific truth' and therefore politically neutral, closer examination reveals conventions of representation that support wider sociocultural and political assumptions and objectives. The body in such textbooks is nearly always that of a young White male, suggesting that this type of body is the 'real' or 'normal' human body, against which other bodies (those of women, people of non-White ethnicity, or the elderly) are considered 'abnormal'.

For conceptual purposes, the anthropologists N. Scheper-Hughes and M. Lock (1987) have defined 'three bodies' at three levels of sociocultural analysis. The first is the *individual body*, or the lived experience of the body as an everyday reality for the individual. Sociologists and other social scientists who are interested in how people understand and experience aspects of **embodiment**, including health and illness states, focus their

embodiment The lived experience of both being a body and having a body.

public health/public health infrastructure Public policies and infrastructure to prevent the onset and transmission of disease among the population, with a particular focus on sanitation and hygiene, such as clean air, water, and food, and immunisation. Public health infrastructure refers specifically to the buildings, installations, and equipment necessary to ensure healthy living conditions for communities and populations.

attention on this conceptual body. The second is the *social body*, or the representational use of the body as a symbol to stand metaphorically for other phenomena and vice versa. This notion has been taken up particularly by anthropologists, who are interested in the ways that cultural groups conceptualise features of human bodies as signifying wider meanings for society, and how in turn metaphors derived from the body are used to describe society. An example is the way that the idea of cancer is used to represent a serious social problem, such as in the statement 'crime is a cancer within society'. The third conceptual body is that of the *body politic*, which refers to the social regulation, surveillance, and control of groups or populations of bodies. This concept has been useful for sociologists interested in exploring the ways in which medicine and **public health** have attempted to regulate and control social groups. While all three levels of conceptualising the body are important and useful, this chapter focuses in particular on the lived experience of the individual body and the ways that medical knowledge and practices serve to define and distinguish between social groups.

Lay beliefs about health and the body

One way that sociologists have explored individuals' understandings and experiences of their bodies is to elicit their beliefs about the causes of health and illness states. Several studies have pointed to the importance of lay health beliefs in people's understandings of the body (see, for instance, Blaxter & Paterson 1982; Crawford 1984; Herzlich & Pierret 1987; Radley 1993; Williams 1990). In these studies it is noted that lay people often adhere to concepts of health, illness, disease, and the body that may differ dramatically from the orthodox medical position. Recent research involving interviews with older African–American women living in a southern State of the USA, for example, revealed a common belief that a blow to the breast could cause a 'bruise' or a 'knot' that could result in breast cancer. As a result of this belief, some of the women thought that a mammogram could predispose them to developing breast cancer because they found the procedure painful (Wardlow & Curry 1996).

Embodiment is a central theme of both the illness experience and the medical encounter. When illness occurs, aspects of the body that were previously taken for granted and never noticed as part of everyday bodily functioning are brought into sharp relief. As the medical anthropologist Byron Good notes, for the person who is experiencing illness or pain, 'the body is not simply a physical object of physiological state but an essential part of the self. The body is subject, the very grounds of subjectivity or experience in the world, and the body as "physical object" cannot be neatly distinguished from "states of consciousness" '(1994, p. 116).

Illness is, above all, an embodied experience, bringing us down to earth by reminding us that we are neither invulnerable nor immortal. For those people who experience chronic illness or disability, permanent changes to the body may be constant reminders of their status as 'outsiders', as people whose bodies may look different from what is considered to be the **norm**, or as people who are not capable of the range of bodily movements expected of 'healthy' or 'normal' people. These experiences may also serve to make them feel as if they are separate from their body. Disease or pain are often described as 'it'—as something that is not the self, that is uncontrollable and has its own **agency** and sense of purpose, and that is foreign from the self and destructive of one's body. An example is the vivid description that a young man gives of the chronic pain he experiences: 'Sometimes, if I had to visualise it, it would seem as though … there's a … demon, a monster, something very horrible lurking around banging the insides of my body, ripping it apart' (quoted in Good 1994, p. 121). He also describes his experience of pain and illness in terms of alienation from his own body: 'I'm outside myself, this whole I've got to deal with is ah, a decayed mass of tissue that's just not any good … I don't feel integrated. I don't feel like a whole person' (quoted in Good 1994, p. 125).

Sociologists and anthropologists have pointed out that the meanings of embodiment are dynamic. There are manifold bodily experiences that appear to be acknowledged and found in some social groups but not in others. The phenomenon of menopause, for example, is experienced and dealt with differently in Western cultures compared with Japan. The Western notion of menopause includes not only the permanent cessation of menstruation in older women but also a constellation of symptoms such as depression and hot flushes, which are believed sometimes to require medical advice and treatment. However, there is no consonant Japanese concept of menopause. While it is acknowledged that menstruation inevitably ceases in older women, most women tend not to report experiencing symptoms associated with this event, and there is no word for menopause. In Japan, middle-aged women are viewed as entering their prime as 'good wives and mothers'. The identification of menopausal symptoms has been a postwar phenomenon in Japan, and menopausal problems are still largely viewed as a 'luxury', largely confined to particular types of women, especially those who are middle-class and urban (see Lock 1993). As this suggests, social expectations about the causes of health and illness are associated with people's experiences of their bodies.

norms Expectations about how people ought to act or behave.

agency The ability of people, individually and collectively, to influence their own lives and the society in which they live.

Even within the same cultural context, notions of the body, health, and disease have shifted and changed over time. In Western societies, for example, a number of conditions or diseases such as chlorosis and hysteria, which were once regularly diagnosed, no longer exist as diagnostic categories, and there are now categories of disease, such as chronic fatigue syndrome, that have only been identified and named in the past few decades. The medical historians Roy and Dorothy Porter (1988) provide a fascinating account of the ways in which people living in Great Britain in the two centuries between 1650 and 1850 conceptualised embodiment in the context of health and illness. They note that, in this era, illness was ever-present; indeed, it was far more unusual to experience prolonged periods of feeling well. There was, therefore, a preoccupation with preventative health, but this was understood somewhat differently from today. For instance, many people believed that, to 'fuel' the body (note the mechanical metaphor to describe embodiment) and to 'replenish the blood', the individual needed to eat rich and strong foods, including meat and wine. As the Porters note, 'the Englishman's devotion to roast beef was not mere patriotic gloating, gluttony or fantasizing, but, according to the folklore of good health, positively therapeutic' (1988, p. 48). There is a marked contrast with contemporary health advice on diet, in which rich, fatty foods and over-consumption of alcohol are almost demonised as 'bad for health'.

The medical encounter, power, and the illness experience

In exploring the relationship between medicine, knowledge, power, and the body, several sociologists of health and illness have taken up the work of Michel Foucault (1926–84), a French historian and philosopher, who wrote about the discourses and practices related to the body in scientific medicine as it developed in Europe from the eighteenth century onwards (see, for example, Armstrong 1983; Lupton 1994; Turner 1992; Turner 1995). Foucault argued that medical knowledge had a major role in constructing notions of the body. In early modern Europe it was considered a sacrilege to cut into dead bodies. The desire to look inside the body in the pursuit of medical knowledge, however, impelled anatomists to dissect dead bodies in order to understand their innermost workings. As a result of this new knowledge about the inside of the body, notions of the body began to change.

According to Foucault in his book *The Birth of the Clinic* (1975), an important shift in the medical approach to the body emerged at the end of the eighteenth century, when the clinical examination began to be important for diagnosis and treatment. Previously, doctors often diagnosed illnesses by relying on patients' own accounts of their symptoms, and did not necessarily undertake a physical examination of their bodies. The clinical examination, however, involved the doctor's close attention to various parts of the patient's body and the documentation of what was observed as a guide to diagnosis: 'the core task of medicine became not the elucidation of what the patient said but what the doctor saw in the depths of the body' (Armstrong 1984, p. 738).

clinical gaze A term originally used by Michel Foucault (1975) to refer to a doctor's direct focus on a patient's body. It is a characteristic feature of doctor–patient interaction, and tends to ignore the patient's emotions, psychology, and personality.

Foucault (1975) refers to what he calls 'the **clinical gaze**', which he regarded as being a central dimension of the doctor–patient relationship in scientific medicine. Doctors may use instruments such as stethoscopes to listen to the patient's body, X-rays to view the bone structure of the patient's body, and surgical incisions to open up the patient's body to look inside. In return, patients do not have the same access to their doctors' bodies. Indeed, sometimes they are completely unconscious—under anaesthesia or in a coma, for example—or they may be severely physically disabled and thus unable to express any opinion or preference to counter medical actions and interventions (Armstrong 1984).

For Foucault (1975), the ability of doctors to gain this access to patients' bodies, along with their superior knowledge about other people's bodies, is the primary source of medical power. He calls this power 'disciplinary power', because he views medicine as having the ability to make pronouncements about how individuals should conduct themselves and treat their bodies through self-regulation. Disciplinary power rarely involves direct punishment or coercive control of people. Rather, it encourages people to behave in certain ways 'for their own good'. Those individuals who are positioned as 'experts' or 'authorities', as those who possess superior knowledge, are placed in the position of making pronouncements about how others should behave. In the case of medicine, the belief that 'good health' is vital to human functioning and happiness supports the notions that medical practitioners should be treated as authorities, and that their actions and advice are legitimate and should generally be heeded. We allow doctors and other health care professionals access to our bodies based on their authority. They are permitted to touch and invade the body in ways that no others are allowed. The gynaecological examination is an example.

Therefore, not only do medical knowledges contribute to ways of seeing the body, but they also intervene directly upon the body through medical practice. The doctor's or nurse's touching of the patient's body in the clinical encounter, the drawing of blood for tests, the prescription of medicines and drugs, and surgical incisions all serve to influence and shape the patient's experiences of the body, for better or for worse. Patients who are hospitalised are involved in a medical regime that dictates many, if not all, of their bodily experiences, from the time of awakening in the morning, to meals, to the expulsion of bodily wastes. Such individuals are constantly under medical surveillance, with little opportunity to engage freely in bodily movement. This may result in feelings of dependence, embarrassment, anxiety, frustration, and vulnerability, and in the need to invest trust in the medical and nursing staff upon whom these patients are dependent.

Health care workers may also be permitted to ask patients 'personal' questions about their intimate lives if they are thought to be relevant to the condition for which the patient is seeking advice or treatment. For example, it is generally accepted that nurses should not only 'know' the patient's body but should also seek to encourage patients to reveal their innermost thoughts and feelings as part of holistic patient care (May 1992). In other contexts, this could be regarded as an invasion of an individual's privacy, but in the context of medical care it is generally accepted as appropriate and even important.

There are a number of established rituals of medical care and treatment in relation to the body that serve symbolic functions. Z. Wolf (1988), for example, observed and recorded a number of nurses' rituals in relation to washing patients' bodies in hospital. She argues that these rituals act to maintain a semblance of order in a highly disordered environment by maintaining the boundary between cleanliness and dirtiness. In his participant-observation study of an operating theatre, S. Hirschauer (1991) notes that the procedures carried out to prepare a patient for surgery tend to reduce the patient to an objectified, segmented, depersonalised body. These include the anaesthetising of the patient, hooking up the patient to various machines and tubes, marking off the sections of the body that are to be operated upon and painting them orange-brown with disinfectant, covering other parts of the body with blue linen, and obscuring the face from the operating surgeons. The life signs of the patient become visualised through the technical equipment to which the patient is affixed: the electrocardiogram (ECG), the respirator, the laboratory results from regular blood analysis. As Hirschauer notes, 'One must read all these values to see how the patient is "feeling", what s/he "needs": water, blood, oxygen' (1991, p. 291).

While these procedures may appear to be brutalising or objectifying, they are necessary to preserve both the patient's health and the patient's feelings. Hirschauer argues that:

> A body cut open and laid bare internally—with organs hanging or dragged out—is more than naked. Its inhabitant would be seized with fear and dismay, but would also react with a different social affect already required for states of lesser disarray of one's appearance:

shame. Patients may lose all sorts of organs in the operating theatre; without narcosis they would lose their face. So what seems to sever patients as persons from the social situation also serves to protect them as persons (1991, p. 305).

Health care professionals, for their part, must approach the task of bodily care bearing in mind the sociocultural meanings attached to certain body parts and functions. Nurses, in particular—who are charged with the responsibility of dealing with the more intimate aspects of bodily care for hospitalised patients— must negotiate the highly sensitive issues of washing the patients' bodies, helping them with excretion, cleaning up bodily wastes that are considered highly polluting or disgusting, and dealing with dead bodies. Nursing, therefore, is conceptualised not only as 'caring work' but also as 'dirty work'—something that it is difficult to talk about with outsiders because it is seen as socially unacceptable (see Wolf 1988; Lawler 1991).

A discussion of embodiment in relation to medicine need not focus only on the bodies of patients, but also on those who care for them. The work of medical practitioners, nurses, and other health care professionals requires an ability to objectify patients' bodies to a certain extent, for to allow one's emotions to intrude too far into the medical encounter can prove disabling. Just as the ritualised procedures in the operating theatre serve to protect patients' feelings, they also protect the surgeons from feelings of shame, disgust, or guilt that may arise from cutting into the patients' bodies and thereby causing them injury. If patients were not rendered anonymous, turned into bodies rather than maintained as people, it would be more difficult to operate upon them (Hirschauer 1991, pp. 305–6).

One of the most confronting experiences faced by medical students face is their encounter with the cadavers they are required to dissect as part of their training in anatomy. For many aspiring doctors, this encounter is a profoundly shocking experience (Good 1994, p. 73). Health care professionals must train their own bodies to avoid the shrinking back, the disgust, fear, guilt, and anxiety that accompanies dealing with others' bodies at such an intimate level and in a potentially harming way. They must also learn to 'see' the human body in a different way from lay people, reconstructing it through the lens of medical perception so that they can deal effectively with patients.

Body maintenance and the disciplined body
It is not only the patient in hospital or in the doctor's surgery who is the subject of disciplinary power in relation to medicine. Less directly, medical and public health knowledges and practices influence the ways in which individuals in Western societies con-

ceptualise and experience embodiment. These knowledges have played a central role in regulating the body by prescribing bodily practices through which health should be accomplished and illness avoided (Lupton 1995).

In Western societies, the ability to exert control over one's body—to regulate it and engage in strategies of self-discipline—is regarded as highly important. This is related to other taken-for-granted assumptions about rationality and the need for the mind to have control over the potentially unruly body. There is a distinct moral underpinning to these distinctions between rationality and irrationality, between mind and body, and between control and unruliness. Those who appear to be unable to exert this self-control—who seem to lack rationality—have been regarded as inferior. In medical and public health discourses, as well as in **commodity culture**, bodies that are overweight, flabby, disabled, aged, or sick are considered to be highly undesirable and socially deviant (see chapter 10).

commodity culture The world of advertising and commercial marketing.

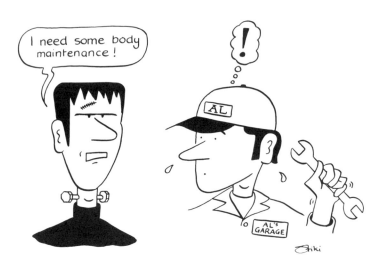

Body maintenance

People with disabilities, for example, are constantly relegated to the margins, becoming the subjects of repulsion and fear. If not treated as 'freaks' and openly subjected to discrimination, they are dealt with as if they were invisible by the able-bodied—they are subjected to the averted gaze (see Davis 1995). Likewise, the bodies of older women and men are virtually absent in popular representations of the body. Few characters in television drama, for example, are older people, and if they are shown, older people are often depicted as frail, ill, pathetic, and dependent. In a society in which older people are treated with pity, disgust, fear, condescension, and neglect (Featherstone & Hepworth 1995), it is perhaps not surprising that early signs of ageing may be a source of consternation. The horror of ageing in Western societies is such that people entering middle age may experience a disjunction between the older self they see in the mirror and the eternally youthful body that they feel themselves to remain 'inside'. Ageing, like obesity and disability, represents an inability to keep one's flesh unsullied and signals the inevitability of mortality (see chapter 12).

Similarly, people who are overweight or obese are thought to lack personal control. Their excess of flesh is read as a potent sign that they 'overindulge'—that their greed overcomes their powers of rationality. In contrast, the thin body bespeaks its owner's ability to maintain strict discipline over the consumption of food. It is not solely the issue of 'health' that is important here; there are also intertwined notions of physical attractiveness and moral assumptions about control of the body. The emphasis in public health and commodity culture in Western societies upon the importance of maintaining a slim body is such that many people feel guilt, anxiety, remorse or lack of control when they feel that they have 'overindulged' in food (see Bordo 1993; Lupton 1996). Since ancient times, diet and exercise have been linked to health states. In contemporary Western societies, medical and public health prescriptions about the deportment and care of the body abound. Perhaps more so than in any other era, individuals living in contemporary Western societies are expected to devote a great deal of time and attention to their bodies, whether for the sake of their physical appearance or for their health. How much food people should eat, what types of food their diet should consist of, how much they should weigh in proportion to their height, how much exercise they should do, how they should engage in sexual activity to avoid pregnancy and infection with sexually transmissible diseases such as AIDS, how much alcohol they should imbibe, how many hours of sleep they should have each night—medicine and public health provide precise recommendations for each of these bodily requirements.

Mike Featherstone has described these requirements as 'body maintenance' (1991, p. 182). This term again suggests the currency of the mechanical metaphor for understanding the human body. Just as cars and other machinery require regular maintenance to keep them working well, it is assumed that human bodies need regular care and attention to prevent malfunction. The discourses of body maintenance do not only draw on medical knowledges for their authority, but are also derived from commodity culture. In Western societies, health, physique, youth, and attractiveness are all seen as contributing to the 'ideal body'. The slim, young body is physically fit and healthy but also conforms to notions of sexual attractiveness. As a result, health promotion campaigns often seek to prevail upon people's desire to achieve or maintain sexual attractiveness and to prevent signs of ageing, while advertising for commercial com-modities ranging from jogging shoes to low-fat or low-salt foods frequently uses health and physical fitness as selling points.

Distinctions between bodies

Throughout the history of scientific medicine, medical and pub-lic health knowledges have been employed to distinguish and differentiate between 'normal', 'healthy' bodies and those that are regarded as 'abnormal', 'diseased', or 'deviant' (Lupton 1995). The male European body has been represented as the archetypical normal, healthy body, at least for heterosexual men and those from elite social groups. By way of contrast, the female body, the bodies of the working classes or the poor, non-White bodies, and homosexual bodies have been singled out as diseased, passive, con-taminating, dirty, and lacking self-control (Petersen & Lupton 1996, ch. 3). There is a symbiotic relationship, therefore, between identifying the bodies of particular social groups (such as women, non-Whites, the working class, or homosexuals) as being uncon-trolled, dirty, and as a result, more susceptible to illness, disease, and early death, and the reproduction of the notion that such groups are inferior to the dominant social group (that is, well-off, White, heterosexual men). The tendency for medicine and public health to emphasise self-control has reproduced and intensified many of these distinctions between social groups.

The bodies of non-European peoples have also been typically represented in Western medicine and public health as far less capable of self-regulation than those of Europeans. Since the eighteenth century, Africa has been portrayed as the breeding ground of disease—a place of dark, dank pestilence, where White travellers should be ever-vigilant. It has been argued that the 'dirty', 'greasy' bodies of Black Africans are a major source of infection for Europeans in Africa (Comaroff 1993). The 'Orient' has also been regarded as an exotic place where health risks lurk, and has been seen to be peopled by unruly 'coloured' bodies that fail to exercise proper control in order to avoid the spreading of disease. In contemporary Western public health discourses, this tendency remains. Certain countries—such as Thailand, for example—are represented as 'danger sites' for Western men because of the possibility that they might contract AIDS through having sex with local sex workers. There is little concern about the possibility that the male clients themselves may infect the sex workers, who are considered to be less worthy and important.

The bodies of women have been the subject of far more medical and public health attention than have the bodies of men (Petersen & Lupton 1996, ch. 3). Compared with the male body, the female body has been represented as sickly, weak, and susceptible to illness. Women are typically described in the legal, medical, and early social scientific literature as possessing problematic and unruly bodies, with their sexual and reproductive capacities requiring constant surveillance and regulation (see chapter 8). Particularly in the nineteenth and early twentieth centuries, medical assumptions about women—for example, that they were prone to uncontrolled emotional outbursts, which in turn were produced by the uterus, or that their natural place was in the home rather than participating in the public sphere—have contributed to the control of women and their confinement to the domestic sphere (Ehrenreich & English 1974).

Not only are women expected to care for their own, physically 'inferior', bodies, but they must also look after the bodies of those individuals for whom they are expected to take responsibility: their husbands or partners, their children, and older members of the family. To use a telling example from the popular media, advertisements for cold and 'flu' remedies typically feature the wife and mother as the caring figure, doling out cough mixture or other remedies to her sniffling husband and (often male) children. In such advertisements, very rarely, if ever, is a women depicted as ill and receiving the caring ministrations of her husband. There have been a number of public health campaigns over the years that have been exclusively directed at women, from the late nineteenth-century campaigns that exhorted women to keep their homes free of flies and dirt in order to prevent the spread of disease, to contemporary campaigns that attempt to persuade women to avoid smoking and drinking alcohol when pregnant and to attend for breast cancer and cervical cancer screening programs. The proponents of such campaigns generally contend that women should engage in such preventative practices not simply for themselves, but also for the sakes of those for whose health they are responsible.

By comparison, men's bodies have rarely been the direct subject of medicine's attention, for they have been assumed to be 'normal' and 'healthy', requiring less in the way of medical advice or intervention, unlike the 'weak', 'sickly', 'less controlled' bodies of women. The male body is culturally represented as ideally invulnerable, disciplined, strong, physically able, and machine-like. As a result, illness, disease, ageing, or disability may undermine or destabilise masculinity (Connell 1995, pp. 54–5; Petersen & Lupton 1996, pp. 80–3). One result of this link between masculinity and physical health and prowess is that issues of **men's health** are only now slowly being recognised in medical and public health forums, and in the popular media. It is only very recently that public health campaigns have been directed specifically at men, and that an emphasis on the vulnerability of men's bodies has emerged.

men's health Running parallel to women's health initiatives, the men's health movement recognises that certain elements of masculine identity and behaviour can be hazardous to health.

More and more news stories are directing attention towards men's health. For instance, in the late 1990s a Sydney newspaper reported the findings of an Australian Institute of Health and Welfare report, which noted that men are three times more likely to die young than women, are four times more likely to commit suicide, and are three times more likely to die in vehicle accidents (reported in Sweet 1996). So, too, there has been increasing attention directed towards men's physical appearance. One example is a cover story that was published in the *Australian* newspaper's Weekend Magazine in July 1996. The heading on the front cover of the magazine read, 'Man Maintenance: Jill Margo's Guide to Men's Health'. The cover featured a close-up of a young man's superbly muscled and toned body, suggesting that 'health' equals 'youth' and 'physical fitness' (note also the use of the word 'maintenance' to describe preventative health endeavours). A glossy magazine entitled *Men's Health* is published monthly in Australia, which again focuses not only on health issues but also on men's physical appearance, their sexuality, and their sporting activities. What is more, in Australia and elsewhere, advertisements are now appearing for clinics offering cosmetic surgery techniques aimed at men. In one such advertisement, published in an Australian women's magazine in 1995, a centre for 'aesthetic surgery' in Sydney claimed that 'All in the aim for [*sic*] better self image and greater self esteem, cosmetic surgery has a lot to offer the "average" male'. The advertisement went on to list procedures such as nose reshaping, eye-lifts, liposuction, and penis enlargement.

Conclusion

This chapter has emphasised that, in order to understand how people perceive and experience their bodies, we must understand the ways that embodiment is shaped through sociocultural processes and contexts. It has been argued that medical and public health—as knowledge systems that are considered to be authoritative in relation to the body, health, and illness—have made a central contribution to representations and understandings of the human body.

Summary of main points

- The human body is not simply a biological or anatomical phenomenon; it is shaped and experienced through social and cultural processes.
- In Western societies, medical and public health knowledges have played a major part in contributing to people's understandings and experiences of embodiment, health, and illness.

- Knowledges, understandings, and experiences of embodiment in relation to health and illness have changed over time and are culturally contextual.
- The Foucaultian critique argues that the source of medical power is the 'clinical gaze', or doctors' focus on patients' bodies.
- Doctors and other health care workers, such as nurses, have privileged access to others' bodies.
- Illness is above all an embodied experience, forcing us to confront the physical reality of our bodies.
- The illness experience and medical treatment may serve to objectify or segment the patient's body.
- Health care workers must exert control over their own bodies as part of their work.
- Medicine and public health have drawn, and continue to draw, distinctions between different types of bodies. These distinctions are often based on moral judgments and assumptions.

Discussion questions

1   Why is the notion of embodiment so important in understanding how people conceptualise and experience health and illness states and medical care?
2   What are some of the lay health beliefs that circulate in relation to the body? How might these health beliefs influence the way people behave?
3   What are some of the dominant metaphors that are used to describe the human body in relation to illness and disease? What do these metaphors convey about how we conceptualise embodiment?
4   How are the bodies of different actors in the health care setting (for example, patients, medical practitioners, nurses) viewed and treated differently by other actors in this setting?
5   How are the distinctions between various actors maintained (for example, with the use of clothing, hospital regulations, and so on)?
6   Why have medicine and public health tended to direct more attention towards monitoring and controlling women's bodies than men's bodies? Why might this difference in emphasis be changing?

Further investigation

1   What are the major similarities between the ways in which nurses engage with patients' bodies and the ways in which doctors do so? What are the major differences, and why do these differences exist?
2   How do medical practices and knowledges that are related to the body reproduce and perpetuate medical power?

Further reading and web resources

Featherstone, M., Hepworth, M., & Turner, B. (eds) 1991, *The Body: Social Process and Cultural Theory*, Sage, London.

Nettleton, S. & Watson, J. (eds) 1998, *The Body in Everyday Life*, Routledge, London.

Scott, S. & Morgan, D. (eds) 1993, *Body Matters: Essays on the Sociology of the Body*, Falmer Press, London.

Shilling, C. 1993, *The Body and Social Theory*, Sage, London.

Turner, B. 1996, *The Body and Society*, 2nd edn, Sage, London.

Web sites

BodyIcon: <http://nm-server.jrn.columbia.edu/projects/masters/bodyimage>

Body Image and Health: <www.rch.unimelb.edu.au/BIHInc>

Eating Disorders: <www.eating-disorders.net>

10

Health Promotion Dilemmas[1]

Katy Richmond

Overview

* *What dilemmas arise in relation to programs that give information about health to individuals and groups?*
* *What are the differences between individualist and structuralist health promotion programs?*
* *How can individualist health promotion programs further the medicalisation of everyday life?*

Health promotion is a relatively recent concept, although public health programs in the broader sense date back to the nineteenth century. While a range of international documents in the last two decades have stressed a broad agenda for health promotion, most Western countries approach health promotion in a very restricted way. The World Health Organization approach suggests that we should not only give health information to individuals and groups, but also make attempts to improve living standards and to involve local communities in constructing their own health agendas. This chapter refers to the limited information-giving approach as the 'individualist health promotion model' and to the broader model as the 'structuralist-collectivist model'. The individualist model is firmly backed by politicians and bureaucrats (because it is easy), and most health professionals, and psychologists (because their jobs are tied to this approach). This chapter provides a number of criticisms of the individualist model and provides some examples of a structuralist-collectivist approach.

Key terms

class	lifestyle choices	social control
consumerism	materialist analysis	social model of health
discourse	medicalisation	social support
epidemiology	new public health	structuralist-collectivist health
health promotion	'race'	promotion (SCHP)
healthism	risk/risk discourse	victim-blaming
individualist health promotion	risk society	
(IHP)	social construction	

---

1   Revisions to this chapter for the second edition were made by John Germov.

Introduction

social model of health A model of health that focuses on social determinants such as the social production, distribution, and construction of health and illness, and the social organisation of health care. It directs attention to the prevention of illness through community participation and social reforms that address living and working conditions.

individualist health promotion (IHP) IHP is a set of programs that provide health education about health risks to persuade people to change their lifestyles. A wide group of professionals are involved in these programs, including doctors, nurses, allied health professionals, psychologists, educators, and media and marketing experts.

structuralist-collectivist health promotion (SCHP) SCHP encompasses a wide range of interventions, including participatory community programs, legislation, and bureaucratic interventions. The latter range from needle exchanges to the enactment of laws restricting industrial pollution, fireworks, flammable nightwear, cigarette advertising, and smoking in public places.

My argument about health promotion is best expressed metaphorically. The medical profession spend their time caring for the sick. The sick can be likened to people near the mouth of a rapidly flowing river, having been thrown into the river from a cliff further upstream. Instead of rescuing people from drowning, we should focus our efforts upstream to find out who is throwing people into the river in the first place. We might perhaps build a few fences. Even better, we might do something about assisting people to change direction, helping them to travel towards a tropical paradise or a cool mountain stream, away from the dangerous cliff face. In other words, doing some planning upstream at the cliff face—working towards structural change to promote good health—is, in the end, more effective than saving people from drowning one by one (metaphor adapted from McKinlay 1994, pp. 509–10).

Health promotion aims to improve the health of whole populations. Before the 1970s, there was a three-pronged approach to health and illness: providing communities with basic public health facilities (clean water, sewerage); providing doctors and hospitals; and providing 'top-down' health education. The new philosophy of health promotion reflects a **social model of health**, and has commonly come to be known as the new public health approach. It was intended to change the health agenda in a modestly radical direction towards community participation and empowerment, and structural and environmental change. But in Australia and elsewhere, health promotion has essentially remained committed to old-style 'top-down' health education. This chapter provides a critique of this approach and offers some examples and suggestions for the future.

The health promotion field is at an early stage, at which theoretical perspectives have not been well developed and emerging debates have received little systematic clarification or critical comment (Baum & Sanders 1995 pp. 153–4). The pathway through the health promotion story is complex, since health promotion practices range along a broad continuum. However, these practices can be simplified by categorising them into two polar 'types'. The conservative end of health promotion can be termed **individualist health promotion (IHP)** and the more radical end **structuralist–collectivist health promotion (SCHP)**. IHP is, in essence, health education about lifestyle. SCHP, on the other hand, encompasses participatory health programs at the community level, legislation, and bureaucratic interventions, which range from small local programs such as the provision of needle exchanges to more significant measures such as laws restricting tobacco advertising and the creation of smoke-free environments.

History

health promotion Any combination of education and related organisational, economic, and political interventions designed to promote behavioural and environmental changes conducive to good health. This promotion may cover a variety of strategies, including legislation, health education, community development, advocacy, and so on. Health promotion has usually, however, been restricted to interventions focusing on the behavioural end of the spectrum.

The major driving force behind **health promotion**—a term first used in 1974—is the World Health Organization (WHO), a United Nations organisation. WHO has hosted a series of important international health conferences, out of which have emerged a number of highly influential health policy documents. These include the Alma Ata Declaration of 1978 (WHO 1978), which was released at its International Conference on Primary Health Care held at Alma Ata in the USSR, the 1981 report entitled *Global Strategy Health for All by the Year 2000*, and the Ottawa Charter for Health Promotion of 1986 (WHO 1986). The tenor of all these publications is a movement away from a focus on illness towards the promotion of health. These documents urge health professionals and policy-makers not only to educate people about health matters, but also to change the environments in which people live and to involve the community in projects to improve health.

The Ottawa Charter was subtitled 'The move towards a new public health' and has been the dominant influence over health promotion approaches to this day. The model is a novel attempt to integrate health education and individual behaviour-change strategies, with broader structural strategies that aim to fundamentally reorient health care services and public policies to address the social determinants of health. As Figure 10.1 (p. 198) depicts, the new public health approach highlights the need to:

- strengthen community action (through community consultation and participation in priority setting, planning, decision-making, and implementation processes)
- develop personal skills (health education to enable behaviour/lifestyle change)
- create supportive environments (in terms of environmental sustainability and wider support systems that ensure social life is safe and satisfying)
- reorient health services (towards prevention, holistic and culturally appropriate care, and power-sharing between health professionals, community groups and individual users of health services)
- build healthy public policy (interventions beyond the health system that aim to make living and working conditions conducive to health and equity).

Stimulated by international debate, the Australian federal government established the Better Health Commission in 1985, and has authorised several health promotion policy documents, including *Looking Forward to Better Health* (1986), *Health for All Australians* (1988), and *Goals and Targets for Australia's Health in the Year 2000 and Beyond* (1993) (O'Connor & Parker 1995,

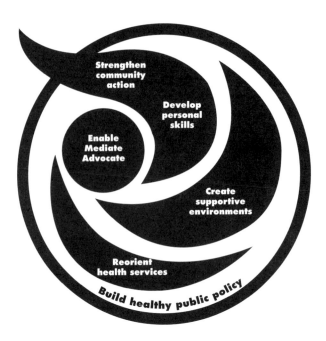

Figure 10.1 Ottawa Charter for Health Promotion

pp. 57–64). Despite the developments at the national and international level in support of making social environments conducive to health, most health promotion activity in Western countries such as Australia has continued to be very narrowly focused around educating people to change their lifestyles. Such programs argue that people put their health at risk by smoking cigarettes, eating unhealthy food, drinking too much, and not exercising enough. In this **discourse**, the problem of illness is conceptualised in terms of individuals' non-compliance. Some people are said to have 'failed' to give up full-cream milk or butter, for instance. Smokers are said to have 'failed to understand' that lung cancer and coronary heart disease are major risks of smoking (Borland et al. 1994, p. 369).

discourse A domain of language-use that is characterised by common ways of talking and thinking about an issue (for example, the discourses of medicine, madness, or sexuality).

Criticisms of individualist health promotion

Individualist health promotion programs of these kinds are difficult to challenge because they are couched in rhetoric that seems so manifestly benevolent (Lupton 1995, p. 433). They are generally promoted as both successful and cost-effective. However, adequate evaluations have rarely been attempted because of a variety of methodological weaknesses in the studies themselves and because the effect of any particular health message cannot be easily isolated from other social changes occurring in the community (Byde 1995, p. 312; Engleman & Forbes 1986, p. 445).

Criticisms of IHP start by pointing out that few programs succeed for any length of time, and that many are 'strikingly unsuccessful' (Beattie 1991, p. 169; Mechanic 1994, p. 472). A. Beattie goes so far as to claim that, on some occasions in the United Kingdom, news of the lack of success of these programs is politically suppressed (Beattie 1991, p. 169). Anti-smoking campaigns in Australia seem to be working with men (albeit slowly), but are less successful with women, and seem to be failing at the teenage level. A big study of cholesterol education in New South Wales achieved some success in imparting information, but almost no success in changing long-term behaviour (Van Beurden et al. 1993, pp. 114–15). In any case, successes are often limited to that segment of the population that is highly motivated to change, and the people who arguably really need to change are often impervious to health messages (Van Beurden et al. 1993, p. 114). In a Newcastle study of cardiovascular disease, those who did not respond to invitations to be involved were more likely to be overweight or obese, or to have had raised triglycerides than those who did respond (Elliott 1995, p. 208).

These individualist health programs continue despite their lack of long-term success because they are supported by a range of powerful interest groups, not least a range of medical and allied health professionals. As Alan Petersen argues, '[h]ealth promotion is not a value free enterprise. It is enmeshed in power relations' (Petersen 1996, p. 56). The IHP model has widespread support because it makes governments look authoritative and active, while at the same time it avoids confrontations that might prove politically costly (Lupton 1995, p. 125). For bureaucrats, this model seems the easiest option because the sort of targets it sets—such as getting 50 per cent of the population over the age of 40 years to exercise three times a week—sound manageable and measurable. IHP has the support of the medical profession because it expands medical turf and it provides work for **epidemiologists**, allied health professionals, psychologists, and educationalists, to the extent that the area has become overcrowded (Beattie 1991, pp. 185–6). IHP meshes well with psychological models of behaviour and is widely supported by media and marketing experts, who circulate its attendant slogans. Drug companies also do well out of some IHP campaigns. For example, fears about heart disease at the onset of menopause have sent thousands of women in their fifties off to pharmacies with doctors' prescriptions to buy packets of oestrogen and progesterone.

Lifestyle choices, promoted by IHP propaganda, are constructed around notions of **risk** or what has been termed the **risk discourse**. Risk used to be a mathematical term, but now it has so changed its meaning that now it simply means 'danger'. The word 'risk' is now an important cultural construct (Lupton 1995,

epidemiology/ social epidemiology The statistical study of patterns of disease in the population. Originally focused on epidemics, or infectious diseases, it now covers non-infectious conditions such as stroke and cancer. Social epidemiology is a sub-field aligned with sociology that focuses on the social determinants of illness.

risk or risk discourse 'Risk' refers to 'danger'. Risk discourse is often used in health promotion messages warning people that the lives they lead involve significant risks to their health.

risk society A term coined by Ulrich Beck (1992) to describe the centrality of risk calculations in people's lives in Western society, whereby the key problem of society today is unanticipated hazards, such as the risks of pollution and environmental degradation.

medicalisation The process by which non-medical problems become defined and treated as medical issues, usually in terms of illnesses, disorders, or syndromes.

healthism The extreme preoccupation with personal health that is evident within the general population.

pp. 425–30). Ulrich Beck talks about the **risk society**, which is negative and defensive and centred around 'preventing the worst' (Beck 1992, p. 49). The study of risks has escalated in medical journals, and the struggle to reduce or eliminate risk factors has become an activity of considerable importance and prestige within the health professions (Skolbekken 1995, p. 297). Thus, what was essentially a medical discussion about the probabilities of getting a particular disease has now entered our daily discourse—a striking example of the **medicalisation** of everyday life.

The social construction of risks is not confined to medicine, of course. Max Weber spoke a hundred years ago about the increasing 'rationality' (or emphasis on calculable goals) of modern industrial society. So it is not surprising that the importance of each of us taking account of health risks is explained to us in terms of good financial management. Governments face economic pressures because of the costs of hospital-based medicine. People must therefore take responsibility for their own health and well-being. As part of this process, people are taught how to 'read' symptoms and to watch for changes in bodily behaviour (Pinell 1996, pp. 13–14). Women, for example, are taught to examine their breasts for symptoms of cancer, and more recently men have been urged to watch for early signs of prostate cancer. Deborah Lupton suggests that the body is now regarded as 'a site of toxicity', which therefore requires a high degree of personal surveillance (Lupton 1995, p. 433).

However, this anxious surveillance of our bodies is paradoxical because our lives are, overall, increasingly under control, and our life expectancy has greatly increased. There are, of course, human-made risks such as acid rain and plutonium boxes that drop from rogue satellites, but overall the risks from our environment are reducing (Skolbekken 1995, p. 291). Yet we regard these risks as overwhelming, and it is as if our anxieties condense around our bodies—almost as if the rest of our problems might become manageable if we could only get our bodies under control (Williams & Calnan 1996, p. 1614). Robert Crawford describes this as **healthism** and says that this extreme concern with personal health has now become a national preoccupation (Crawford 1980, p. 365). In fact, it can be argued that our preoccupation with bodily health is unhealthy. The hazards that we face are often rare, and the risks are so small they should be ignored (Skolbekken 1995, p. 302).

Healthism has generated a consumer culture in which health has become a market commodity. We are all exhorted to make use of aerobics classes, gymnasiums, exercise bicycles, health-food shops, and new diet foods. We watch television programs discussing 'the healthy lifestyle', and we read magazines telling us what to eat (Nettleton 1995, p. 36). The lifestyle choices that we make are each

consumerism The processes and institutions by which individuals satisfy their needs by purchasing goods and services in a market. Mass consumerism refers to post-war consumer practices, whereby the reduction of the cost of commodities and the extensive use of advertising and new credit arrangements created a mass market. It is often argued that consumerism has less to do with the satisfaction of wants than with the desire to be different and distinctive.

social control Mechanisms that aim to induce conformity, or at least to manage or minimise deviant behaviour.

given a moral value, and how we consume these various commodities helps to constitute our sense of self (Johanson et al. 1996, p. 398). The sign of being normal is to have a healthy body. So what emerges from the new **consumerism** based on health is a set of status distinctions that become elaborated into a system of **social control** (Crawford 1980, pp. 382–3).

IHP programs are based on highly simplified psychological models that exaggerate the ease with which behaviour can be changed based on the assumption of a direct connection between health knowledge and behaviour modification (see, for example, Bennett & Hodgson 1992). In fact, little is known about how people choose between various courses of action in relation to their health. No one has ever found clear links between 'knowing' and 'doing', and much ordinary, everyday behaviour is not easily changed (Kaplan 1988, p. 221; Kassulke et al. 1993, p. 56). This is particularly true for the most disadvantaged (Siskind et al. 1992, p. 319). As one respondent in a Sydney study said, the healthy choice is 'not that easy to do even if you know it, believe in it and want to do it' (Ritchie et al. 1994, p. 101). David Mechanic is a particularly strident critic. He argues that 'health actions that must depend on persistent conscious motivation' are unlikely to be successful in the long run (Mechanic 1994, p. 487). Weight loss, dietary modification, and quitting smoking are all difficult to achieve. Individual aspects of behaviour are integrated into a person's sense of self and of belonging to a particular social group (Giddens 1991, p. 121). Social isolation is something that people quite reasonably consider when they consider making changes in their daily lives. If the people all around them smoke, they would place themselves in a marginal position if they stopped smoking. As Byde says, 'individual behaviour change is extremely hard if it requires social isolation as well' (Byde 1995, p. 314).

The limits of epidemiology

It is only recently that the medical approach to health promotion, and in particular epidemiology, has been challenged on its claims to scientific objectivity (Crawford 1980, p. 372). The job of epidemiologists is to research the statistical risks of acquiring particular diseases, but their language is the language of probability, not certainty. We are a long way from being able to perfectly predict illnesses. Some associations between risks and outcomes are strong and others are weak, yet the community is encouraged to think of risks in all-or-none terms. For example, there is a proven link between smoking and lung cancer (though not all people who smoke get the disease). Yet the links between fat consumption and heart disease, or between exercise and heart disease, are not of the same order of risk, and it has been argued that it is dishonest and counterproductive to suggest otherwise (Davison et al. 1992, p. 108; Germov & Williams 1996; Kaplan 1988, p. 231; Skolbekken 1995, p. 302).

Coronary heart disease, for example, can only be partly explained by orthodox behavioural risk factors. Genetic factors are also significant in explaining why some people get heart disease and others do not (Tannahill 1992, p. 99; McKinlay 1996, p. 13). There is now considerable debate about whether cholesterol should be seen as a coronary risk factor for whole populations or, rather, a risk factor for certain small sections of the community. Even when we know more about cholesterol, the story will be very complex: far too complex to peddle to the community in a simple message (Rieger 1996, p. 1232).

However, critics go further than simply maintaining that the messages of the epidemiologists have been misapplied. Critics argue that there should be far more criticism of epidemiological research itself (see chapter 3). There are two sets of arguments here. First, critics point to methodological flaws in epidemiology where (unwittingly, no doubt) fake risks have been created. These include cases in which epidemiological studies have selectively cited supportive trials and ignored non-supportive data (Skolbekken 1995, p. 300). The second set of criticisms surround the social construction of the statistical data upon which epidemiology is based. In an important study, John McKinlay (1996) argues that the statistics about women and heart disease are (like all scientific 'facts') socially constructed, and that a rereading of basic coronary heart disease data indicates that, in each age category, women's risk of heart disease is about the same as, or slightly lower than, men's. Risk does not rise suddenly at the time of menopause. One of the major flaws in the statistical data, so McKinlay argues, is the lack of recognition that a sizeable proportion of women arriving at hospital in their 50s with heart attacks have experienced unrecognised coronary 'incidents' earlier in their lives. McKinlay also points to inaccuracies in cause-of-death attribution, which minimise the number of early coronary heart disease deaths in women before menopause.

The complexities of epidemiological research data are largely ignored by IHP programs, the basic currency of which are simple slogans that frequently go well beyond the evidence (Le Fanu 1986, p. 118). How would people respond to waves of stories about scientists changing their minds about risk factors such as cholesterol? The lay population experience illness as sets of events related to people they know or read about. Some smokers they know may live to a ripe old age, and some people who jog regularly drop dead (this is described as the 'prevention paradox' by Williams & Calnan 1996, p. 1614). If people then observe health scientists changing their minds about health risks, they will inevitably come to treat health messages with some cynicism (Tannahill 1992, p. 97; Davison et al. 1992, p. 108). There is some evidence that this is, in fact, already occurring. Ritchie and others, in their Sydney study, report that their respondents indicated that health messages, especially relating to food, generated confusion: 'One minute red meat is bad for you, chicken is good. The next thing you know chicken is bad and pork's the thing' (Ritchie et al. 1994, p. 100).

The structuralist approach

Critics writing from the structuralist perspective argue that the ineffectiveness of the lifestyle approach to health promotion wastes community resources. But more importantly, they argue that these programs are fundamentally misconceived. The failure of individuals to comply with health warnings is not the problem; the problem is with governments and powerful corporate interests, such as the tobacco lobby, who do not accept responsibility for major diseases in the community. Putting pressure on people to change their lifestyles is, in effect, **victim-blaming**, and does nothing to correct the structural causes of ill health (Waitzkin 1983, p. 215). Structuralists argue that '[t]o focus on individual life-styles is to assume an independence and freedom of the individual that is an illusion' (Navarro 1986, p. 35). Health promotion policy should instead do something about the social situations that frame the decisions that individuals make about their health, especially situations such as inadequate incomes and lack of choice of employment and housing.

victim-blaming The process whereby social inequality is explained in terms of individuals being solely responsible for what happens to them in relation to the choices they make and their assumed psychological, cultural, and/or biological inferiority.

There are also material impediments to people's ability to put health messages into practice. One example comes from a study of food-buying in Canada, which looked at five low-income women and how they budgeted for food for their families (Travers 1996). It was found that they were not adhering to a 'live-for-today' mentality, and what determined their food purchases was their low income, which reduced their capacity to select appropriate foods or to shop at more distant locations, where food was cheaper. Another significant factor was the pressure that the women faced from their children, who saw food advertised on television. Travers argued that 'good food' messages are phrased in dogmatic terms and list unfamiliar, often expensive, and not easily available foods. He concluded that teaching someone to budget does not address the structural inequity created by inadequate welfare allowances (Travers 1996, pp. 551–2). In relation to diet, '[h]ealthy choices are not usually easy choices for the socially disadvantaged' (McMichael 1991, p. 10).

class (or social class) A position within a system of structured inequality based on the unequal distribution of power, wealth, income, and status. Class membership is determined by three characteristics: ownership and control of scarce economic resources; ownership of marketable skills and qualifications; and wage labour. People who share a social-class position typically share similar life chances.

materialist analysis An analysis that is embedded in the real, actual, material reality of everyday life.

The structuralist perspective provides two sets of arguments about why working-**class** people suffer more ill health than middle-class people. The first is a **materialist** explanation: working-class people do not have access to the same range of choices as middle-class people (Whitehead 1992, pp. 432–3). They live in suburbs close to toxic waste; their houses are overcrowded, and in some rural communities sanitation may be poor. Many working-class jobs are associated with health hazards, and generate illnesses and disabilities, such as deafness, that only become apparent years or even decades after employment has ceased. There are also a range of occupationally induced cancers, asbestos-related diseases, and respiratory illnesses associated with industrial chemicals. Neil Burdess argues that 'occupational diseases are of much greater significance in explaining the low health status of the working class than official figures suggest' (Burdess 1996, p. 175). Some industrial pollution also affects those who live in suburbs nearby. And industrial chemicals adhering to men's clothing can cause illnesses among women washing this clothing. People with material wealth, on the other hand, have cars and access to jobs with good working environments, and they live in pleasant suburbs a long distance from industrial pollution (Burdess 1996, pp. 175–6).

The second set of explanations relates to cultural factors that limit people's ability to purchase appropriate health care, and that promote differences not only in behaviours relating to diet, smoking, alcohol, and exercise, but also in attitudes to taking risks. These cultural factors often have their basis in material circumstances. There are, for example, important emotional consequences of working in jobs with considerable surveillance, low levels of personal fulfilment and creativity, and the stress that accompanies the constant threat of unemployment (Link & Phelan 1995, p. 83; Burdess 1996, pp. 180–1).

The basic reason, however, for the lack of a connection between 'knowing' and 'doing' lies in the power to choose. The rhetoric of individualist health promotion is that, if you know the health risks of a particular form of behaviour, then you have some choice and some power in your life. Yet this vastly exaggerates the options for the poor and economically vulnerable. Individuals in the middle class may well have some control over their lives, and therefore some capacity to care for their own bodies, but such messages often simply create anxiety for those with fewer material resources.

Health promotion practitioners, by definition, see health as a top priority. However, some people see health differently. Though this 'difference of opinion' might appear to be a cultural matter, ultimately our views about life's priorities depend on material resources. Living healthily, according to individualist health promotion wisdom, means acknowledging risks. But these risks are framed in the way that middle-class people (the health promoters) see the risks (Nettleton 1995). When faced with health promotion relating to lifestyle, people undertake what is essentially a cost–benefit analysis. They look at what they will lose by undertaking healthy lifestyles and think about what the health promoters tell them about their future 'gains' (Tannahill 1992, p. 101; Engleman & Forbes 1986, p. 445). If they believe that their lives are dominated by things they cannot do anything about, then the pleasures that they gain from the so-called unhealthy aspects of their life are not worth giving up. Most people with little choice about their lives regard their immediate comfort to be of far greater importance than end-stage health (Ritchie et al. 1994, p. 101): 'It is because of the operation of this simple model that giving up smoking is a different proposition to someone who works in the polluted atmosphere of a petrochemicals plant and someone who spends their day in an air-conditioned suburban office block' (Davison et al. 1992, p. 99).

A survey of 1000 people in the Hunter Region of New South Wales found that drugs, crime, and road safety were major concerns, and that health was of far less importance. Cancer came sixth on the list of concerns, and fears of heart disease were placed even further down the list. Respondents in this study thought that heart problems were almost inevitable when you got older and could be dealt with appropriately when the time came through drug therapies or surgery (Higginbotham et al. 1993, p. 319).

The structuralist perspective also criticises IHP programs for targeting their health messages to particular groups in the community, and especially for their use of generalised class and '**race**' categories. The apparently value-free activity of giving people health messages can become an important form of discrimination (Thorogood 1992, p. 54). To target 'the working class', for example, is to claim that this social category is well defined. But, in fact, it is not, and there are hidden values involved in pretending that it is. There is a strong possibility that stigmatisation and a sense of failure will emerge in the targeted group. Such stigmatisation will be accentuated in the case of marginalised groups, such as drug-takers or sex workers. For example, the 'Grim Reaper' AIDS campaign in 1986 swamped diagnostic and pathology services with 'worried well' low-risk individuals, and also extended socially divisive attitudes towards homosexuals (Bray & Chapman 1991, pp. 112–13).

There is, in fact, a strong class dimension to IHP activity. IHP programs work within a set of concepts that are familiar to middle-class people. These include the need to plan for the future,

'race' A term without scientific basis that uses skin colour and facial features to describe allegedly biologically distinct groups of humans. It is a social construction that is used to categorise groups of people and usually infers assumed (and unproven) intellectual superiority or inferiority.

and the importance of self-improvement and self-control (Crawford 1984, p. 78; Beattie 1991, p. 175). In essence, health promotion messages are created by the middle class and visited upon the working class, who are then castigated for their 'failure to hear'. Some have argued that health promotion is essentially social regulation and surveillance by the rich of the poor, and that it must be seen in the context of new forms of social regulation (Nettleton 1995, p. 234; McKinlay 1994, p. 512). Crawford, for example, suggests that health is a moral discourse, which allows the middle class to visibly demonstrate their capacity for self-discipline—to 'strut the turf' and to display not only their control over themselves, but also their control over others (Crawford 1984, p. 80).

There is a strong possibility that working-class people resist messages from the middle class. One reason that IHP programs fail is that they are, at best, paternalistic, and at worst, authoritarian. People do not like being told what to do, and many of them resist. Painting what seems to be a quintessentially accurate picture of the average IHP worker face to face with a client, Anthony McMasters, an Aboriginal health worker, has commented:

> as a professional health worker, our work involves giving advice to people about how things are affecting them and what might be contributing to their poor health ... [but] it can be difficult to give advice in this way ... It can sometimes be interpreted as interfering and telling people what to do, or, even worse, as a personal criticism. If that happens, clients will respond quickly: they may get angry, walk away or just ignore the health worker (McMasters 1996, p. 319).

Moving towards a structuralist-collectivist approach

The SCHP approach should work towards both small-scale local interventions and broader legislative change. But further than that, it is difficult to prescribe exactly what a structuralist–collectivist approach to health promotion should be, and in fact, some argue that the approach should be about processes and not about end results (Baum & Sanders 1995, p. 156).

Broad legislative change is complex and requires long-term commitment. Australia has already been successful in enacting a wide range of health-related legislation. Laws include those outlawing industrial pollution, fireworks, flammable nightwear, cigarette advertising, and smoking in public places, and requiring water fluoridation, compulsory car seat belts, and the labelling of poisons. Some of these legislative changes have emerged through debate within the major political parties, but others have been the result of pressure from groups of individuals who have worked outside conventional political processes, sometimes within environmental groups and sometimes from within the 'not for profit' health and social welfare sectors.

Legislation rarely brings about radical change. Some legislation that looks good on the surface may be no more than symbolic because, in the end, 'weak-kneed' politicians compromise with powerful interest groups. Simon Barraclough argues that tobacco legislation in Victoria is, at least in part, no more than ritual legislation because tobacco companies are still free to advertise goods with the same names as well-known brands of cigarettes, and they are still able to advertise at some 'incidental' events, such as the Grand Prix (Barraclough 1992, p. 207). Furthermore, legislation is not always effective. One famous example is the failure of the prohibition of the alcohol consumption in the USA in the 1920s (Hart 1989, p. 422). Ensuring that legislation is acted upon is a difficult matter.

The following four examples provide a good explanation of the differences between the IHP and the SCHP approaches. They are not intended to be comprehensive, but merely illustrative. Several of the suggested approaches listed here are already being utilised in some areas of Australia.

Example 1: Smoking

Smoking is a major cause of heart disease and lung cancer. Rather than continue IHP programs 'advising' people not to smoke, energy would be better expended on some structural change. For example, there is a need for more laws that outlaw remaining forms of tobacco advertising in Australia (Barraclough 1992, p. 207). Other possible measures against smoking include comprehensive legislation for cigarette packet health warnings and measures to prevent the discounting of cigarettes in larger pack sizes (Hill & White 1995, p. 308; Hill et al. 1995, p. 448). Given the fact that community hostility towards smoking is increasing, further attempts should be made to increase taxes on smoking, as the cost of cigarettes can be a particularly effective tool to prevent the onset of habitual smoking in teenagers (Crowley et al. 1995, p. 341). And enforcement of already existing legislation at the point of sale needs to be improved from its present very low level. Store-owners need to be given more vigorous warnings in relation to selling cigarettes to minors, and more could be done to improve police and court action when store-owners break the law in this respect (Girgis et al. 1995, p. 32; Sanson-Fisher et al. 1992).

Example 2: Diet

Governments have a great deal of power in relation to food. They can control the ingredients and labelling of processed food and can create incentives for primary producers of meat and grain. And they can ban inappropriate food produce, such as little drink packages that look like orange juice but that, in fact, contain alcohol (McMichael 1991, p. 10). Rather than trying to change individual behaviour in relation to adding salt to food (the IHP approach), it would be more effective and economical to change food processing laws to reduce the salt content of tinned and frozen foods (a SCHP approach) (Jamison 1995, p. 523).

Example 3: Immunisation

Immunisation levels (which have dropped substantially in recent decades) would seem particularly amenable to SCHP rather than IHP measures (Hawe 1994, p. 241). Governments could require regional computerised immunisation records to be kept. Alternatively, general practitioners could be required to keep their own immunisation registers and to have recall systems whereby parents are notified when immunisations are required for their children (Rixon et al. 1994, p. 260; Salmond et al. 1994, p. 257). Already some Australian State governments are utilising primary schools to achieve improved immunisation levels in children through a requirement that parent-held immunisation records be routinely assessed at primary school entry. In 1997, the federal government announced a major program of immunisation for babies and young children, whereby the parents of non-immunised children are financially penalised through a reduction of the family child allowance.

Example 4: Aboriginal health

Baum and Sanders argue that good health is determined outside the health sector, and this is especially true of Aboriginal health, which is at Third World standard (Baum & Sanders 1995, p. 150). There have also been suggestions that the Australian army should be employed to improve Aboriginal living conditions, especially in relation to access to water and sewerage (*Age*, 14 November 1996), and this is precisely the sort of structural change that is required. More modest structural change is also needed. For example, more Aboriginal health workers need to be trained and utilised as community consultants (O'Connor & Parker 1995, p. 201). Aboriginal diets are generally unhealthy, largely because of extreme poverty. Modest but effective structural interventions in relation to diet could include efforts to improve the stocking of stores where Aboriginal people purchase food (Lee et al. 1994, p. 283; Lee et al. 1996, p. 214; Scrimgeour et al. 1994). Problem drinking among Aboriginal people might also be tackled through structural means. Aboriginal people themselves want more stringent controls on alcohol, but they are often ill-informed about their right to oppose increases in the number and the location of liquor outlets. Administrative procedures for making these statements of opposition also need to be radically improved to facilitate such protests (Gray et al. 1995, p. 181).

Community-based approaches

It is conventional to suggest that SCHP should be community based. Much of what has occurred so far in the name of community-based health promotion is, however, not structural change at all but health education in disguise (Beattie 1991, p. 177). Where health education has been imposed on communities, there has been some negative reaction, especially with regard to matters such as quitting smoking and controlling alcohol intake (Brown & Redman 1995, p. 268; Flaherty et al. 1991, p. 305). This suggests that community-based SCHP programs clearly need to be 'bottom up' rather than 'top down'. But making this a reality is not as easy as it sounds.

There is a great deal of unrecognised hostility within community health promotion programs. Conflict usually emerges when community gatekeepers 'bite the hands that feed them' by challenging existing health services and policies, or the ongoing domination of local medical and allied health personnel (Beattie 1991, p. 178). Sometimes this conflict is suppressed, and control stays in the hands of doctors, hospitals, and some special interest groups (Brownlea 1987, p. 612). Sometimes the hostility is so intense that the community program is denied funding. Since one of the major stumbling blocks in community health promotion programs is professional intransigence, one of the most obvious concerns of SCHP programs should be the restructuring of professional groups, at least at the local level, so that they are less rigid and more cooperative (Beattie 1991, p. 188). Some critics, however, doubt that empowerment of community groups is a real possibility given 'the imbalance of participatory capacity between participants' (Kelly & Van Vlaenderen 1996, p. 1245) (see chapter 18 for more discussion on community health).

Future directions

SCHP programs should focus on creating new avenues for structural change. Current workplace health programs are largely limited to safety issues, and much more could be done to influence employers to provide a range of health-related facilities. In one study, workers complained about canteen food because it was 'loaded with fat and oil ... we know it's not good for us ... but what can you do to get something else when you've only got half an hour for lunch break' (Ritchie et al. 1994, p. 101). Employers could be encouraged to provide walking tracks, better canteen foods, and longer lunch periods so that workers can take advantage of available facilities.

New advocates for structuralist health promotion also need to be found. Trade union leaders have focused heavily on worker health and safety, yet they are particularly well placed to encourage a broader structural approach to health in the workplace (Brownlea 1987, p. 607). Local councils might also be encouraged to extend health promotion efforts through their health officers, a strategy used successfully in the United Kingdom (Acton & Chambers 1990).

A problem facing SCHP is to decide what practical benefits might be provided at the community level alongside efforts to promote structural change. One such benefit might be targeted clinical care, such as help for young mothers (Redman et al. 1992, p. 180). Another might be access to health-screening programs (but there are some difficulties in deciding the overall benefits of these programs) (Engleman & Forbes 1986, p. 454). Additionally, self-help programs need to be considered, especially in relation to quitting smoking, though modest levels of **social support** might still be required (Brown & Owen 1992, p. 190). Furthermore, health-education programs should be widened from their present predominantly Anglo-Saxon base to provide interpreters for non-English-speakers and with suitably translated and widely disseminated documentation (Turnbull et al. 1992, p. 74).

Finally, new SCHP approaches should reassess current health promotion programs, which are at present mostly IHP-based. First, this might mean abandoning attempts to utilise general practitioners, on the grounds that they operate only with individuals, and mostly in a patronising, advice-giving mode (Nettleton 1995, pp. 230–1). Second, supermarket programs designed to educate people about good nutrition are trivial and of limited, short-term value (Scott et al. 1991, p. 53). Third, school education about health issues may well be wasted effort if no attempts are made to reach parents at the same time (Gore et al. 1996, p. 193).

Whatever the structural changes required to improve health, people still need some sort of critically based education about health matters—not information *per se*, but information about how to utilise health services and health resources, and how the social and geographical environment impinges on people's health (Beattie 1991, p. 164). People have a right to good health education, and certainly there is evidence that people are anxious to obtain it (Richmond 1995, p. 55). They do not need lists of the latest epidemiological risk factors for heart disease. Instead they need information about how to evaluate sources of health knowledge. Perhaps new computer technology, especially the Internet,

social support The support provided to an individual by being part of a network of kin, friends, or colleagues.

could be a vehicle for improved access to good information. However, lack of access to the Internet for those who cannot afford computers or computer training means that many people are likely to remain 'information poor'.

Conclusion: towards an integrated and global perspective

At the beginning of this chapter, it was noted that health promotion practices range along a broad continuum, but for simplification, they could be categorised into either IHP or SCHP 'types'. Table 10.1 compares the key areas of focus of the two types against the new public health approach. The novel feature of the new public health is its attempt to bridge the gap between IHP and SCHP approaches. While the argument in this chapter suggests that the new public health has relied primarily on individualistic approaches in practice, such a conclusion must acknowledge the difficulty in overcoming political, economic, and organisational obstacles in attempting to translate the model's rhetoric into reality.

	Individual	Community	Nation	Globe
New Public Health model	✔	✔	✔	✔
Individualist health-promotion model	✔		✔	
Structuralist-collectivist model		✔	✔	

Table 10.1 Key focal points of three approaches to health promotion

While the philosophies that underpin individualist and structuralist approaches to health promotion cannot always be easily reconciled, there is some ground for convergence. As we have seen in the examples discussed above, health promotion can involve culturally appropriate individualistic methods of health education and lifestyle change, coupled with structural and collective methods aimed at producing wider social change. The future of health promotion clearly needs to head in this direction.

In conclusion, we need to see health promotion in Australia from a world perspective. Currently Australian policy has a 'health-in-one-nation approach'. But many argue that Australian policy should be also concerned with global problems (Baum & Sanders 1995, p. 157). There is widespread hunger and malnutrition in many parts of the world, and many regions experience recurring outbreaks of diseases such as cholera, which are unknown in Australia (Mechanic 1994, pp. 485–6; Van Bergen 1996, p. 93). Though Australia is relatively free of industrial pollution, many non-Western countries lack even the most basic industrial controls. What is good health promotion for the Western world may be bad for the non-Western world. As soon as we outlaw polluting industries, they move to countries with fewer regulations or fewer agents to do the regulating. As soon as we control smoking, tobacco companies move to new markets in Asia. One of the most obvious pieces of urban decoration in modern Ghangzhou (formerly known as Canton) are the giant Marlboro advertisements that Australia outlawed years ago. In the global context, the Western world's preoccupation with diet and exercise is aptly described as 'a luxury problem of the richest part of the world' (Skolbekken 1995, p. 300). It is as well not to be too smug about our successes.

Summary of main points

- Health promotion can be categorised into two types: individualist health promotion (health education about lifestyle change) and structuralist-collectivist health promotion (health programs involving the community, legislation, and bureaucratic interventions).
- Criticisms of individualist health promotion programs involve their general lack of success in terms of changing behaviour long-term, and their tendency towards victim-blaming.
- Much individualist health promotion is based on risk discourse and healthism, and has encouraged such a massive preoccupation with health—often linked to beauty and youth—that health has become a commodity in the marketplace through gyms, health-food shops, and diet foods.
- Examples of structuralist-collectivist health promotion can be found, but much more can be done. It may even be possible for some convergence of IHP and SCHP via the new public health approach.

Discussion questions

1 How effective are health education messages? Have they influenced you?
2 Can health education messages have a negative impact?
3 What is healthism? In what ways can healthism have negative implications?
4 What are the major criticisms that can be made of individualist health promotion?
5 What are the major barriers to structuralist-collectivist health promotion?

6 Are individualist health promotion programs easier to implement than structuralist programs? Why might some people be opposed to structuralist-collectivist approaches, and who might these people be?

Further investigation

1 'Public health has, over time, lost its broad gauged approach and moved into a phase of medical dominance and concern for behavioural epidemiology, preventive medicine and health education. It has individualised social and cultural patterns by concentrating on disease categories and risk factor causation principles (heart disease/high blood pressure/less fat/health behaviour change)' (Kickbusch 1989, p. 266). Discuss.

2 What are the differences in how health promotion is understood by the biomedical model compared to the social model of health? Why do these differences exist? Are the limitations of one model addressed by the other? Can the two models be reconciled?

Further reading and web resources

Ashton, J. & Seymour, H. 1988, *The New Public Health: The Liverpool Experience*, Open University Press, Milton Keynes.

Ashton, J. (ed.) 1992, *Healthy Cities*, Open University Press, Buckingham.

Baum, F. 1998, *The New Public Health: An Australian Perspective*, Oxford University Press, Melbourne.

Baum, F. & Sanders, S. 1995, 'Can Health Promotion and Primary Health Care Achieve Health for All Without a Return to Their More Radical Agenda?', *Health Promotion International*, vol. 10, pp. 149–60.

Beattie, A. 1991, 'Knowledge and Control in Health Promotion: A Test Case for Social Policy and Social Theory', in J. Gabe, M. Calnan, & M. Bury (eds), *The Sociology of the Health Service*, Routledge, London, pp. 162–202.

Blaxter, M. 1990, *Health and Lifestyles*, Routledge, London.

Bunton, R., Nettleton, S., & Burrows, R. (eds) 1995, *The Sociology of Health Promotion*, Routledge, London.

Crawford, R. 1980, 'Healthism and the Medicalization of Everyday Life', *International Journal of Health Services*, vol. 10, pp. 365–88.

Lupton, D. 1995, *The Imperative of Health: Public Health and the Regulated Body*, Sage, London.

—— 1999, *Risk*, Routledge, New York.

Marmot, M. & Wilkinson, R. G. (eds) 1999, *Social Determinants of Health*, Oxford University Press, Oxford.

McKinlay, J. 1994, 'A Case for Refocussing Upstream: The Political Economy of Illness', in P. Conrad & R. Kern (eds), *The Sociology of Health and Illness: Critical Perspectives*, 4th edn, St Martin's Press, New York, pp. 509–23.

Petersen, A. & Lupton, D. 1996, *The New Public Health: Health and Self in the Age of Risk*, Allen & Unwin, Sydney.

Williams, S. & Calnan, M. 1996, 'The "Limits" of Medicalization? Modern Medicine and the Lay Populace in "Late" Modernity', *Social Science and Medicine*, vol. 42, pp. 1609–20.

World Health Organization 2000, *World Health Report 2000*, World Health
    Organization, Geneva.

Web sites

Healthy Cities Illawarra:
International Public Health Watch: <www.ldb.org/iphw/index.htm>
Noarlunga Healthy Cities project: <www.softcon.com.au/nhc/>
Public Health Association: <www.phaa.net.au>
Public Health Resources (University of Sydney):
    <www.health.usyd.edu.au/research/index.html>
Public Health Resources on the Internet (QUT):
    <www.hlth.qut.edu.au/ph/phlinks/useful.htm>
Public Health Virtual Library: <www.ldb.org/vl/index.htm
WHO Health Promotion Declarations:
    <www.phs.ki.se/whoccse/Declarations.htm>
World Health Organization: <www.who.org>

11

The Human Genome Project

A Sociology of Medical Technology

Evan Willis

Overview

* *How can we apply the sociological imagination to explain the likely implications of the Human Genome Project for society?*
* *How might we understand such developments in terms of the treatment of disease from a sociological point of view?*
* *How will the knowledge and possibilities that such a project provides shape the sort of society in which we live?*

This chapter is a case study in the sociology of medical technology. It analyses the implications of developments in molecular biology associated with the Human Genome Project. The project is a research program to identify the 30 000–35 000 genes in the human body. The most controversial aspect of the project is the search for genes that are thought to be likely to affect behaviours such as depression, alcoholism, homosexuality, and obesity. This chapter considers the question of how the knowledge and possibilities that such a project provides might shape the sort of society in which we live. How can a sociological perspective begin to understand, even predict, what the future implications of such developments will be? Analysing the sociological and related social policy implications of the project involves considering the tension between the individual and collective uses to which emerging genetic biotechnologies are put.

Key terms

ageism	ideology
biological determinism	immigrants
biotechnology	modernism
ethnic group	racism
eugenics	social control
geneism	social Darwinism
genetic manipulation	social justice
genetic reductionism	sociobiology

Introduction: the Human Genome Project

> Future scientific advances enabling parents to genetically improve their offspring should be subsidised by government to ensure that the children of poor people were not further disadvantaged compared with the rich, who could not afford to pay for it themselves … I do not think that we have grounds for concluding that a genetic supermarket would harm either those who choose to shop there or those who are created from the material they purchase. (Bioethicist Professor Peter Singer, as quoted in the *Age*, 22 August 2000)

On a visit to Melbourne, Peter Singer gave an address entitled 'Shopping at the Genetic Supermarket' which outlined some of the social and ethical issues associated with rapid developments in molecular genetics that have collectively become known as the Human Genome Project. How can a sociological perspective help us to understand, even predict, what the future implications of the Human Genome Project will be? When sociologists study health and illness, what sorts of features do they concentrate on and analyse? These questions are addressed in this chapter in the context of a sociology of medical technology.

The Human Genome Project (HGP) is an international research program in molecular biology (centred in the USA) to identify and map the 30 000–35 000 genes on the 23 different human chromosomes, and sequence the approximately three billion nucleotide bases from which these genes are composed. Funded initially through the United States Department of Energy, some US$3 billion are involved, the largest scientific project since the Moonshot. It has been a joint effort between the US National Institutes of Health, the US Department of Energy, the Wellcome Trust in the UK, US venture capitalist **biotechnology** company Celera, and universities around the world including in Australia. Since it began in 1988, rapid progress has been made, and in late June 2000 the completion of the basic mapping project (akin to a 'first draft') was announced.

biotechnology The use of molecular biology and genetic engineering to modify plants and animals, including humans, at the molecular level.

Although some of the genetic discoveries predated the formal establishment of the project, two directions of research have arisen out of this basic mapping expedition. The first direction is what could broadly be called 'disease genetics'. This is the search for specific gene mutations thought to cause particular ill-health conditions: on the one hand, single gene disorders such as Huntington's disease, and on the other, a predisposition to common diseases such as, for example, certain types of breast and ovarian cancer. The second and much more controversial direction has been in the area of 'behavioural genetics'. This has involved a search for genes that are thought to be likely to affect behaviours that some define as socially undesirable and therefore potentially amenable to 'alteration' such as depression, alcoholism, homosexuality, obesity, and the 'holy grail', intelligence.

All the social sciences are concerned with studying the relationship between the individual and society, but arguably it is to sociology that this relationship is most central. The relationship between the individual and the group is often cast as a tension. How can maximum individual liberty be reconciled with the need for people to get along together in the interests of social harmony? The HGP has resulted in rapid discoveries in the genetic basis of disease. Understanding the social (including the legal, ethical, and political) impact of these findings, however, lags far behind. By way of analogy, if we think of the project as a 400-metre race, the molecular biology aspect, having streaked away, is nearing the home straight, while the social understanding has only just left the starting blocks. This is despite the fact that 5 per cent of the project's funds have been committed for what has come to be called the ELSI (ethical, legal, and social implications) part of the project. The tension between the individual and collective uses of the biotechnologies that are resulting from the project are well illustrated by an example given at a recent genetics conference: a (non-Australian) airline pilot has consistently refused to be tested for Huntington's disease, even though, on the basis of family genetic history, he has a 50-50 chance of having inherited the genetic mutation, and irrational psychotic behaviour is a known symptom of the disease. The question is one of the balance between individual and collective uses of the biotechnologies.

There are both sociological and social policy aspects to be investigated here. The study of sociology, as Anthony Giddens (1983) has argued, is the search for alternative futures—the study not only of what *is*, but of what might be. So a concern with social policy, or 'what is to be done', is an important part of the sociological enterprise. In other words, we are interested in social phenomena not only for their own sake, but also for their social policy implications. So the social policy question that arises out of the sociological analysis is 'how can the benefits be maximised and the drawbacks be minimised?' If we take the example of the genetic supermarket outlined above (originally coined by Nozick 1975), to illustrate that if it does eventuate that parents are able to make choices about their offspring, do we need social policies, as Professor Singer argues, so that the ability to choose does not only become available to the wealthy?

In the case of the HGP, it should be noted from the outset (lest this chapter be considered hostile to the attempts to reduce the individual and community toll of genetically caused illness) that benefits will flow from the project to lessen the human burden of suffering (morbidity) and death (mortality) that result from genetically caused illness. In some cases, the benefits are relatively clear—for instance, where there is the possibility of intervention to delay the development of clinical disease, as with polycystic kidney disease. With other cases, such as myotonic dystrophy, intervention can avoid life-threatening complications. Or in other cases—such as familial colonic polyposis, a syndrome that runs in families—surgery can be curative. Where screening for the presence of genetically caused conditions can be done prenatally (of the foetus *in utero*), then the possibility exists (at least for those whose values and beliefs support abortion) to terminate the pregnancy. So there are some benefits for individuals that should be maximised. However, already there are drawbacks to be minimised, which are more the subject of this chapter.

After a slow start, a specifically sociological literature analysing the HGP and the 'new genetics' has begun to appear, some of it Australian. Most of the effort has been in a few areas: an overview of the main issues for social scientists (e.g. Davison et al. 1994; Conrad 1997; Rothman 1998; Conrad & Gabe 1999); an analysis of how the project has been reported in the media (e.g. Henderson & Kitzinger 1999; Petersen 1999, 2000); and the implications for other areas of health care such as public health (Petersen 1998; Willis 1998). There is also the beginning of a literature on the sociological issues surrounding particular genetic illnesses (Cox & McKellin 1999; Hallowell 1999).

The sociological analysis in this chapter follows the general framework established for this book—a framework that takes account of the four sensibilities: historical, cultural, structural, and critical. How does an understanding of each of these elements improve our understanding of the opportunities and dangers of a project as important as the HGP? And how does its analysis reveal what a sociological explanation has to offer?

There is one other important proviso. The relationship between technology and society—which this chapter deals with in the context of biotechnologies resulting from the HGP—is what is called a dialectical relationship; that is to say, each influences the other. Most studies of new technologies focus upon their impact on society—how the introduction of a particular technology (say, mobile phones) has an impact on the society into which it is introduced. But that is only half the question. As important to the sociology of technology is the study of the impact of society on the technology—that is, how a particular society shapes the technology that it develops and uses. This is called the social shaping of technology. This chapter is presented as a case study of the sociology of medical technology in both its social impact and social shaping aspects.

History

eugenics The study of human heredity based on the unproven assumption that selective breeding could improve the intellectual, physical, and cultural traits of a population.

ideology In a political context, ideology refers to those beliefs and values that relate to the way in which society should be organised, including the appropriate role of the state.

ethnic group A group of people who not only share an ethnic background but also interact with each other on the basis of their shared ethnicity.

immigrants The overseas-born population in a society. The term is sometimes extended to refer to the descendants of immigrants through the terms 'second-generation' and 'third-generation immigrants'. However, this usage tends to confuse the term, as it obscures the important fact that those born overseas have a set of immigrant experiences that their descendants do not.

As far as the use of genetic information is concerned, what are the 'lessons from history'? An adequate answer to this question would require a much lengthier treatise than is possible here, but a few points can be made. The first concerns **eugenics**. There has been a systematic attempt to avoid the use of this highly controversial term in discourses surrounding the HGP but the shadow of eugenics hangs over the project. Although the Nazis are most often and most obviously associated with the abuses of genetic knowledge, the history of misuse predates them by half a century. The term 'eugenics' (meaning 'well born') was coined by Englishman Francis Galton in 1883 as 'a brief word for to express the science of improving the stock' (Galton 1883, p. 24). Eugenics can be understood as an **ideology** in the sense that it is a set of ideas that justifies a course of action. Historically, two sorts of social engineering eugenic programs have been advocated: positive eugenics (to encourage the 'fit' to have more children) and negative eugenics (to exclude the 'unfit' and, through the use of sterilisation, to prevent them from having children). Eugenics has been embraced by 'progressives' from across the political spectrum as holding the promise of human betterment. The Nazis' process of selection and eradication—first of people labelled as having mental and physical disabilities, and then later of other 'inferior types', such as Jews, homosexuals, and gypsies—drew directly on eugenic programs that had been developed in the United Kingdom and the USA (see Caplan 1992). This was especially the case with the United States Immigration Restriction Act 1924, which was designed to limit immigration into the country of 'defectives' from southern and eastern Europe. These **ethnic groups** were felt to have a much higher proportion of 'mental defectives' than **immigrants** from the United Kingdom and northern Europe.

After the World War II, interest in eugenics declined, partially in revulsion from the Nazi practices and partially because advances in genetics changed the understanding of dominant and recessive conditions (Hubbard & Wald 1997 p. 23). But eugenicist ideology remains, though the word itself is consciously shunned because of its history. Positive eugenicist policies have been in force for some time in the state of Singapore, for instance, where well-educated couples are encouraged to have more children (see Duster 1990). A current example of negative eugenics comes from the People's Republic of China, where Article 38 came into operation on 1 January 1995. It bans the marriage of anyone diagnosed with a serious genetic disease that is considered medically inappropriate for bearing children, unless the couple agree to be sterilised or undertake long-term permanent contraception. The aim is to prevent the transmission of genetic illnesses from one generation to the next, which is, of course, partly what the Nazis were trying to do. The classic problem is always how to define what is 'inappropriate'.

This has been the stumbling block for eugenics in the past. There have been two problems: the knowledge basis required to achieve the desired ends, and the value judgments about how to define good and bad genes. What are the positive genes and what are the negative? Arguably what the HGP does is provide a much better knowledge base on which to make decisions, but the issue of what is considered 'defective' remains as problematic as it has ever been (see Duster 1990).

So, although, as Hubbard and Wald argue, the earlier forms of eugenics have died out; the root concepts remain, especially:

> the idea that it is more beneficial for certain people to have children than others, and that a vast range of human problems can be cured once we learn how to manipulate our genes ... Testing prospective parents to see if they are carriers of genetic 'defects' leads to the labelling of large groups of people as 'defective'. Not only the people who manifest the condition but also the carriers are likely to be less than perfect. Such tests are usually considered to be altogether helpful because they increase people's choices, but it would be a mistake to ignore the ideology that almost inevitably accompanies their use ... Any suggestion that society would be better off if certain kinds of people were not born puts us on a slippery slope (1997, pp. 24–5).

The second 'lesson of history' relates to the first: that political conservatives have often used biology to explain the social order, including structured forms of social inequality, and thus legitimate their own privileged position in the social order. A historical example is the disease pellagra, which reached epidemic proportions in the American South in the early part of this century. Pellagra is a chronic condition involving skin lesions, nervous and muscular disturbances, and eventual mental deterioration, and eugenicists assumed that its causation was hereditary and therefore irremediable by social programs. However, in 1919, an epidemiologist discovered the condition to be the result of a dietary deficiency of niacin, a member of the vitamin B complex group, which is commonly found in vegetables and grains that were missing from the diet of many sufferers (see Hubbard & Wald 1997, p. 17). Yet conservative Republican administrations resisted the funding of nutrition programs until the Democrats introduced the New Deal in 1933.

The third lesson is that the unintended consequences of using genetic information cannot be predicted easily in advance. Sickle cell anaemia is a genetic condition that disproportionately affects people of African descent. In the 1970s it was supposed (wrongly as it turned out) that altitude posed a hazard to people who were susceptible to sickle cell anaemia (they were thought less able to withstand the stress of low oxygen at high altitude). This was used as grounds for excluding, for instance, African Americans from employment in the US Air Force (see Hubbard & Wald 1997, pp. 33–4).

The final lesson to be learnt here is that, once developed, a technology can be put to uses not at first envisaged. An example is the development of amniocentesis to predict birth defects in the foetus. This technology could also be used to determine sex, and then could become widely used to practise selected female infanticide in cultures that traditionally favour male children (including affluent countries). Likewise, the genetically engineered human growth hormone (HGH) was first developed to treat pituitary dwarfism (see Hubbard & Wald 1997, pp. 69–70). However, the number of people who suffer from this condition, and hence the market for the product, is relatively small. In an attempt to improve the market for the product, HGH has been marketed to (wealthy) parents of children who are at the short end of the normal height range but who understand the social advantages of height, especially for men. There is also an emerging 'black market' in body-building circles, where HGH is the latest performance-enhancing substance, replacing anabolic steroids. Because it is naturally occurring, this latest form of cheating cannot be detected by any drug test and is therefore attractive to sportspeople. Another looming consequence is the controversial suggestion that HGH might slow some of the ageing processes (Wilkie 1994, pp. 62, 136).

In the same way, advances in prenatal genetic diagnosis is enabling parents to make decisions in the genetic supermarket, not only about how 'perfect' the child has to be ('Shall we abort this foetus, which has been shown to carry the gene for baldness?'), but also about what sort of child they want to bear. An example is the couple, both of whom were dwarfs, who chose to abort a foetus because it was not also a dwarf but was expected to be within the normal height distribution (Fisher 1996, pp. 19–20). The apparent discovery of a gene for obesity (the so-called 'fat gene') and the likelihood of the development of a gene therapy to treat the condition may well have similar consequences. For those in the population who are medically defined as 'morbidly obese', the discovery may well have benefits for health and longevity (so long as they can afford the technology), but it is likely also to be used by some who are within the normal weight range but who will attempt, through self-starvation, to be extremely slender for social reasons.

Culture

A cultural sensibility is the second feature of a sociological analysis. It enables a consideration of the social context into which technologies are introduced and through which they are shaped. These technologies are linked to the cultural preoccupations of those societies. This is seen most clearly in the USA, where the gene has become a cultural icon that:

> intersects with important American cultural values. Genetic explana-
> tions appear to locate social problems within the individual rather
> than in society, conforming to the ideology of individualism. They
> are thus a convenient way to address troubling social issues; the
> threats implied by the changing roles of women, the perceived
> decline of the family, the problems of crime, the changes in the racial
> and ethnic structure of American society and the failure of welfare
> programs (Nelkin & Lindee 1995, p. 194).

In the USA, for instance, the claim has been made in the behavioural genetics field that the HGP will provide a 'cure' for much homelessness. According to one of the staunch advocates of the HGP—the editor of the journal *Science*, Daniel Koshland (1989, p. 189)—since many homeless people suffer from mental disorders, which the HGP will show have a genetic basis, then the knowledge gained from the project will lead to a cure or treatment for homelessness (see Beckwith 1991, p. 6).

In a similar vein, it is asserted that the main potential benefit of screening tests is that they permit the avoidance of transmitting the 'problematic' gene to future generations. The technology used to achieve this benefit is termination of pregnancy following pre-natal diagnosis. The politics of abortion in different countries, especially the USA, will affect the social acceptability of benefit-ing from prenatal diagnosis. Certainly, the social and political process makes for interesting conflict, with both feminist groups and 'pro-life', anti-abortion groups involved. The implications of advances in the genetic understanding of diseases, and therefore of the HGP itself, are inextricably linked with the issue of abortion (Schwartz-Cowan 1992, p. 246).

Another cultural issue relates to how particular genetic diseases are more commonly associated with particular ethnic groups. Cystic fibrosis is most common among people of Caucasian descent, thalassemia among those of Mediterranean and South-East Asian descent, Tay-Sachs disease among the Jewish population, and sickle cell anaemia among those of African descent. This raises the possibility of culturally specific solutions to these problems. One such community solution—to combat Tay-Sachs disease in the Jewish communities in New York and Israel—is a mate selection organisation called Chevra Dor Yeshorim (the Association of an Upright Generation). Tay-Sachs disease is a particularly unpleasant genetically transmitted disease that causes children to die at an early age. The service operates as a premarital genetic screening agency.

When a person begins to date someone from within the community, that person is able to dial up this agency, provide a six-digit code, which will identify the other person, and be told if that other person has genes not only for Tay-Sachs but also for cystic fibrosis and Gaucher's Disease. It functions as a sort of genetic roadworthy test and apparently enjoys a high degree of community support as an effective means of avoiding the transmission of major genetic defects. Would such agencies be likely to occur on a wider scale in society as a whole? Is it considered culturally appropriate only because it occurs in a community in which arranged marriage is not unknown? Certainly it raises the possibility of creating 'genetic wallflowers', whom nobody may want to marry because of their genes.

Structure

A structural sensibility involves considering the aspects of social organisation that influence both the social impact and the social shaping of emerging biotechnologies. How do different societal contexts affect the ways in which technologies are introduced and used? These result from the differing characteristics of the various societies into which these biotechnologies are introduced. A couple of examples will illustrate this point. In the USA, the lack of a universal health insurance scheme funded through taxation (as exists in most other developed countries) means that there is a greater likelihood that developments in molecular biology will result in abuses of genetic knowledge. Medicare in Australia—like the National Health Service in the United Kingdom—will shield 'genetically impaired' people from many of the adverse consequences faced by those Americans who rely on their employment for health insurance. Hence the likelihood of discrimination on the basis of an individual's genetic make-up is a greater fear for Americans than it is for Australians.

A second example involves different attitudes to the patenting of discoveries, which have been a source of conflict between the different countries involved in the project (see Cook-Deegan 1994). It has traditionally been thought that scientific activity necessarily involves cooperation between scientists in order to maximise progress. The patenting of individual genes to allow biotechnology companies, funded through venture capital, to 'cash in' on these discoveries has been considered more acceptable within the political economy context of the USA than elsewhere. The latter stages of the project indeed have become a race to complete the genome sequencing process, characterised by considerable public squabbling. On one side, private venture capitalist firms, notably Celera Genomoics, hope to become the Microsoft of the biotechnology industry by selling its information. On the other side, government agencies aim as much as possible to keep the knowledge in the public domain. In other cultural contexts, the response has been different. The European Community has decided not to allow contractors in the HGP to exploit on an exclusive basis any property rights arising from discoveries (Commission of the European Communities 1989, cited in Kevles & Hood 1992, p. 314). It has been suggested that United States investment in the HGP has been directed at giving the USA a competitive edge in the burgeoning biotechnology marketplace (see Rose 1994). So, throughout the HGP so far, something of a contradiction has existed between international cooperation, which has traditionally been one of the norms of scientific activity, on the one hand, and national interest, in the form of enhancing competitiveness through private control, on the other. The challenge is to maintain international competitiveness in the face of high commercial stakes (Kevles & Hood 1992, p. 315).

genetic reductionism An assumption that people are simply the sum of their individual genes, so that the causes of disease are reduced to an individual's genes rather than the social, economic, and political context in which they live. See 'biological determinism'.

The politico-economic context is important in understanding the HGP. The project was conceived under the Reagan administration, during which the causes of disease were held to be based in an individual's genes rather than the wider social context. This is **genetic reductionism**, a form of biological reductionism. According to this view, individuals are the sum of their genes and represent the latest version of the 'biology is destiny' scheme—a sort of 'genes–R–us' approach. It is a new twist to social Darwinism and **sociobiology**. In the past, the search was for 'germs'. The Rockefeller Foundation, for instance, funded research into germs for laziness in the 1930s in the American South (see Brown 1979). Now it is genes. The move from germs to genes focuses attention away from the social environment. As Hilary Rose (1994, p. 173) argues, '[t]his new genetics, a product of an alliance between an aggressively entrepreneurial culture and life sciences, fused the conservatism of biology as destiny with the modernist philosophy of **genetic manipulation**'. It is a **modernist** project in the sense that it is based on a belief that the problems faced by humanity can be solved by rational applications of science and technology.

sociobiology A theory of evolutionary biology, associated with E. O. Wilson, that seeks to explain the evolution of social organisation and social behaviour as based on biological characteristics.

genetic manipulation Alteration of the genetic material of living cells to perform new functions (by rearranging or deleting existing genes), including the transferral of genetic information from one species to another.

modernism A view of the possibilities and direction of social life that is grounded in a faith in rational thought. From a modernist perspective, truth, beauty, and morality exist as objective realities that can be discovered and understood through rational and scientific means. These themes are rejected by postmodernists.

Criticism

A critical sensibility involves asking 'how could it be otherwise?' It involves paying attention to the social policy implications of these technological developments. There are a number of biotechnologies that have been mooted as arising out of the HGP. Gene therapies, long mooted as a hoped-for technological development are still largely at the potential, 'cautious optimism' stage of development. A recent technology assessment report from Norway found that although there have been several thousand articles published on gene therapy, with between three and four thousand people treated with different gene therapy strategies, in more than 400 clinical studies, with the exception of a treatment for eye infections in AIDS patients, gene therapy is not yet an established treatment modality for any disease today (Kolberg 2000).

The most widespread technology being developed by the project is genetic screening tests. These are the main commercial products being developed by biotechnology companies on the basis of their patented discoveries. A screening test can tell if the individual has the 'defective gene' and is therefore at a higher than normal risk of developing an ill-health condition. In social policy terms, the crucial question is 'under what circumstances is the knowledge gained on the basis of screening likely to be oppressive or liberating for the individual?' The relationship between 'oppressive' and 'liberating' should be thought of as a continuum rather than a dichotomy; there are likely to be degrees of each. Would one want to know if one carried the genes for a particular condition? The social policy aim is to maximise benefits and minimise drawbacks. There are likely to be elements of both; there are some conditions that appear to have a heritable basis, for which the benefits of screening are relatively clear. Phenylketonuria (PKU) is an example, for which mandatory screening (using 'the heel-prick test') has operated effectively with community support in many countries. With this condition, a course of action is available that benefits the individual. However, with other supposedly genetically caused phenomena, the benefits are very mixed. An example is the so-called (hypothetical) gene for homosexuality (see Hubbard & Wald 1997, pp. 94–8; *Time* 13 November 1995, p. 67). If homosexuality is genetically determined, then it must be 'natural', so any form of discrimination on the basis of sexual preference would be clearly inappropriate. In that sense its discovery would be liberating. But there are also drawbacks. If it is genetically determined, then the likelihood of having a homosexual child can also be screened for. I would hazard a guess that there are still a significant number of parents who would choose to abort such a foetus and try again. This outcome would hardly be liberating for the gay community or for the child itself. James Watson, the first director of the HGP, stirred controversy when he was reported as advocating the right of parents to abort their unborn babies if they were found to be carrying a hypothetical gene for homosexuality (*Age*, 17 February 1997). However, a more basic and immediate problem is that, with many conditions (for which the gene has been located), nothing can be done for the person. Huntington's disease is an example of this: onset of the disease occurs in the mature adult, and people die unpleasantly over a long period of time. In this case, a legitimate question is 'why would people want to know?' Is knowing that you are likely to develop Huntingdon's disease in your forties or fifties likely to be liberating or oppressive? (see Cox & McKellin 1999).

There appear to be two types of relationship between the presence of genes and the health outcomes that those genes suggest. One is direct, as occurs with the heritable cancers. The presence of the gene brings a considerably enhanced probability of the onset of cancer. The second is more indirect, with the presence of the gene implying only a predisposition to certain diseases—in effect, a recognition of the complex interaction between genotypes and environmental factors.

Similar issues exist, of course, with all screening. It needs to be asked, 'if screening is the answer, what is the question?' For what purpose is screening being done? There is a classic tension in sociological terms between the individual and society. How can the individual ends be reconciled with the collective ends? The collective ends are public health ends, and this tension is, of course, the basis of the controversy surrounding eugenics. What level of coercion of individuals is acceptable in the interests of public health? This has been a big issue in terms of managing public health over a very long period of time. Some degree of compulsion is accepted—as, for example, with recent community controversies over the immunisation of children. But what is already occurring is that screening is increasingly being used for the societal purposes of **social control** and surveillance of populations. Often nothing can be done for the individual concerned, but there are lots of benefits to others in knowing an individual's genetic make-up. Screening may have liberating consequences in the future, but it is already having oppressive consequences. It opens the way for the individual to be discriminated against in various ways. **Geneism** is starting to take its place alongside other forms of discrimination, such as **racism**, sexism, and **ageism**. What they have in common is the allocation of social rewards on the basis of ascribed rather than achieved status; on the basis of what an individual is born like rather than what that person achieves in life. This goes against the whole thrust of social policy in recent decades, especially social justice policies, according to which social rewards should be allocated on the basis of achievement.

Geneism has becoming apparent, especially in the USA, as information about people's genes is increasingly being used for social-control purposes. It is used to deny access to certain socially desired ends, such as life and health insurance, employment, and even driver's licences (see Billings et al. 1992). In Australia, there

social control Mechanisms that aim to induce conformity, or at least to manage or minimise deviant behaviour.

geneism A form of discrimination—like racism, sexism, and ageism—in which people are judged on their ascribed, rather than achieved, status. In this case, their genetic make-up is used as the basis for determining access to social rewards such as employment or health insurance.

racism Beliefs and actions used to discriminate against a group of people because of their physical and cultural characteristics.

ageism A term, like 'sexism' and 'racism', that denotes discrimination, in this case, discrimination based on age.

has been some evidence of this form of discrimination emerging. David Keays, a law researcher at the University of Melbourne, has uncovered several cases, including:

- A 34-year-old ophthalmologist refused a bank loan to buy equipment unless he obtained income insurance. He was refused cover unless he passed a genetic test for myotonic dystrophy, a muscular disease that runs in his family. He took the test, found he didn't have the gene, and obtained the loan.

- An 18-year-old school-leaver denied a public service job unless he passed a genetic test for Huntington's disease, a severe condition that hits in middle age. He had a 50-50 chance of having the gene but, having seen his mother suffer, preferred not to know. At times he threatened to kill himself if he ever found out. On a second appeal, he was offered the job—with reduced superannuation.

- A 37-year-old quality manager refused an increase in a preexisting income insurance policy after a research project genetic test revealed he had Charcot-Marie-Tooth disease—a physical condition that, even if it progressed from its mild state, would not affect his ability to earn income in his deskbound work (Button 2000).

So geneism is a current phenomenon, not simply something that may occur in the future. Furthermore in countries like Australia, it will probably not be very long before immigration authorities propose genetic screening to exclude potential immigrants as a means of avoiding future impost on the country's health system, in the same way that HIV testing has been mandatory for potential immigrants for some time.

Moreover, there appears to be a clear political program attached to the HGP, which helps to explain how it is funded, given the blanket influence of neo-conservative economics around the globe and the hegemony of post-Cold War American values. This context is important in relation to the project's role in providing a rationale and a justification for inequality. The emphasis is upon a genetic form of **biological determinism**: people are the way they are because of their genes rather than the sort of society in which they live. Therefore, government programs are not likely to have any impact, as inequality is determined by nature, not by culture. As is occurring in the USA, social justice and welfare programs can legitimately be abolished, and tax cuts can be made that will disproportionately benefit the rich. Social policy considerations of equity issues feature largely here, especially equity of resource allocation. In the context of the USA, for instance, these changes are occurring at a time when, in the absence of a universal health insurance scheme, 40 million

biological determinism The unproven belief that people's biology determines their social, economic, and health statuses.

American citizens have no health insurance at all and major illness can expose these people to financial ruin. The issue is even more apparent on a world scale, where many more people die of simple preventable diseases, such as malnutrition and infectious diseases, than of genetic diseases. Individual treatments based on genetic therapies will probably never be affordable by the majority of the world's population. Furthermore, the deterioration in the world environment is likely to take a greater toll on human health than genetic disease ever will. Access to basic nutrition and basic medical care is likely to remain a greater priority for most people, with the promised benefits of the new genetic medicine remaining out of reach for all but an affluent few in the richest countries (see Beardsley 1996).

Future directions

The ramifications of the HGP on the sort of society in which we live are likely to be considerable. Understanding these implications from a sociological point of view involves considering the four core sensibilities of sociological explanation: historical, cultural, structural, and critical sensibilities. I have outlined how these sensibilities illuminate the sociological issues, as well as the related social policy question of how the benefits can be maximised and the drawbacks minimised. How can the tensions between individual and collective uses of the technologies arising from the new genetics be reconciled? If there are to be benefits flowing from widespread genetic testing, then, arguably, considerably more attention will need to be given to the social implications and consequences of this testing for those benefits to be realised.

But there is one other benefit flowing from a sociological awareness of these issues, and it acts as something of an antidote to the daily hype surrounding developments in biotechnology. A sociological perspective with the inherent reflexivity or scepticism, which is a key feature of a sociological imagination, demands that the 'technophoria' with which many developments are reported be taken with a metaphorical grain (even lump) of salt. It enables, even requires, questions to be asked, such as:

*   Who benefits from these developments?
*   Is the knowledge generated likely to be oppressive or liberating for the individuals concerned?
*   What are the likely societal implications arising out of this development?
*   Are there likely to be drawbacks associated with this knowledge, and if so, what can be done about them?

Articulating questions of this sort is what sociology, in its search for alternative futures, seeks to do.

Summary of main points

- Rapid developments have occurred in the understanding of the genetic basis to ill health. Understanding the social impact of these findings, however, lags far behind.
- There is an emerging tension between individual and collective uses of the biotechnologies being developed.
- Considering the social impact of new medical technologies is only part of the sociological task. The other part concerns understanding the social shaping of those technologies.
- In social policy terms, the focus is upon how to maximise any benefits that may flow from these biotechnologies, as well as how to minimise any drawbacks.
- Consideration of the historical, cultural, structural, and critical elements that together comprise a sociological perspective provides something of a balance to the 'technophoria' surrounding many of these developments.

Discussion questions

1 What is the difference between the social-shaping and the social-impact aspects of the relationship between (medical) technology and society?
2 In what ways are advances in genetic medicine linked to issues about abortion?
3 What is geneism? How can we as a society prevent genetic testing being used as the basis for discrimination?
4 What are the social implications of theories alleging the genetic basis of human behaviour?
5 What are the social policy considerations that are important to understanding the HGP?
6 In your view, how can any tension between individual and collective uses of genetic biotechnologies be reconciled?

Further investigation

1 What can sociology offer to an understanding of the likely implications of the Human Genome Project for society?
2 'Analysing the relationship between technology and society requires a consideration not only of the impact of new technologies on society, but also how the technology is shaped by society.' Discuss in relation to the Human Genome Project.

Further reading, web, and film resources

Hubbard, R. & Wald, E. 1997, *Exploding the Gene Myth*, revised edn, Beacon Press, Boston.

Nelkin, D. & Lindee, S. 1995, *The DNA Mystique: The Gene as a Cultural Icon*, Freeman and Co., New York.

Richards, M. P. M. 1993, 'The New Genetics: Some Issues for Social Scientists', *Sociology of Health and Illness*, vol. 15, no. 5, pp. 567–86.

Wilkie, T. 1994, *Perilous Knowledge: The Human Genome Project and Its Implications*, Faber & Faber, London.

Web sites

Centre for Law and Genetics—based mainly at the University of Tasmania, this site focuses on the legal and ethical aspects of the HGP and has a searchable database of materials: <www.lawgenecentre.org>

Council for Responsible Genetics—a United States activist organisation, this site contains a number of position papers on issues of relevance: <www.gene-watch.org>

National Human Genome Research Institute—a body of the United States National Institute of Health, this is close to being the 'official' HGP web site. Details of the ELSI program (ethical, legal, and social aspects of the project) may be found here: <www.nhgri.nih.gov>. See also <www.ornl.gov/hgmis>

Film

Gattaca, 1997, Columbia Pictures. Written and directed by Andrew Niccol. 102 minutes. Borrow the film from the local video store. View it as a means of thinking about the social and ethical issues associated with the new genetics, especially pre-implantation genetic diagnosis from 'the genetic supermarket'. The film's rather negative and sensationalist view has been analysed in an essay by Colin Gavaghan entitled 'Off-the-peg offspring in the genetic supermarket', which can be found at: <http://www.philosophynow.demon.co.uk/offspring.htm>

12

Ageing, Dying, and Death as the Twenty-first Century Begins

Maureen Strazzari

Overview

✱ *What are the prevailing social attitudes towards death and dying?*
✱ *How are ageing, death, and dying experienced in Western society?*
✱ *What is ageism?*

This chapter is concerned with the social construction of ageing, death, and dying in contemporary Australia. Experts are involved in institutional policy decisions, some arguing that the aged are a 'social burden', placing a strain on health and other resources as they become frail and immobile. While death, statistically, is postponed until old age for non-Indigenous Australians, there is an increased awareness of the risks associated with contemporary living and of ever-emerging new risks, which generate fears of death and suffering, even among the young. Medical life and death decisions have become complex as the boundaries between life and death have become blurred. Significantly, these decisions are being made within an environment of economic rationalism, with pressure on medical and health professions to cut health care costs. Medical, legal, and other discourses associated with the process of dying have provided a contemporary language for discussing death, but these discourses do not address 'ontological insecurity' (Giddens 1991); that is, existential concerns that are likely to emerge in the experience of dying.

Key terms

ageism	globalisation
class	ideology
collective conscience	individualism
discourse	medicalisation
ethnicity	public health
economic rationalism	social construction
euthanasia	social death
gross domestic product (GDP)	state
gender	

Introduction

social construction/

constructionism Refers to the socially created characteristics of human life based on the idea that people act-ively construct reality, meaning it is neither 'natural' nor inevitable. Therefore, notions of normality/abnormality, right/ wrong, and health/illness are subjective human creations that should not be taken for granted.

globalisation Political, social, economic, and cultural develop-ments—such as the spread of multinational companies, infor-mation technology, and the role of international agencies—that result in people's lives being increasingly influenced by global, rather than national or local, factors.

Biological life and death are not of themselves the reality that people experience and to which they respond. What is perceived as real and normal about events and processes such as ageing, dying and death is **socially constructed**, and depends on the historical, social, and cultural contexts in which they occur and are given meaning. At the beginning of the twenty-first century in Australia, for example, the death of a young person is considered tragic because it is 'premature'. Not too far back in history, however, it was normal for the young to die; to reach old age was extraordinary.

Age structures are shifting radically as populations age, and it is predicted that this phenomenon will continue to have profound implications within the areas of health and medicine, as well as in the broader social, political, and economic spheres. These social processes are deeply connected with people's lives. Anthony Giddens (1991) argues that a characteristic of 'late modernity' (which is what he calls present-day society) is the interconnection of individual experiences with **globalisation**. People may have little, if any, personal contact with death, but television brings into their homes graphic and selected images of death and dying from around the globe—'bringing the world back home'. At the insti-tutional level, international agencies influence national policies, which affect individuals. Recommendations of the World Health Organization (WHO), for example, become translated into Australian health policies. These policies are reflected in health promotion and education activities, which assist people to main-tain their health into old age. These are contemporary resources and strategies, which have become available, and which are replacing traditional relationships (Giddens 1991). In times of per-sonal crisis, for example, severe illness or bereavement, modern experts—doctors or counsellors—are more likely to be sought for guidance than is a priest. The terms 'life span' and 'life cycle' are representative of changes in life and death meanings. Once the life cycle linked the generations, and resonated with the seasonal cycles of nature. The cyclical notion of renewal following death provided death with meaning. No effort was required to believe in life after death, as it appeared to be perfectly natural that this was so. The life span, by contrast, is linear. It has a definite begin-ning and end. What can and ought to be done to improve the quality of the life span, and how it can be extended, are empha-sised. Differences, even conflict, between generations are highlighted, for example between the baby boomers and genera-tion X. The baby boomers, stereotypically, are accused of spending their children's inheritance or conversely of becoming the 'sand-wich' generation, 'caught between parents who are living longer and children who won't leave home' (Sampson 2000). As Giddens (1991) argues, life in late modernity is profoundly different from life in earlier times. In his analysis the contemporary social world is forever changing, with an array of novel resources, previously unimaginable, becoming available to individuals to create their own lifestyle, while traditional linkages, such as close family ties, lose significance. Giddens (1991) acknowledges that disadvantaged groups are marginalised or excluded from the new opportunities. Moreover, death, he argues, has been sequestered from social life. Not only has it physically been removed to the hospital, but questions and anxieties arising from the universality of human finitude have, at least until very recently, been repressed.

The health and medical care that elderly people can expect to receive is the result of institutional planning and strategies. Other social responses to the ageing population come from those experts who contribute to bodies of knowledge that affect experiences of ageing and old age. Expert knowledge informs health and medical practices, and influences or directly advises government policy-makers. In Australia people continue to die in hospitals, but hospices and palliative care have come to be associated with dying. **Euthanasia**, although illegal in Australia, is receiving support as an alternative 'good death', while also generating controversy. Opinions concerning euthanasia are deeply divided among health and medical professionals. This may affect relationships between professional carers who are sharing the care of patients. The wider social context within which health and medicine are practised—especially economic and political concerns about escalating public health and medical costs—cannot be excluded from consideration. What are the consequences of all these conditions for the ways that ageing, death, and dying are experienced?

euthanasia Meaning 'gentle death', the term is used to describe voluntary death, often medically assisted, as a result of incurable and painful disease.

Historical overview

In Australia the average life expectancy at birth in 1997 was 75.9 years for males and 81.5 years for females (AIHW 2000). It is estimated that there will be dramatic increases in the numbers of people aged 65 years and over living in Australia when the so-called baby boom generation (those born between 1946 and 1965) reach the age of 65 years and over. With people living longer, the number of people in their eighties and over is also expected to grow significantly (see Table 12.1). The baby boom generation is so named to describe the spate of births during the above years. It is perhaps surprising to learn that 20 per cent or more of Australian women born between 1861 and 1913 did not have children. The baby boomers were produced by women born in the 1930s and 1940s, of whom only 8–10 per cent did not have children (ABS 1994). The current trend towards a lower birth rate is therefore a reversion rather than a new phenomenon, but it needs to be borne in mind that there are specific social conditions in any historical era that shape birth patterns. Children of post-World War II migrants contribute to the baby boom generation, for example. Their migrant parents, such as those from Italy and Poland, are now aged and ageing cohorts and this is reflected in their high mortality rates.

Table 12.1   Australia's ageing population

	Aged 65 and over	Aged 85 and over	
	% of total population	% aged 65 and over	% of total population
1901	4.0	2.8	0.1
1998	12.2	10.0	1.2
2051 (projected)	24.2	18.8	4.5

Source: Adapted from ABS 1999a

Every country in the world is experiencing a trend towards ageing, but there are still large discrepancies both between and within countries. In some poor countries, most people still live only to about 45–50 years of age, and large numbers of children do not reach their fifth birthday (World Bank 1993). Death still occurs at an earlier age for many Australian Aborigines and Torres Strait Islanders than is normal for the rest of the population. The life expectancy for Aboriginal and Torres Strait Islander males is 57, and for females it is 62 (ABS 1998).

Throughout Western history, until relatively recently, it was uncommon for people to live into old age. Little could be done to control epidemics, diseases, infections, and childbirth complications. Historian Philippe Aries (1981) suggests that, because of this, death remained 'tame' throughout most of the long history of Western civilisation; it had to be accepted as fate. Fate offered the solace of a better existence in the next world for those who righteously accepted life in this world as a 'vale of tears'. Slowly people became aware that life conditions were not completely out of their control and that action could be taken to improve some situations. The Enlightenment—an eighteenth-century intellectual movement—marked the beginning of a growing optimism that there were secular answers to life's problems. Causes, and therefore prevention and cures, of illness and disease could be discovered. Medical interventions such as vaccinations and antibiotics have generally been credited with the decline in mortality that has occurred in Western societies. Against this, it has been argued that public health measures, introduced earlier through quarantine and sanitary reform, were the reason for decline in disease. No doubt both public health measures and medical treatments have contributed to people living longer. Better standards of living—including working conditions, accommodation, availability and affordability of nutritious food, and education—have also made a significant contribution.

The medical profession came to occupy a position of dominance in the health area, symbolised and institutionalised by the establishment of the prestigious modern hospital. Fighting to save lives became a central task of hospitals, which also became the sites at which deaths occurred when the battles were lost. Dying and death were thus removed from the homes and neighbourhoods where they had always resided, thereby becoming separated from everyday life. The idea that death can be avoided or postponed indefinitely is fostered as people live increasingly longer lives, and younger deaths are seen as premature and abnormal. Optimism is invoked by claims that quality of life can be enhanced or maintained by healthy living. A steady stream of media reports inform people of the promising results of new curative or preventative research findings. Medical technology has become very sophisticated and expensive. People can be kept alive through surgical procedures such as heart bypasses, organ transplantations, as well as continually updated pharmaceutical drugs and technological therapies. The mapping of the human genome has produced radical promises for the elimination of hereditary diseases.

Somewhat paradoxically in the light of these actual and potential achievements aimed at conquering death, together with the institutional sequestering of death, dying and death are returning to everyday life. The limitations of medical technology's endeavour to eliminate diseases are apparent in the chronic, sometimes debilitating, ailments associated with ageing. Also, technology blurs the distinction between life and death: is chemotherapy, for instance, prolonging life or prolonging the dying process? With increasing awareness of risk, and of ever-emerging new risks, life seems dramatically less secure. Death may be lurking in unprotected sex, contaminated food, the very air we breathe.

The social construction of old age

There are considerable differences in social and cultural responses to old age and hence in meanings and experiences associated with old age, some of which are discussed in this chapter. Subjectively, people have very different views of when old age begins. Thirty years of age can seem old to children, but in today's society, where everyone is encouraged to lead a healthy, active lifestyle, many aged people may not feel old. Nevertheless, the loss of a youthful appearance may be difficult to accept in today's society where youthful bodies that are 'taut and terrific' are displayed in the media as the norm to be desired and achieved. The following excerpt is from a tongue-in-cheek reply, in the *Sydney Morning Herald*'s magazine, *Good Weekend*, to a reader's question asking whether it is wrong to lie about her age. Despite its humour, the question and response illustrate prevailing attitudes regarding age:

> ... [it] makes sense in theory [that] if women aren't willing to stand up and have their crow's feet counted, then society's obsession with youth and firm upper arms continues unchallenged. But, in practice, things are not so clear-cut. 'Age modification' is not just about vanity, it's about survival, too. For men as well as women.
>
> Growing old is now a luxury most of us just can't afford ... These days, we're 40, but our kids are still in preschool, we've topped up the mortgage to pay for renovations, cashed in our super to start a new career, and watched while our parents squander our inheritance on state-of-the-art hip replacements and 'lifestyle condominiums'. Who's got the cash to turn 50?
>
> Of course, it's no accident, M.S., that your 'age enhancement' began at work. In an ageist corporate culture, midlife birthdays are less likely to be celebrated with a cheesecake at morning tea than acknowledged with a package over lunch—a retrenchment package! (Sayer-Jones 2001, p. 9).

When do people become old?

For much of the twentieth century, the legal age for male retirement from the workforce has been 65 years, and this age became the hallmark of a socially defined 'old age' in countries such as Australia. From the latter part of the twentieth century there have been dramatic changes that have confused meanings of old age. Economists continue to assume that 65 years marks the start of old-age dependence (National Commission of Audit 1996, p. 126), and national aged populations are defined as those 65 years of age and over. Moreover, the statutory age for women to receive an age pension has been progressively rising from 1994 and from 2004 will be 65 years, the same as the retirement age for men. These classifications are in contradiction with the marked shift that has been occurring in the requirements of the labour market. Modern and constantly developing technology and computerisation require fewer workers with different types of skills. Workers are now referred to as resources—human resources—who become redundant as their skills become outdated and as companies 'downsize'. Within this process people are finding themselves unemployed in their forties or fifties with no prospect of further employment, as employers all too often consider that people of this age are too old to be retrained. Australian men aged between 55 to 59 years are particularly affected by this trend. 'Early retirement', rather than redundancy or involuntary retirement, is often used to describe the decline in the labour force participation rates for older males, giving the false impression that leaving work has been their personal choice. No distinction is made between the relatively few who leave work with substantial pay-outs from superannuation funds and/or 'separation packages' from their employers, and who have opportunities for future employment, and the many who are simply given notice that their employment is terminated, with no prospect of employment ahead of them.

Retirement incomes in transition: changing experiences of old age

After Federation in Australia a national provision for a flat-rate age pension was introduced, and the age pension has remained the retirement income of most Australians, although this is now changing. The pension income in Australia is low in comparison with that in other major developed countries such as Canada, Germany, Japan, the Netherlands, New Zealand, and the USA, and extremely low in comparison with that in France and Italy, where citizens can expect to maintain incomes at a similar level to their working wage, owing to the historical arrangements in those countries of a universal flat-rate pension, combined with an earnings-related system (King, Walker, & Harding 1999). Australia also has the lowest amount of public spending on pensions as a proportion of **gross domestic product (GDP)**. Table 12.2 illustrates these comparisons.

gross domestic product (GDP)
The market value of all goods and services that have been sold during a year.

King, Walker, and Harding (1999) state that Australia's system, by relying less on public spending on pensions as a proportion of GDP than other comparable countries, will be more sustainable over time, minimising the economic burden of expected large

Table 12.2   Pension income as proportion of non-pension income and public spending on pensions as a proportion of GDP—selected countries

Country	Income of couple pensioners as proportion of income of all non-pensioners (%)	Public spending on pensions as a proportion of GDP, 1995 (%)
Australia	68	2.6
Canada	85	5.2
France	103	10.6
Germany	92	11.1
Italy	81	13.3 (including 2.1% on disability pensions)
Netherlands	84	5.9
United Kingdom	83	4.5 (pensions, plus 1.1% means-tested benefits)
USA	85	4.1 (plus 3.5% on Medicare and means-tested programs)

Source: Adapted from King, Walker, & Harding 1999

numbers of aged baby boomers. European countries, however, have been experiencing ageing populations for a longer period of time than has Australia, without crisis, at least thus far. Figure 12.1 provides a comparison of the proportion of population older than 65 in selected countries for 1995, and their projections into 2050, and shows that ageing populations will continue to increase over that period. It should be noted that there may be projection variations, owing to differences in assumptions and methodology.

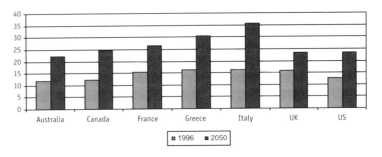

Figure 12.1 Proportion of population aged over 65 years and over—selected countries

Source: Adapted from ABS 1999d

Although the Australian pension is low by international comparisons, because most Australian retirees have relied solely on the aged pension, their income, until recently, has been more equitably distributed than in other countries. There have been exceptions. Public service employees, for example, historically, have been covered by generous superannuation schemes. Nevertheless, throughout the industrial era Australians perceived their modest, non-contributory pension as an acknowledgment of them as citizens who had contributed to the country by their years of hard work and taxes paid. Old age had a different meaning then, when most Australians relied on the pension, which they saw as their due, and when consumerism, **individualism** and **economic rationalism** had not yet become dominant.

At present the Australian retirement system is in a state of transition. Concerned about the demographic wave of old age that is approaching and its impact on the public purse, the government is seeking to limit the age pension to a safety net for those most in need, while others are expected to provide for their own retirement. A compulsory Superannuation Guarantee scheme, introduced in 1992, requires employers whose employees earn $450 a month or more to make superannuation contributions on behalf of their employees to private superannuation funds. The level of superannuation under this scheme commenced at 3 per cent, is currently at 7 per cent, and will increase until it reaches 9 per cent

individualism/individualisation
A belief or process supporting the primacy of individual choice, freedom, and self-responsibility.

economic rationalism or economic liberalism Terms used to describe a political philosophy based on 'small-government' and market-oriented policies, such as deregulation, privatisation, reduced government spending, and lower taxation.

in 2002. Australians are also encouraged to make voluntary savings towards their old age, and are given taxation deductions for taking out their own superannuation. The government's assumption is that Australians are individually responsible for planning their own future, and that they have a wide range of choices in making decisions to maximise their retirement (Bishop 1999).

Given these changes, in contrast to much of the twentieth century, it seems likely that experiences of old age in the twenty-first century will be individualised, as the greater the disposable incomes that individuals have, the more chance they have of investing their money, or paying higher levels of superannuation, in order to maximise their retirement income. Greater disparity between retirement incomes is likely between those with the resources to plan ahead and save for their retirement and others unable to do so. Low paid workers and those with limited participation in the workforce, for example many women, and workers in industries where there is a practice of employing labour on a casual basis, will remain dependent on the age pension.

The Superannuation Guarantee scheme is theoretically mobile but a lack of coordination means that people who can find only a series of casual occupations may have to keep track of their savings in a number of private funds, which are then eroded by administrative costs and transfer fees. Also, people whose wages may be barely adequate are forced to regularly forfeit a portion in order to save for their old age without a **state** guarantee that their savings are safe. Government does not guarantee workers' entitlements, including employer contributions to superannuation. Entitlements can be lost, for example when companies set up a shelf company—that is, a legal, but nonetheless bogus, company—which becomes the employing firm, and which is liquidated with no assets to pay workers' entitlements, or when their employer does not comply with the law to pay regular superannuation contributions on behalf of employees. Retirement income is inherently risky as private trustees may lose their clients' savings through the volatility of the share market or make poor investments of their funds. Whereas young people are now held responsible to save for security in their old age, for many people, saving for old age is beyond their control.

state A term used to describe a collection of institutions, including the parliament (government and Opposition political parties), the public-sector bureaucracy, the judiciary, the military, and the police.

Ageism

ageism A term, like 'sexism' and 'racism', that denotes discrimination, in this case, discrimination based on age.

Ageism, according to Hepworth (1995, p. 177), is 'prejudice against older people collectively stereotyped as a section of the population disqualified by reason of the chronological age from making a full contribution to society'. A popular belief is that derision of old age is a characteristic of modern Western society, whereas in earlier times, or in other cultures, the elderly were or are respected for their wisdom, but historical studies have revealed ambivalent attitudes towards the elderly—that is, attitudes that fluctuate between being favourably and unfavourably disposed (Bytheway 1995). The significant question is how ageism is constructed in today's society. An example has already been mentioned above—Australian males, especially, are excluded from the workforce in their forties and fifties and considered too old for retraining, thus experiencing ageism at an early age. Memory loss, incontinence, lack of cleanliness, making mistakes, slowness, becoming argumentative or withdrawn, or acting childishly are all associated with being old. Old age is considered something to be feared, as it is increasingly associated with becoming demented.

Given these embedded stereotypical views of old age, it is perhaps not surprising that younger people manifest ageist attitudes towards older women and men by seeing them, first and foremost, as old. In the modern era, youth, health, and fitness are highly valued. Having these attributes enables individuals to be flexible about the multitude of choices that present themselves in their daily lives: what to eat, what to wear, whom to meet in an evening out, and so on. When younger people interact with the aged it may remind them that one day they will no longer be young and fit, and that there will be restrictions on the choices that they can make. Even though they cannot know what it feels like to be old, their perception of what it will be like may feel threatening. Moreover, aged people may themselves internalise ageist views, their feelings of self-worth diminished by their loss of youth, fitness, and choice.

The mass media, in their variety of forms—television, magazines, advertising, and films—provide stereotypical images of age. Elderly people may be presented as incompetent. Consider, for example, Eddie's mother in *Absolutely Fabulous* or Maggie in *Mother and Son*. On the other hand, advertisements promoting retirement finance or housing are often accompanied by images of a smiling and contented older couple. People endeavouring to make sense of what old age means in today's society have to contend with stereotypical images such as these. Such oversimplified images contribute to ageism. They cannot capture the diverse situations of older people, or the effects that their different gender and cultural backgrounds, or their **class** positions, have on their lives.

Ageism can result in the progressive exclusion of elderly people from the social world, a situation for which Mulkay (1993) has coined the term '**social death**', and which can occur well before biological death. Many people's lives become more restricted as they retire and have less income. Over a period of time they become frail, are marginalised by family members, are visited

class (or social class) A position within a system of structured inequality based on the unequal distribution of power, wealth, income, and status. Class membership is determined by three characteristics: ownership and control of scarce economic resources; ownership of marketable skills and qualifications; and wage labour. People who share a social-class position typically share similar life chances.

social death The marginalisation and exclusion of elderly people from everyday life, resulting in social isolation.

less frequently, and become socially isolated. Finally they cease 'to exist as an active agent in the ongoing social world of some other party' and become a 'non-person' (Mulkay 1993, pp. 33–6).

Stereotypical and ambivalent images of ageing and old age are also constructed by experts, through bodies of knowledge that are generated in order to provide ways of understanding ageing and old age. Specialised forms of knowledge inform the practices of medical and health professions, as well as the practices of bureaucrats and others involved with making policies that affect the aged or aged care. Experts define the problems and solutions connected with old age, and policies are developed from the ways that experts define old age. The construction of age by experts establishes images of what is 'normal' for particular age groups. The result is contradictory. On the one hand, old age is presented as a burgeoning social problem, as the numbers of people living longer increase and become an economic and social burden. On the other hand, the aged are perceived as being responsible for their own quality of life, and having the potential to remain healthy and active participants in society. Both approaches are ageist constructions, contributing to stereotypical views.

Old age as a 'social burden'

Nationally and internationally, rather than longevity of populations being appreciated as an achievement to be applauded, this trend is being viewed increasingly with dismay. Indeed, current concern about the perceived burden of the aged is said to be reaching the level of hysteria, with a 'sense of impending crisis' pervading several international reports (Walker 1990, p. 378). Key economic advisers to the Australian federal government present the aged as an expanding group of unproductive people who, as they age further, will require increasingly high levels of health care and other resources (National Commission of Audit 1996, pp. 124–33). It is hardly surprising that older Australians have more health problems than younger Australians and that this is reflected in higher health care expenditure. Data from the Australian Institute of Health and Welfare (1999) show, for example, that 35 per cent of the total health services expenditure in 1993–94 was used by Australians aged 65 years and over, although they comprise only 12 per cent of the total Australian population.

The above, and similar, data should be interpreted carefully. The authors explain that over the period they were studying, 1982–83 to 1994–95, costs associated with an ageing population contributed to only 0.6 per cent of the growth in health expenditure. New technologies and increasing pharmaceuticals costs were major contributing factors. Apart from that, total health services expenditure does not refer simply to government spending but includes non-government spending, more than half of which is individuals' own spending on their health services. Total health service expenditure includes, as well, health insurance, which is comprised of individuals' contributions. Added to this, the source of Medicare funding is individual contributions through taxation. Much of the health care costs attributed to older Australians act- ually refers to accommodation expenses in nursing homes for the very old. It needs to be borne in mind, too, that older Australians paid taxes over the years of their employment and that many con- tributed to health insurance schemes during the years when they were younger and healthy, but in their old age, when they are likely to be in most need of health services, many can no longer afford to pay the high premiums required of them. It may well be asked whether health insurance companies are taking advantage of many older Australians by taking their money through their young and healthy years, but providing services only to the aged who can continue to pay high premiums.

Another argument for the aged being a social burden is that they are perceived as constituting the major unemployed, and therefore economically dependent, group. National age dependency ratios are calculated as the ratio of people 65 years and over to those between 18 (or sometimes 15 or 16) and 64 years of age. The assumption underlying this method of estimation is that people aged between 18 (or 15 or 16) and 64 years are the nation's working population, while those below 18 years and those 65 years and older are un- employed and therefore economically dependent. As the result of an expected huge increase in the numbers of people 65 years and over, it is projected that economic dependence in Australia will increase dramatically during the twenty-first century.

These calculations and projections are questionable. Projections 40 to 60 years into the future can be based only on present trends and on present interpretations of prevailing and perceived future conditions, yet usually there is little, if any, admis- sion of uncertainty. Also, in calculating national dependencies purely on the basis of age, no account is taken of people who are excluded from the workforce because of factors that have little to do with age, such as the sick, prisoners, home-makers, those with disabilities, tertiary students, and those unable to gain employ- ment because there are too few positions available. Nor do these estimates take account of the fact that a portion of retired people over the age of 65 years is wealthy and independent. Nearly 28 per cent of Australia's invested wealth is owned by males 65 years and over and females 60 years and over (National Commission of Audit 1966, p. 139). This reflects, at least in part, the historically high rate of home ownership in Australia, although the bulk of the wealth is likely to be confined to a small number of very wealthy older Australians. It can also be argued that the definition of economic dependency is too narrow for other reasons. Older people's past contributions to the economy during working life, taxes paid during that time, unofficial caring and financial assistance provided to adult children and grandchildren, and other voluntary work are all discounted. Further, stereotyping the aged as a collective social burden has sexist implications as well as being ageist because the majority of older people are women. Finally, anxiety about the baby boomers becoming a bourgeoning social burden neglects the growing influence of aged people with disposable income as a market sector for a range of services (ABS 1999f). Employment is likely to be generated in the tourist industry, for example, to cater for growing numbers of retired travellers.

The situation is complex, as power, wealth, and health are unequally distributed among the aged. Social class, status, **gender**, and **ethnicity** may be contributing factors in determining whether people retire with chronic health problems resulting from long years of repetitive or heavy manual work, or whether they retain positions of power for many more years as members of boards of directors or as consultants. The recent policies and strategies that have been set in place for differential retirement incomes will exacerbate these inequalities. It is well to remember that terms are never neutral. While experts warn that the ageing masses are likely to be a social burden, this term is not directed at, say, ex-politicians, many of whom retain costly benefits throughout their retirement at public expense.

> **gender/sex** This term refers to the socially constructed categories of feminine and masculine (the cultural values that dictate how men and women should behave), as opposed to the categories of biological sex (female or male).

> **ethnicity** Sociologically, the term refers to a shared cultural background, which is a characteristic of all groups in society. As a policy term, it is used to identify migrants who share a culture that is markedly different from that of Anglo-Australians. In practice, it often refers only to migrants from non-English-speaking backgrounds (NESB migrants).

'Successful ageing'

Recognition of the discriminatory effects of ageism, especially in a world that is rapidly ageing, has prompted resistance to the notion of the aged as a 'social burden'. Theoretically this cause has been assisted through Laslett's identification of a stage in life that has become known as the 'third age'. Laslett states that nearly all elderly are, or have the potential to be, healthy and active, and many are highly productive. Conceivably the length of this period could be extensive, as the biological limits of the human life span are uncertain, with predictions ranging as high as 120 years, or even well beyond (Laslett 1989, p. 13). Health promotion focuses on the healthy elderly, who age 'successfully', and offers advice to encourage individual responsibility for maintaining healthy lifestyles into old age. Age is no longer perceived as a barrier to health promotion activities. It is possible for older people to achieve measurable health improvements and fitness levels. To be healthy has become a moral imperative; to age 'successfully' is a moral duty.

Within this positive view of ageing, the continuing rise in life expectancy poses the possibility of life continuing indefinitely. Illness, deterioration, and death do not fit into the construction of 'positive health'. Death cannot—in the end—be denied, but with medical cures and disease prevention, death may be postponed, avoided, or resisted. Individuals are encouraged to concentrate on daily healthy living (choosing and eating healthy foods, making time for daily exercise, coping with stressful situations as they arise). They are reassured by the continuing advancement of medical techniques to combat disease (for example, bypass surgery, transplantations, chemotherapy, and so on) and, more recently, by the potential of genetic intervention. The result of the construction of 'positive' or 'successful' ageing is the idea of an indefinitely extended and healthy middle age, with death coming quickly at the end of a satisfactory life.

In reality, however, people do not necessarily exit life in this way. The 'fourth age'—which, according to Laslett (1989), is the final stage of life and is one of 'decrepitude and dependency'— appears to be a lingering rather than a short, abrupt period of time. He suggests that the repercussions are profound: for personal relations (in terms of time and effort), especially for families, and for national budgets (in terms of supplying hospital and medical care) (Laslett 1989, p. 13). It is during this final stage, then, that old age is perceived as a social burden. That the last years of life are represented by the term 'social burden' says much about the way old age is constructed by experts in today's society. Measuring and discussing chronic illness and dependence on the services of others in terms of cost not only merely disregards personal experiences of ageing, but also must surely have an effect on experiences of becoming old and ill and needing care.

Services for the aged

Most aged, even frail aged, manage to remain at home rather than go into institutional care. Institutional care is expensive and takes people, in their declining years, away from all that is familiar to them. Budgetary restraints and ageing populations in Australia and other Western countries mean that residential services are restricted to those who are assessed—in Australia, by Aged Care Assessment Teams—as being unable to be appropriately supported at home.

Basic daily care fees and accommodation charges for aged residential care (nursing homes and hostels) in Australia increased from 1 April 1999. Federal government legislation enables proprietors of hostel facilities, from October 1997, to charge each new resident a bond if the resident has assets worth more than $23 000. From the bond money, residential care proprietors will keep $13 000 over a period of five years, as well as the interest earned from the bond money, as a contribution to capital costs—that is, for repairs, upgrades, or extensions to facility buildings. After five years, the residue, if there is any, is to be returned to the resident or to the deceased resident's estate. A similar scheme for nursing homes was not, in the end, adopted, but licensing procedures have been altered so that nursing homes and hostels now have a common licensing arrangement, blurring the distinction between them.

Senator Bronwyn Bishop, former Minister for Aged Care, was subject to intense public questioning in relation to the quality and quantity of aged care accommodation, with descriptions of 'nursing homes from hell' reported in newspaper articles (for example, Horin 2000). According to the executive director of Catholic Health Australia, the Commonwealth Government does not adequately fund nursing homes and hostels at a level to ensure services are sustainable (Sullivan 2000). The Aged Care Amendment Bill 2000 gives the government more power to implement sanctions against nursing homes but such punitive measures may have the effect of silencing the concerns of residents and their families when there is no other accommodation available, as nursing home beds are insufficient to meet current needs. It is, in any case, government policy to reduce nursing home accommodation and increase hostel accommodation and community care packages, but the reduction in nursing home accommodation has been greater than the increase in hostel accommodation (Australian Bureau of Statistics 1999c).

Aged people who are dependent and frail, especially if they are poor and unable to contribute to their care, have, in a very real sense, become captives in institutions—nursing homes and hostels. Many of these institutions, in many ways, resemble workplaces rather than homes. The quality of services—including availability of privacy, leisure activities, timing of meals, and so on—is determined by staffing needs and salary awards (Fine 1988, p. 71). This can mean, for example, that aged residents must consume their three daily meals within an eight-hour period, that patients who cannot feed themselves may remain unfed, that patients with 'behavioural problems' may be physically, or medically restrained, and that bed-bound patients may develop unnecessary and untreated bedsores.

The provision of care to assist aged people to remain at home is the preferred option for the frail aged, and funding is available through the Home and Community Care (HACC) program for support services, such as assistance with housework, shopping, respite care, and so on. All such services are subject to the HACC National Fees Policy, that is, clients are charged for services according to their income and the level of services they require. An

ideology In a political context, ideology refers to those beliefs and values that relate to the way in which society should be organised, including the appropriate role of the state.

ideology of 'community' has accompanied governmental decisions to rely more on non-institutional, rather than institutional, care. Notions of 'community' care carry connotations of neighbourhoods in which people have the time and motivation to help one another, and especially to be willing to care for the sick and needy in their midst. Instead, modern suburbia can be isolating, with people being divided by traffic, urban developments, and poor public transport. Acutely ill people remain in hospital for only a short time as a result of prevailing budgetary constraints; they are discharged before being able to resume their own care and consequently may require intensive home support services. This means that there is less funding available for HACC services for the frail aged with chronic problems. They must fend for themselves, pay for services if they can afford it, or rely on voluntary assistance or family support. The burden of home or 'community' care, to a very large extent, falls back on the family, and in particular on those in the family who are willing to take up and maintain the responsibility of caring for their elderly relatives. Table 12.3 shows that the largest source of 'community' assistance is informal, being provided by family and/or friends, and that to a large extent individuals pay for the formal services they receive.

Table 12.3   Informal and formal assistance for persons 65 years and over, 1998

Source of assistance	65–79 years (%)	80 years and over (%)	65 years and over (%)
Informal	82.9	84.2	83.3
Family*	76.1	76.6	76.3
Partner	42.9	16.7	34.5
Adult child	26.7	33.8	28.9
Friends	13.8	15.7	14.4
Formal	55.9	66.9	59.4
Private for-profit	39.7	43.8	41.0
Private not-for-profit	6.5	13.5	8.7
Government	24.1	35.8	27.8

* People may receive assistance from more than one source and therefore components do not add to totals.

Source: Adapted from ABS 1999c

Dying and death

Most people in Australia die after the age of 65. In 1998, for example, 78 per cent of all deaths were of Australians aged 65 years and over—an increase from 63 per cent in 1968 and 72 per cent in 1988—while a quarter of all registered deaths in 1998 were of persons aged 85 years and over, which is double the proportion of such deaths in 1968 (ABS 1999b). The health and social problems of Aborigines and Torres Strait Islanders are reflected in the fact that they die twenty years earlier than the rest of the population. While the death of old people is accepted—they are said to have had their 'good innings'—young deaths are perceived as premature, and therefore problematic. Some deaths are not caused by disease, for example, accidents, motor vehicle traffic accidents, suicide, and homicide, but cancer and ischaemic heart disease are the main causes of death in Australia.

Death has become an ambivalent process, rather than an event. Brain death has become the accepted criterion for death so that an apparently live patient whose heart is still beating but whose brain no longer functions is declared dead, thus becoming a source of fresh body parts for patients who would otherwise die. Medical intervention can retard the advancement of many diseases, which once would have killed more quickly, so that it is possible for individuals to continue their normal social activities for months, or even years, after having been diagnosed with a terminal illness, albeit often in a state of uncertainty about how much future they have. Patients are now likely to be informed of their dying status, and urged to make preparations for the time when they may no longer be competent to make decisions. They can discuss their preferences for their final stages of life and for their death, for example their medical treatment and funeral. Living wills or advance directives can be drawn up and/or an enduring power of attorney given to a trusted person to ensure, as much as possible, that the dying maintain control over their lives. The underlying assumption is that all people want to be informed that they are dying, that they all have the knowledge, and the will, to plan ahead—to consider their potential future circumstances, and choose possible alternative ways of dying—and that their wishes will be adhered to.

New ethical issues have arisen in relation to death and dying for which there is often no easy solution. People are encouraged to donate organs in order to save lives, but executed prisoners in China have their organs *taken*. In some countries there is a black market in organs. In Australia the kidney supplied to Kerry Packer by his employee raises the question about the meaning of 'donation'. There is also the question as to how patients are selected as organ recipients. How many Aboriginal people, for example, have received organ transplantations? Challenging ethical questions arise in relation to dying, such as, in relation to the withdrawal of treatment, at what stage should patients be taken off ventilators? Who decides, and when, whether the lives of patients who have suffered severe brain trauma will continue to be worthwhile? Is it ever ethical to withdraw nutrition and fluid from a patient? Should euthanasia be legalised in Australia, and if so, what should be the conditions of its legalisation? Should priority be given, in terms of health care costs, research and expertise, to more sophisticated technology and treatment, or to palliative treatment for the chronically ill and dying?

A good death

medicalisation The process by which non-medical problems become defined and treated as medical issues, usually in terms of illnesses, disorders, or syndromes.

The ideal 'good death', before its **medicalisation**, and before the secularisation of society, was to die at home, surrounded by friends and neighbours, accepting this last earthly suffering as a preparation for eternal life after death. Death often came early and relatively quickly, as there was little medicine could do. In the face of the inevitable the doctor retreated, leaving the priest to perform the last rites. When the hospital became the place where people were sent to be cured, or to die, no longer was the dying person, or the person's family, in charge of the dying process. The patient became the property of the hospital, with visiting hours restricted and subject to hospital rules for the convenience of hospital organisation and staff. The image of dying in hospital became that of patients attached to an arsenal of equipment in a futile attempt to defeat death, and resulting only in the unnecessary prolongation of their suffering. This is likely to have contributed to prevalent fears of experiencing suffering, degradation, and loss of control during a drawn-out dying period. People are made more fearful by descriptive media accounts of dying with cancer, HIV/AIDS, and dementia.

Palliative care, and more recently euthanasia, may be thought of as providing contemporary ideals of a 'good death'. A good death may be envisaged as having a period of time during which the dying individual and relatives prepare for their forthcoming separation, for affairs to be put in order, and for the spiritual side of death to be approached. The aim of palliative care is to alleviate suffering in order to allow for these opportunities. Others may wish to die suddenly and painlessly after living a healthy, active life in old age, and when nature does not oblige, euthanasia, or physician-assisted suicide may appear to offer a good death.

Palliative care

Palliative care is usually associated with care offered to the dying within a hospice. Hospices are not available to all the dying in Australia, for example to those living in rural areas, or the elderly in nursing homes. While local medical and health workers can provide palliative care, doctors and nurses in hospices specialise in palliative care. The word 'hospice' derives from the hospice of medieval Europe, which offered refuge to pilgrims as well as to the sick and destitute. Cicely Saunders is regarded as the founder of the modern hospice movement at St Christopher's Hospice, London, in 1967. Hospices can provide both inpatient care and care to patients in their own homes. The aim is to offer comprehensive support by controlling pain and other symptoms, as well as addressing the psychological, social, and spiritual needs of the dying person.

In recent years limitations of palliative care have been pointed out. Individuals have their own particular needs and it is argued that, especially as hospices have become more medicalised and institutionalised, tension has developed between the maintenance of the ideal of a good death and the maintenance of the hospice organisation (McNamara, Waddell, & Colvin 1994). Hospices have tended to focus on patients with cancer, and more recently HIV/AIDS, while excluding other types of illness. Palliative care may be restricted to achieving pain relief, which is not always possible without rendering patients unconscious. While palliative care has become the professional domain of nursing and medicine, the professor of palliative care at La Trobe University is sociologist, Professor Allan Kellehear. Kellehear (1999) argues that palliative care is underdeveloped and should be available to those with life-threatening illness, rather than only to those in the later stages of terminal illness. It should be concerned with promoting the health of the ill as well as wider social aspects of illness. Palliative carers have traditionally been opposed to views supportive of euthanasia, aiming neither to hasten death nor prolong dying. Yet, while such views continue, they are becoming less than universal.

Euthanasia

Euthanasia and physician-assisted suicide provide the medical means of ending life that is perceived as being unbearable, usually, although not necessarily, in relation to terminal illness. These actions are illegal in most countries. The Netherlands is a well-known exception, and physician-assisted suicide has been allowed in the US State of Oregon since 1997. For a short time in Australia euthanasia and physician-assisted suicide for the terminally ill were permitted in the Northern Territory. This was during the period from July 1996 until March 1997 when the Commonwealth Government overturned the Northern Territory's legislation.

The 'requested death' movement, which, through groups such as the Voluntary Euthanasia Society and the Hemlock Society, advocate for the legalisation of euthanasia and physician-assisted suicide, appears to be strongly supported by the public, according to public opinion surveys. McInerney (2000), however, discusses the uncertainty of meaning that can be attached to such surveys as survey results may be contradicted by voting results.

The word 'euthanasia' literally means a 'good death', or 'dying well', but within the complex debate that has emerged there are conflicting opinions about what constitutes the practice of euthanasia. The very definition of the term, therefore, is in dispute, and this can cause much confusion when posing the question 'What is euthanasia?' The injection of a lethal drug dose by a doctor, with the explicit intention of terminating life at the request of a patient who is competent to make decisions, is voluntary euthanasia, sometimes referred to as 'active' euthanasia. When a doctor does not directly cause death, but prescribes or provides the substance that causes death, it is regarded as physician-assisted suicide. This is closely aligned with voluntary 'active' euthanasia in that the intention of the doctor and patient is to actively cause the patient's death, but in physician-assisted suicide, the patient self-administers the fatal dose.

The withdrawal of medical treatment from the terminally ill when it is considered to be useless, and the provision of drugs to the terminally ill to relieve pain knowing that this may result in death, have traditionally been accepted as good medical practices. These measures are sometimes referred to as 'passive' euthanasia. It has generally been accepted that while death may be the side effect of pain relief, the intention is to relieve pain, not end life, and also, that if individuals die after the withdrawal of useless treatment, they are merely being allowed to die naturally from their disease, without having their lives artificially prolonged. Within the current euthanasia debate, however, euthanasia supporters may argue that these practices cannot be divorced from 'active' euthanasia, because the end result is the same—death.

Euthanasia can also be non-voluntary, as was the case in Nazi Germany where killings, sanctioned by the state under Nazi rule, were carried out by doctors (Morgan 1996, pp. 12–14). Euthanasia intentionally administered to patients who are incapable of making decisions (such as the severely demented), or those unable to make their wishes known (for example the unconscious), is referred to as involuntary euthanasia. Supporters of voluntary euthanasia (for example Baume 1995, p. 14) suggest that the problem of involuntary euthanasia can be overcome by competent people leaving clear instructions of their wishes in a living will or advance directive, as well as appointing an enduring power of attorney to act on their behalf in the case of their becoming incompetent. Against this is the argument that even if these measures become widespread, people may change their mind over time. As well, from a legal perspective, written instructions must be extremely precise and do not guarantee medical compliance (Hoffenburg 1996, pp. 94–5).

Supporters of euthanasia usually focus on arguments for voluntary euthanasia by appealing to the right of individuals to control their own death. The reasoning is that legislation upholding this right will have no impact on others, who can simply refrain from exercising this prerogative. According to this view, legalised voluntary euthanasia provides justice for all. A law that denies choice is unjust and oppressive to those who decide that life has become unbearable for them, or that it has lost any qualities that would make it worthwhile. Opponents of legalised voluntary euthanasia often evoke what is called the 'slippery slope' (or 'thin edge of the wedge') argument to support their case. They assert that it is not simply a matter of individual rights, but that changing attitudes resulting from the legislation will eventually lead to the acceptance of some forms of non-voluntary euthanasia whereby the quality of life of those considered too socially burdensome may be perceived as being not worthwhile. While the debate continues, ethical decisions about whether to continue treatment are being taken daily in hospitals.

Future directions: death and dying

The euthanasia debate has highlighted, and probably provoked, attitudinal divisions among medical and health professionals, but what they have in common is a paramount aim to relieve the suffering of dying patients. While pain relief is only one factor driving the euthanasia debate, it is a serious factor for those dying patients who suffer uncontrolled pain, and for others who fear that this will be their fate. The interest of researchers and funding bodies, as well as of appropriately trained medical and health practitioners, is required to bring adequate and sustained pain relief to the dying, which at the same time allows them to retain some control over their lives.

Euthanasia and physician-assisted suicide are morally wrong, according to the main religions in Australia, most notably the Catholic and Anglican religions. Religion, according to Émile Durkheim, provides a **collective conscience**, that is, a moral framework that transcends any individual conscience or morality (Durkheim 1984). Many people, however, no longer accept moral answers based on traditional authority. Giddens (1991) suggests that, although traditional authority, including religion, continues to exist, there are many other competing authorities in the modern world of expertise (Giddens 1991, p. 195). The modern world is characterised by expert systems in all areas of life. Individuals are presented with choices from a wide range of contested and changing bodies of expert knowledge and techniques (Giddens 1991, pp. 18, 121). When making life-and-death decisions during times of illness, medicine, rather than religion, is likely to be regarded as more significant because of the high value that is placed on medical knowledge and technology that can save or maintain life. Alternative healing methods have become popular for some, either to complement medical treatment or to replace it when treatment is not achieving a cure or reprieve (see chapter 16). Medicine, however, remains the area of

collective conscience A term used to describe shared moral beliefs that act to unify society.

expertise that controls the knowledge, the drugs, and the technology associated with health and illness, and the dying process.

Medical and health professionals are under increasing pressure to consider the economic outcome of their practices, as the Australian government, following world trends, is seeking methods to achieve cost-efficiencies in distributing funds and in setting priorities for the allocation of health services. Medical life-and-death decisions are being made within this environment, and are no doubt influenced by it. Perceived quality of life is an important factor in making such decisions, but 'quality of life' is not a neutral term.

Historically religion has provided a language for speaking about death to the dying but from the time death was transferred from home to hospital, and for the first half of the twentieth century, death became something of an embarrassment. It was felt that dying persons should remain unaware of their fate, and instead be kept in a state of hopefulness of a medical cure. Now there are new ways of speaking about death, derived especially from medical and legal **discourses**. Individuals can decide whether they wish to become an organ donor, to appoint an enduring power of attorney, discuss medical treatment such as chemotherapy, and so on. Such language encourages discussion of end-of-life decisions, but does not encourage discussion of existential questions and anxieties that may emerge when individuals are facing their mortality. For the dying, the reality and taken-for-grantedness of everyday life may be called into question, and they may face questions about the meaning of their existence, experiencing what Giddens (1991) calls 'ontological insecurity'. Sociologists tend not to speak intimately about death, but Kellehear (1999) recognises the importance of understanding the significance of death's meaning for the dying. He states that although many people, especially the well-educated from professional classes—the experts—believe life begins and ends with material embodiment, most people believe in personal survival after biological death. Perhaps all individuals are seekers of immortality in some way. The better educated and the wealthy may simply pin their hopes on achieving secular, rather than, or even as well as, spiritual, immortality, as they have more chances of leaving something of lasting material value after their death.

discourse A domain of language-use that is characterised by common ways of talking and thinking about an issue (for example, the discourses of medicine, madness, or sexuality).

Summary of main points

- It is often taken for granted that death and dying are associated with old age. For most of human history, however, it has been uncommon for people to reach old age. This continues to be the case in many Third World countries, although this is changing.

- In all countries in the world, people are living longer, although there are differences both between and within countries. Australian Aborigines and Torres Strait Islanders, for example, have a lower life expectancy than the rest of the Australian population.
- Health, fitness, and youth are dominant values in modern society, and this contributes to ageist attitudes towards those who display characteristics associated with old age.
- Expert bodies of knowledge have constructed conflicting stereotypical views of old age. Within these constructions, the aged are either a 'social burden' draining scarce resources, or proof that the ills associated with old age can be avoided.
- Within the bioethical construction of euthanasia, the proponents of legalised voluntary euthanasia argue that it will enable individual autonomy in life-and-death decision-making. Those opposing legalisation argue that it will lead inevitably to some form of non-voluntary euthanasia and to disregard for human life.
- Medical experts control the knowledge, drugs, and technology associated with health and illness, but life-and-death decisions are being made by medical and health practitioners at a time when they are under pressure to cut costs.
- The dying may experience 'ontological insecurity', raising questions about the meaning of life and death.

Discussion questions

1 What examples of ageism can you think of?
2 How do you distinguish between people who are old and people who are not old?
3 Why are health, fitness, and youthfulness so highly valued?
4 What does death mean in today's society?
5 Which groups of people do you think are more likely to agree with legalised voluntary euthanasia? Which groups are more likely to disagree? Why?
6 Why is it important to understand the economic and political factors that affect health and medical care?

Further investigation

1 Extending on the information in this chapter, critically analyse policies that affect the aged in Australia.
2 Are the ethical dilemmas that have emerged in relation to dying and death, new dilemmas? Critically discuss this question.
3 Critically discuss whether a 'good death' is possible? What is the meaning of death in the sense of a 'good death'?

Further reading and web resources

Arber, S. & Ginn, J. (eds) 1995, *Connecting Gender and Ageing: A Sociological Approach*, Oxford University Press, Oxford.

Chapman, S. & Leeder, S. 1995, *The Last Right?*, Mandarin, Melbourne.

Featherstone, M. & Hepworth, M. 1991, 'The Mask of Ageing and the Postmodern Life Course', in M. Featherstone, M. Hepworth, & B. Turner (eds), *The Body: Social Process and Cultural Theory*, Sage, London.

Kellehear, A. (ed.) 2000, *Death and Dying in Australia*, Oxford University Press, Melbourne.

McInerney, F. 2000, '"Requested death": A New Social Movement', *Social Science and Medicine*, vol. 50, no. 1, 147–54.

McNamara, B. 2001, *Fragile Lives: Death, Dying and Care*, Allen & Unwin, Sydney.

Web sites

Australian Institute of Health and Welfare—Aged Care: <www.aihw.gov.au/agedcare/index.html>

Sociology of Death and Dying: <www.trinity.edu/~mkearl/death.html>

SocioSite —Death and Dying: <www.pscw.uva.nl/sociosite/ TOPICS/health.html#DEATH>

Part 3

The Social Organisation
of Health Care:
Professions, Politics,
and Policies

That any sane nation, having observed that you could provide for the supply of bread by giving bakers a pecuniary interest in baking for you, should go on to give a surgeon a pecuniary interest in cutting off your leg, is enough to make one despair of political humanity.

George Bernard Shaw 1908, The Doctor's Dilemma, preface

The chapters in this part of the book are concerned with the social organisation of health care: the role of health policy, political ideology, and the health professions in shaping the institutional features of the Australian health care system. A common theme among the chapters is an analysis of the medical profession's influence on health policy, on other health professions, and on the delivery of health services. The chapters examine the key features of the health system—its history, its structure, and the changes under way—to understand why the health system is organised the way that it is and how it could be otherwise.

Part 3 is divided into six chapters:

* Chapter 13 discusses the politics of health care by examining the role of the state in providing access to health services through health insurance.
* Chapter 14 traces the development of medicine's dominance of health care and how this dominance is continually the source of challenge and resistance.
* Chapter 15 explores the changing role of nursing in the health system and the practical insights sociology can offer in understanding the changes taking place.
* Chapter 16 deals with alternative medicine in terms of its effectiveness, popularity, and future.
* Chapter 17 reviews the position of allied health practitioners, highlighting the complexity and diversity of health care provision, as well as the struggle for survival and legitimacy that these professions face.
* Chapter 18 considers the historical development, philosophy, policies, and outcomes of community health services in Australia.

13

Power, Politics, and Health Care

Helen Belcher

Overview

* *What is the nature of health policy in Australia?*
* *What are the major health interest groups, and what influence do they have?*
* *What role does politics, power, and ideology play in shaping the health system?*

This chapter provides an analysis of the nature of Australia's health policy. The financing and organisation of Australian health policy are products of a clash between the ideologies of compulsion and freedom of choice. Ideological differences between the major political parties remain the principal reason for the frequent changes in policy direction. These are the result of competing beliefs over the role of the state, the individual, the community, and the market. The major players are politicians and doctors, with hospitals and the insurance industry playing supporting roles. After providing a brief overview of the Australian health care system, the chapter examines the role of politicians and doctors with reference to the impact of ideology, politics, power, and structural interests on health insurance arrangements.

Key terms

economic rationalism	pluralism
gross domestic product (GDP)	ruling class
ideology	social liberalism
individualism	social structure
liberalism	socialisation
life chances	socialism
market	state
medical dominance	trickle down

Introduction

In 1963 Sir Theodore Fox described the Australian health care system as 'private practice publicly supported' (*Lancet* 1963, p. 875). The comment remains an apt description of the organisation, financing, and delivery of health services in Australia today. The term 'health care system' refers to the institutions, arrangements, and activities involved in providing health care services (Palmer and Short 1994, pp. 5–6). Such a definition, however, can obscure the fact that health care is concerned with more than just health. As other chapters have shown, social conditions such as unemployment and poverty also affect health (AIHW 2000, pp. 218–23). What is more, the activities of various interests—described by Sidney Sax (1984) as 'a strife of interests'—affect financial and organisational arrangements. The Australian health care system—or for that matter any health system—then is the product of responses not only to bodily malfunction but also to vested interests and influences, many of which are seemingly unrelated to health (Sax 1990, pp. 1–5). For instance, the *First Report—Public Hospital Funding and Options for Reform* recently noted:

> In addition to (the) high level of interest of the community in health-related issues, it is notable that health policy is dominated by vested interests. Governments are self-evident participants, as are groupings of health practitioners, while others include industry groups, academics, commentators, patients and the community generally. Although the community funds the health system, ostensibly for the benefit of the community, much of the debate and commentary often seems to focus on the requirements of funding agencies such as governments and the needs of practitioners. The voice of the patient is often lost among this 'strife of interests' as the participants in health policy debates have been labelled by Dr Sidney Sax (2000, clause 1.9, p. 3).

A comprehensive analysis of the health care system is beyond the scope of this chapter; therefore, it will concentrate on health insurance. Sax argues that the financing and organisation of Australian health insurance is fundamentally a clash of **ideology**. This clash is not so much over the need for medical and hospital insurance but over the issue of compulsion or freedom of choice. He identifies two major players—politicians and doctors—with hospitals and the insurance industry playing supporting roles (Sax 1984, p. 29). Gray extends this argument by claiming, 'the competing ideological perspectives of Australia's major parties are the principal reasons for the frequent and major changes in policy direction' (1991, p. 184). These changes are marked by competing ideological understandings over the role of the **state**, the role of the individual/community and the role of the **market** (Crichton

ideology In a political context, ideology refers to those beliefs and values that relate to the way in which society should be organised, including the appropriate role of the state.

state A term used to describe a collection of institutions, including the parliament (government and Opposition political parties), the public-sector bureaucracy, the judiciary, the military, and the police.

market Any institutional arrangement for the exchange of goods according to economic demand and supply. This term is often used to describe the basic principle underlying the capitalist economy.

1990; Sax 1984; Duckett; 1995). This chapter, after a brief overview of the Australian health care system, examines the role of politicians and doctors with reference to the impact of ideology, politics, power and interests on health insurance arrangements.

The Australian health care system

Key features of the Australian health care system are its federal structure and a public/private division of responsibilities. These two characteristics provide a backdrop for the organisation of the Australian health care system.

Federal structure

In 1901 six Australian colonies accepted the need for a national and central authority. They agreed to the passing of an Act for the establishment of the Commonwealth of Australia known as the *Commonwealth of Australia Constitution Act*. As a consequence the people of New South Wales, Victoria, South Australia, Queensland, Tasmania, and Western Australia were united in a federal Commonwealth under the name of the Commonwealth of Australia. The founding fathers were, however, anxious to balance the needs of the Australian people as a whole against the rights of the individual States. Hence they adopted a federal structure for the Constitution. It provides for the operation of a national government (the Commonwealth) in parallel with six State governments. A third tier of government, local government, was not included in the Constitution, relying for its existence instead on its respective State or Territory. Each State, together with the Australian Capital Territory, the Northern Territory and the Commonwealth Government has its own constitution, parliament and public service (for a fuller discussion of the Australian political system see Jaensch 1988; Gardner 1995).

The Constitution of Australia divided responsibilities between the Commonwealth government and the State (and eventually Territory) governments but, as Jaensch notes, 'the division of powers was more complex' (Jaensch 1988, p 30).

1   The national parliament was given the power to legislate 'for the peace, order, and good government of the Commonwealth' in regard to the forty subjects named in Section 51 of the constitution.
2   There were also concurrent powers on which both the national and State governments had the authority to pass laws, but in the event of a conflict between the two, the national legislation would prevail.
3   The national government was granted some powers exclusively, including customs and excise, defence, currency, external affairs and territories.

4 Some areas of potential legislative activity were prohibited to both national and State governments …

5 All other powers remained with the States (Jaensch 1988, p. 30).

This division of responsibilities, although designed to protect the interests of the States against the dominance of the national government, has created problems for the adequate management of health services, not the least being overlapping responsibilities.

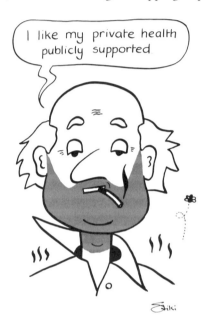

Shared responsibilities

The responsibility for the organisation and delivery of health services is shared between the three tiers of government (Richardson, 1998, pp. 192–213). The federal government has a leadership role in policy making, particularly in national issues like public health, research, and national information management (McGuinness 1999). It funds most hospital medical services, which amounts to 19.3 per cent of recurrent health services expenditure (AIHW 2000, p. 404). The universal, public health scheme known as Medicare is a Commonwealth responsibility. It provides for:

- access to free treatment in public hospitals, including
- medical treatment—as 'hospital' in-patients or out-patients, through agreements between the federal and State or Territory governments, which compensate for loss of income as a result of the free, public hospitalisation of those electing to be treated as 'public hospital' patients (Grant & Lapsley 1993)
- universal insurance against the cost of private medical services (Deeble 1991).

In addition to this the Commonwealth manages the Pharmaceutical Benefits Scheme, which accounts for 12.1 per cent of recurrent health services expenditure (AIHW 2000, p. 404).

The source of Commonwealth Government funds is revenue collected via general taxes and specific taxes such as the compulsory Medicare levy. These are then distributed to the States and Territories as financial assistance grants and special purpose payments. Funds are also provided to non-government bodies including private hospitals, doctors, allied health practitioners, pharmacists, and community health services. Whereas the federal government is not responsible for the direct provision of health services, its financial responsibility has an impact on the provision of health services, and consequently upon the providers and consumers of health services.

The States and Territories deliver public acute and psychiatric hospital services and a wide range of community and public health services including school health, dental health, maternal and child health and environmental health programs. They are also primarily responsible for the delivery and management of public health services and for maintaining direct relationships with most health care providers, including the regulation of health professionals (McGuinness 1999).

The Commonwealth shares with the States and Territories the costs of public hospitals. In 1997–98, the latest figures available, public hospital operating costs amounted to 58.6 per cent of the total health expenditure by the States and Territories whereas capital expenditure amounted to 12.7 per cent and capital consumption 4.9 per cent of their total health expenditure (AIHW 2000, p. 404). It also shares the costs of community-based services, aged care, and public health with the States and Territories. Residential aged care is financed and regulated by the Commonwealth Government, representing 7.5 per cent of recurrent health services expenditure (AIHW 2000, p. 404), but is largely provided by non-profit and for-profit providers. The Commonwealth, States and Territories jointly fund and administer community care such as meals on wheels, home help, and transport (McGuinness 1999).

The State and Territory governments directly fund a broad range of health services including public hospitals, public and mental health services, disability, and aspects of community, residential aged care, and rehabilitation services (AIHW 2000, pp. 240, 404; Bloom 2000, p. 24). As a percentage of total health expenditure, however, State government expenditure inclusive of local government expenditure declined from 25.8 per cent in 1984–85 to 23.4 per cent in 1997–98. This can partly be explained by the introduction of Medicare, which raised the

Commonwealth's share of expenditure from 38 per cent in 1983–84 to 45.8 per cent in 1984–85, to a reduction in the number of acute and psychiatric beds, and to an increase in the number of people treated in the community (AIHW 1996a, p. 126; AIHW 2000, p. 235).

Local government is responsible for aspects of environmental control, some personal preventative services, and for home care services (AIHW 1996a). As a minor but nevertheless important player in health service provision, it draws its funding from its respective State or Territory government and from the levying of its own taxes and charges (AIHW 2000, pp. 233–40; Bloom 2000, p. 25).

Public/private division of responsibilities

There is a clear public/private split in the organisation and financing of health care. In 1997–98 private sources accounted for 31.4 per cent of total health expenditure, in contrast to expenditure of 23.4 per cent from the States and local governments, and 45.2 per cent from the federal government (see Figure 13.1). Since 1984–85 total government funding has fallen from 71.6 to 68.6 per cent, while private funding has increased from 28.4 per cent to 31.4 per cent. Although the total government fall in expenditure and the private increase in expenditure has not been even across the intervening years, the trend is evident (AIHW 2000, p. 235). Private sources include payments by health insurance funds and compensation schemes, as well as payments made by private individuals.

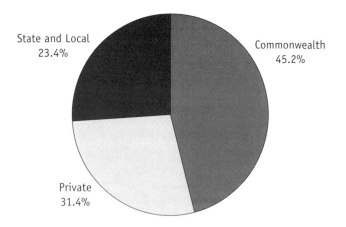

Figure 13.1   Percentage of health expenditure according to source of funds, Australia, 1997–98

Source: Adapted from AIHW 2000, p. 235

The importance of the public/private division is highlighted by the degree of influence exerted by private providers—most notably doctors—upon the organisation and financing of health care services. This influence is well documented (Thame 1974; Sax

1984; Gillespie 1991; Scotton 1998; Alexander 2000). It is most obvious in Australia's continuing reliance on fee-for-service medicine and in the 'grudging acceptance' of Medicare and universal health insurance by the Australian Medical Association (AMA) and more recently their suspicion, if not resistance, to the introduction of managed care. Doctors in cooperation with insurance funds and private hospitals have exerted, and continue to exert, significant influence upon health insurance arrangements (Sax 1984; Crichton 1990; Gillespie 1991; Richardson 1998).

Health insurance

The purpose of insurance is to provide protection against loss. This involves 'a contract whereby, for a stipulated consideration, called a premium, one party undertakes to indemnify or guarantee another against loss by a certain specified contingency or peril, called a risk, the contract being set forth in a document called a policy' (Titmuss 1974, p. 90).

Generally, insurance is a market commodity, but health is unlike other goods and services. The need for health care is largely uncertain; the costs of health care are high, and most consumers do not have the knowledge that enables them to make an informed choice in relation to treatment. What is more, illness can restrict others, either through the risk of the spread of infection, through emotional and psychological suffering, or through the loss of productivity (McClelland 1991). Health insurance, then, requires more than just protection against loss. It must also incorporate 'the social objectives of access and equity' (Scotton & Macdonald 1993, p. 2). Therefore it cannot be left entirely at the mercy of market forces. It requires some level of collective responsibility, which may be satisfied either though private or public provision, or through a mix of public and private funding.

The purpose of health insurance, be it public or private, is to provide protection against the financial loss of unpredictable health care costs. It does this by eliminating or reducing out-of-pocket expenses through the pooling of costs. It generally incorporates a redistributive element in the form of cross-subsidisation of the sicker and poorer members of society by the healthier and wealthier members. This is known as 'community rating' (Scotton & Macdonald 1993).

There are various health insurance models, and these range across two continuums: selective–universal coverage and public–private provision. Selective coverage is targeted, usually by means testing, so that only those considered unable to provide for themselves receive benefits and/or services. Universal coverage seeks to provide benefits and/or services for the whole population. Public provision is largely defined as provision of goods and services by the state. Private provision generally refers to goods and services that are provided in the market, and is dependent on the efforts of individuals, families, and communities to provide for their own needs.

Selective coverage assumes that the majority of the population will be responsible for their own health care needs and hence favours private health insurance. Universal coverage assumes collective responsibility and is usually financed through taxation. At the very least, universal coverage requires some level of government involvement. Public financing of health insurance is likely to be more equitable, as ability to pay is taken into consideration, with payments or contributions being calculated as a proportion of income; for example, the Medicare levy is calculated on the basis of 1.5 per cent of taxable income. Private financing, however, is likely to result in the sicker and poorer members of society bearing increased health costs. They are also likely to face increasing difficulty in meeting those costs because of their poor health status. The adoption of community rating seeks to address these problems.

International comparisons

The Australian health care system can best be described as 'mixed'. The financing, organisation, and delivery of health services are drawn from a combination of public and private sources. Services are largely delivered by private practitioners in public institutions on a fee-for-service basis. These are financed by government and/or private health insurance and by individual contributions. The American system, by way of contrast, is largely dependent on the private sector (Ham et al. 1990; Starr 1982), while the British system is largely public in character (Ham 1992).

The United States system of health insurance is largely the result of a movement sponsored by the providers of health care services (Bates 1983). The need for hospitals, combined with a political philosophy that emphasised individual responsibility, resulted in a largely private health care system. Almost all services are provided on a fee-for-service basis and are supported through public and private insurance arrangements. The majority of Americans rely on private insurance taken out through employers under group policy arrangements, but there are also two public insurance programs: Medicare and Medicaid. The federally funded Medicare program covers the elderly and some disabled groups, while Medicaid draws on federal and State funds to provide cover for low-income families. As well as being selective, none of these private and public insurance programs provide comprehensive coverage against the risks of illness. Consequently gaps have emerged in health insurance coverage, with approximately 41 million Americans having no health insurance and another 28 per cent of the population being under-insured (Ham et al. 1990; Callahan 1990; Hehir 1996; Ross et al. 1999, pp. 73–4).

British health insurance began as 'a movement run by consumers for their mutual benefit' (Bates 1983, p. 104). The fact that
this movement was backed by a strong working class partly
explains the British adoption of a more collectivist, and hence
public, approach. The government, through the National Health
Service (NHS), provides health care services for everyone in need
of care and treatment, free at point of delivery. Funds to support
this service come from three sources, 'the largest of (which) is
general taxation, followed by national insurance contributions,
charges and miscellaneous sources' (Ham 1992, p. 60; Ross et. al.
1999, p. 67).

Hospital doctors are salaried employees of the NHS, although
they do retain their clinical autonomy. General practitioners (GPs)
are paid on the basis of capitation or are salaried (Ham 1992).
Reforms introduced by the Conservative Government in 1989
opened up health care provision to market forces by introducing
purchaser–provider splits, hospital trusts and fund holding in
general practice. The purpose of these changes was 'to separate
purchasers and providers, promote competition within the system
(thus reducing outlays by government and increasing consumer
choice) and devolve decision making and accountability to the
local level' (Ross, et. al 1999, p. 70). Some of the larger GP practices
have been given a budget by government, out of which they purchase certain hospital services for and on behalf of their patients.

The same reforms organised hospitals and other individual
providers of health care into semi-autonomous 'trusts'. They compete for the patients of the GP fund holdings, now known as
primary care groups, (PCGs) on the basis of the range of services
offered, and their fee structures. Income is derived from long-
term contracts with the PCGs, activity-level-based contracts with
a regional health authority, income from extra contractual referral, that is, patients from outside the health authority catchment
area, patient payments, and non-medical services such as catering
(Ross 1999, p. 68).

During the years of Conservative government under Margaret
Thatcher and John Major, the general tax basis of health services
financing remained largely unchanged, although, in an effort to
promote market principles, the development of private insurance
and the private provision of health services was encouraged.
Approximately 11 per cent of the population is covered by private insurance (Ross, et. al 1999, p. 67). Consequently, the private
sector has emerged as a relatively small but important player in the
organisation and delivery of health care services in the United
Kingdom (Ham 1992).

The Australian public health insurance system, Medicare, falls
somewhere between the systems in place in the USA and the
United Kingdom, combining both a belief that all people have a

right to basic health care, and the principle of non-interference in the doctor–patient relationship, which is embodied in the catch-phrase 'doctor of choice'.

Differences between the three systems are reflected in the percentage of **gross domestic product** (**GDP**) expended on health (see Figure 13.2). In 1997 Australian health expenditure, as a percentage of GDP, was 8.3 per cent, compared with approximately 6.8 per cent for the United Kingdom and 13.9 per cent for the USA (AIHW 2000, p. 408). This higher health expenditure has not resulted in better health for United States citizens (see Tables 13.1 and 13.2). In fact they experience glaring gaps in health care coverage and, as a result, in access to health care services (Callahan 1990). On the other hand, those living in Australia and the United Kingdom experience good health while supporting and maintaining universal, comprehensive health insurance coverage.

gross domestic product (GDP)
The market value of all goods and services that have been sold during a year.

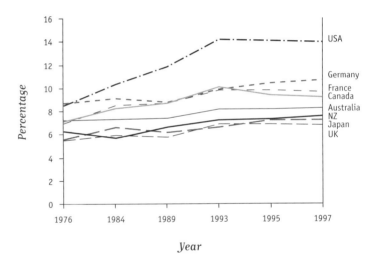

Figure 13.2   Health expenditure for Australia and selected OECD countries as a percentage of GDP, 1976–97

Source: AIHW 2000, Table S45, p. 408

Table 13.1   Neonatal, postneonatal and infant mortality rates* for Australia, the United Kingdom and the USA, latest available year per 1000 live births

Country	Males			Females		
	Neo-natal	*Post-neonatal*	*Infant*	*Neo-natal*	*Post-neonatal*	*Infant*
Australia (1998)	3.7	1.8	5.5	3.0	1.5	4.5
United Kingdom (1996)	4.5	2.3	6.8	3.6	1.8	5.3
USA (1995)	5.3	3.0	8.3	4.4	2.4	6.8

* Neonatal: less than 28 days; Postneonatal: 28 to 364 days; Infant: less than one year

Source: AIHW 2000, Table S9, p. 370

Table 13.2 Life expectancy at selected ages, for Australia, the
United Kingdom and the USA, latest year

Country (latest year)	Life expectancy (years of age)					
	At birth		At 15 years of age		At 65 years of age	
	Males	*Females*	*Males*	*Females*	*Males*	*Females*
Australia (1995–97)	75.9	81.5	61.3	66.9	16.1	19.8
United Kingdom (1996)	74.3	79.5	60.0	65.1	14.8	18.3
USA (1995)	72.5	78.9	58.4	64.7	15.6	18.9

Source: AIHW 2000, Table S12, p. 372

History of health insurance in Australia

The emergence of 'private practice publicly supported' has its origins in the white settlement of Australia. In the beginning, the
colony's administration was the only source of health care. This situation was partly attributable to the government's responsibility
for all the needs of the convicts and their gaolers, but is also partly
explained by the absence of two traditional sources of support:
families and the Church (see Sax 1984). Throughout the nineteenth century, the emphasis of health care was on self-help.
Friendly societies embodied this ideal. Payment of regular amounts
entitled members and their families to the services of a 'lodge
doctor', who entered contracts with the societies in exchange for
a capitation fee (Green & Cromwell 1984; Gillespie 1991).

Throughout the nineteenth century, growth in medical
knowledge and medical status led to increased demand for medical and hospital care, not only among the poor but also among
those considered able to pay. Government, however, opted for a
'hands-off' policy, leaving hospital funding to voluntary charit-
able organisations. This led to funding problems for the voluntary
sector and to the consequent emergence of a three-tiered system:

1   The better-off in the community sought private medical ser-
    vices. They were also expected to contribute to charities for
    the support of the poor (Crichton 1990).
2   Friendly societies catered for the working man and his
    dependents (Green & Cromwell 1984; Gillespie 1991).
3   Those who could not afford private medical services or
    friendly society contributions either went without or attended
    public hospital out-patient clinics. The poor depended on
    charity (Sax 1984; Crichton 1990; Daniel 1995).

The question of who could be treated free of charge created
a dilemma for medical professionals and for the state, reaching
crisis points between the two world wars. James Gillespie argues

that this dilemma provided the climate for the development of hospital insurance schemes that 'epitomised the two major tendencies of the organisation of interwar medical practice—the move towards collective responsibility for the costs of health care and the hegemony of the hospital' (1991, p. 27).

By 1949 a clear division had developed between conservative and labour forces over health insurance arrangements. Doctors, who were aligned with conservative forces, pushed for:

1   fee-for-service medicine financed by private contribution
2   the maintenance of subsidies for those unable to provide for themselves or their families (Crichton 1990).

Working-class leaders, aware of the strain placed on the friendly societies by the economic depressions of the 1890s and the 1930s, identified with the Labor Party and its push for universal, non-contributory health care schemes. Tensions between the two major parties and their supporters were particularly evident in the debates over the several unsuccessful Labor attempts to introduce a comprehensive 'free' national health scheme (Dewdney 1972). Doctors—partly influenced by the experiences of their British colleagues with National Health Insurance and by their fear of loss of autonomy (Gillespie 1991)—combined with conservative politicians. Together they depicted Labor's attempts as a communist threat. The failure of the Chifley government to adequately counter medical and Opposition tactics thwarted any changes that would threaten doctors' control of the health care system (Crichton 1990). In fact, doctors' influence was extended, most notably through the addition of paragraph xxiii(A) to section 51 of the Constitution.

In 1945, the Victorian Attorney-General, acting on behalf of the Victorian branch of the British Medical Association (BMA), challenged the *Pharmaceutical Benefits Act 1945* (Cwlth) in the High Court. This Act allowed patients to receive pharmaceutical benefits only if the doctor's prescription was written on a government-supplied form. The court ruled that the Commonwealth did not have the power to provide or finance health services and that, therefore, its request that doctors use a prescribed form was unconstitutional (Gillespie 1991). Alarmed by this 1946 ruling, the Labor Government sought to amend the Constitution by referendum. Paragraph xxiiiA, section 51 of the Constitution empowered the Commonwealth to make laws with respect to '[t]he provision of maternity allowances, widows' pensions, child endowment, unemployment, pharmaceutical, sickness and hospital benefits, medical and dental services (but not so as to authorise any form of civil conscription), benefits to students and family allowances'. Robert Menzies moved to include the bracketed words at the suggestion of the BMA president, who believed that the original wording would result in the nationalisation of medical and dental services.

The addition was accepted by the federal Attorney-General, Herbert 'Doc' Evatt. Consequently the bracketed words were included in the amendment and became law (Dewdney 1972; Sax 1984; Gillespie 1991). The amendment has allowed governments to provide a wide range of welfare services (Bloom 2000), but it has also enabled doctors to forestall or prevent any attempts that might subject doctors to non-medical control (Sax 1984).

Following the defeat of the Chifley Government in 1949, the new conservative Menzies Government introduced a voluntary health insurance scheme known as the 'Page Plan', which was largely drawn up by the Australian leaders of the BMA (Crichton 1990). The scheme combined patient contributions with government subsidisation of hospital and medical costs. This satisfied the government's desire to introduce a 'National Health Scheme that would have a wide cover, but at the same time preserve the uncontrolled doctor–patient relationship' (Menzies, as quoted in Dewdney 1972, p. 38). The Plan, however, was not successful. It became increasingly clear, over the years, that the voluntary health care insurance arrangements introduced by the Menzies Government were not serving the needs of many sections of the Australian community (Crichton 1990). This was accompanied by increasing disquiet in medical ranks regarding Liberal–Country Party attempts to bring more order to the administration of the voluntary health insurance scheme (Crichton 1990). Not the least of these attempts was the introduction of the common fee, which had originally been canvassed by the AMA (formerly the BMA) as a means of updating medical benefits payable to patients (Dewdney 1972). Many doctors, however, saw the introduction of the common fee as a step towards nationalisation or, at the very least, a government attempt to restrict the doctors' rights to set their own fees (Sax 1984). At the same time, State involvement in hospitals was being extended, and there were calls for the integration of health care services (Crichton 1990). Pressures on the health system were mounting, not the least being the need to address rising health insurance costs and the lack of insurance coverage for increasing sections of the Australian community.

The election of a Labor government in December 1972 offered an opportunity to address these health problems. One solution was the introduction, in July 1975, of the universal health insurance scheme, Medibank, which provided universal cover for free public hospital accommodation and treatment, and 85 per cent of the schedule fee for medical services, with a maximum $5 gap payment (Willcox 1991). It was, however, strongly resisted by doctors, private hospitals, and private health insurance providers, who cited unwarranted interference in the market and in the relations between doctor and patient as the reason (Sax 1984).

The Coalition's return to power in December 1975, only months after the introduction of Medibank, marked a gradual move away from universality and a return to selectivity, all in the name of choice and competition. Over a period of several years Medibank was slowly dismantled. This process culminated in the Fraser Government's 1981 abandonment of the goal of universal coverage and the re-establishment of a private insurance scheme in which financial insecurity and the debt collector again became features of the Australian health care system (Scotton & Macdonald 1993).

The reintroduction of universal health insurance, renamed Medicare, followed the Australian Labor Party (ALP) win in the 1983 election. Old animosities between the medical profession and the ALP soon re-emerged, finding expression in the New South Wales specialists' strikes of 1983 and 1985. Ostensibly these strikes were over section 17 of the *Health Insurance Act 1983*, which sought 'to safeguard the balance between the private and public sectors within public hospitals, to restrain the rates of growth of diagnostic services, and to protect the interests of patients by ensuring the appropriateness of fees charged where publicly funded facilities were used to provide services' (Committee of Inquiry into Rights of Private Practice, as quoted in Sax 1990, p. 75).

Doctors, however, perceived section 17 as unnecessary interference in their right to practise and as an attempt to nationalise the health care system (Sax 1990; Crichton 1990). An ideological clash between doctors and politicians erupted, with the doctors arguing for freedom of choice and the government arguing for the right to control practice in the interest of economic stability. The federal government eventually backed down, but Medicare survived and grew in popularity. Private health insurance, however, declined—from 50 per cent in June 1984 to 34.3 per cent in December 1995 (AIHW 1996a)—prompting grim predictions that the public hospital system would collapse under the weight of public admissions. Doctors and conservative politicians argued that this could only be avoided by increasing the numbers of privately insured individuals and/or the dismantling of Medicare, which they argued promoted overservicing and inefficiency.

The election of the Coalition in March 1996 again shifted the focus of the health insurance debate. While the government promised to maintain Medicare, moves have been made to increase the attractiveness of private health insurance. These incentives are based on the right of individuals to choose how to meet their health care needs, and on the assumption that increased levels of private health insurance will reduce pressure on public hospitals, and hence government funds. In the 1996 Budget, two moves were announced to encourage the purchase of private health insurance. The first entitled those with private health insurance to an annual tax rebate worth $450 for families and $125 for individuals. The second increased the Medicare levy by 1 per cent for individuals earning more than $50 000 and for couples earning more than $100 000. Both provisions were consistent with the ideology of individual responsibility, which underpins Coalition policies.

Following the introduction of the above measures, levels of private insurance did not increase, but rather continued to fall, reaching the lowest level in December 1998 with 30.1 per cent having some level of private health insurance. Following its re-election in 1998 the Liberal–National Party Government replaced the 1996 rebate with a 30 per cent tax rebate for individuals with private health insurance. The Medicare surcharge was retained for those individuals with taxable incomes higher than $50 000 and families with taxable incomes higher than $100 000 without private health insurance. The government also introduced 'lifetime community rating', which penalises individuals who take up private health insurance later in life. This is a significant modification of the community rating principle that has characterised private health insurance arrangements in Australia until 2000. As a consequence of this move, combined with the 30 per cent rebate, private health insurance cover increased to 44.9 per cent of the population by the end of December 2001 (PHIAC 2002).

The adoption of these measures runs the risk of 'white-anting' the universal nature of Medicare by improving the attractiveness of private health insurance, which in turn increases the pressure to introduce 'opting out' provisions similar to those that marked the end of Medibank. The ideological nature of the measures is reflected in the $1.6 billion cost of the 30 per cent health insurance rebate. The government has opted for 'propping up' private health insurance rather than increasing investment in public hospitals and the public health care system. As the Friends of Medicare note, 'private health insurance does not buy health services—it buys insurance ... There is no guarantee that public hospital demand will fall as a result' (Friends of Medicare 1999). The *First Report—Public Hospital Funding and Options for Reform* noted:

> Most participants viewed recent Commonwealth Government initiatives on private health insurance with some concern. This was particularly the case with regard to the 30 per cent rebate which most participants believed was unlikely to relieve demand on public hospital services, despite costing in excess of $2 billion per annum. Arguably, the 30 per cent rebate can be seen to run counter to the Medicare principles of universality, equity and access. Little evidence was presented showing benefits for public hospitals from the rebate (Community Affairs References Committee 2000, 3.1).

The history of Australian health care financing reveals that, after an initial period of government responsibility, there was a gradual evolution 'from a private entrepreneurial-philanthropic way of providing care towards a government funded and controlled service organisation' (Crichton 1990, p. 7). Government involvement remains a contested issue, especially as it relates to the question of compulsion versus freedom of choice. The need for medical and hospital insurance is not the issue; rather, the debate centres on the role of the state, the role of the individual (versus that of the community), and the role of the market (Crichton 1990; Sax 1984; Duckett 1995). All the major players—political parties, doctors, and their private health allies—have acknowledged the role of private health insurance in the Australian health care system (Sax 1990). All acknowledge that there are funding problems—notably cost-shifting between the States and Commonwealth, and patient queuing—but the responses to these problems are shaped by the underlying ideological perspectives of the particular parties. The Coalition has, so far, opted for assistance to private health insurance, while the ALP had opted for the retention of universal health insurance and the reform of delivery arrangements through the introduction of managed care, 'whereby an organisation assumes responsibility for all necessary health care for an individual in exchange for a fixed payment' (Duckett 1996, p. 10). In order to understand these different responses, it is necessary to examine both the philosophical principles underpinning the competing ideological perspectives, and the role of power and structural interests in the organisation and financing of health insurance arrangements.

Ideology

The meaning of 'ideology' is contentious (Abercrombie et al. 1988), but it generally refers to 'a set of beliefs and values which express the interests of a particular social group' (Haralambos & Holborn 1991, p. 21). Ideology shapes judgments about fairness and justice, which are often characterised as contests between freedom and equality—between the right to 'do as I choose' and the need to ensure that societal benefits are fairly distributed. Discussions of the merits (or faults) of health insurance revolve around these principles of freedom and equality, but the difficulty with these two principles is that they can and do conflict.

The concept of 'liberty' or 'freedom' refers to the ability of the individual to make choices independently of outside interference. It assumes individual responsibility. The concept of equality relates to equality of outcome and, as such, implies some level of collective responsibility. Conflict emerges over the question of fairness or equity. In cases in which liberty assumes importance, questions of fairness are decided on the basis of merit. Access to goods and services must be 'earned'. When this system fails, targeted welfare services may be provided. However, these services are linked to demonstrations of willingness to work. Welfare provision is residual—available only as a last resort (Gardner 1995).

If equality of outcome is perceived to be more important, then it is more likely that fairness will be determined on the basis of need. Satisfaction of that need is more likely to be seen in terms of a collective responsibility requiring public and universal provision: an institutional approach. Rather than holding the individuals responsible for their predicament, this approach acknowledges structured inequality and opts for institutional provision in order to ensure equality of outcome (Dalton et al. 1996; Gardner 1995).

From Left to Right

Traditional understandings of freedom and equality stretch along a political continuum from Left to Right, from **socialism** to **liberalism**. The history of politics in Australia has tended to be a history of liberalism rather than of socialism. This can be attributed to the predominance of **ruling-class** values and elites, and to the relative weakness of the working class: 'Liberalism, the "official ideology" of the ruling class, has had a pervasive and persistent influence on social policy. The classic values of individualism, competition, individual freedoms and inequality, have combined with an acceptance of a minor role for government in protection for the "really needy" ' (Tulloch 1983, p. 255). Working-class initiatives have been constrained by these dominant values, resulting in a residual view of welfare that reinforces, rather than challenges, the status quo (Beilharz et al. 1992).

Equality is generally associated with the socialist end of the continuum, and freedom with the liberal end. While this understanding is too simplistic (see Kymlicka 1990), it does provide a useful guide to the impact of the principles of liberty (freedom) and equality upon the health insurance policies of the major political parties and their supporters.

Liberalism

Attitudes to liberty find expression in the ideology of liberalism. Understandings of liberty range from 'freedom from' coercion to 'freedom to' benefit. Both understandings acknowledge the concept of rights, but the former views these rights as negative—freedom from interference—whereas the latter sees rights as positive—the right to services and benefits that enable participation in society.

socialism/communism Political ideology with numerous variations, but generally refers to the creation of societies in which private property and wealth accumulation are replaced by state ownership and distribution of economic resources. Communism represents a utopian vision of society based on communal ownership of resources, cooperation, and altruism to the extent that social inequality and the state no longer exist. Both terms are often used interchangeably to refer to societies ruled by a communist party.

liberalism An ideology that regards the interests of individuals and their place in the market-place as being of primary importance.

ruling class This is a hotly debated term used to highlight the point that the upper class in society has political power as a result of its economic wealth. The term is often used interchangeably with 'upper class'.

Rights

One person's 'right' entails another's obligation. It also creates expectations. In the case of health, a positive right entails an obligation to provide appropriate care and an expectation that such care will be forthcoming. A negative right entails an obligation not to interfere in the actions of another (Beauchamp & Faden 1979). The splitting of rights into negative and positive types, however, is simplistic, as rights are 'complex, containing both negative rights and positive rights' (Beauchamp & Faden 1979, p. 120). There is, for example, a tension between the right not to insure and the right of the community not to have to support the non-insured in times of adversity. Simplistic as it is, the division into negative and positive broadly defines two types of liberalism.

Proponents of negative rights generally argue for non-interference, which is linked to their advocacy of the libertarian variety of liberty—freedom from coercion. The state may only intervene to limit the liberty of an individual when and if the exercise of that liberty will harm others. This justification is a feature of narrow and conservative social health programs. Rights and expectations are framed within an individualistic perspective, which argues for the satisfaction of health access through private provision. Public provision should be limited to cases in which harm may flow from the actions of others, such as quarantine of contagious diseases, or to the provision of those public goods for which individuals are unlikely to pay. Inequality is inevitable because people have unequal levels of intelligence and different skills and abilities. The solution, however, lies not in the public provision of goods and services, but rather in the operation of the market. Unfortunately some will fail, but eventually the rewards will **trickle down** and they will receive some benefit. Failing that, they can turn to charity. The moral justification of this outlook lies in the proposal that libertarianism is grounded in free choice. Libertarianism extends its defence of individual freedom to the assertion that taxation is inherently wrong because it violates people's rights to dispose of their wealth as they see fit (Kymlicka 1990). When all is said and done, individuals 'earn' access to goods and services.

Such a belief underpins the concept of **economic rationalism**, or economic liberalism, which refers to the capacity of the market to allocate resources efficiently (Beilharz et al. 1992). Economic efficiency drives not only economic policy but also health and social policy. It requires the cutting back of government responsibilities, the introduction of private sector competition, and the promotion of independence, all in the name of economic efficiency (Rees & Rodley 1995). The privatisation of government functions is necessary in order to return responsibility to the indi-

trickle down The theory that everyone benefits by allowing the upper class to prosper relatively unfettered. If wealthy capitalists are allowed and encouraged to maximise their profits, it is believed that this increased wealth will eventually 'trickle down' to the workers.

economic rationalism or economic liberalism Terms used to describe a political philosophy based on 'small-government' and market-oriented policies, such as deregulation, privatisation, reduced government spending, and lower taxation.

vidual, thereby ending the culture of dependency. People should be free to make their own choices and their own mistakes. In the case of health, this idea finds expression in the call for individuals to finance their own health care needs through the purchase of private health insurance, thereby leaving the public health care system to care only for those who cannot afford private health care.

Social liberalism, by way of contrast, views rights as positive: liberty means 'freedom to' benefit. This ideology acknowledges that compensation is needed to counteract the excesses of the marketplace. This is done by assuming some degree of collective responsibility for improving access to health care services, which in turn enables individuals to participate fully in society. State intervention, through either the levying of taxes, legislation, or public provision, is expected, even if not always welcome (Beilharz et al. 1992).

The influence of socialism, with its emphasis on equality, is evident in social liberalism. Equality extends beyond equality of opportunity to equality of conditions and outcomes. Hence the emphasis is not on 'the abstract individual' who exists before his or her social situation (Forder et al. 1984, p. 16), but upon the **social structure** that either limits or enhances the condition of the individual and hence his or her **life chances**. Resources, then, are allocated according to need, not merit. Reliance on the idea of individual, negative rights is insufficient. These rights must be supplemented by positive rights, which allow for the 'freedom to' benefit. The state needs to be involved so that those obstacles that hinder individual development can be addressed (Beilharz et al. 1992). Universal health insurance enables access to health care services and benefits, and so enables individuals to participate in society. By definition, it impinges on personal liberty in the interest of equality.

social liberalism An ideology that is based on individual freedom but that acknowledges the need for state intervention to overcome the inadequacies of the market, which can act to limit the freedom of individuals to fully participate in society.

social structure The recurring patterns of social interaction through which people are related to each other, such as social institutions and social groups.

life chances A term derived from Max Weber that refers to the opportunities available to people in society. People with different social-class locations have different life chances, including different opportunities with regard to education, wealth, and health.

Politics, power, and structural interests

Australian health insurance arrangements reflect the ideological struggle between social and economic liberalism (Beilharz et al. 1992), which has found political expression in the two major political parties: the Liberal–National Coalition and the Australian Labor Party (ALP). Generally speaking, the working class, through the trade unions, has aligned itself with the ALP, whereas doctors, private hospitals, and the insurance industry have supported the Coalition. The strength of the differences between the two political parties, however, can be overestimated. In fact, there has been a tendency to strike compromises between the two views, and over time these compromises have been embedded into health care arrangements (Green & Cromwell 1984; Gillespie

1991; Sax 1984). Nevertheless, there have been significant ideological disputes, and the reforms to health insurance are a political expression of such disputes.

Politics

Politics is the process of resolving conflict between rival interests, and of the allocation of scarce resources. Politics is about power. While there are several definitions of power, ranging from elitist through pluralist to radical theories (see Gardner 1995), **pluralism** is dominant. The pluralist view maintains that health policy outcomes are a consequence of compromise between the interests of government and the interests of various interest groups, the most significant of which are those groups representing doctors. This is a legitimate exercise of power.

pluralism A theory whereby state power is shared with a large number of pressure or interest groups.

A contrasting view is provided by Stephen Lukes (1974), who identifies three dimensions of power. The first dimension is equivalent to pluralism and is evident in issues over which there is observable conflict. The second dimension refers to those occasions on which decision-making is confined to safe issues through the process of non-decision-making. The use of power suppresses conflicts so that this use becomes covert. Issues are kept out of the political or decision-making process by removing them. Tactics used include transferring a contentious issue to a committee for examination and co-opting opponents to the committee, knowing full well that nothing will happen or that the dissenting voices will be neutralised (Lukes 1974). The third dimension offers a radical critique of power by highlighting the actual shaping of interests and preferences, usually without individuals being aware that they are being shaped. Lukes maintains that people's expressed preferences and interests are shaped by **socialisation**, education, and the media, thereby creating a system of dominant values and beliefs: ideology. Conflict is latent—sleeping until woken—because people are unaware of their real preferences and interests. This enables those who exercise power to protect their interests at the expense of the powerless.

socialisation The process of learning the culture of a society (its language and customs), which shows us how to behave and communicate.

Lukes's theory of power can be combined with the 'structural interest perspective' developed by Richard Alford (1975). He maintains that health policy and the organisation of health care are the products of the social, political, and economic forces that exist at a particular time. Vested or structural interests are formed. These may be classified as dominant (professional monopoly), challenging (corporate rationalism), or repressed (equal health advocacy). Interests are dominant if they have achieved ideological status—that is, they do not have to organise to defend their interests because other institutions do that for them. Challenging interests seek the overthrow or modification of the dominant interests, while repressed interests are kept under control by the dominant interests.

Pluralist accounts of health insurance reforms assume too level a playing field. They ignore the role of ideology in shaping the context within which decision-making occurs, as well as the dominance of some interests over others. Pluralism also ignores the unequal distribution of resources, although this inequality impedes the effective mobilisation of competing interests (Gardner 1995). More satisfying explanations are provided by Lukes and Alford.

By far the most powerful group within the health care system are doctors—the professional monopolists. **Medical dominance** is derived not through a natural process but, rather, through scientific medical knowledge, which then enables the doctor to 'construct the demand for his or her services. Put simply, patients depend on their doctor to define their malady and propose the alternative treatments available. This monopoly of therapeutic knowledge has been the key to the political strength of the medical profession' (Gillespie 1991, p. 16). In the case of health insurance, this dominance has been seriously challenged by politicians and governments, most notably Labor politicians and governments.

The introduction of Medibank in 1975 and Medicare in 1984 was strongly resisted by doctors, who clung to the old bogey that it would mark the fall of medicine to a socialist, nationalist scheme. In particular, they raised concerns related to 'fees, conditions of service in public hospitals, a perceived threat to private hospitals and the pernicious threat that could be exerted by a single government-directed paymaster' (Sax 1984, pp. 109–10). Resistance also came from the health insurance funds. In conjunction with doctors, they developed arguments that advocated 'the virtues of freedom of choice through subsidised insurance and the retention of an element of market activity' (Sax 1984, p. 112). Drawing on the ideology of economic liberalism, they argued that any reduction in freedom of choice would result in a deterioration in the quality of health care. In this, they were supported by the Coalition—a combination that was sufficiently powerful to achieve modification of both schemes (Sax 1984). The fact that universal health insurance was introduced and remains, means that they have not been entirely successful in maintaining control of health matters, largely because of the combined efforts of the two challenging interests who espoused the ideology of social liberalism. Stephen Duckett (1984) notes that the bitter struggle over the introduction of Medibank was marked by a convergence of interests between the corporate rationalisers and equal health advocates. Together they challenged the dominance of the medical monopolists, but this has only dented

medical dominance A general term used to describe the power of the medical profession in terms of its control over its own work, over the work of other health workers, and over health resource allocation, health policy, and the way that hospitals are run.

medical control. Doctors retain professional and economic control. Their continuing resistance to universal health insurance means that the maintenance of universal coverage depends on the strength of support for Medicare, the strength of its advocates in relation to its opponents, and the willingness of government to support its retention. The return of a Liberal–National Party government that strongly espouses the value of freedom of choice and its willingness to 'prop up' private health insurance strengthens the position of doctors and their ally, the private health insurance sector. This is not to argue that relations between government and private health insurance providers and doctors is all rosy. Indeed there is considerable dispute between the players. The Howard Government, in view of the popularity of Medicare with the Australian public, has been forced to commit itself to Medicare's retention. At the same time its ideological commitment to freedom of choice has required it to reach an accommodation between support for government funding of health care and encouragement of individual responsibility.

Future directions

The core issue in relation to health insurance concerns not health itself but private enterprise and freedom of choice. It is generally agreed that medical care should be available to all those who need it. Differences emerge regarding how this should be achieved, with the solutions being framed according to the decision-maker's view of reality. While no party can claim a monopoly on any one view, doctors and conservative politicians—influenced by economic liberalism's emphasis on self-help and individual responsibility—have generally opted for restricted state intervention when the market and the family break down. On the other hand, the ALP and its supporters—influenced by social liberalism—have tended to opt for the expansion of state intervention in the belief that this will allow citizens not only to enjoy the fruits that society can offer but also to participate in the shaping of society. The purpose of compulsory, universal health insurance, then, was to ensure universal access to medical and hospital care, and to fund that access more equitably in order that all citizens might participate fully in society (Sax 1984).

There remain fundamental differences of opinion that are largely ideological. Adherents of economic liberalism argue that the public provision of health tends to blunt 'the personal thriftiness that used to influence patients, doctors and administrators' (Sax 1984, p. 193), and the personal responsibility for one's own health. Social liberals counter that public provision breaks down barriers to health care. Generally there is acceptance of the need for medical and hospital insurance, but conflict remains over how that might best be achieved. There is acceptance of some level of state involvement, but differences occur over the terms of state intervention and over the question of freedom of choice.

Conclusion

The value of the sociological imagination applied to health policy is that it reveals its complexity. At the same time it enables analysts to identify the impediments to change and may assist in the identification of solutions. This chapter has outlined the historical and cultural influences upon the development of health policy, in this case health insurance. Australia's penal origins, her smallness, and isolation has produced a citizenry that unlike her American counterparts looks to the state for some measure of collective responsibility for the welfare of her population. At the same time she has been suspicious of 'big brother', also attributable to our origins, our size, and isolation.

Structural factors that have shaped the way health policy and more particularly health insurance has been organised include the federal organisation of the Australian health care system, the role of ideology, and the relationship between and power exercised by the various structural interests, namely the professional monopolists, the corporate rationalisers and the equal health advocates. The present health insurance arrangements are not a 'natural' part of Australian health policy. Rather they are a consequence of historical, social, political, economic, ideological, and cultural factors, which together with vested interests have produced the public/private mix. The dominant interest, although under challenge, remains professional monopoly. As Cormack and Hindle note, 'Retention of private practice, fee-for-service payment and voluntary health insurance is not so much a consequence of government's unresponsiveness or the personal beliefs of ministers, but because they are symbols of success for perhaps the most powerful constituency—the organised medical profession' (1999, p. 6).

Understanding the role of the first three blocks of the sociological imagination is important for any decision on how things might be improved for the benefit of all Australians. The 30 per cent private health insurance rebate will be difficult to remove as it achieves 'taken-for-granted' status among those who receive the benefit. At the same time the high level of community acceptance of Medicare (Cormack & Hindle 1999, p. 5; Blewett 2000, p. 11) also makes its dismantling unlikely. Therefore Australia seems set to retain both private and public health coverage at least into the foreseeable future. Problems, however, continue, not the least being protection of vested interests. As Blewett notes in relation to the links between the private sector:

> The providers of care (the private specialists) want to maximise their independence and their incomes; the payers for care (the private health funds) want to minimise the costs; and the private hospitals want reasonable bed occupancies (and are therefore dependent on the private specialists to provide patients) and want a reasonable recovery of their costs (and are therefore dependent on the private funds). The dependency of the private hospitals and the wimpishness of the funds have tended to mean that the private medical specialists have called the shots despite the efforts of governments of both political persuasion to strengthen the hands of the private funds and the private hospitals (2000, p. 14).

Similar comments can be made in relation to the public sector. The alliance between doctors, private health insurance, and private hospitals, although under tension, is underpinned by the belief in individual responsibility, the restriction of government activity, and the operation of market forces—a belief shared by the Liberal–National Party Government. As already noted, Australians tend to look to government for solutions, but at the same time retain a suspicion of too much interference. Solutions that fail to take account of these tendencies will either falter or face a stormy passage. They should, however, take note of the advice of four leading health economists, Evans, Reinhardt, Maynard, and Preker: 'First, important decisions on health must not be left to the market. Second, competition and markets are not worthwhile ends in themselves and should be used only when it is safe to do so. Third, it would be destructive to encourage commercial health insurance' (Cormack & Hindle 1999, p. 5).

Summary of main points

- Health policy and the organisation of health care is the product of the social, political, and economic forces that exist at a particular time.
- An understanding of health policy and of the organisation of health care requires an examination of the role of politicians and doctors; an examination of the impact of ideology, politics, and power; and an examination of the role of the state, of the individual and community, and of the market.
- Government involvement in health care is a contested issue, related as it is to the question of compulsion versus freedom of choice, and of the rights of the individual versus the rights of the community.

- Health policy and the organisation of health care reflect an ideological struggle between economic and social liberalism. This struggle has found political expression in the two major political parties: the Australian Labor Party and the Liberal–National Coalition.

Discussion questions

1 What are the attitudes of Australians to the role of the state? Place your response in a historical context.
2 What are the key principles that underpin attitudes to health policy?
3 What is the role of structural interests in the formation of a health policy?
4 How does health policy reflect the relationship between politics, power, ideology, and structural interests?
5 What is economic rationalism? Discuss in relation to health insurance.
6 What is meant by the term 'community rating'? What is its significance?

Further investigation

1 Evaluate the role of ideology in the development of health policy. Illustrate your answer with examples of specific health policies.
2 Discuss and analyse the health policies of the Liberal–National Party Coalition, the Australian Labor Party, and the Australian Democrats.

Further reading and web resources

Beilharz, P., Considine, M., & Watts, R. 1992, *Arguing about the Welfare State: The Australian Experience*, Allen & Unwin, Sydney.

Bloom, A. L. 2000, *Health Reform in Australia and New Zealand*, Oxford University Press, Melbourne.

Duckett, S. J. 2000, *The Australian Health Care System*, Oxford University Press, Melbourne.

Gardner, H. (ed.) 1995, *The Politics of Health: The Australian Experience*, 2nd edn, Churchill Livingstone, Melbourne.

Gardner, H. (ed.) 1997, *Health Policy in Australia*, Oxford University Press, Melbourne.

Gillespie, J. A. 1991, *The Price of Health: Australian Governments and Medical Politics 1910–1960*, Cambridge University Press, Melbourne.

Hancock, L. (ed.) 1991, *Health Policy in the Market State*, Allen & Unwin, Sydney.

Leeder, S. R. 2000, *Healthy Medicine: Challenges Facing Australia's Health Services*, Allen & Unwin, Sydney.

Mooney, G. & Scotton, R. (eds) 1998, *Economics and Australian Health Policy*, Allen & Unwin, Sydney

Sax, S. 1984, *A Strife of Interests: Politics and Policies in Australian Health Services*, Allen & Unwin, Sydney.

Web sites

Australian Democrats (AD): <http://www.democrats.org.au/>
Australian Department of Health and Aged Care:
     <http://www.health.gov.au/
Australian Greens: <http://www.greens.org.au/>
Australian Labor Party (ALP): <http://www.alp.org.au/>
Australian Medical Association: <http://www.ama.com.au/>
Doctors Reform Society of Australia:
     <http://www.drs.org.au/drshome.htm>
Friends of Medicare:
     <http://www.pha.org.au/friends_of_medicare/frame_friends_of_
     medicare.html>
Liberal Party of Australia (LPA): <http://www.liberal.org.au/>
National Party of Australia (NPA): <http://www.npa.org.au/>
Public Health Association of Australia: <http://www.pha.org.au/>

14

Challenges to Medical Dominance

John Germov

Overview

* ✳ *What is medical dominance?*
* ✳ *How did medicine become the dominant health care profession?*
* ✳ *In what ways are challenges to medical dominance affecting the medical profession and the organisation, delivery, and use of health services?*

There is a significant sociological literature that critiques the dominance of the medical profession in the health system. In fact much of health sociology can be viewed as based in an analysis of the role, influence, and misapplications of medical power in society more generally. This chapter provides an overview of how medicine established its dominance in the health care system. It briefly discusses how medical dominance was established, outlines some of the problems of such dominance, and then examines the effectiveness of various challenges to the medical profession. While medical dominance has never gone unchallenged and has often been resisted in formal and informal ways, in recent decades challenges have proved more effective and medical power appears to be in steady decline, though it is likely that medicine will remain the dominant health profession.

Key terms

agency	managerialism	professional bureaucracy
biomedical model	McDonaldisation	rationalisation
class	medical dominance	risk society
clinical governance	medical-industrial complex	sexism in medicine
commodification of health care	medicalisation	social control
deprofessionalisation	negotiated order	social structure
empirical	patriarchy	state
evidence-based medicine	professionalisation/profes-	trait approach
health promotion	sional project	women's health movement
ideology	proletarianisation	

Introduction

> There would never be any public agreement among doctors if they
> did not agree to agree on the main point of the doctor being always
> in the right.
>
> George Bernard Shaw (1908), *The Doctor's Dilemma*, preface

medical dominance A general term used to describe the power of the medical profession in terms of its control over its own work, over the work of other health workers, and over health resource allocation, health policy, and the way that hospitals are run.

The term **medical dominance** refers to the fact that medicine is clearly the most powerful profession in the health system. Despite this, doctors comprise only 16 per cent of the total health professional workforce, compared with nurses who make up 65 per cent, and allied health practitioners (dietitians, occupational therapists, physiotherapists, pharmacists, radiographers, speech pathologists, optometrists, and podiatrists) who collectively constitute 15.5 per cent (AIHW 1998). This chapter briefly explains what medical dominance is, how it was established and the problems it poses to the delivery of optimal health care. The chapter then focuses on the various challenges to medical dominance that are said to be undermining medicine's influence over health care delivery, other health professions, and patients. It is argued that medical dominance has always been contested, and that medicine is likely to face continued assaults on its legitimacy and occupational territory, including challenges that may also undermine health care delivery and patient outcomes.

What is medical dominance?

According to Eliot Freidson (1970), a key author in the field, the 'professional dominance' of medicine is due to doctors' clinical role of diagnosis and treatment; the ability of doctors to exert control over the knowledge base and occupational territory of other health professions; the requirement that doctors request and supervise the work of other health practitioners; and the unequal public status of medicine compared to other health professions. Furthermore, Mintzberg states: 'The professional's power derives from the fact that not only is his [*sic*] work too complex to be supervised by managers or standardized by analysts, but also that his services are typically in great demand ... which enables him to insist on considerable autonomy in his work' (1979, p. 357).

The medical profession dominates every aspect of health care delivery, particularly other health professions such as nursing and allied health, in the following ways:

- Only doctors can formally diagnose disease, sign birth and death certificates, and they have significant control over access to non-medical benefits, such as sick leave, workers' compensation, and early retirement due to health reasons.

- Doctor's control of diagnosis and treatment means that they effectively have administrative and financial authority over other health professions. The decisions of doctors set in train the work of nursing and allied health professionals who are either directly or indirectly responsible to doctor authority, particularly within the hospital system. This means that doctors can control access to a range of therapies through the requirement of a doctor's referral before other health professions can treat a patient.
- Doctors are over-represented on hospital management boards, the registration boards of most other health professions, health policy advisory bodies, and the bodies that fund health research. Such a situation limits the ability of alternative, nursing and allied health practitioners to produce evidence to support their work and expand their occupational role, which could potentially challenge the legitimacy of medical expertise if their treatments were proven to be particularly effective.

As Freidson points out, the key feature of medical dominance is autonomy, which he defines as the 'authority to direct and evaluate the work of others without in turn being subject to formal direction and evaluation by them' (Freidson 1970, p. 135). Mary Elston (1991) makes a useful distinction between three forms of medical autonomy that highlights the basis of medicine's dominance:

1   *economic autonomy*: the right of doctors to determine their pay rates (fee for service)
2   *political autonomy*: the right to make policy decisions as the legitimate experts on health matters
3   *clinical autonomy*: the right to set professional standards about treatment, which dictate hospital expenditure and the work of other health care workers (enacted through licensing laws, which protect medicine from occupational encroachment).

The notion of autonomy helps to explain why many other occupational groups have achieved limited success in attempting to mimic medicine's attributes by adopting a strategy of **professionalisation** (see chapters 15, 16 and 17 for further discussion). Professionalisation assumes that professional status can be gained by simply meeting a set of criteria or traits that, once acquired, function collectively to transform an occupation into a profession. Such a **trait approach** to professionalisation reflects functionalist theory (see chapter 2), which views professions as performing essential 'functions' for society by possessing certain attributes from which they derive their high status and rewards. The assumption behind such an understanding is that, if any occupation acquires similar attributes or traits (such as university qualifications, highly specialised knowledge and skills, or a code of

professionalisation (professional project) The process of becoming a profession, whereby an occupational group attains publicly recognised and government-legitimated monopoly and autonomy over its area of work. Professional status is usually associated with certain traits (see 'trait approach').

trait approach A general theory that assumes that professional status can be achieved by meeting a set of criteria (usually defined as specialised expertise and training), by having the exclusive right to practise in a particular field, by self-regulation (based on a code of ethics), and by charging a fee for service.

ethics) they can also become a profession. Despite their professional projects, nursing and allied health professions have not achieved the same level of power or status as medicine because they have been unable to acquire the essential characteristic of autonomy. They have also been deprived of the special historical and political advantages that provided the medical profession with its exclusive professional status, as the following section describes.

Medical dominance: a brief historical overview

Medical dominance was secured and has been maintained by political means. It was not until the nineteenth century that medicine as a science began to develop and that medicine became a full-time occupation. A number of significant works have examined the issue of professions, particularly the rise of the medical profession (see Freidson 1970, 1994; Johnson 1972; Larson 1977; Starr 1982; Larkin 1983; Willis 1983, 1989b; Abbott 1988; Gillespie 1991; see also Porter 1997; Duffin 1999; and Le Fanu 1999 for general histories of medicine). In Australia, the landmark text on the rise of the medical profession remains Evan Willis' *Medical Dominance* (1983, 1989b), on which much of this section's content is based.

Medical dominance is less than a century old. During most of the nineteenth century and even the early twentieth century, most people did not consult a doctor when they were sick, but rather visited the more affordable, accessible, and respectable homoeopaths, chemists, Chinese herbalists, and midwives. In the early nineteenth century, doctors had few cures and little scientific understanding of disease. Most doctors serviced the wealthy, who resided in the major cities and could afford their fees. The general population was highly sceptical of medicine, particularly surgeons, because of the high death rate from post-operative infection (antiseptic only came into use in the 1880s).

Doctor numbers in Australia were also small, with only 18 doctors for Melbourne's 20 000 residents in 1841, rising to more than 500 by 1863 (Willis 1989b). As their numbers increased, mostly because of an oversupply in the United Kingdom, doctors used two political strategies to gain a competitive advantage over unqualified practitioners (the 'quacks', as some doctors refer to them) (Willis 1989b). The main way to achieve this advantage was for doctors to expand their client base by establishing a health care monopoly. First, medical associations were formed to unify doctors against their competition, and second, the associations lobbied the **state** to ban 'quacks'. In 1862 the Victorian government (with other colonies to follow) became the first to pass

state A term used to describe a collection of institutions, including the parliament (government and Opposition political parties), the public-sector bureaucracy, the judiciary, the military, and the police.

legislation giving doctors significant advantages, such as the exclusive use of medical titles, and the right to sign death certificates, hold government appointments, and sue for non-payment of fees. Because of the dominance of a *laissez-faire* **ideology**, most governments were unwilling to ban 'quacks', viewing this as a curtailment of people's freedom of choice.

ideology In a political context, ideology refers to those beliefs and values that relate to the way in which society should be organised, including the appropriate role of the state.

The major legal development that firmly entrenched medical dominance was an amendment to the Australian Constitution. Doctors have traditionally been aligned with conservative political forces, which favour free enterprise and private health insurance arrangements, and support the development of medical dominance. However, in 1946 it was the federal Labor government that secured medical dominance by allowing a minor constitutional amendment of section 51, paragraph xxiiiA by referendum. The primary purpose of the referendum was to enable the federal government to make laws on a range of welfare services such as maternity allowances, pensions, unemployment benefits, and medical services. The Australian branch of the British Medical Association (BMA)—a separate Australian Medical Association (AMA) would not be formed until 1962—believed that the wording of the referendum would result in the nationalisation of medicine (as had occurred in the United Kingdom). On behalf of the BMA, Robert Menzies (the leader of the Opposition at the time) introduced an additional phrase, which forbade any form of civil conscription of medicine (Gillespie 1991). The Labor Government acceded to this request to lessen opposition to the referendum, which was passed by popular vote (one of only eight successful referendums in Australia to date). The constitutional amendment allowed federal governments to provide a wide range of welfare services, but it effectively enshrined medical autonomy in the Constitution—medicine being the only profession to be granted freedom from civil conscription. It is worth mentioning that the exact meaning of the amendment with respect to medicine has never been challenged or clarified. Rather, it has been accepted as the hallmark of medical dominance in Australia and is now regarded as a naïve slip on the part of the then Labor government. The rise of medical dominance, therefore, was primarily a result of its political organisation and lobbying.

class (or social class) A position within a system of structured inequality based on the unequal distribution of power, wealth, income, and status. Class membership is determined by three characteristics: ownership and control of scarce economic resources; ownership of marketable skills and qualifications; and wage labour. People who share a social-class position typically share similar life chances.

As Willis (1989b), among others, argues, the development of the medical profession's monopoly was guaranteed by the state through the support of fee-for-service, self-regulation, medical education (particularly the independent specialist colleges), and the suppression of competition from other health practitioners. State support was partly achieved through **class** allegiances between the profession and conservative political forces. Moreover as Connell argues, state support of a self-regulated and profit-oriented medical profession 'assimilated medicine to the economic and ideological patterns of capitalism' (1988, p. 214). This has resulted in a commonality of lifestyles and interests between doctors and the upper class to the extent that 'doctors as a group, and medical organisations as institutions, have particular political and economic interests they do not share with most of their patients: interests in maintaining a sharp division of labour in health care, in a substantial amount of public ignorance about health, and in seeing that self-help arrangements for health care remain marginal or ineffective' (Connell 1988, p. 214). It is indeed an irony that while the state helped to establish medical dominance, a large segment of the medical profession opposes significant forms of public health care, as shown by the Australian Medical Association's (AMA) continued opposition to the Medicare system.

Maintaining dominance

Willis (1989b) describes four methods by which medicine has exerted control over its competition in an attempt to maintain its dominance:

1   *subordination*: ensuring that some health workers, such as nurses, midwives, and allied health practitioners all work under the direct authority of doctors, especially within the hospital system
2   *limitation*: legally restricting the occupational territory of other health workers—such as physiotherapists, dentists, and optometrists—particularly through doctor representation on registration boards
3   *exclusion*: denying legitimacy to alternative health practitioners—such as acupuncturists, chiropractors and homoeopaths—by excluding them from registration, state-supported education, research, and public health insurance (Medicare) coverage
4   *incorporation*: the absorption of occupational territory into medical practice (such as doctors practising 'spinal manipulation').

Male-dominated medicine played a significant part in the subordination of women as health practitioners. Barbara Ehrenreich and Deidre English (1973) were among the first writers to highlight the patriarchal and oppressive role of medicine in the persecution of women healers, who were often accused of being witches. Furthermore, medicine played a role in denying women access to medical education to become doctors. It also effectively opposed the professionalisation of female-dominated occupations such as nursing by opposing the establishment of state-supported nurse registration, education, and practitioner autonomy (see chapter 15).

Despite using incorporation, subordination, limitation, and exclusionary practices, medicine has never completely dominated health care. In fact, other health professions have resisted medical dominance, with varying degrees of success (see chapters 15, 16, and 17). The introduction of Medibank and then Medicare (see chapter 13) is evidence that governments can introduce policies to which many doctors are opposed, despite overwhelming public support for such policies. Medicine's dominance over other health therapies has also been incomplete.

In 1978, after a long struggle against medicine, chiropractors were able to gain formal recognition as a profession by the state through registration and funding of a university degree course (Willis 1989b). Willis argues that the success of chiropractors in challenging medical dominance resulted from public support and a record of successful treatment. Chiropractors are still unable to hold positions in public hospitals and are not covered by Medicare; however, all workers' compensation schemes recognise chiropractors as primary practitioners (patients do not need a doctor's referral). Therefore, it is important to note that the achievement and maintenance of medical dominance does not mean that doctors have total control, and there have been, and continue to be, effective forms of resistance.

biomedicine/biomedical model The conventional approach to medicine in Western societies. It diagnoses and explains illness as a malfunction of one of the body's biological mechanisms. The biomedical approach of most health services focuses on the treating of individuals, and generally ignores social, economic, and environmental factors.

Problems with medical dominance

medicalisation The process by which non-medical problems become defined and treated as medical issues, usually in terms of illnesses, disorders, or syndromes.

Many of the chapters in this book deal with specific issues arising from medicine's dominance in the health system. The main criticisms of medical dominance are briefly discussed here and include:
- self-regulation
- fee-for-service
- medicine's monopoly over clinical decision-making
- the tendency towards the **medicalisation** of social issues and the limitations of the **biomedical model**
- **sexism in medicine**.

sexism in medicine Refers to discriminatory and harmful treatment of women by doctors in terms of ignoring women's health concerns in medical research and intervention, not informing women about alternative treatments or the side effects of drugs/therapies, and labelling women's problems as 'psychosomatic' rather than 'real'.

Medicine has often been criticised for being self-serving—placing self-interest over patient or public interest—in the delivery of health services and the treatment of disease. The profession has been accused of not being open to self-criticism, with self-regulation being unable to effectively address issues of fraud, negligence, misconduct, or incompetence among its members. Media exposés of medical fraud and negligence have made the public increasingly aware of the potentially damaging effects of medical treatment and of some practitioners' exploitation of patients (Illich 1977; Germov 1994; 1993). Various forms of fraud have been exposed over the years—particularly scientific fraud in the form of biased medical research (La Follette 1992), pharmaceutical fraud such as the promotion of thalidomide (Braithwaite 1984), and medical technology fraud such as the marketing of the Dalkon Shield (Cashman 1989). The patient deaths and abuses at Chelmsford Hospital and the Auckland Women's Hospital further demonstrate that self-regulation can result in the unwillingness of health professionals to engage in 'whistle-blowing' (see Daniel 1998) even in the face of allegations of gross negligence (see Bromberger & Fife-Yeomans 1992; Coney 1988).

The problems of self-regulation have often been linked with the issue of fee-for-service and the pursuit of profit, which have raised concerns over whether clinical or financial concerns determine appropriate courses of treatment (Navarro 1976; 1986; 1992). Doctors' clinical autonomy means that their decisions significantly shape resource usage in the health system, making it difficult for hospital administrations and governments to control health expenditure or evaluate the effectiveness and quality of the health care provided. Claims of overservicing and quality problems are given credence by studies showing significant variations in surgery rates between practitioners, hospitals, and regions within a country (Renwick & Sadkowsky 1992), as well differences in the diagnosis rates of certain mental health conditions,

social control Mechanisms that aim to induce conformity, or at least to manage or minimise deviant behaviour.

which can vary substantially between countries (see Turner 1995). Medicine's monopoly over clinical decision-making in terms of the diagnosis and treatment of disease has marginalised the role of other health therapies, to the possible detriment of providing optimal health care. Moreover, the limitations of the biomedical model have displaced a concern with the social origins of disease (see chapter 1) and have led to the medicalisation and **social control** of particular social groups (see chapter 8).

patriarchy A system of power through which males dominate households. It is used more broadly by feminists to refer to society's domination by patriarchal power, which functions to subordinate women and children.

Medicine's monopoly has often been considered **patriarchal** for much of the last century, with many writers accusing the medical profession of various forms of sexism in the research, diagnosis, and treatment of disease and in terms of discrimination against female doctors (see Broom 1991; Fee and Krieger 1994; Pringle 1998). Although women initially were not allowed to study medicine at university, there was a gradual entry of women into the profession during the second half of the twentieth century. Women now make up around 50 per cent of medical school enrolments in Australia, but still comprise only 26 per cent of medical practitioners, with the number of qualified practitioners expected to rise to 42 per cent by the year 2025 (AIHW 1996d). The **women's health movement** and the increasing numbers of female doctors provide circumstantial evidence to show that medical dominance can be effectively challenged in this domain (see chapter 5; Pringle 1998; Broom 1991).

women's health movement
A term used broadly to describe attempts to address sexism in medicine by highlighting the importance of gender in health research and treatment. Achievements include women's health centres and the National Women's Health Policy.

Challenges to medical dominance: countervailing powers

It is important to point out that medical dominance has never been absolute and has also been the subject of resistance and contestation. Light's (1993; 2000) concept of countervailing powers attempts to convey this situation, whereby: 'The central idea is to regard the medical and other health professions as one of several major countervailing powers in society ... consisting of the state, patient groups, the medical–industrial complex, alternative therapies—each of whom pursue their interests resulting in power struggles ...' (2000, p. 203). Most doctors work in some form of **professional bureaucracy** (Mintzberg 1979) and have always been subject to bureaucratic and budgetary constraints (Abbott 1988; Light 1993, 2000; Barnett, Barnett, & Kearns 1998). For example, a number of authors have written about how the organisation of hospitals reflects a constant tension between the power structures of bureaucratic authority and medical autonomy (Turner 1995). Therefore, while the medical profession has considerable power over the provision of health care, there are countervailing powers that constrain and even oppose medical influence.

Many authors have highlighted a range of factors that imply that medical dominance is in decline, such as the professionalisation strategies of allied health practitioners (see chapter 17); new models of health that focus on prevention, social factors, and community care (see chapters 1, 10, and 18); and the increasing popularity of alternative therapies (see chapter 16). However, in the remainder of this chapter we will discuss three broad social trends that represent the major challenges to medical dominance:

- **deprofessionalisation**: the undermining of doctors' political autonomy due to increasing public scepticism of medical authority in the face of media reports of medical fraud and negligence, and the patient rights movement
- **proletarianisation**: the increasing numbers of doctors employed on salaries in private and public sectors, resulting in doctors being subject to corporate or bureaucratic goals and regulations that limit their economic and clinical autonomy
- **McDonaldisation**: the intensive use of performance monitoring of the quality, cost, and effectiveness of medical care through sophisticated protocols and regulations that guide doctors' clinical judgments and daily work practices.

professional bureaucracy Mintzberg's (1979) term for an organisation that relies on staff with specialised knowledge and expertise to deliver complex services that require decision-making autonomy at the point of service delivery.

proletarianisation A theory that predicts the decline of medical power as a result of deskilling and the salaried employment of medical practitioners. This results in a loss of economic independence, whereby doctors lose control over their work because of managerial authority and bureaucratic regulations.

McDonaldisation A term coined by George Ritzer to refer to the standardisation of work processes by rules and regulations. It is based on increased monitoring and evaluation of individual performance, akin to the uniformity and control measures used by fast-food chains.

Deprofessionalisation

Deprofessionalisation is the process by which medicine's monopoly over knowledge, and its authority over the patient, is reduced as a result of increased public knowledge and influence over the health system (Haug 1973; 1988). According to Marie Haug,

health promotion Any combination of education and related organisational, economic, and political interventions designed to promote behavioural and environmental changes conducive to good health. This promotion may cover a variety of strategies, including legislation, health education, community development, advocacy, and so on. Health promotion has usually, however, been restricted to interventions focusing on the behavioural end of the spectrum.

increasing rates of education and the emphasis on **health promotion** have produced a vast health literature as well as increased self-awareness of health issues, meaning that the power and mystique of medical practice is in decline. The media have contributed further to the demystification of medicine through exposures of medical fraud and medical negligence, leading to a decline of medical status (see Germov 1995a; 1995c; Gabe et al. 1994).

Medical fraud

The extent of medical fraud has been estimated at 7 per cent of health expenditure, which in 1995 placed the cost of fraud at more than $500 million (Germov 1995c). Medi-fraud can take a number of forms, such as:

* charging for work never done or for services more extensive than those provided
* overservicing (unnecessary treatment, testing, and hospitalisation)
* unnecessary referrals to other specialists as a result of fee-splitting arrangements
* treating so many patients per day that adequate treatment would be impossible
* unfairly giving private patients priority over public patients in public hospitals because of the increased revenue they provide.

Overservicing may not only result from conscious attempts to defraud, but may also be the consequence of improper clinical practices, negligence, or the lack of alternative forms of treatment. However, where overservicing results in direct financial gain to the practitioner, overservicing is a form of fraud (see Box 14.1 for a recent example). Reports of the Health Insurance Commission (1993) and the Auditor-General (1992) state that part of the overservicing problem, apparent in significant variations in surgery rates (Renwick & Sadkowsky 1992), results from fraudulent practices. While attempts to explain medi-fraud can easily lead to the 'demonisation' of doctors, the key issue is that the present health system allows self-regulation, which provides an incentive for some doctors to pursue profit at patient and public expense.

Box 14.1 The MRI scan scam: anatomy of a medical fraud

In 1998 the federal government approved Medicare rebates for MRI (magnetic resonance imagining) scans for private practices to address waiting lists. At around $3 million, the cost of MRI machines limited their use in the private health sector, meaning that most scans were done in public hospitals. After lobbying by the radiology profession, the then federal Minister Dr Wooldridge approved rebates of $475 per scan for private practice, with the proviso that it would only apply to practices that already owned MRI machines or had them 'on order' when the scheme was officially announced (to avoid profiteering). However, news of the policy leaked and there was a surge in orders for MRI machines just before the announcement. Such a large number of orders could not be accounted for by chance or justified by need and suggested the possibility of over-servicing and profiteering, at great cost to the public purse. The poorly thought-out policy meant that for highly used machines, the rebate could amount to $1.5 million per year, per machine—a good return for a one-off outlay of $3 million. The scandal, known as the 'scan scam', was widely reported in the media in 1999 and resulted in an official inquiry that cost $450 000. The inquiry found that around 250 radiologists had been suspected of being involved in ordering 46 machines just before the announcement (many had fraudulently backdated their orders or had contracts of sale that would only be filled if the rebate scheme went ahead). However, the inquiry was a white-wash as no charges were laid due to insufficient evidence to sustain prosecutions. The 'scan scam' case is an example of how health policy decisions can be influenced by the political lobbying efforts of health professions, and can lead to profiteering and the potential waste of public funds. It further undermined public confidence in the medical profession, and particularly damaged the reputation of radiology (Wilkinson 2000; Metherall 2000).

Medical negligence and adverse events

An Australian report, The Quality in Australian Health Care Study, found that each year there are 470 000 'adverse events' (as they are called), including 18 000 deaths, and 50 000 permanent disabilities arising from medical complications, error, and negligence (TQAHC 1996; see also Wilson et al. 1999). While this is an alarming figure, the numbers partly reflect the known risks and chance of human error that can occur when undergoing some medical procedures. Nonetheless, the figures for adverse events are four times higher than those reported in the USA and warrant investigation as a significant number are likely to be the result of medical negligence and preventable error. Despite the conclusions of the report, the federal government never endorsed or systematically acted on its findings (Wilson et al. 1999).

In Australia each year a few thousand cases of negligence are filed, but because of the high legal costs, only 2 per cent of cases make it to court, with many claimants settling out of court. Approximately 60 per cent of claims fail, with the successful claimants paying out 40 per cent of their financial compensation in legal fees (see Germov 1995b). The cost of justice is prohibitive for many, and the small numbers of medical specialists mean that few doctors are willing to 'blow the whistle' on their colleagues for fear of retribution (Daniel 1998; Germov 1995a). In such cases, self-regulation—the crux of medical autonomy—can clearly work against the public interest by subverting patient rights.

Patient rights

The deprofessionalisation trend is also reflected in the organised efforts of the women's health movement and the consumer health movement (such as carers and illness-specific interest groups), which have both emphasised patient rights. The acknowledgment of patient rights represents a clear displacement of medical autonomy in favour of patient autonomy, and they are increasingly being recognised by the courts and governments. For example, a South Australian magistrate set a precedent by awarding in favour of a patient who was taken to court by an anaesthetist for not paying the component of the bill that was above the scheduled fee. The patient had not been informed of the extra expense involved, and thus the magistrate found in favour of the patient and established the notion of informed financial consent (Consumers' Health Forum 1994). In *Rogers v. Whitaker* (1992), the High Court of Australia also set a precedent by establishing the right of patients to full disclosure of information about treatment (see Germov 1995b). Moreover, the introduction of health rights charters and the establishment of health care complaints commissions by State governments are further evidence of a shifting balance of power between doctors and patients.

The focus on patient rights can often involve a conception of an 'ideal' health consumer who is assertive, knowledgeable, critical, and prepared to shop around for the best deal. Treating patients as consumers tends to replace concerns about access and equity with a more individualistic model, in which the emphasis on meeting consumer demands ignores all those 'consumers' who find it difficult to make demands, such as the elderly, the chronically sick, and the disabled (Hindess 1987). The assumption of the 'ideal consumer' pervades the discussion of patient rights, according to which decisions and actions are based on maximising the satisfaction of

social structure The recurring patterns of social interaction through which people are related to each other, such as social institutions and social groups.

individual wants and desires, ignoring the possibility that choices may be manipulated or determined by an individual's social location or by inequalities in **social structure**, particularly in the case of marginalised groups (Stretton & Orchard 1994).

The recognition of health rights and the establishment of independent complaints mechanisms in Australia represent significant examples of deprofessionalisation, with the medical profession no longer being the sole arbiter of what constitutes appropriate and ethical care, undermining medicine's political and clinical autonomy. However, as Peter Lloyd and others (1991) found in their study of health consumers, doctor–patient interaction still reflects the traditional relationship of trust and dependence: patients tend not to invoke their rights as 'active' consumers, rarely question doctors even when they have not understood what they have been told, and are generally unable to evaluate whether medical services are good or bad. Such findings dampen the enthusiasm surrounding patient rights and highlight the limits of the deprofessionalisation challenge to medical dominance.

The deprofessionalisation thesis also predicted that medicine's monopoly over health care delivery would be undermined by competition from alternative practitioners. In chapter 16, Gary Easthope notes that the popularity of alternative health care is increasingly challenging medicine, leading some doctors to incorporate alternative therapies such as acupuncture and spinal manipulation into their own practice. However, such a development means that doctors can practice therapies like acupuncture with minimal training and receive Medicare payments (with no cost to the patient) under the pretence of a normal consultation, giving them an unfair advantage over qualified acupuncturists (who are not covered by Medicare). In this way, medical dominance is actually reasserted as alternative therapists suffer a market disadvantage by having to charge patients full fees for service or primarily rely on patients who have private insurance, which may cover some of the costs of alternative therapies.

Proletarianisation

The proletarianisation thesis is derived from a neo-Marxist perspective (see chapter 2) and has been particularly used to explain developments in the United States health system, in which profit-motivated health companies have transformed the way that medical services are delivered (McKinlay & Arches 1985; McKinlay & Stoeckle 1988; Salmon 1990; 1994). According to this view, corporations are increasingly controlling the provision of health care, with doctors employed on salaries and thus subject to corporate goals and organisational regulations that serve to diminish their clinical and economic autonomy. John McKinlay and John Stoeckle (1988) nominate seven areas in which medical dominance is being curtailed by the process of proletarianisation:

1   entrance criteria into the medical profession (education and registration)
2   content of the medical curriculum
3   autonomy over the work that doctors perform
4   the way that patients are treated
5   the way that medical technology is used
6   the way that hospitals are designed and organised
7   the rate of remuneration (fee schedules and wage levels).

empirical Describes observations or research that is based on evidence drawn from experience. It is therefore distinguished from something based only on theoretical knowledge or on some other kind of abstract thinking process.

The proletarianisation thesis encounters **empirical** problems when applied to countries like the United Kingdom and Australia, which both have substantial public sectors that have always had salaried doctors. For example, the British National Health Service represents almost five decades of nationalised medicine, but has proven that 'salaried status and state intervention are not incompatible with a high level of some aspects of professional autonomy and dominance' (Elston 1991, p. 66). In the United Kingdom, medicine has still retained self-regulation and control over the use of health resources through clinical and political autonomy. Australia is similar, in that under Medicare, doctors have retained self-regulation, fee-for-service, and the right to treat private patients in public hospitals.

Part of the federal Labor Government's political deal with doctors to gain their compliance in establishing Medicare in 1984 allowed doctors a specific 'job perk': the right to treat private patients in public hospitals. In effect, Medicare subsidises the fee-for-service system. It sets a schedule fee, which doctors and hospitals can charge for public patients, but the schedule is not compulsory for private patients since most doctors are private contractors to the public system. The system provides an incentive for doctors and hospitals to treat private patients because of the greater revenue private patients provide. Such an open-ended system—ensuring little accountability with regard to doctor and hospital practice—has sustained doctors' economic autonomy under Medicare.

A study of doctors' earnings from Medicare found that in 1991–92, payments to doctors represented 18 per cent of total Medicare expenditure, with the majority earning between $150 000 and $200 000 a year from Medicare income alone (Lawson & Forde 1995). These figures do not take into account substantial amounts of private income earned through direct payments from patients and private insurance companies. Compared with other taxpayers, most doctors are in the top 12 per cent of income earners. Furthermore, many medical specialists are in the top 1 per cent of income earners. While Lawson and Forde conclude that the incomes earned by most doctors from Medicare are fair and reasonable (once business costs are taken into account), they also state that incomes from Medicare higher than $500 000 are difficult to justify. While such earnings are received by a minority of doctors, this minority includes 5.4 per cent of dermatologists, 3.8 per cent of obstetricians and gynaecologists, 4.4 per cent of ophthalmic surgeons, and 5.8 per cent of cardiologists (Lawson & Forde 1995).

The corporatisation of general practice

In recent years there has been a growing trend towards the corporatisation of general practice in Australia, which may lend further weight to the proletarianisation thesis. A number of large companies have expanded their presence in the field of general practice by taking over the ownership and management of existing clinics (see White 2000). Corporate ownership is likely to place constraints on doctors' clinical autonomy through restrictive work practices and revenue quotas as corporations seek to increase shareholder value through significant yearly returns on investment. Not only may this have negative implications for the quality of patient care, but 'corporatised doctors' would be required to use company specialists and diagnostic services (pathology and radiology clinics), intensifying the **medical–industrial complex** and potentially providing an incentive for overservicing.

The medical-industrial complex, originally coined by Vincente Navarro and colleagues in the late 1960s (see Navarro 1998) and popularised by Arnold Relman (1980), describes the role of large profit-oriented corporations in health care. It highlights what Connell (1988) describes as the **commodification of health care**, whereby health services become governed by the pursuit of profit-maximisation: a goal that often contradicts the task of meeting the health needs of the community. This has been an especially important insight in the USA, which has a significantly under-funded public health system, whereby more than 41 million Americans have no public or private health cover (Hehir 1996; Ross et. al. 1999).

While the corporatisation of general practice may have proletarianising effects, corporate ownership in the health system is not new, and thus it is unclear to what extent such a development is a challenge to medical dominance, particularly as doctor incomes remain high and many become shareholders in these new corporate ventures. Despite some evidence to indicate a trend towards proletarianisation in medicine, it is difficult to agree with the assertion that doctors are becoming as powerless and exploited as the average worker. Navarro (1988) argues that the use of the word 'proletarianisation' is misleading and should be abandoned because it carries with it Marxist connotations of allegiance with working-class interests. The mere fact that more doctors are salaried and subject to corporate or bureaucratic regulations has not led to a substantial

medical-industrial complex
The growth of profit-oriented medical companies and industries, whereby one company may own a chain of health services, such as hospitals, clinics, and radiology and pathology services.

commodification of health care
Treating health care as a commodity to be bought and sold in the pursuit of profit maximisation.

decline in medical autonomy to date, primarily because clinical autonomy has remained intact. However, recent developments suggest that this aspect of medical dominance is also under threat.

McDonaldisation: managerialism and clinical governance

rationalisation The standardisation of social life through rules and regulations (see also McDonaldisation).

A neo-Weberian perspective (see chapter 2) on challenges to medical dominance highlights the increasing **rationalisation** of doctors' work, in which new managerial strategies have been introduced to constrain doctors' clinical autonomy. George Ritzer (1993) conceptualises these attempts as part of a wider social trend towards the McDonaldisation of society—his term for rationalisation—in which the characteristic features that govern the work organisation of fast-food restaurants are coming to dominate increasing areas of society. Ritzer (1993, pp. 9–11) identifies four interrelated features of McDonaldisation:

1   *calculability*: the quantification of medical work through continual performance measurement, such as measuring patient through-put and expenditure
2   *efficiency*: an overriding concern with using the cheapest means to deliver services
3   *predictability*: the use of detailed regulations to ensure the delivery of health services uniformly operate irrespective of the practitioner
4   *control*: the use of technology to replace human judgment and labour, such as medical databases and the Internet in which a qualified practitioner may not be physically present with the patient for their diagnosis or treatment.

Ritzer suggests all four processes are combining to place constraints on medical practice. As an example, he cites the new generation of 'McDoctors', who work in 24-hour fast-food-type clinics that are 'based on rules, regulations, and controls so that what physicians do in them will be highly predictable' (1993, p. 97). The new McDoctors have limited autonomy as a result of increased monitoring and evaluation of their daily work performance. However, in Australia such private chains have had a limited impact to date, but this may be changing in light of the trend towards the corporatisation of general practice discussed above. A more substantial development has been the rise of **managerialism** in the public health sector.

managerialism The introduction of private-sector management techniques into the public sector.

Managerialism

Recent reforms to the public health systems of many countries, broadly referred to as managerialism, indicate that the state presents an increasing challenge to medical dominance, as attempts are made to exert control over health planning and funding. The main features of managerialism are: 'a focus on management, not policy, and on performance appraisal and efficiency; the disaggregation of public bureaucracies into agencies which deal with each other on a user-pay basis; the use of quasi-markets and contracting out to foster competition; cost-cutting; and a style of management which emphasises, amongst other things, output targets, limited-term contracts, monetary incentives and freedom to manage' (Rhodes 1991, p. 1).

A wave of managerial practices has been introduced into the Australian public health sector, such as 'best practice' and Total Quality Management (TQM). Such strategies have involved highly specified performance criteria, sometimes in the form of contractual relations, performance targets and measures, and work-specific protocols, which have attempted to reign in doctors' clinical autonomy.

An extensive literature has examined the impact of managerialism in the health sector, with a particular emphasis on its impact on medicine (see Gabe, Kelleher, & Williams 1994; Coburn 1988; Exworthy & Halford 1999; Clarke & Newman 1997; Clarke, Gewirtz, & McLaughlin 2000). To varying degrees, there is an emerging consensus in the literature that managerial strategies are making inroads into constraining medical autonomy. The success of the new public sector managers cannot be judged by the profits they earn (as with their private-sector counterparts); rather, they are judged by the 'savings' they can accrue. The focus on management is to 'do more with less'. It is important to note that the 'management turn' in the public sector is not without its critics, with the potential for cost-cutting to over-take a concern for quality. Nonetheless, managerialism has been one of the key trends affecting the work of all health professionals, particularly doctors.

One of the first applications of managerialism in the health sector in Australia occurred in Victoria through the introduction of a competitive funding model for hospitals based on 'casemix' and Diagnosis Related Groups (DRGs). Casemix is a funding system that relates hospital resource use to specific treatments given to patients and makes possible the comparison of hospital performance. DRGs are a casemix classification system based on the grouping of patients of similar clinical conditions to determine treatment costs. Concerns have been raised that competitive funding models in the health sector may be leading to the premature release of patients to keep costs down (discharging patients 'quicker and sicker'), with hospitals shifting responsibility for continued care onto the community (Draper 1992; Jackson 1993).

Clinical governance

clinical governance A term to describe a range of quality assurance measures that control doctors' clinical decision-making through standardised work protocols and performance measurement at the clinical level.

Clinical governance is a term that has gained currency in the United Kingdom as part of the Labour government's reforms of the health system. It is often used as an umbrella term to describe a range of quality assurance measures at the clinical level, but its exact meaning and the measures it refers to remain the subject of some debate (Flynn 2001). Donaldson (1998; 2000), one of the original architects of clinical governance measures in the UK, views them as a means to address variations in medical practice, prevent unnecessary errors and ensure clinical practice reflects state-of-art **evidence-based medicine**. Clinical governance essentially refers to attempts to control doctors' clinical autonomy through the standardisation of their clinical practices using various types of performance measurement, work protocols, and benchmarking. It involves the measurement, comparison, and standardisation of medical practitioners' individual and team performance in hospital settings, and represents the extension of the rationalisation process to clinical activity. For example, 'critical pathways' are commonly being developed to direct doctors' treatment decisions. A critical pathway is a set of clinical practice guidelines that map the provision of services in a chronological manner in terms of diagnosis and treatment for a specific condition. The pathway also serves to identify and remove variance in patient treatment and aims to achieve optimal patient care.

Clinical governance refers to the systematic introduction of such measures in an effort to improve the quality and efficiency of delivering health services. In essence, they involve attempts to micro-manage the daily clinical decisions and work practices of health professionals. In this sense they are a direct response to the issues of rising health care costs, fraud, negligence, and error as well as an attempt to address patient rights in terms of public accountability. Clinical governance heralds an era where the performance of individual doctors and hospitals can be publicly comparable in terms of cost, timeliness, and clinical standards of effective treatment outcomes. Clinical governance is clearly an attempt by the state to gain control over the medical profession at the clinical level—the last bastion of medical dominance. Since the establishment of clinical protocols and their measurement requires the cooperation of clinicians, it remains to be seen how effective a challenge they will be to medical dominance.

Managerialism in its general and clinical modes may represent the most effective challenge to medical dominance to date. In confronting managerialism at the clinical level, the medical profession is likely to be hoist with its own petard, since such policies appeal to the *laissez faire* currents within medical ideology. In a sense, such reform is cushioned from severe medical resistance because it is difficult to object to the pursuit of accountability and comparability of performance, although they represent a significant threat to the clinical and economic autonomy of medicine. However, like all predictions of the imminent demise of medical dominance, caution should be adopted. One factor that has often been overlooked in the debate over managerialism is that the measurement

evidence-based medicine (EBM)
An approach to medicine arguing that all clinical practice should be based on evidence from randomised control trials (RCTs) to ensure the effectiveness and efficacy of treatments.

and comparability of performance can lead either to collusive and secretive behaviour or to outright manipulation of performance indicators, meaning that many of the alleged benefits are imagined rather than real—see Box 14.2 for an example.

Box 14.2 Loopholes and new games in response to managerial reforms

With every new system of rules arise attempts to subvert them. In 1996, a special report by the *Age* newspaper (8 October) revealed that decreased waiting lists for elective surgery in Victoria were illusory. On paper, Victorian public hospitals had achieved remarkable decreases in waiting lists for cases defined as 'urgent'—and had achieved this during a period of cutback to public hospital funding. The then Victorian Liberal–National Party State Government claimed that the improvements were the result of financial incentives and improved measurement of waiting lists. However, public hospitals and various health practitioners had simply found ways to 'play the game' and rig the waiting lists so as to attract extra funding. This was done by admitting patients to 'phantom-wards', effectively booking patients into a ward 'on paper' (but not in reality), or by reclassifying less urgent cases to receive full funding. In essence, there were two lists: the official waiting list and the unofficial 'booking list' that showed the true number of patients awaiting treatment. An example of the lengths to which game-playing has gone can be found in the employment of administrative staff known as 'coders'— that is, medical records staff whose task it is to comb through patient records in search of cases that could be reclassified in favour of funding guidelines.

Future directions: continuing challenges to medical dominance

Despite predictions of the decline of medical dominance in the context of increasing bureaucratic and corporate constraints, Freidson (1994) maintains that the medical profession has been able to respond to changing social circumstances and has been able to stave off the major threats to its power. Freidson (1986; 1994) agrees that individual doctor autonomy is increasingly constrained by consumer, bureaucratic, and corporate requirements, but discounts these developments and maintains that the collective autonomy of the medical profession remains relatively intact. He argues that the medical profession has been able to maintain its power by becoming internally stratified between 'rank-and-file professionals', who continue to deliver clinical services to patients, and 'supervisory professionals' who 'are accountable for the aggregate performances of the workers ... [and who] tend to have an organizational perspective' (Freidson 1994, p. 142). Dent (1998, p. 221) comes to a similar conclusion, arguing that '[m]edical autonomy can be seen to be under revision and the *individual* autonomy of the physician is giving way to a *group* version.' According to this view, the medical profession is going through a process of re-stratification (Riska 1993).

Coburn and Willis (2000) point out that it is now difficult to write about 'the' medical profession as a single group because it is increasingly fragmented into diverse and sometimes competing factions, such as the various specialities, GPs, and salaried doctors, meaning that the medical profession no longer speaks in a unified voice and disunity among doctor ranks is not uncommon. For example, the two most active medical representative bodies—the AMA and the DRS (Doctors Reform Society)—are diametrically opposed on many key issues such as Medicare and private health insurance reform (see chapter 13). Furthermore, the increasing entry of large corporate entities into health care delivery is likely to only further lead to fragmentation and division in the medical profession.

While the autonomy of individual physicians may be in decline, Coburn, Rappolt and Bourgeault (1997) argue that the re-stratification hypothesis underestimates the extent to which the extension of state control, through various managerial and financial measures, is constraining medical autonomy. They argue, in their Canadian study, that medical 'incomes, numbers, and modes of representation have all been affected' (Coburn, Rappolt and Bourgeault 1997, p. 18). Yet, such conclusions also need to be treated with caution. It has long been observed that the complex and indeterminate nature of medical work means that it is not easily subjected to control and rationalisation (Strauss 1978; Mintzberg 1979; Freidson 1994). As Dent notes, 'clinical decision making is a complex process which can not be standardised because patients are not standard and disease processes are themselves highly variable' (1998, p. 207).

The indeterminacy of much health care work along with the contributions of nursing and allied health professionals has always meant that medical dominance has been the product of a '**negotiated order**' (Strauss et al. 1963; Strauss 1978; Fine 1984). The concept of a negotiated order stems from the symbolic interactionist perspective (see chapter 2) and highlights the importance of understanding the daily interaction between health professionals, whereby nurses and allied health professionals regularly challenge and undermine medical dominance in direct and indirect ways (see chapters 15 and 17). While this perspective has been criticised for implying that everything is 'open to negotiation' and

negotiated order A symbolic interactionist concept that refers to any form of social organisation in which the exercise of authority and the formation of rules are outcomes of human interaction and negotiation.

agency The ability of people, individually and collectively, to influence their own lives and the society in which they live.

thus downplaying the unequal distribution of power within an organisation like a hospital (Day and Day 1977), it exposes the need to take into account the **agency** that nursing and allied health professionals do exert in their experience of medical dominance; something that Marxist and Weberian accounts have tended to neglect.

Conclusion

Challenges to medical dominance such as deprofessionalisation, proletarianisation and McDonaldisation, and the medical profession's responses to such challenges reflect the dynamic nature of the health system. Medical dominance will continue to be the subject of formal and informal challenge, and it remains to be seen how long-lasting these trends will be in eroding the professional autonomy of medicine. What appears certain is that at all three levels—political, economic, and clinical autonomy—medical dominance is being challenged and steadily undermined. The recent development of clinical governance, though still in its infancy in Australia, may prove to be the most significant challenge yet. It has always been the case that the clinical decisions of doctors determine, to a large extent, health expenditure and the work of other health practitioners. While the McDonaldisation of medical practice represents new forms of accountability and constraint over the medical profession, it is not without inherent problems and may undermine the flexibility and quality of health care provided if the primary concern becomes one of cost-cutting and rule-following. With increasing pressure on governments to find innovative ways to control increasing health expenditures, the future of medical dominance will continue to be contested. Freidson (1994) asks what the alternative to medical dominance might be. His answer is that medicine needs to be 'liberated' from 'material self-interest'; only in this way will the negative aspects of medical dominance be quashed.

Summary of main points

- Medicine monopolises health care delivery, health policy, and the nature of health practice.
- Medical dominance was achieved through political means and was granted and guaranteed by the state through legislation and constitutional amendment.
- Medical dominance has always been the subject of resistance and challenge, however recent challenges may result in the most significant curtailment of medical autonomy to date.
- The main challenges to medical dominance are deprofessionalisation, proletarianisation, and McDonaldisation.

- It has been argued that managerialism, particularly clinical governance, offers the potential to significantly undermine the clinical autonomy of medicine and, as such, present a significant challenge to medical dominance.

Discussion questions

1   How would you define medical dominance?
2   How was medical dominance achieved?
3   What are some examples of deprofessionalisation? To what extent does it represent a challenge to medical dominance?
4   What are some examples of proletarianisation and corporatisation? To what extent do they represent a challenge to medical dominance?
5   What might be some of the positive and negative outcomes of McDonaldisation in the health sector?
6   What could be done to further address the problems related to medical dominance?

Further investigation

1   There is considerable debate over whether the power of the medical profession is being undermined by the trends of deprofessionalisation, proletarianisation, and McDonaldisation. What do these trends involve and to what extent have they curtailed the political, economic, and clinical autonomy of the medical profession?
2   Examine the impact of medical dominance on one other health profession such as nursing or an allied health profession (e.g. dietetics, occupational therapy, physiotherapy, pharmacy, and so on). How is the profession you have chosen challenging medical dominance and has this been or is it likely to be effective?
3   Discuss the challenge that managerialism and corporatisation pose to medical dominance in Australia.

Further reading and web resources

Annandale, E. 1998, *The Sociology of Health and Medicine: A Critical Introduction*, Polity Press, Cambridge, ch. 8, pp. 223–50.

Coburn, D. & Willis, E. 2000, 'The Medical Profession: Knowledge, Power, and Autonomy', in G. L. Albrecht, R. Fitzpatrick, & S. C. Scrimshaw (eds), *Handbook of Social Studies in Health and Medicine*, Sage, London, pp. 377–93.

Daniel, A. E. 1998, *Scapegoats for a Profession: Uncovering Procedural Injustice*, Harwood Academic, Amsterdam.

Elston, M. A. 1991, 'The Politics of Professional Power: Medicine in a Changing Health Service', in J. Gabe, M. Calnan, & M. Bury (eds), *The Sociology of the Health Service*, Routledge, London, pp. 58–88.

Exworthy, M. & Halford, S. (eds) 1999, *Professionals and the New Managerialism in the Public Sector*, Open University Press, Buckingham.

Freidson, E. 2001, *Professionalism: The Third Logic*, Polity Press, Cambridge.

—— 1994, *Professionalism Reborn: Theory, Prophecy and Policy*, Polity Press, Cambridge.

Gabe, J., Kelleher, D., & Williams, G. (eds) 1994, *Challenging Medicine*, Routledge, London.

Leeder, S. R. 2000, *Healthy Medicine: Challenges Facing Australia's Health Services*, Allen & Unwin, Sydney.

Pringle, R. 1998, *Sex and Medicine: Gender, Power and Authority in the Medical Profession*, Cambridge University Press, Cambridge.

Walby, S. & Greenwell, J. 1994, *Medicine and Nursing: Professions in a Changing Health Service*, Sage, London.

Walton, M. 1998, *The Trouble with Medicine: Preserving the Trust Between Patients and Doctors*, Allen & Unwin, Sydney.

Wearing, M. 1999, 'Medical Dominance and the Division of Labour in the Health Professions', in C. Grbich (ed.), *Health in Australia: Sociological Concepts and Issues*, 2nd edn, Longman, Sydney, pp. 197–216.

Willis, E. 1989, *Medical Dominance*, revised edn, Allen & Unwin, Sydney.

Witz, A. 1992, *Professions and Patriarchy*, Routledge, London.

Web sites

Australian General Practice Accreditation Limited (AGPAL): <www.agpal.com.au/site/index.asp>

Australian Medical Association (AMA): <www.ama.com.au>

Australian Medical Workforce: <http://amwac.health.nsw.gov.au/>. See also: <http://www.health.gov.au/workforce/index.htm>

Centre for Clinical Governance Research in Health: <www.med.unsw.edu.au/clingov>

Consumers' Health Forum: <www.chf.org.au>

Doctors Reform Society (DRS): <www.drs.org.au/drshome.htm>

Health Insurance Commission: <www.hic.gov.au>

National Health and Medical Research Council (NHMRC)—the major funding and advisory body for health and medical research and policy in Australia: <www.nhmrc.gov.au>

National Institutes of Health (NIH)—the United States equivalent of Australia's National Health and Medical Research Council, the NIH is a key site for providing access to medical research on the prevention, diagnosis, and treatment of disease and disability: <www.nih.gov>. Also includes the Images from the History of Medicine (IHM) site: <http://wwwihm.nlm.nih.gov/>

National Library of Medicine (USA)—part of the NIH (see above) and the producer of MEDLINE, the online index of articles in medical and health-related journals: <www.nlm.nih.gov/nlmhome.html>

Public Health Association (PHA): <www.pha.org.au>

Royal Australian College of General Practitioners: <www.racgp.org.au>

15

Nursing and Sociology

An Uneasy Relationship

Deidre Wicks

Overview

* *Why is nursing often depicted in a negative light?*
* *What is the 'New Nursing'?*
* *What are some of the new developments in nursing in Australia and overseas?*

This chapter reviews some of the more recent sociological writings on nursing and discusses them in relation to the practical insights they have to offer for nursing. Recent reforms to nursing in Australia and the United Kingdom are analysed to see how these might be interpreted through a sociological lens. Implicit in this analysis will be a focus on the tension between the structure of the health system (particularly the influence of medicine) and the agency of nurses in these different accounts of nurses and nursing work.

Key terms

agency
biological determinism
biomedical model
class
discourse
doctor/nurse game
empirical
essentialism
ethnography
feminism/feminist

gender
horizontal violence
materialist analysis
medical dominance
meta-narratives
nurse-practitioner
patriarchy
phenomenology
post-structuralism
primary health care

professional project
racism
sexual division of labour (SDL)
social institutions
social structure
state
structure/agency debate
theory

Introduction

In the period following World War II, nursing training in Australia was broadened to include both the technological and clinical advances that had occurred as a result of nursing experiences in war. Further expansion of nursing curricula occurred during the 1960s and 1970s to include input from the social sciences, namely psychology and sociology. This was based on a view of nursing that held that nurses needed an understanding of the social context of health care delivery as well as the individual, psychological needs and perceptions of their patients. The sociology introduced at that time, with few exceptions, revolved around the concept of 'roles' and role relationships, such as 'the role of the doctor and nurse in health care delivery' and 'the role of the patient in hospital care'. As such, it encouraged an acceptance of existing social relationships and their hierarchies of power and authority. It did, nevertheless, encourage nursing students to think about social relationships and the impact of these relationships on nursing work and on patient care. As the 1970s progressed, the popularity of more radical approaches within sociology began to be taken up and applied to sociology courses within nursing education. New interpretations of nursing history and practice, based on feminist **theory** in particular, began to appear, especially in the new diploma and later degree courses within universities. These courses encouraged a more critical examination of nursing history and practice, as well as a more critical interpretation of the relationship of nursing to other health occupations, especially medicine.

At the same time as broadening the ways of understanding nursing, these more radical approaches had the unintended effect of presenting nursing in a much more negative light; so much so that in recent years, sociological writings about nursing have presented an almost uniformly negative picture. Repeatedly, nursing has been presented as a 'subordinated' occupation, and nurses themselves as passive victims of medical power. While there have been differences in the way that various sociological perspectives view nursing, it is also possible to see a consistent theme running through all the interpretations, from social histories of nursing through to more radical feminist accounts. In the historical accounts, it is argued that many of the enduring characteristics of nursing have their roots in nineteenth-century **gender** relations and associated ideas regarding the appropriate behaviour for women in Victorian society. This argument has become the 'holy grail' of nursing history and is trotted out whenever a potted history of nursing is required as an introduction to current trends in nursing. For instance, it has been argued that '[t]hese [strategies] replicated within the hospital the existing gender relationships of Victorian society, and did not challenge prevailing

theory A system of ideas that uses researched evidence to explain certain events and to show why certain facts are related.

gender/sex This term refers to the socially constructed categories of feminine and masculine (the cultural values that dictate how men and women should behave), as opposed to the categories of biological sex (female or male).

class (or social class) A position within a system of structured inequality based on the unequal distribution of power, wealth, income, and status. Class membership is determined by three characteristics: ownership and control of scarce economic resources; ownership of marketable skills and qualifications; and wage labour. People who share a social-class position typically share similar life chances.

ethnography A research method that is based on direct observation of a particular social group's social life and culture—of what the people actually do.

horizontal violence A concept derived from Paolo Friere that describes a behaviour common to all oppressed groups, whereby, because of their powerlessness, the oppressed are unable to direct their anger towards their oppressor and so turn it towards each other, with various degrees of violence and negativity.

social structure The recurring patterns of social interaction through which people are related to each other, such as social institutions and social groups.

male notions of womanly behaviour. Deference to doctors and acceptance of the "handmaiden role" was a cornerstone of this strategy' (Beardshaw & Robinson 1990). And in an Australian version, it is explained that '[s]ince 1868, when the first Nightingale graduate arrived in Australia, nursing as an occupation has tended to attract relatively passive and subordinate women from middle and lower **class** backgrounds who have accepted that their occupation was inferior and subordinate to male-dominated medicine' (Short & Sharman 1995, p. 236).

In all of these potted historical overviews, and in the analyses that follow, there is a theoretical and logical flaw. It is assumed that the political strategy of those in charge and the real-life behaviour of the nurses in question were one and the same. Victorian doctors and administrators may well have desired the nurse to be 'restrained, disciplined and obedient, [carrying] out the orders of doctors in a suitably humble and deferential way' (Davies 1977). But this did not mean that matrons, nurses, and sisters always cooperated in this way. There is ample evidence to show that they frequently did not. For instance, in the earliest era of modern nursing in London, there was an important dispute at Guy's Hospital between Mrs Burt (the matron) and the doctors (Abel-Smith 1960), and there were also the disputes at St Thomas's Hospital over the timing of medical rounds ('The Doctors versus the Nurses' 1962, pp. 783–4). In Australia, the disputes between Lucy Osborn, the doctors, and the lay administrators at the Sydney Infirmary were so intractable that the government of the day had to resort to a Royal Commission to settle (in the matron's favour) the struggle for authority (Wicks 1995b). In addition, labour history has documented various forms of industrial action taken collectively by nurses over the past century. Finally, **ethnographic** studies have revealed numerous examples of negotiation, disagreement, subversions, and open conflict as constant elements of nurse–doctor interactions within hospital settings (Game & Pringle 1983; Hughes 1988; Porter 1995; Svensson 1996; Wicks 1999). Against this evidence, an orthodoxy has developed within both mainstream and more radical approaches that has focused on the power of doctors, hospitals, and medicine more generally. Nurses were thought to have inherited a tradition of passivity and powerlessness, and worse, a tendency to engage in **horizontal violence** (Roberts 1983). Indeed, given these characteristics and the twin edifices of class and gender, the position of nurses was considered to be all but hopeless (Short & Sharman 1995). The common thread running through these accounts has been an emphasis on the power of **social structure** to shape and control nurses' work, identity, and behaviour.

More recently, theoretical developments in feminist theory, and within sociology more generally, have promoted a re-examination

structure/agency debate A key debate in sociology over the extent to which human behaviour is determined by social structure.

post-structuralism (and postmodernism) Often used interchangeably with postmodernism, it refers to a perspective that is opposed to the view that social structure determines human action, and that emphasises the local, the specific, and the contingent in social life.

social institutions Formal structures within society—such as health care, government, education, religion, and the media—that are organised to address identified social needs.

of the debate concerning individual choice versus determination by outside forces (**structure/agency debate**), and of the need to understand an issue that has such important implications for politics and social life. Through the influence of **post-structuralism**, there has been a re-emphasis on individual choice and action in the making and re-making of **social institutions**. While some authors think that this trend has gone 'too far' (Walby 1992), others see it as liberating, challenging the 'grand narratives' that characterised groups such as women as being oppressed by strong and unchanging social structures (Barrett 1991). I shall begin with a brief review of some earlier feminist approaches to nursing, of what they had to offer, and of what they missed. I will then go on to examine nursing responses to these, new sociological approaches to nursing and an examination of recent developments and directions for nursing practice in Australia and Great Britain. Finally, I will address the question of how nursing and sociology might have a more mutually productive relationship in the future.

Earlier feminist approaches

In the early 1970s, two writers from the USA—Barbara Ehrenreich and Deirdre English—turned conventional theories on their head with their pamphlet *Witches, Midwives and Nurses: A History of Women Healers* (1973). Their work, with its strong feminist perspective, was a breath of fresh air in a field dominated by conventional histories of medicine. And yet its widespread influence in the decades since its publication has also had a detrimental effect on feminist sociological analyses of nursing. This stems from the way that Ehrenreich and English view the struggle within health care as something that took place in an earlier period between traditional women healers and formal male practitioners. According to their analysis, the defeat of the women healers ushered in an epoch of widespread subordination to organised, scientific male medicine. For instance, they are critical of middle-class reformers, such as Florence Nightingale, and of nineteenth-century feminists who 'did not challenge nursing as an oppressive female role' (1973, p. 38). This analysis overlooks much that is crucial to a dynamic analysis of the historical relationship between nursing and medicine. By viewing the nineteenth-century formation of modern nursing only in terms of capitulation and defeat, the work has had the unintended effect of devaluing contemporary nurses and nursing work.

The most influential piece of writing on nursing and its relationship to medicine is Eve Gamarnikow's 'Sexual Division of Labour: The Case of Nursing' (1978). In this important paper,

sexual division of labour This refers to the nature of work performed as a result of gender roles. The stereotype is that of the male breadwinner and the female home-maker.

biological determinism The unproven belief that people's biology determines their social, economic, and health statuses.

materialist analysis An analysis that is embedded in the real, actual, material reality of everyday life.

patriarchy A system of power through which males dominate households. It is used more broadly by feminists to refer to society's domination by patriarchal power, which functions to subordinate women and children.

Gamarnikow challenges accounts of the **sexual division of labour (SDL)** that are based on 'naturalism' or **biological determinism** (that is, the idea that it is 'natural' for women to be nurses in the same way that women are 'naturally' maternal). She argues, rather, for a **materialist analysis**, which locates the SDL as a *social* relationship that is not inevitable or natural but that has been socially constructed This was such a significant break-through, in an area typified by naturalist explanations, that sociological analysis to this day continues to refer to it to establish a position that runs counter to biological or naturalist accounts of the nurse–doctor relationship (see, for example, Game & Pringle 1983; Hazleton 1990; Russell & Schofield 1986; Short & Sharman 1995; Willis 1983). It is still widely regarded as the nec-essary foundation on which any critical sociological account of nurse–doctor relations must be built.

However, upon closer examination, it is evident that Gamarnikow's account is located squarely within a 'modernist' feminist theoretical model, with its attendant problems of overgen-eralising and universalising. In this case, Gamarnikow generalises the structural oppression of all nurses by all doctors through a patriar-chal ideological structure. While Gamarnikow's approach provides a crucial sense of the strength and pervasiveness of social structure in explanations of the SDL, it does so at a price. Both Bob Connell (1987) and, more recently, Anne Witz (1992) make the point that this approach ignores or at least minimises the importance of patri-archal practices within the labour market and the workplace itself. What is the point of resistance in the workplace if gender (and/or class) relations are determined elsewhere? The effect of this empha-sis on patriarchal ideology and structure in Gamarnikow's account, and other accounts derived from this analysis, has been the repre-sentation of nurses as an undifferentiated bloc of subordinated women. Individual or collective acts of resistance have either been ignored or minimised, being characterised as insignificant or as yet another variant of 'complaint' among nurses (see Turner 1986b). The emphasis on an all-pervasive ideological structure has also had the effect of denying nurses subjectivity (their own identity), for in accounts based on the power and pervasiveness of structure, the voices of nurses have rarely been heard. (There are some exceptions, however: notably the work of Game & Pringle 1983).

Gamarnikow's contribution was pivotal for a critical reassess-ment of the conventional literature on nurse–doctor relations. Indeed, the emphasis on power relationships in general, and **patriarchy** in particular, opened up the traditional nurse–doctor relationship to a sophisticated and long overdue sociological critique. Nevertheless, an emphasis on structural oppression, and on an inferred passivity on the part of nurses, also runs the danger of indirectly contributing to the status quo by emphasising the inevitability and hopelessness of the situation.

Nursing backlash?

medical dominance A general term used to describe the power of the medical profession in terms of its control over its own work, over the work of other health workers, and over health resource allocation, health policy, and the way that hospitals are run.

phenomenology Its main aim is the analysis and description of everyday life. It is the study of the ways in which individuals construct the daily realities of their social world through interaction with others.

professionalisation (professional project) The process of becoming a profession, whereby an occupational group attains publicly recognised and government-legitimated monopoly and autonomy over its area of work. Professional status is usually associated with certain traits (see 'trait approach').

Given these theoretical directions and assumptions, there was certainly potential for academics, students, and intellectual leaders in nursing to develop an ambivalent attitude towards sociology and towards feminist sociology in particular. Why are sociology lecturers so surprised when student nurses appear hostile to their lectures on **medical dominance** and begin, in their postgraduate work, a mass exodus towards **phenomenology**? Why, indeed, are academics surprised that students do not enthusiastically embrace the notion that, on graduation, they are to be dominated and oppressed as both women and nurses? Is it any wonder that they prefer to believe their nursing mentors, who make use of the more comforting language of professionalism, with its associated characterisation of nurses as authoritative, autonomous practitioners? Interestingly, this is not the case with those working, clinical nurses who enter universities on a part-time basis as mature-age students. They have neither an investment in an idealised future career nor an investment in the practical and political realities of a **professional project**. They have, rather, the direct experience of both the restrictions and the rewards of the complicated work process of nursing. They generally enjoy feminist analyses of medical dominance, which give a name to many of their own discontents, and yet at the same time they are also quick to point out the contradictions and the reversals of power that arise in specific work situations. In other words, they frequently feel that both Marxist and feminist analyses (defined in chapter 2) of nursing work are 'good' but make things out to be 'too black and white'. At the same time, these working nurses have little time for nurse academics whom they see as 'feathering their own nests' and ignoring the concerns of working nurses in their preoccupation with developing nursing theory.

It can be seen that feminist sociology has had both a beneficial and also a less positive effect on nursing. At the same time, these particular views of nursing have had a less than beneficial effect on sociology. The assumed realities of the daily oppression of nurses by doctors that are implicit in the accounts discussed above have served to reinforce certain tendencies within sociology—in particular, within Marxist sociology and radical feminist theory. Specifically they have reinforced the notion that social structure is set in concrete, rather than being the continually constructed outcome of human practice (Connell 1987). As a result, and despite the goodwill on the part of individual sociologists and nurse academics, the relationship between academic nursing and sociology has, on the whole, been a troubled one. While health sociologists continue to research and write on nursing, other more central areas of sociology (class and gender analyses, cultural studies, theory construction) rarely rate nursing a mention; what could nursing possibly contribute to the development of sociological theory? At the same time, nursing has, for some time, been losing interest in sociology and has turned towards various forms of interpretive sociology or philosophy that appear more sympathetic to the quest of nursing for a rationale and an underpinning for professional authority and autonomy. In the second part of this chapter, I discuss some recent developments within sociology that could provide a basis for a useful bridge between nursing and sociology. Finally, I discuss some recent developments within nursing in Australia and the United Kingdom that may have the potential to contribute to developments within sociology.

Paradigm shift in feminist theory

Over the last two decades there has been what some writers have referred to as a 'paradigm shift' within the founding theoretical principles of modern **feminism** (Barrett & Phillips 1992). Central to this 'shift' has been a questioning of at least three of the basic assumptions of '1970s feminism'. These are:

1   the notion of women's oppression
2   the assumption that it is possible to specify a cause for the oppression
3   consensus that the cause lies at the level of social structure, be it patriarchy, class, ethnicity, or a combination of any or all of the above (Barrett & Phillips 1992).

feminism/feminist A broad social and political movement based on a belief in equality of the sexes and the removal of all forms of discrimination against women. A feminist is one who makes use of, and may act upon, a body of theory that seeks to explain the subordinate position of women in society.

This is not to say that these authors (and others like them) are arguing that women do not experience oppression. Rather they are attempting to acknowledge that different women experience different types and different degrees of oppression in specific circumstances. It allows for the possibility of resistance to the operation of power and for the exercise of counter-power. It also allows for the possibility that some women may experience oppression at the hands of other women. It recognises the uneven nature of human experience, the fact that individuals and groups can shift from being oppressed to inflicting oppression over others, the fact that even the most dominated and powerless groups work away at clawing back whatever autonomy and freedom they can. In the end it recognises the 'contingent' and 'fluid' nature of power itself (Barrett 1991).

This approach (or, more correctly, collection of approaches) has been heavily influenced by the work of the French philosopher and social theorist Michel Foucault, through what Rosemary Pringle

(1995) has called 'the Foucault effect'. Pringle argues that Foucault's emphasis on power as productive (and not merely coercive) has opened up the space for a view of women as active agents rather than the passive recipients of orders from above: 'Women actively produce the forms of femininity through which they are also controlled: they are never merely victims' (Pringle 1995, p. 207). Pringle also clearly states that, in her view, the use of the term 'patriarchy' is more of an obstacle than an aid to understanding specific operations of power. Rather than treating patriarchy as a social system, Pringle—in her work on secretaries (1988), and more recently on women doctors—has emphasised the more fluid and local contexts in which gender and power operate (Pringle 1995).

This and other similar approaches have not been without their critics. Feminist theorist Sylvia Walby has argued that the shift away from 'structure' and towards **discourse** has resulted in a conceptualisation of power as highly dispersed rather than as concentrated in identifiable places and groups. She argues further that the concepts of 'woman' and 'patriarchy' are, in fact, essential if we are not to lose sight of the power relations involved and if we are to understand the gendered nature of the social world. In particular, she points out that an analysis of the new international division of labour shows clearly the need to maintain the use of the structural concepts of patriarchy, class, and racism (Walby 1992). While Walby agrees that there were problems with 'the old **meta-narratives**' based solely on class, she holds that the answer is not to discard the concept of social structure. Rather, the answer is to develop better, theoretically richer concepts that are more capable of 'catching' and explaining the theoretical and practical complexities of the operation of power in the social world. In fact, she argues that a solution to this problem is to develop a theory of patriarchy that is based on six structures rather than one. She sees the six main structures that make up a system of patriarchy as:

1   paid work
2   housework
3   sexuality
4   culture
5   violence
6   the state.

It is the inter-relationships between these that create different forms of patriarchy (Walby 1992).

In his work on gender and power, Connell has grappled with the same issues; he has kept hold of the concept of social structure and has developed a theoretical concept of gender relations that is based on three sub-structures: labour, power, and cathexis (or emotional attachment) (Connell 1987). The important point about these theoretical developments and debates is not that there are

discourse A domain of language-use that is characterised by common ways of talking and thinking about an issue (for example, the discourses of medicine, madness, or sexuality).

meta-analysis and meta-narratives The 'big picture' analysis that frames and organises observations and research on a particular topic.

disagreements, but that feminist theory in the twenty-first century is marked not by orthodoxy and homogeneity but rather by debate, openness, and heterogeneity. Directly or indirectly, these developments have encouraged a revival in sociological analyses of nursing and of the division of labour with medicine. Rather than accept old-style assumptions about the patriarchal oppression and medical dominance that are implicit in the **doctor/nurse game**, recent writers, working from a variety of sociological perspectives, have re-examined nurses' and doctors' working relationships and come up with some fascinating and important findings.

doctor/nurse game A concept that derives from an article by L. Stein (1967), who describes a 'game' that, he claims, is played out between doctors and nurses. The main feature of this game is that the nurse must be assertive and make positive suggestions regarding patient care while not appearing to do so. In other words, nurses must couch suggestions regarding patient care in such a way that doctors can pick them up and act on them as though they were their own initiatives.

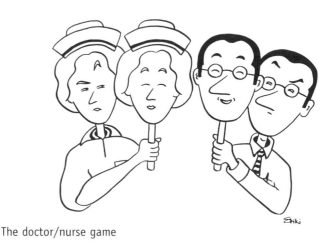

The doctor/nurse game

New sociological approaches to nursing

empirical Describes observations or research that is based on evidence drawn from experience. It is therefore distinguished from something based only on theoretical knowledge or on some other kind of abstract thinking process.

Many of the more interesting contributions to the sociological literature on nursing have resulted from small-scale **empirical** studies. In his study of a casualty ward in a British hospital, David Hughes (1988) demonstrates that there are many specific circumstances in which the nurse's influence is strengthened in relation to the doctor's. More recently, Christopher Tye (2000) has also looked at nurse–doctor relations in an accident and emergency department, in this case to examine (among other themes) the blurring boundaries between doctors and the new staff category of emergency nurse-practitioner. Sam Porter (1992) reached similar conclusions to Hughes in a study of nurse–doctor interactions in an Irish hospital. He reported that neither doctors nor nurses behaved in the ways that Leonard Stein (1967) predicted (in the 'doctor/nurse game'), but that nurses often openly directed doctors to particular actions and decisions, and that doctors frequently appeared to welcome their suggestions. These results have gained further support from a large study of the relations between nurses and doctors in British hospitals, which supplied numerous instances of nurses having direct influence over patient care (Mackay 1993; Walby & Greenwell 1994). Jocelyn Lawler (1991) used observation and interviews to reveal the way in which nurses actively construct rules about dealing with bodies, and with normally taboo bodily functions, in a way that avoids embarrassment to both themselves and their patients. In another study based on interviews, this time from Sweden, Roland Svensson reported that 'nurses' position on their wards has been altered in a significant manner. The nurses have increased their influence over decisions which affect the patient, and they can influence the norms for interaction and work performance to a greater extent than previously. On the wards covered by this study, the voice of nursing clearly makes itself heard in more areas and with greater strength than it did before' (Svensson 1996, p. 396).

Finally, this author further developed the approach outlined above by drawing on extended observations and one-to-one interviews in a hospital setting to explore incidents that reveal both cooperation and contestation with doctors and their medical goals and priorities. In my book, an examination is made of the ways that nurses call on their knowledge and formal/informal authority to influence healing outcomes in the areas of pain relief, wound healing and care of the dying patient (Wicks 1999).

None of these studies attempts to ignore or gloss over impediments to nursing authority and action. Svensson points out that one area in which it is difficult and sometimes impossible for nurses to negotiate change is the actual division of work: much of the traditional service work remains with nurses. However, what all of these studies have in common is an openness to the practical and theoretical possibility of nurses exercising various degrees of direct authority and power.

The second sociological approach that has developed the theme of 'active nursing' has come from an unlikely quarter. It has come from the sociology of the professions. This has historically been an area that has provided little joy for nurses. In its traditional form, the sociology of professions set up an (ever-changing) 'checklist' of criteria for what constituted a profession. It will come as no surprise to the reader to learn that nursing (like every other female-dominated occupation) never made it to the 'A' list and, therefore, was relegated to the nether world of the 'semi-professions' as a 'stunted occupational subspecies' (Salvage 1988, p. 517). The response of many nursing theorists was to develop yet another set of criteria or 'traits', which could then be used to demonstrate that nursing did, in fact, meet the criteria and should therefore be recognised as a true profession (see, for example,

Smith 1981). It was clearly an uncomfortable position for nursing, whose spokespeople were constantly on the defensive in a theoretical world seemingly dominated by 'gatekeeping' sociologists.

Recent work by Ann Witz has broken with this mould. She has grappled with the issue of gender and the professions directly, and has developed a very different approach to interpretations both of the past and of analyses of the present and future (Witz 1992; 1994). She puts the case for a theory of professionalisation 'that can cope with the fact that women as well as men have engaged in professional projects' (Witz 1992, p. 37). In terms of the history of modern nursing, she has analysed the various political strategies of nursing leaders as strategies of 'dual closure'. This term refers to the double focus of the strategy: on the one hand, members of the group resist domination from above and seek to extend their territory; on the other, they seek simultaneously to close off the occupation and to restrict entry to its ranks (Witz 1992, p. 201). She goes on to argue that, while there are elements of historical continuity in nursing's occupational strategy, there is also an important new element. This is the emphasis on the content of nursing work, which, she argues, represents a bid to establish practitioner autonomy in the daily practice of nursing work (Witz 1994). This strategy, and the type of practice that is envisaged for nursing, has come, at least in the United Kingdom, to be called 'the New Nursing'.

New Nursing

The origins of New Nursing can be found in the United Kingdom in the 1970s, as new departments of nursing in universities and polytechnics generated interest in nursing theory (Salvage 1992). In the publications that emerged from these academic environments, several clear themes were evident. Salvage expresses these succinctly when she notes that:

> [i]n these publications, the key to the New Nursing is held to be its clinical base. The bureaucratic occupational model must be replaced by a professional one, with the practitioner as its linchpin; preparation for this demanding role is to be achieved via education. This 'new animal' ... should have greater autonomy at the centre of a new division of labour; no longer should a position of seniority mean leaving direct patient care (Salvage 1992, p. 11).

biomedicine/biomedical model

The conventional approach to medicine in Western societies. It diagnoses and explains illness as a malfunction of one of the body's biological mechanisms. The biomedical approach of most health services focuses on the treating of individuals, and generally ignores social, economic, and environmental factors.

The other central point about the New Nursing is that the theoretical base for its practice moves away from the **biomedical model**, towards a holistic approach that enables—indeed, requires—the patient's active participation in their own care. The advocates of the New Nursing have met with a significant, though

nurse-practitioner The title given to nurses with an enhanced and extended role, such as the ability to prescribe certain drugs and undertake procedures such as Pap smears and minor surgery. In some countries (such as the USA) it may also refer to the nurse's ability to charge a fee for service.

primary health care Both the point of first contact with the health care system and a philosophy for delivery of that care.

uneven, degree of success so far. There are at least four outcomes in the United Kingdom, which can be traced to successful lobbying on the part of New Nursing advocates. First, there have been innovations regarding the **nurse-practitioner** role in **primary health care**. Second, professional nursing bodies have made successful efforts to encourage the government to introduce a new clinical career structure for nurses (though this is certainly not regarded as a great success—indeed, it has been dubbed 'the biggest con that ever was') (see Beardshaw & Robinson 1990). Third, there have been the proposals contained in the Project 2000 report. At the time the Project 2000 report was published, it was heralded as an important reform, which would give nurse education priority over the needs of health service delivery systems. The aim of Project 2000 was to change the 'learning on the job' system to one in which nurses became full-time students in either diploma or degree courses at universities. It was hoped that this would make nursing a more attractive option for those of a more reflective and academic bent. As well as the older universities, such as Manchester, Edinburgh, and Nottingham, which had been offering nursing degrees since the mid-1960s, degree courses proliferated among the newer universities.

And yet this important reform was seemingly sabotaged in its implementation. Now many years on, it is clear that the funding of the degree courses contained built-in mechanisms to discourage students and to direct them towards the lower status diploma courses. Diploma students receive a non-means-tested annual bursary of £4500 (about A$13 000), as well as a travel allowance, and they have their fees paid. Degree students, on the other hand, receive a means-tested grant from their local authorities and no travel allowance. To cap it all off, both diploma and degree nurses start their careers at the same grade and pay (*Guardian*, 17 December 1996). Clearly dissatisfaction with both the clinical career structure and the system of nurse education will need to be addressed in the future, especially in the light of massive nurse shortages in the United Kingdom, with some London hospitals currently experiencing a 20 per cent vacancy rate for their nursing staff (*Guardian*, 17 December 1996).

The fourth practical outcome of the New Nursing ideology has been the establishment in the United Kingdom of nursing development units (NDUs). Of the original two units, the Burford unit was established in 1981 and the Oxford unit followed in 1985. A key aim of the units was to emphasise the therapeutic role of nursing, and the need to establish hospital beds specifically for patients with nursing problems. To this end, a system of primary nursing was developed, which used only qualified nurses in the delivery of care (Pearson 1988). The establishment of these units should really be seen as an extraordinary achievement. For instance, the Oxford NDU, which functioned between 1986 and 1989, contained 16 nursing beds, to which patients were admitted by the senior nurse. Nurses worked as autonomous practitioners, admitting and discharging patients who would normally have been situated in acute care wards. Nurses administered drugs and sought to implement the ideology of partnership between nurse and patient (Witz 1994). Jane Salvage, who spent time in the unit as well as analysing its reports, notes that interpersonal contact between nurses and patients was encouraged and was seen as central to the nurse's work. In addition, staff attempted to offer patients genuine informed choice in their care, and to respect the choices made (Salvage 1992). Witz (1994) notes that the Oxford NDU provides an example of how primary nursing redefines the traditional division of labour between doctors and nurses through the development of an exclusive nurse–practitioner–patient relationship. In the end, the unit was closed, partly because of the opposition of doctors who declared that the unit was 'medically unsound', who would not refer patients, and who were reluctant to provide emergency cover.

On the basis of this and other experiences, Witz has developed a useful distinction between the aspiration of nurses to either an extended or an enhanced role. She argues that nurses are more likely to encounter opposition from doctors when they attempt to enhance their role by emphasising their own authority and autonomy. On the other hand, they are less likely to encounter medical opposition when they limit their aspirations to extending their work by taking on the more routinised tasks traditionally done by doctors, especially junior doctors (Witz 1992). Witz contrasts the experience at Oxford with the experience at Worthing Hospital. Here the NDU was welcomed, rather than opposed, by doctors. This unit is a day ward as well as a 'drop-in' centre for patients with cancer and leukaemia. Nurses perform a range of tasks, from administering toxic chemotherapy drugs and blood transfusions to dealing with a range of issues at the drop-in centre. Witz concludes that the reason that the doctors did not oppose the NDU here was because the nurses were seeking only to extend their role—in this case, by performing routine medical tasks normally performed by doctors (Witz 1994, p. 36).

In evaluating the success of New Nursing thus far, it is important to note the gains, as well as the limitations and retreats. It is, for instance, important to remember that the New Nursing represents a coherent philosophy, which has been successfully combined with a model for practice in the NDUs. The question to be asked is 'can the genie be put back in the bottle?' NDUs have been fully evaluated (see Pearson 1988, pp. 67–72 for details) and are now part of nursing experience and the history of public policy. Much will clearly depend on proof of their cost effectiveness, as initiatives arising from a nursing agenda have historically been successful only when they have coincided with wider political and administrative concerns (Dingwall et al. 1988). As we shall see, this qualification also applies in Australia. For example, in an environment of increasing cost pressures, there are indications that concerns about impediments to efficiency and productivity in health care may provide sections of the state with reasons to support nursing goals in certain areas. These areas include changes to work organisation, to skill development, and to occupational demarcations, especially the removal of restrictive work practices on the part of doctors, which have been identified as a barrier to efficiency in health care settings. This could well be pivotal for the long-term success or failure of New Nursing (see Audit Commission 1991 for the United Kingdom; and Green 1992 for Australia).

Another area where there is potential congruence between the aspirations of nurses and the economic interests of the state is in the opening up of portals of entry into medicine. An access to medicine course, started in 1993 in Britain and which aims to encourage mature students to enter medical training, reports that most of its intake are nurses and that numbers applying are on the increase. The one-year, full-time course at West Anglia College, King's Lynn, costs £780 and consists of physics, chemistry, and biology up to A level standard. The director of the course has stated that while the course is 'very tough' and that students have to get a distinction in all subjects, they have had 'an amazing response' from nurses (Snell, 2000). In the year 2000, there were seven nurses and two midwives out of a class of 16, who, between them, won 23 offers from medical schools. Snell argues that the popularity of this course among nurses is a further development in the process of the two professions of nursing and medicine moving closer together. Wicks (1999) offers a different perspective on the same theme when she argues for a three-year generic course for all health workers before students undertake specialist, graduate courses in medicine, specialist nursing, or other health professions.

New directions for nursing in Australia

Although it can be said that New Nursing is making uneven advances in Australia (though the term itself does not appear to have wide usage in Australia), it can also be said that, overall, the advances here are actually more substantial than in the United Kingdom. There are at least five areas in which it is possible to see changes— where the philosophy of New Nursing has provided the theoretical or ideological impetus behind political pressure that has at least contributed to change. This is especially apparent in areas in which there has been congruence between nursing and state or administrative agendas. The first area of change has been the transfer of nurse education to the university sector. The move began in New South Wales in 1985 and is now complete across Australia. While the courses began as diploma qualifications, they have now all been upgraded to degree level, and so the damaging split between graduates with diplomas and those with degree qualifications has been avoided here. It is true to say that a major factor in the transition from 'on the job' training and university education was economic considerations. In an inspired move, the New South Wales Nurses Education Board (NEB) changed its arguments concerning the need for change, moving away from the perceived advantages for nurses and towards its cost-cutting potential. In a carefully argued piece of research, the NEB argued that, once established, it would be 'cheaper and more efficient to staff hospitals with fully trained nurses' (NEB 1980, p. 70). The change in nurse education was announced within three years of the release of this document.

It is a widely held view, and one held by many sociologists, that economic considerations were the sole reason for the transfer. Elizabeth Herdman, for instance, states that 'it is difficult to perceive the decision in other than economic terms' (1995, p. 65). While economic considerations were clearly central to the decision, recent theoretical insights from within sociology concerning the nature of the state can further enrich this analysis. Over the last decade there has been some important work published on what might be summarised as the dynamic and contradictory nature of the state in terms of gender and other relations. Susan Franzway and others make the point that: 'the state is culturally marked as masculine and functions largely as an institutionalisation of the power of men, especially heterosexual men. In that sense it is patriarchal ... Yet this institutionalisation is uneven and generates paradoxical reversals, in which the state participates in constituting antagonistic interests in sexual politics and can become a vehicle for advancing those interests' (1989, p. 41).

This view can be seen as one in which the state is regarded less as a monolith of class or patriarchal power than as a constellation of competing interests, with outcomes that are historically and nationally variable (Witz 1992). In this light, it is possible to see this and other achievements of the New Nursing as the result of the changing nature of the state, which can no longer ignore the interests of a large group of working women. It also acknowledges the central role of nurse leaders, who successfully harnessed the appropriate arguments at the right time. This, surely, is the nature of effective political action. Rather than detracting from their achievement, the successful linking of nursing interests with the interests of sections of the state might also be seen as evidence of clever political acumen.

Second, the implementation of the New Nursing in Australia has also created a clinical career path for nurses, as part of the Public Hospital Nurses (State) Award (1986), which includes the creation of 'specialist' and 'consultant' positions. These positions carry not only enhanced status but also financial recognition. Third, the category of 'women's health nurse' has been created. In 1987 the New South Wales Department of Health decided to prepare family planning health practitioners (who had received a very positive response from consumers) for a broader primary health care role. In addition to providing a wide range of services—including Pap smear collection, vaginal and pelvic examination, the fitting of diaphragms, pregnancy testing, and the issuing of oral contraceptives (under authorisation)—women's health nurses would receive additional training, which would allow them to provide services in the fields of counselling and health education (Short et al. 1993). As a result of vociferous opposition from some sections of the medical profession, the autonomy of these nurses was encroached upon, but not removed.

The fourth area of achievement that can be related to New Nursing has been the establishment of con-joint chairs of clinical nursing at teaching hospitals and universities. There are now over 67 chairs of clinical nursing in Australian universities, and a significant number of these are con-joint with teaching hospitals. One of the earliest of these appointments was that of Professor Judy Lumby to the E. M. Lane Chair of Surgical Nursing, Faculty of Nursing, at the University of Sydney, Concord Repatriation Hospital. Lumby comments:

> my work with surgeons to develop an interdisciplinary skills labora-
> tory in which nurses, doctors and allied health professionals can learn
> together is evidence of a joint commitment to a paradigm shift
> regarding individual and joint roles. This reconceptualisation places
> the patient in the centre of a web of professional care coordinated for
> the best possible outcomes. When the focus moves from the needs of
> a professional group to the needs of patients then we will know that
> the shift is beginning (Lumby 1996, p. 5).

While Lumby also talks about opposition to role changes, even in areas that have been assessed and have been found to be successful in terms of health outcomes, the fact that surgeons are sitting down with nurses and talking about joint learning opportunities is a huge achievement, and one that would have been unimaginable 25 years ago.

Finally, the establishment of an independent nurse-practitioner role is advancing apace in Australia. The National Nursing

Organisations define the nurse-practitioner as 'A registered nurse working in an advanced clinical role the characteristics of which will be determined by the context in which they are authorised to practice and which includes legislative authority to exercise clinical functions not currently within the scope of nursing practice' (National Nursing Organisations, 2000).

In 1999, New South Wales was the first State in Australia to pass legislation to enable nurses to work at this advanced level in order to provide a new and additional health service for people in rural and remote areas (NSW Department of Health 2000). The nurse-practitioner program provides specialist nurses with greater clinical powers, including the power to prescribe certain medications and order diagnostic tests, without the approval of a doctor. There is an accreditation process, and nurses with more than 5000 hours of clinical experience are eligible to apply. The title 'nurse-practitioner' is protected and it is an offence for anyone to use the title without authorisation by the Nurses Registration Board. Similar initiatives are also under way in the states of Victoria, South Australia, and Western Australia, and in the Australian Capital Territory and Northern Territory.

Despite extensive consultation, and in New South Wales the requirement for 'a local agreed need' to be present from all relevant stakeholders (including GPs), before a nurse-practitioner can be appointed to an area, medical organisations continue to complain about the role and the placement of nurse-practitioners. In a joint statement, the NSW AMA, the NSW faculty of the RACGP, and the Australian College of Rural and Remote Medicine have called on the NSW government to allow nurse-practitioners only where there is a locally agreed need and only where a doctor cannot be found. This is clearly an attempt to limit the allocation of nurse-practitioners to those areas where doctors do not wish to be located. How this situation develops in future years will depend on the ability of nurse-practitioners to deliver high quality, cost-effective care in a way that brings them significant public support. Whatever happens in the future, the establishment, in law, of this expanded role for the nurse is a highly significant achievement for nursing in Australia.

Conclusion: towards a more productive relationship?

For nursing, recent developments in sociology—notably the concern with **agency** and practice in connection with the formation of social structure, the incorporation of ideas from post-structuralism into feminist theory, and the integration of theories of gender into analyses of occupational strategies such as professionalisation—have created the potential and rationale for some

agency The ability of people, individually and collectively, to influence their own lives and the society in which they live.

theoretical bridge-building across the two disciplines. But it is important to note that this need not be a one-way relationship. In the same way that nursing stands to gain greater clarity and understanding by looking at various aspects of nursing through a sociological lens, sociology has much to learn from nursing. Nursing is a complex and fascinating occupation, which is at an exhilarating and yet dangerous moment in its history. For sociologists, nursing exemplifies several significant social issues of the late twentieth century: the issue of human agency, the role of gender in occupational strategies, the role of the state in constructing gender relations, the issue of the uses and dangers of **essentialism** (which in nursing is inherent in the attempt to valorise care at the expense of cure), and the nature of power. These are just some of the central issues that are encapsulated by nursing and its problematic relationship with medicine, with other health occupations, and with patients. Nurses are at the cutting edge of gender relations in health care. As they will tell you, it is not a comfortable position in which to be. In practice, nurses are working out political solutions to many of the theoretical conundrums facing sociology. Given the potential for mutual enlightenment, it might be worth working a little harder on this relationship.

essentialism An approach based on the assumption that there is an essential core or essence to identity that is inevitable and stable over time (for example, that women are essentially caring and nurturing).

Summary of main points

- Historical developments in sociological theory have affected sociological views of nursing.
- 'Classic' sociological and feminist interpretations of nursing have emphasised the overwhelming power of social structure at the expense of an account of nursing agency. This has led to an uneasy relationship between nursing and sociology.
- Recent developments within sociology in general, and feminist theory in particular, have led to a refocus, away from structure and towards nursing agency and resistance.
- At the same time, there has been a shift within nursing to focus on the content of nursing work in order to establish a case for practitioner autonomy.
- These developments illustrate that the time could not be better for both disciplines to reassess what they might fruitfully learn from each other.

Discussion questions

1 How do you understand the term 'agency' in the context of nursing work?
2 Describe the rules of the doctor/nurse game.
3 What is 'dual closure', and how does it relate to nursing?

4   What is new about 'New Nursing'? How far has it come in Australia?
5   Discuss nursing development units and outline their key features.

Further investigation

1   Outline two different approaches to nursing history and analyse their implications for a sociological understanding of nursing today.
2   Discuss and apply the sociological theory or theories that best enable us to understand the current position of nurse-practitioners in Australia.

Further reading and web resources

Ehrenreich, B. & English, D. 1973, *Witches, Midwives and Nurses*, Old Westbury Feminist Press, New York.

Gamarnikow, E. 1978, 'Sexual Division of Labour: The Case of Nursing', in A. Kuhn & A. M. Wolpe (eds), *Feminism and Materialism*, Routledge, London.

Roberts, S. J. 1983, 'Oppressed Group Behaviour: Implications for Nursing', *Advances in Nursing Science*, vol. 5, no. 4, pp. 21–30.

Salvage, J. 1992, 'The New Nursing: Empowering Patients or Empowering Nurses?', in A. Robinson, A. Gray, & R. Elkan (eds), *Policy Issues in Nursing*, Open University Press, Buckingham.

Wicks, D. 1999, *Nurses and Doctors at Work: Re-thinking Professional Boundaries*, Allen & Unwin, Sydney.

Web sites

Australian Nursing Federation (ANF): <www.anf.org.au>
NSW Health Department: <www.health.nsw.gov.au>
NSW Nurses' Association: <www.nswnurses.asn.au>
NSW Nurse Practitioners: <www.health.nsw.gov.au/nursing/npract.html>

16

Alternative Medicine

Gary Easthope

Overview

* *Why is alternative medicine alternative?*
* *Why is alternative medicine increasingly popular?*
* *Does alternative medicine work?*

Orthodox medicine is the dominant form of medicine because, historically, its practitioners organised themselves to lobby governments for a special status. However, alternative forms of medicine are becoming increasingly popular, especially among those with higher education and higher incomes. The reasons for this popularity are related to people's search for meaning, a distrust of science, the preponderance of chronic rather than acute illness, a 'personal' relationship between healers and their clients, and the search for control over one's life. Users of alternative medicine do not reject orthodox medicine but use both modalities. Alternative medicine can 'work' by changing the relationship of a person to his or her illness, or by producing a change in a set of symptoms. There have been few scientific demonstrations of the efficacy of alternative practices, but this is also true of most orthodox medical practices. Some alternative practices are being incorporated into orthodox medicine, and such alternative medical practices are being reclassified as complementary to, rather than alternative to, orthodox medicine.

Key terms

allopathy	postmodern society
biomedicine	randomised control trials (RCTs)
complementary medicine	risk factors
convergence	risk society
empirical	social closure
lifestyle choices	social support
orthodox medicine	state
placebo	theodicy

Introduction

empirical Describes observations or research that is based on evidence drawn from experience. It is therefore distinguished from something based only on theoretical knowledge or on some other kind of abstract thinking process.

orthodox medicine The medical practices and institutions developed in Europe during the nineteenth and twentieth centuries that are legally recognised by the state. Central to these practices is the teaching hospital, where all new doctors are inducted into laboratory science, clinical practice, and allopathic biomedicine. These practices and institutions are now dominant in all parts of the world.

In this chapter you will be introduced to the major arguments about alternative medicine and the **empirical** research conducted on alternative medicine. By the time you have completed reading the chapter, you should be aware that the simplistic distinction between the two medicines that sees the orthodox as scientific and the alternative as 'quackery' is wrong. It will also become clear that the distinction between orthodox practice and alternative practice has more to do with the relative political power and organisation of the two types of medicine than it has to do with any characteristics of their modes of treatment.

The chapter is structured around three questions. These questions are those frequently asked by anyone—layperson, doctor, or sociologist—who is at all interested in alternative medicine. The first question—why is alternative medicine alternative?—explores what distinguishes alternative medicine from **orthodox medicine**. The answer given provides a historical and political explanation, rather than an explanation in terms of modes of treatment. The next question—why is alternative medicine increasingly popular?—is answered by looking at empirical research on the clients of alternative practitioners in the context of changes in society and the nature of illness today. An answer to the last question—does alternative medicine work?—requires a discussion of what it means for a treatment to work. The conclusion to the chapter draws attention to the increasing usage of alternative treatments by orthodox practitioners, and to the re-labelling of alternative medicine as **complementary medicine**.

Why is alternative medicine alternative?

complementary medicine A term used to describe those alternative medical practitioners and practices that do not stand in opposition to orthodox medicine but that collaborate with orthodox practice.

allopathy A descriptive name often given to orthodox medicine. Allopathy is the treatment of symptoms by opposites.

Orthodox medicine is a recent social invention. Early last century, it was just one among a range of medical practices. Its theoretical base was that disease was a result of an imbalance in the body. To restore balance something must be given or taken away. To decide what was given or taken, the doctor observed the symptoms and prescribed something to produce an opposite effect to those symptoms (a process known as **allopathy**). For example, a patient whose face was suffused with blood would be bled to reduce the blood in their body. Allopathic physicians were also committed to treating the body (biomedicine), not the minds or spiritual aspects of their patients.

The practice base of orthodox medicine was broader than its theory. Its practice was developed in the clinic or hospital. Here doctors observed large numbers of patients and began to develop classificatory schemes that grouped sets of symptoms into categories.

Initially such groupings were based upon immediately observable characteristics, and nosological schemes were developed that, for example, grouped fevers into different types, dependent on such symptom characteristics as their incidence over time, to produce the categories of continued, intermittent, or remittent fevers. Later such classifications became more sophisticated, and symptoms were used as indicators of underlying theoretical entities called 'diseases'.

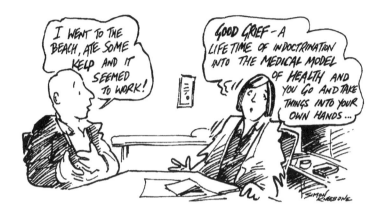

Source: Simon Kneebone, reproduced with permission

state A term used to describe a collection of institutions, including the parliament (government and Opposition political parties), the public-sector bureaucracy, the judiciary, the military, and the police.

The hospital, as well as providing doctors with large numbers of patients to observe, gave them much more control over their practice. Society physicians were employed by patrons, and had to defer to their patrons' views and treat them accordingly. In the hospital, the doctor was employed by the hospital or the **state** and had to defer to his fellow doctors' clinical judgment rather than that of his patient. In these circumstances, the empirical success of a treatment *as judged by fellow doctors* was more important than its congruence with allopathic theory.

Allopathy received a great boost when Louis Pasteur discovered micro-organisms. Allopathic theory was vindicated: toxic organisms invaded the body, upsetting its balance and causing symptoms that needed to be treated by attacking the invaders. Following Pasteur's lead, the application of laboratory science to medical practice was an outstanding feature of the development of orthodox medicine in the latter half of the nineteenth century and during the early twentieth century. Modern medicine was thus created from a combination of allopathic theory, a focus on the body, empirical clinical experience, and laboratory science. This scientific, clinical, allopathic **biomedicine** became the orthodox medicine in the late nineteenth century.

biomedicine/biomedical model The conventional approach to medicine in Western societies. It diagnoses and explains illness as a malfunction of one of the body's biological mechanisms. The biomedical approach of most health services focuses on the treating of individuals, and generally ignores social, economic, and environmental factors.

It did not become the orthodox medicine because it had a better cure rate than other forms of medicine. It became the orthodox medicine because its practitioners were better organised and more politically astute than practitioners in other forms of medicine, such as homoeopathy. In the United Kingdom, from which Australian doctors took their lead, this organisation took the form of a coalition between three disparate and competing groups of healers:

1   *local apothecaries*: who sold drugs and gave advice on treatment, much as drugstores continue to do in the Third World. These developed into provincial general practitioners (GPs) and were the driving force behind the development of the British Medical Association (BMA), upon which the Australian Medical Association (AMA) is modelled (Vaughan 1959)

2   *society physicians*: who dealt with the health needs of the upper classes and were not supposed to sell drugs

3   *surgeons*: who were the only healers licensed to practise surgery. This coalition created a national medical association, which lobbied governments to grant 'doctors' (a term that now included surgeons, physicians, and GPs) the legal right to practise their trade. There has been some variation between countries in the form that this historical development took (for the USA, see Starr 1982), with some variation in outcome. In some countries it has meant the exclusion of all other forms of medical practice as illegal. More commonly it has meant that only certified doctors could act to verify illness for work absence, insurance purposes, and other bureaucratic needs. Despite minor variations, the overall effect has been to produce an orthodox medicine supported by the state in all countries in the world. The status of orthodox medicine was further boosted by the improved morbidity and mortality rates of the twentieth century. Orthodox medicine took credit for these improvements, although we know now that they were primarily the result of clean drinking water, improved sewerage, and better nutrition rather than medical intervention (Szreter 1988).

Today, orthodox medicine and alternative medicines exist side by side, as they did last century. The dominant mode of medicine is the orthodox. From its position of strength, it can deal with its competitors in three ways. First, it can exclude them by seeking to categorise them as poorly trained quacks compared with orthodox doctors. This was the position taken by the president of the RACGP when she stated, 'It is to nobody's advantage that alternative medical providers with varying levels of qualifications and experience, can position themselves at the luxury end of the health care market' (Mercury 2000, p. 5). Second, it can reformulate the alternative practices so that they sound as though they are 'scientific' medicine; the empirical basis of clinical practice provides doctors with this option. Thus mesmerism was reformulated in the United Kingdom as hypnosis in the early years of this century, and was allowed so long as it was practised solely by certified doctors. More recently in Australia, chiropractic manipulation has become redefined as spinal manipulation by some GPs. Finally, doctors can incorporate the alternative practice into their normal repertoire, as has happened with acupuncture, which was once an exotic alternative but is now a clinical practice for which a Medicare rebate can be claimed (Easthope et al. 1998; 2001).

Those practising alternative medicine are not passive actors in this situation. Many alternative medical associations have observed how the doctors achieved their pre-eminence and seek to emulate them. Chiropractic has been particularly successful in this. It has set up colleges to train and certify its practitioners. It has practised usurpatory **social closure** by limiting chiropractic to these certified chiropractors, and has achieved this with the support of private health insurers and the state (O'Neill 1994; 1995, Dew 2000). Alternative therapists have also sought, usually unsuccessfully, to stop doctors using their techniques. For example, Judy James, the executive officer of the Australian Acupuncture association, echoing doctors' critique of alternative medicine, accuses doctors of being poorly trained: 'There are doctors who go out and do a weekend course in acupuncture and think they are qualified to practise. Unfortunately, the public are led to believe that because these practitioners are doctors they know what they are doing' (cited in Derkley 1998, p. 21).

The dominance of orthodox medicine is, however, so secure that alternative medicines, even such strongly organised alternatives as chiropractic, can only be said to exist in its shadow. Nonetheless, that shadow is very broad and has spread over a wider area. In the next section I look at the phenomenal growth of alternative medicine before asking why this has happened.

social closure A term first used by Max Weber to describe the way that power is exercised to exclude outsiders from the privileges of social membership (in social classes, professions, or status groups).

Why is alternative medicine increasingly popular?

During the 1980s and 1990s in Australia, alternative medicine became accepted by the general public, with spending on such alternative therapies in 1993 (extrapolated from a South Australian study) standing at A$309 million and expenditure on alternative medicines estimated at $621 million (compared with the $360 million contribution patients made for pharmaceutical drugs in the same year) (MacLennan et al. 1996). The National Health Survey of 1995 (ABS 1997) reported that 30 per cent of the Australian population were using a vitamin or mineral supplement. A study using a national random sample of adults undertaken for the RACGP found 44 per cent of respondents had used an alternative medicine provider in the past (Wirthlin 2000). Similar figures are reported in the USA (Eisenberg 1998), Canada (Verhof & Sutherland 1995), the United Kingdom

(Zollman & Vickers 1999; Ernst & White 2000), and Europe (Vincent & Furnham 1998), with Japanese expenditure on medicinal herbs estimated to have increased fifteen-fold between 1974 and 1989 (WHO 1996).

The demand has led to a growth in the number of therapists registered with the Australian Traditional Medicine Society (the ATMS claims to represent 65 per cent of all alternative therapists) from 3200 in 1994 to 7253 in 1999, and the number of colleges affiliated with the ATMS that are training therapists has grown from 17 in 1986 to 69 in 1998 (Doran 1999). It has also led to increased demand for alternative medicines, with Blackmores reporting a 21 per cent increase from 1995 to 1998 (Norman 1998) and Mediherb, the main supplier to alternative therapists, reporting sales of over $8 million in 1997 (Eccleston 1997).

Such therapies have also found favour with medical insurance companies. Private medical insurance is held by more than a third of the Australian population. In a bid to attract clients, insurance companies have competed by offering, often as extras, access

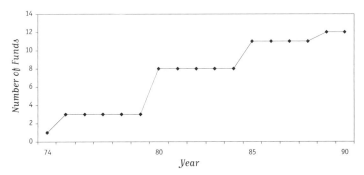

Figure 16.1   Number of funds offering complementary therapies by year of introduction

Source: Doran, 1999

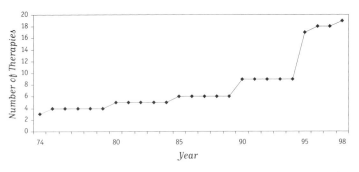

Figure 16.2   Number of different complementary therapies covered by private health insurance in Australia

Source: Doran, 1999

to complementary therapies (Easthope 1993). In recent years the number of insurance companies offering alternative therapies and the variety of therapies offered has dramatically increased (see Figures 16.1 and 16.2). One company, Grand United, has even bought a share of two of Sydney's natural health clinics (Ragg 1997).

During the 1980s and 1990s complementary therapies gained acceptance by being offered as courses in higher education institutions. The leaders in this area were the chiropractors who, by imposing a levy on each chiropractor, were able to set up a course at Preston Institute of Technology (later Phillip Institute of Technology) to train chiropractors and to confer degrees. This obtained federal funding in 1982 and ultimately became part of RMIT, a university-level tertiary institution. In 1992 Victoria University of Technology began offering a bachelor's degree in acupuncture. In 1994 the University of Technology in Sydney began offering a bachelor of health science in acupuncture and in 1997 a degree in Chinese herbal medicine, both within the (orthodox) Department of Health Science. In 1995 Southern Cross University in New South Wales began offering a degree in Naturopathy. In 2000, Monash University opened a new Institute of Public Health, which, along with health economics, medical informatics, and clinical effectiveness, also has a segment on complementary medicine.

Recently there has also been growing interest in research on the efficacy of alternative medicines and therapies. Orthodox peer-reviewed medical journals now carry papers on the testing of alternatives. Furthermore, centres of alternative medicines and therapies have been established within traditionally orthodox institutions such as universities (for example the Herbal Medicines Research Centre at Sydney University in 1997 and the Centre for the Evaluation of Complementary Health Practices at the University of Queensland in 2000) and hospitals (for example the Natural Therapies Unit at the Royal Women's Hospital in Sydney).

Governments have also been important in legitimating complementary medicine. In Australia the federal government, as part of its control of therapeutic goods, has set up an Office of Complementary Medicine to oversee complementary medicines; its committee has input from members of the industry. In Victoria, after financing a study of traditional Chinese medicine (Bensoussan and Myers 1996), the government has moved to set up registration of practitioners in that State, and a bill to achieve this is currently under debate. In the USA the government has set up and funded an Office of Alternative Medicine at the National Institutes of Health to evaluate alternative practices.

It is impossible to give a full list of alternative therapies as the number is vast and growing. Some of the major therapies are listed in Table 16.1. Several arguments have been advanced to explain the increase in usage and provision as shown by the table.

Table 16.1   Alternative medicines

Category	Alternative Medicines
Comprehensive systems	Ayuverdic medicine
	Anthroposophy
	Herbalism
	Homoeopathy
	Naturopathy
Spiritual and Mental	Faith Healers
	Spiritual Healers
	Mental Imaging
	Past-life regression
	Primal regression
	Transcendental meditation
Energy Work	Acupuncture
	Acupressure
	Crystal healing
	Polarity
	Reflexology
	Reiki
	Shiatsu
	Therapeutic Touch
Dietary therapies	Bach flower remedies
	Colonics
	Gerson Therapy
	Macrobiotics
	Pritikin Diet
	Vitamin therapy
Manipulation	Alexander technique
	Chiropractic
	Cranialsacral therapy
	Feldenkrais
	Massage
	Osteopathy
	Rolfing
	Tai Chi
	Trager
	Yoga
Diagnostics	Applied kinesiology
	Biorhythms
	Iridology
	Kirlian photography
	Psionics
	Radionics
Other	Aromatherapy
	Colour therapy
	Hydrotherapy

Sources: Trevelyan & Booth 1994; Murray & Shepherd 1993; Stanway 1979; also see Healey 1996

The search for meaning

Health and illness are fundamental issues that all societies face. Ways of explaining illness, suffering, and death (theodicies) are central to all religions. Such modes of explanation are a central part of any cosmology, or explanation of the universe. In modern Western societies, the traditional religious cosmology that attributed illness to the work of the devil or original sin no longer has institutional support. Orthodox medicine, the main institution to deal with illness, has no developed cosmology to explain illness except allopathy and the theory of germs. In a society in which few become seriously ill through germs, but in which many suffer heart attack or cancer, this has little appeal. Even within the germ theory there is no clear explanation of personal misfortune—why one person gets ill in a 'flu' epidemic and another stays healthy. Under these circumstances, alternative medical cosmologies that explain illness in terms of spiritual forces (spiritualism), the balance of elements in the body (yin and yang, naturopathy), or the development of life force (homoeopathy) have great appeal.

The distrust of scientific experts

Science has lost its gloss, and scientific medicine has declined in status along with science (Gray 1999). Science is no longer seen as the solution but is frequently seen as part of the problem. The **risk society** (Beck 1992) is obsessed with the risks created by scientific actions; the environment is seen to be under constant threat from oil spills, nuclear radiation, and acid rain, all of which are blamed on science and technology. Scientific medicine has produced thalidomide as well as the bionic ear. The technological fix is increasingly mistrusted. Books such as *Bad Medicine* (Archer 1995) document the iatrogenic toll and call upon people to become educated health consumers rather than patients.

> **risk society** A term coined by Ulrich Beck (1992) to describe the centrality of risk calculations in people's lives in Western society, whereby the key problem of society today is unanticipated hazards, such as the risks of pollution and environmental degradation.

The 'personal' healer–patient relationship

Closely related to the previous point is the fact that many, although not all, healers provide a personalised service. They spend time listening to their clients and tailor their treatment to the individual client (Easthope 1985; Lowenberg & Davis 1994). They can do this because their clientele are generally paying for the service themselves. In this way, many alternative practitioners are acting as the society physicians did in an earlier age, but in a society in which many more people can afford to pay for such personal treatment.

The search for control over one's life

In a **postmodern society** much of life is outside the control of the individual. Movements on the international money markets can dictate whether one has a job next week or even if one's

> **postmodern society** A disputed term to refer to a society in which many of the central institutions, including the state, have lost their power to determine social outcomes. There are no longer clear paths for the individual to influence events by participating in such institutions as political parties, unions, or professional bodies.

doctor will be able to treat you because he or she can get mal-practice insurance (Hay 1992). In such a society, people search for areas of control. One such area is the self (Giddens 1991). People seek to control their own bodies through jogging, gymnasiums, vitamins, and alternative medicine. Healers give people the abil-ity to manage their own disease by giving them the ability to reconstruct themselves. As one healer said in a lecture to his students, 'Be a reflection of the person you're treating ... to be a more reliable, more secure part of themselves. So, you're the rock, absolutely dependable, absolutely competent, absolutely sure of everything you do and as you're reflecting them, they too can become sure of themselves' (Easthope 1985, p. 62). The relation between illness and the level of control people have over their life is now also becoming recognised by orthodox doctors (see Marmot et al. 1997).

The nature of illness: chronic and terminal

The success of environmental controls over sewage and water—coupled with immunisation, vaccination, and antibiotics—has meant that most illness in modern societies is either chronic or terminal. By definition, neither of these states can be cured. In these circumstances the traditional practice of orthodox medicine is relatively useless. Furthermore, its procedures and the mode of payment for those procedures—the clinical examination followed by clinical intervention to produce cure—do not allow for treat-ment of chronic or terminal illness, both of which require long-term, intermittent intervention rather than one-stop cures. People are therefore turning to those healers who do offer such a long-term relationship: the alternative practitioners.

Empirical research in Canada (Verhoef et al. 1990), New Zealand (Sawyer 1994), the United Kingdom (Murray & Shepherd 1993; Thomas et al. 1991), and Australia (Lloyd et al. 1993; MacLennan et al. 1996; Yates et al. 1993; Siahpush, 1998) supports most of these arguments, although different studies focus more on one aspect than another. Those using alternative practi-tioners are seeking explanations for their health problems. They are worried about the dangers of medical intervention and prefer alternative medicine because it is seen as drug-free and 'natural'. They very much appreciate the personal attention they get from the alternative practitioners. They also seek control over the meth-ods of dealing with their illness and, when they deal with doctors, want control over treatment decisions. Overall it would appear that it is not dissatisfaction with orthodox medicine that is leading people to look to alternative medicine (Astin 1998) but rather a positive choice of a medicine that offers a natural, holistic approach and a sense of individual responsibility (Siahpush 1999).

However, there is conflicting evidence regarding the characteristics of users. Small-scale studies have found users to be more likely to have chronic or terminal illness, but such studies have frequently selected their sample from such sufferers (Sawyer et al. 1994;Yates et al. 1993). General population surveys and surveys of general practice suggest that it is young and middle-aged people who are using alternative medicine as a **lifestyle choice** (Lloyd et al. 1993; MacLennan et al. 1996; Thomas et al.1991). A small study of the users of alternative medicines, as distinct from users of alternative therapies (Rayner & Easthope in press) was able to distinguish two major types of users (see Table 16.2): 'postmoderns' and 'modified moderns'. Postmoderns, predominantly young women, were committed to postmodern values, were reflexive about their health, and tended to use aromatherapy and homeopathy. Modified moderns were committed to the modern values of technology and expertise but were also likely to engage, for example, in buying evening primrose oil and herbal medicines to control the symptoms of the menopause.

lifestyle choices/factors The decisions people make that are likely to impact on their health such as diet, exercise, smoking, alcohol, and other drugs. The term implies that people are solely responsible for choosing and changing their lifestyle.

Table 16.2 A typology of alternative medicine consumers

	Postmoderns	*Modified moderns*
Positive values	Holism, choice, natural	Technology, expert control
Negative/indifferent values	remedies, individual control	Individual control, natural remedies, choice
Demographics	Female, young, single, highly educated, higher income	Female, middle-aged/ elderly, married, less educated, lower income
Behaviours	Gyms, outdoor activities, meditation, sports, high health reflexivity	Diets, average health reflexivity
Products	Aromatherapy, homoeopathics	Evening Primrose Oil, herbal medicines

Source: Rayner & Easthope (in press)

In brief, it appears that the majority of those who use alternative medicine do so for the reasons cited above—a preference for the 'natural', an appreciation of personal attention, and a desire for control over treatment. However there is also a minority of users who resort to alternative therapies and medicines when orthodox medicine fails to alleviate their symptoms.

Does alternative medicine work?

The question of whether alternative medicine works is much more complex than it would at first appear. An intervention by a healer can be said to 'work' in three analytically distinct ways (although these ways often overlap empirically):

1   It changes the relationship of individuals to their afflictions so that they feel more comfortable, suffer less pain, and are able to manage their normal daily lives.
2   It produces a clinically observable change in a set of symptoms.
3   It produces a change in a set of symptoms that is scientifically demonstrated to be a function of the intervention.

These three ways of 'working' can be observed in both alternative and orthodox medicine. It is important to realise that only a small proportion of orthodox medical interventions—estimated as 15 per cent (Coleman 1994)—have been scientifically tested via **randomised control trials** (**RCTs**), and the Cochrane collaboration (Berman et al. 2000) reports that only 21 per cent of conventional medicine's practices have a clear positive effect.

It is equally important to realise that an even smaller proportion of alternative medical practice has been scientifically tested. Let us look at each of these three ways of working in turn, looking solely at alternative medicine, and speculate on how alternative medicine works in each instance. In the first instance—in which the individual's relationship to their affliction is changed—there is a redefinition of the patient's bodily or mental state as one in which healer and client agree that a healing has taken place. In a study of spiritual healing groups, healings in such groups were seen as 'events that rely on "rhetorics" of healing that encourage persons to define and redefine problems within idioms that are appropriate to healing [and] that healing must be understood in terms of treatment of lifestyle … the realisation of meaning attributed to a symptom … or the awakening into a religious world view … rather than the treatment of a pathology' (Glik 1990, pp. 162, 163). In these terms, healing works by providing a **theodicy**, an explanation for the affliction, which enables the afflicted to deal with it.

There is little doubt that, in terms of clinical efficacy, many alternative healing practices work. Why they work is unclear, but that is equally true of many orthodox healing practices. Two possible explanations of such clinical efficacy have been advanced: the **placebo** effect and the operation of social support (including the activation of the immune response through such support).

The placebo effect is any therapeutic practice that has no clear physiological effect but that nevertheless has an effect on the patient: pain and other symptoms go away ('Sugaring the Pill' 1996). Work on placebo response has demonstrated that the key features that produce a placebo effect are a feeling of uncertainty in the patient coupled with trust in the authority of the healer. People go to a healer—orthodox or alternative—when they are uncertain of their own diagnosis and prognosis, and are seeking expert advice and aid. When that healer presents as an authoritative person who gives

randomised control trials (RCTs) A biomedical research procedure used to evaluate the effectiveness of particular medications and therapeutic interventions. 'Random' refers to the equal chance of participants being in the experimental or control group (the group to which nothing is done and is used for comparison), and 'trial' refers to the experimental nature of the method. It is often mistakenly viewed as the best way to demonstrate causal links between factors under investigation, but privileges biomedical over social responses to illness.

theodicy An explanation of suffering, evil, and death.

placebo/placebo effect Any therapeutic practice that has no clear clinical effect. In practice it usually means giving patients an inert substance to take as a medication. When a patient reacts to a placebo in a way that is not clinically explicable, this is called the 'placebo effect'.

them personal attention, and who is therefore someone that they feel they can trust, a placebo response is very likely. Most alternative practitioners, and many orthodox practitioners, present themselves in precisely this way (Easthope 1985). However, meta analyses of clinical interventions using acupuncture, herbal remedies, manual therapies, and nutritional therapies have found they are more effective for certain conditions than placebos, for example, echinacea for relief of cold symptoms (Barrett et al. 1999) and acupuncture for post-operative nausea (Berman et al. 2000). A placebo response is consequently not an adequate explanation for the success of some alternative therapies.

Social support has been implicated in the sociological view of the causes of affliction since Émile Durkheim (1951) demonstrated in 1897 that apparently individual acts of suicide produced suicide rates that varied according to the levels of such support (what he called 'social solidarity'). A similar finding was made in a comparative analysis of modern societies (Wilkinson 1996), which found that social cohesion is a central factor in producing good health for populations. An extensive summary of the literature argued that 'social relationships, or the relative lack thereof, constitute a major

risk factors Conditions that are thought to increase an individual's susceptibility to illness or disease such as abuse of alcohol or smoking.

risk factor for health—rivalling the effects of well-established risk factors such as cigarette smoking, blood pressure, blood lipids, obesity and physical activity' (House et al. 1988, p. 541).

It is now becoming clear that social support may also be implicated in the relief of affliction. Two studies of the survival rates of women with breast cancer report that social support is an important variable (Waxler-Morrison et al. 1991; Maunsell, Brisson, & Deschenes 1995), and David Ornish, an American physician, uses

social support The support provided to an individual by being part of a network of kin, friends, or colleagues.

social support (along with diet and exercise) in a regimen that produces changes in the hearts of his patients that are demonstrable in angiograms (Ornish 1990; Ornish et al. 1990).

A biomedical, rather than a sociological, explanation of these effects is provided by psychoneuroimmunology (pni). What the theory of pni does is to reduce the social to the biological. Pni proponents argue that social effects cause changes in the immune system of individuals, and that these changes mean that people are less likely to become ill and more likely to recover when they are ill. The evidence for pni effects is ambiguous (Vedhera, Fox, & Wang 1999).

There have been very few scientific tests of alternative medicine. One reason for this is the different world-view held by many alternative practitioners. Many are not concerned with cure, but rather with healing, and thus do not accept the scientific criteria of cure. Further, their strong emphasis on the individual makes them resistant to treating groups of people in exactly the same way, so that a treatment group can not be compared with a control group to test the efficacy of a treatment. However the Research Council on Complementary Medicine in the United Kingdom has argued that conventional randomised control trial methodologies can be used to assess alternative therapies (Berman et al. 2000), and a new journal *Focus on Alternative and Complementary Therapies* (*FACT*) is using similar methods to the Cochrane collaboration to assess the clinical effectiveness of alternative therapies and medications. One of the few studies to conduct a scientific test of an alternative practice was a study of the Bristol Cancer Help Centre in the United Kingdom (Bagenel et al. 1990), where patients are encouraged to use visualisation techniques to reduce their tumours. The study found a better survival rate in the control group than in the treatment group, a difference that was attributed to the extreme vegetarian diet of the treatment group (Richmond 1990), but the scientific status of the study has been contested (Stacey 1991).

Conclusion: future directions

An interesting feature of recent publications on the working of alternative treatment modalities is the increasing interest being shown in them by orthodox practitioners in many countries (Goldbeck-Wood et al. 1996 Astin et al. 1998; Pirotta et al. 2000; Easthope et al. 2000 in press). Both Siegel and Ornish (cited above) are orthodox practitioners, not alternative practitioners. Compare these three quotations:

1   'In summary, then, your mind, body and spirit are all intimately interconnected. Because of this the … program is designed to address all of these levels not just the physical ones' (Ornish 1990, p. 250).

2   'We're so interrelated as human beings, and in different parts of ourselves. Any physical healing may be the first link in the chain … wholeness of body, mind and spirit' (pers. comm.).

3   'We can use our pain—emotional or physical—as a catalyst to begin healing not curing. To me curing means only getting back to the way we were before we became diseased. Healing is when we use our pain or illness as a catalyst to begin transforming our lives—healing our inner pain and our relationships, our hearts and our souls' (Ornish 1990, p. 226).

It is difficult, if not impossible, to discern which quotes are from an alternative practitioner and which from a doctor (in fact, quotes 1 and 3 are from a medical doctor, and 2 is from a healer I interviewed in the 1980s).

Many orthodox doctors are incorporating alternative treatment modalities into their practice of medicine, and making judgments of their efficacy and safety (Easthope et al. 2000a and b). In

Australia, one in seven GPs uses acupuncture (Easthope et al. 1999) and many doctors are using other complementary therapies or referring patients to other therapists, both medical and non-medical for such treatments (Pirotta et al. 2000; Hall & Giles-Corti 2000; Easthope et al. 2000b) In Canada, England, Germany, New Zealand, Scotland, the USA, and the Netherlands, studies of GPs found widespread usage of alternative medical practices and referral to alternative practitioners (Astin et al. 1998). In response to this interest most medical schools in the USA and over half of those in the United Kingdom now teach their trainee doctors about alternative medicine (Lewith 2000). In the United Kingdom the BMA has produced several reports on alternative practice (the most recent being published in 1993).

GPs in particular are looking to alternative practices to re-establish their role, which is being eroded by increased competition for patients among GPs and the development of corporate medicine backed by the state (Strasser 1992, White 2000). Alternative practices, with their emphasis on holism, are a tempting route for those wishing to avoid this fate. In the market-place for medical treatment, as in the commercial market-place, one way to deal with the opposition is to mount a take-over bid (Saks 1994). Nurses, too, have seen advantages in adopting alternative practices: the emphasis on care rather than cure, which is a major aspect of alternative medicine, is a means of extending their professional role (Trevelyan & Booth 1994).

The result is that alternative medicine is becoming less and less alternative. Some (Willis 1989a) have argued that there is a **convergence** between orthodox and alternative medicine but such convergence, if it is occurring, is very weak (Bombardieri & Easthope 2000). Rather, for some practitioners, both orthodox and otherwise, it is being reclassified as complementary medicine—acting as a complement to orthodox medicine. In some instances it is being incorporated into orthodox medicine and becoming part of the orthodoxy. This incorporation can be achieved because of the concept of clinical judgment, which is an essential aspect of medicine as an art rather than as a science. Without the idea of clinical judgment, medicine could not lay claim to professional status, as the essence of professionalism is the ability to exercise professional judgment—judgment based on knowledge and experience. This concept allows the division between orthodox medicine and alternative medicine to become blurred if doctors, in their clinical judgment, see some alternative therapies as efficacious. Some doctors are choosing to blur this division by incorporating some alternative therapies into their practice as they become disenchanted with modern medicine as a means of treating some chronic illnesses, although they retain

convergence The process, which may or may not be occurring, whereby orthodox medicine adopts many of the practices of alternative medicine, and alternative medicine acts to become more orthodox by, for example, seeking to license practitioners and make practitioners subject to training.

scientific diagnosis (Eastwood 2000). It is unlikely that the demarcation will ever disappear, but it will no longer be a clear battle-front; rather, it will be an area of cooperation, in which orthodoxy gradually shades into alternative practice.

Summary of main points

- Orthodox medicine dominates because, historically, it has been better organised politically than other forms of medicine.
- Alternative medicine is increasingly popular because it provides an explanation of illness, more people now distrust scientific expertise, healers appear to cope with chronic and terminal illness better than orthodox medicine, and healers provide more personalised attention. It also helps people to believe that they are in control of their illness.
- Users of alternative medicine commonly also use orthodox medicine.
- Alternative medicine 'works' by changing the relationship of people to their illnesses through the placebo effect (which is also important in orthodox medicine), through the provision of social support, and through other means which are not yet clear (Lewith 1999).
- There have been few scientific tests of the efficacy of alternative medicine, but neither has most orthodox medical practice been subject to scientific testing.
- Many orthodox doctors, especially general practitioners, are incorporating alternative treatment methods into their practices and referring patients to alternative practitioners. Such usage has led to the abandonment of the term 'alternative medicine' and to the increasing use of the term 'complementary medicine'.

Discussion questions

1 Which alternative medical practices are most likely to be accepted into orthodox medicine? Why?
2 Alternative medicine is mainly used by people who have good incomes and can afford to pay the fees. Should the government subsidise some alternative practices so that poor people can use them? If so, which practices should be subsidised?
3 Placebos work even when people know that they are placebos. What are the implications of this for orthodox medical practice and for alternative medical practices?
4 What are the main features of healer–client or doctor–patient interaction that would convince afflicted individuals that they are being treated on a personal level?
5 Does alternative medicine provide practices that could be adopted by nurses or other health workers to improve their practice? If so, which alternative practices would be most useful?

6 What alternative therapies (or medicines) would be attractive to different types of people?

Further investigation

1 Compare any one alternative/complementary medical therapy (e.g. acupuncture) with any one orthodox therapy (e.g. fixing a broken wrist). In making your comparison you should examine the mode of diagnosis, the role of technology in treatment, the types of therapists involved in treatment, and the institutions in which treatment occurs.
2 Compare and contrast the way orthodox medicine and alternative/complementary medicine are portrayed in the media. Make comparisons in only one type of media (television, radio, newspapers, or magazines).
3 Using the Yellow Pages for your area, examine all the alternative/complementary therapists listed. Which are the most common and which the least common? Consider why some are more common than others. (An alternative would be to compare two areas very different in their social or ethnic composition and speculate why there are (or are not) differences in the therapies offered.)

Further reading and web resources

What is alternative about alternative medicine?

Dew, K. 2000, 'Apostasy to Orthodoxy: Debates Before a Commission of Inquiry into Chiropractic', *Sociology of Health and Illness*, vol. 22, no. 3, pp. 310–30.

Why is alternative medicine increasingly popular?

Siahpush, M. 1998, 'Postmodern Values, Dissatisfaction with Conventional Medicine and Popularity of Alternative Therapies', *Journal of Sociology*, vol. 34, pp. 58–70.
——— 1999, 'Why do People Favour Alternative Medicine?', *Australian and New Zealand Journal of Public Health*, vol. 23, no. 3, pp. 266–71.

Does alternative medicine work?

Vincent, C. & Furnham, A. 1998, *Complementary Medicine: A Research Perspective*. Wiley, Chichester.

'Complementary' not 'alternative' medicine

Bombardieri, D. & Easthope, G. 2000, 'Convergence between Orthodox and Alternative Medicine: A Theoretical Elaboration and Empirical Test', *Health*, vol. 4, no. 4, pp. 479–94.

Easthope, G., Tranter, B., & Gill, G. (in press), 'The Normal Medical Practice of Referring Patients for Complementary Therapies Among Australian General Practitioners', *Journal of Complementary Therapies in Medicine*.

Eastwood, H. 2000, 'Why are Australian GPs Using Alternative Medicine? Postmodernisation, Consumerism and the Shift Towards Holistic Health', *Journal of Sociology*, vol. 36, no. 2, pp. 133–56.

Pirotta, M. V., Cohen, M. M., Kotsirilos, V., & Farish, S. J. 2000, 'Complementary Therapies: Have They Become Accepted in General Practice?', *Medical Journal of Australia*, vol. 172, pp. 105–9.

Web sites

Complementary Health Studies at University of Exeter:
    <www.exeter.ac.uk/chs/>
Complementary Therapies in Medicine (journal):
    <www.harcourt-international.com/journals/ctim>
Complementary Therapies in Nursing & Midwifery (journal):
    <www.harcourt-international.com/journals/ctnm/default.cfm>
Guild of Complementary Practitioners (UK):
Society of Homeopaths:

17

In Search of Profession

A Sociology of Allied Health[1]

Lauren Williams

Overview

* *What role does allied health play in the delivery of health care to Australians?*
* *How are allied health professions affected by medical dominance in the health system?*
* *What strategies have allied health practitioners used to seek professional status, and how successful have they been?*

The aim of this chapter is to analyse critically those health professions that provide a diverse range of specialised services directly to patients to help meet their physical, psychological, social, functional, nutritional, pharmaceutical, and informational needs. Collectively known as 'the allied health professions', they arose from an increasing trend towards specialisation within the health system. In attempting to establish domains of practice, and to obtain power and prestige, many of the allied health professions are trying to model themselves on medicine, a strategy likely to achieve limited success. While some professions have made more gains than others, this group generally remains subordinate to medicine. The extent to which the allied health occupations fulfil their professional projects, and survive within the public and private health sector, depends upon the strategies they use, and the extent to which they ally with each other.

Key terms

class
economic rationalism
encroachment (vertical and
  horizontal)
feminisation
gender/sex
health promotion
medical dominance
norms

patriarchy
professionalisation (professionalising project)
sexual division of labour
social closure
social structure
state
trait approach

1 Thanks to Joanne Prendergast for her insightful thoughts on the current status of allied health and for the provision of several key references. The contribution of Jane Potter is noted with gratitude. Thanks especially to John Germov for his patience and valuable suggestions.

Introduction

medical dominance A general term used to describe the power of the medical profession in terms of its control over its own work, over the work of other health workers, and over health resource allocation, health policy, and the way that hospitals are run.

social structure The recurring patterns of social interaction through which people are related to each other, such as social institutions and social groups.

This chapter considers the role and contribution of the health professionals who provide specialised services directly to patients, as distinct from services provided by doctors or nurses. The range of services provided by allied health is broad, addressing the physical, psychological, social, functional, nutritional, pharmaceutical, and informational needs of patients. The aim of this chapter is to describe, and then analyse from a sociological perspective, the role of allied health practitioners, focusing on their development into professions in a health system characterised by **medical dominance**. We will see how allied health professions struggle for power within the health system, in order to be able to deliver effective patient care.

To study the division of labour in what Evan Willis (1989b) calls the **social structure** of health care delivery, we must look at how the various professions operate within the system. This is the purpose of this section of the book. (Other groups are discussed in chapters 14, 15 and 16). If you are a student in an allied health profession, you will find this chapter particularly useful, in that it will give you a perspective on the challenges facing the profession you desire to enter. It should be noted, however, that this chapter is introductory and provides only a broad overview of a group that is really a collection of complex and diverse subgroups. Students interested in more than a generalised introduction should pursue the further reading recommended at the end of the chapter.

Much has been written from a sociological or political perspective about medicine and, increasingly, nursing. This is not surprising since doctors largely control the health system and nurses comprise approximately two-thirds of the health workforce (see Table 17.1 on p. 346). By contrast, allied health professions have been largely overlooked in the literature, which reflects their relatively small numbers and less than powerful position within the health system. It is also likely that few social scientists were exposed to many of these professions as potential subjects of analysis prior to 1989, when college-based training courses became part of the Australian university system. Those authors who have studied this group have commonly focused on physiotherapy, occupational therapy, and speech pathology (previously known as 'speech therapy').

Perhaps more surprising is the fact that the allied health professions themselves have not demonstrated a critical perspective. But, as we shall see, most of the professions align themselves with medical science, largely neglecting to develop a culture that encourages criticism of their own development. These groups may regard a critical perspective as being too negative, but it is a critical perspective that will uncover barriers to success and thereby inform the future direction of the allied health professions. It is the purpose of this chapter to provide such a perspective.

Description of the allied health professions

First, let us look at each part of the term 'allied health professions' in turn. 'Allied' means 'related to' or 'connected with', which, in this context, is traditionally taken to mean 'allied to medicine'. 'Health' refers to the type of care given by these workers and to the system within which this care is delivered. The term 'professions' connotes a specific level of occupation, one that confers a high status. Some authors argue that this group would more correctly be called para- or semi-professionals, but use of the term 'profession' by allied health occupations indicates that these groups individually and collectively regard themselves as meeting the criteria for professional status. Issues related to being defined as a profession will be discussed later in the section on cultural and structural analysis. The previous label for this group was 'paramedical'. This term literally means 'beside medicine' and is defined as 'supplementing and supporting medicine' (*Australian Concise Oxford Dictionary* 1987), demonstrating that allied health professionals are subject to the medical dominance of the health system (discussed later).

'Allied health' can be defined as those professions (other than medicine and nursing) that are involved in patient care. This functionality is reflected in the organisational structures of public hospitals, where these professions are grouped formally or informally under the name of allied health. Some authors, including some of those cited in this chapter, include nursing in a definition of allied health, and indeed nurses have some issues in common with allied health professionals, especially in being subject to medical dominance. However, in the Australian hospital system, nursing is usually structurally separate from allied health and is excluded from the definition used in this chapter (see chapter 15 for a discussion of nursing). Alternative or complementary practitioners, such as chiropractors and osteopaths, are also excluded from this definition since they are not usually employed within the public hospital system (see chapter 16).

The Australian Bureau of Statistics (ABS) groups allied health practitioners into two categories: the health occupations (those with a diagnostic and treatment role, such as doctors, physiotherapists, nurses, and dietitians) and the health-related occupations (including psychologists, social workers, and counsellors) (AIHW 1994). Allied health professions, as defined above, make up 15 per cent of the total numbers of the health occupations as listed in Table 17.1.

Table 17.1   Health personnel in Australia, by occupation, 1996

Health occupations	Percentage of health occupations	Percentage increase 1991–96
Total medical practitioners	16.0	13.8
Dentists	2.8	13.1
Chiropractors and osteopaths	2.7	29.1
Total nurses (registered and enrolled)	65	0.5 (11.5 registered; −38.1 enrolled)
Allied health practitioners		
Pharmacists	4.5	13.1
Physiotherapists	3.2	24.9
Medical imaging professionals*	2.4	41.7
Occupational therapists	1.6	19.2
Speech pathologists	0.8	33.5
Optometrists	0.8	23.9
Podiatrists	0.5	28.2
Other practitioners	1.7	−13.8
Total allied health practitioners	15.5	15.7

*   Previously listed as radiography, this category has changed since the last AIHW report and therefore figures over time are not directly comparable.

Source: AIHW 1998

Allied health workers form a homogeneous group in the sense that, broadly, they have a common role within the health system in supporting patient care. The fact that Australia has national, State, and special-purpose organisations of allied health professions—the work of which includes annual conferences and developmental projects—reflects this commonality. In addition, allied health professions usually operate under the same or similar management structures within the health system, as we will see in the cultural and structural analysis section of this chapter.

A closer analysis of the functions of the individual professions illustrates their heterogeneity, and most have their own professional associations, fostering a specific professional identity. A short chapter such as this is unable to do justice to the diversity of the various allied health groups; it is more important for a sociological analysis to focus on the features common to the group as a whole.

Nature of the work of allied health professionals

Table 17.2 (p. 347) lists the key hospital-based, allied health professions in Australia and describes important features of each. These professions work in multidisciplinary teams in either a hospital or community-health setting.

The patient-care role of an allied health professional within the hospital setting involves the following steps:

1   Individual needs of the patient are assessed to determine the extent of a problem, taking the present and past physical condition and lifestyle of the patient into consideration.

Table 17.2 Characteristics of a sample of allied health professions in Australia

Role in health care delivery	Main place of work	Doctor's referral	Origins
Physiotherapy is the use of physical and manual methods in the treatment and prevention of injury and disease, with the aim of maximising normal movement.	With individual patients in a hospital, out-patient, or private-practice setting.	Not required	Massage therapy in the early 20th century, and university degree training since the 1970s
Occupational therapy attempts to maximise the quality of life of people affected by developmental delay, ageing, physical illness or injury, or psychological or social disability.	With individual patients in hospital, out-patient, or community-health settings	Professional body has no official position on this.	Workers in care of mentally ill in late 18th century. Established in Australia after WWII. University-based training established in 1945 at University of Qld.
Speech pathologists use speech therapy to diagnose and treat problems with communication and with higher brain function involving speech and language.	Community health, rehabilitation, hospitals, and private practice.	Professional body has no official position on this.	Developed as a result of the two world wars and was firmly established in Australia by WWII.
Dietetics is the application of nutrition knowledge in the dietary treatment of disease. Dietitians also advise on dietary changes to prevent illness in groups, communities, and populations.	Half the profession are employed in the public-hospital system, and the others are employed in private practice, the food industry, and public health.	Professional body has no official position on this.	Before the 1930s, dietitians were brought out from the USA (home economics based), or nurses studied dietetics in the UK. University-based training established at Melbourne University in 1938.
Medical radiation science is a term that covers the three distinct professional streams—medical imaging; radiation therapy and non-ionising radiation; and radioactive and stable nuclides—that produce images to assist diagnosis and to treat disease.	Private practice and hospitals	Diagnostic tests and treatment are performed under medical referral and supervision.	This profession arose from male-dominated science and technical background, but was feminised in the 1930s as nurses increasingly gained the necessary qualifications.
Podiatrists (previously known as chiropodists) deal with prevention, diagnosis, treatment, and rehabilitation of medical and surgical problems concerning feet and lower legs.	Private practice and community health	Legal right to diagnose and treat patients without a doctor's referral.	

2   Treatment goals are decided upon, in consultation with the patient, and treatment is provided while the patient is in the acute-care setting. The goals of treatment may be modified as the patient progresses.

3   Records are kept and patient progress is communicated to other members of the health-care team.

4   The patient and his or her family or carers are educated in an individualised treatment program.

5   If the patient needs care beyond the period of the hospital stay, follow-up is organised before the patient leaves hospital, to be provided in an out-patient setting.

Historical analysis of the allied health professions

In examining the issues facing allied health professions today, it is important to be aware of the history of their development.

In the beginning, there were doctors

The dominance of medicine was well established before the development of the allied health professions. These professions have arisen as part of a trend towards increasing specialisation in the delivery of health care. The professions developed areas of specialisation by encroaching on tasks that were previously performed by doctors or nurses. In the development phase of allied health in Australia, these new occupations were mostly staffed by nurses who underwent further specialised training (du Toit 1995), with fully specialised training established in the 1940s.

Table 17.2 lists the origins of some professions. It should be noted that it gives only a brief overview, and each profession has its own complex history of development, which should be referred to for further detail. For example, Phillipa Martyr (1994) outlines the development of those professions involved in the rise of rehabilitation in Australia: physiotherapy, occupational therapy, and speech pathology. Heather Nash (1989) has documented the history of the dietetic profession in Australia. Anne Witz (1992) analyses the **feminisation** of the radiography profession (which had previously been dominated by male scientists and technicians) in the 1930s.

feminisation A shift in the gender base of a group from being predominantly male to increasingly female.

Cultural and structural analysis of the allied health professions

This section examines issues relating to the culture of the allied health professions and/or their location within the health system's division of labour. These topics have been placed together since some issues, such as medical dominance, cross both cultural and structural perspectives.

Working within a medically dominated public health system: 'it is always the doctor's patient'

Cultural and structural issues for the allied health professions are largely defined by the existence of medical dominance, which is outlined in chapter 14. In this discussion, we will examine what impact this dominance has on the allied health professions.

Eliot Freidson (1970) has defined four key dimensions of medical dominance that impact on allied health:

1 control over the work and knowledge base of other health professions
2 the physician role of diagnosis and treatment
3 the need for the work of others to be requested and supervised by medicine
4 the unequal status of medicine and other health professions.

As mentioned above, it is within the context of medical dominance that the allied health professions were established. Evan Willis (1989b) notes that, in Australia, medicine has used strategies of subordination, limitation, exclusion, and incorporation to produce and reproduce medical dominance of the health system (these terms are defined in chapter 14). The strategy that has most characterised the relationship between medicine and the allied health professionals within the hospital system is subordination. Willis (1989b) defines this as a mode of domination in which the occupations work under the direct control of doctors. These non-medical occupations are usually predominantly female, thereby creating a relationship between the **sexual division of labour** and the occupational division of labour.

The medical dominance strategy of subordination affects allied health professionals in several ways:

1 Doctors hold positions of authority within the hospital and health system, and therefore have administrative and financial control over allied health.
2 Doctors have absolute autonomy over their work but control the amount of autonomy available to allied health professionals.
3 Doctors have direct or indirect control of **state** recognition of some allied health professions through representation on registration boards.

First, subordination is implemented by doctors having traditionally dominated the structure of the health system's division of labour, including having power over allocation of funding and resources. Although this situation is gradually changing with the increasing bureaucratisation of the system (Germov 1995c), medicine continues to receive significantly more funding for practice and research than do other health areas. This is mostly because of medical representation on committees that control the allocation

sexual division of labour This refers to the nature of work performed as a result of gender roles. The stereotype is that of the male breadwinner and the female home-maker.

state A term used to describe a collection of institutions, including the parliament (government and Opposition political parties), the public-sector bureaucracy, the judiciary, the military, and the police.

professionalisation (professional project) The process of becoming a profession, whereby an occupational group attains publicly recognised and government-legitimated monopoly and autonomy over its area of work. Professional status is usually associated with certain traits (see 'trait approach').

of funds. Allied health professions have neither the power nor experience to compete with medicine at this level, which, in a continuous cycle, limits their power and prestige.

Second, subordination affects the autonomy of the allied health professions. Autonomy is defined as control over one's own work, and has been identified by Freidson (1970) as the most important feature of **professionalisation**. An important question is the extent to which allied health professionals have autonomy in delivering care to patients. An Australian study looked at issues of dominance, autonomy, and authority for nursing and for four allied health professions (physiotherapy, occupational therapy, speech pathology, and psychology) within the hospital setting (Kenny & Adamson 1992). They found that allied health professionals, on average, believe that they have professional autonomy, but that this was truer for practitioners with more years of experience. A staggering 20 per cent of health workers in their first year of practice felt unable to make recommendations on patient care to referring doctors. This indicates limits to professional autonomy.

A factor limiting real autonomy is that, in the present hospital system, the ultimate responsibility for the care of the patient lies with the doctor. So doctors can simply disregard the recommendations of allied health professionals, or even prevent those professionals from seeing patients. This was illustrated in an American study by M. Mason and L. R. Winslow (1994), which showed that both physicians and dietitians perceive themselves as being responsible for the nutritional care of patients. Yet the physicians in the survey chose to disregard more than 50 per cent of recommendations made by dietitians.

Thus, although allied health professionals may perceive themselves as having high professional autonomy, the real measure of autonomy is a profession's ability to influence the outcomes of patient care. Increasing the scope of allied health professionals to influence patient outcomes would require significant changes in current policy on the delivery of patient care, since it is commonly hospital policy to require a medical request for an allied health consultation. It is important to note that allied health professionals can subvert this system by finding alternative means of seeing patients rather than directly challenging doctors. In addition, cross referral among allied health professionals is a common practice. Even if a medical referral is not officially necessary, the patient remains the responsibility of the doctor who has the power to cease the contact between the patient and the allied health professional.

The situation tends to be more relaxed in community-health settings, and allied health practitioners see patients with or without medical approval. Most professionals in private practice will also see patients without medical referral, which has greatly increased the autonomy of groups, such as physiotherapists, working within this setting. For some professions, such as podiatry, the majority of practitioners are based in private practice.

Finally, subordination is also implemented through medical representation on registration boards for allied health, which is ironic, since many of the professions (for example, occupational therapy and physiotherapy) have invited medicine to play this role.

The question of profession

Authors have referred to the need for allied health occupations to achieve professional status as a struggle for survival (Gardner & McCoppin 1995; Willis 1989b). Use of the term 'profession' by allied health practitioners shows that they themselves perceive their occupation to be of a high status. Some authors argue that allied health professionals would be more correctly called 'semi-professionals', since they lack the autonomy, power, status, and economic remuneration of traditional professions such as medicine (Willis 1989b).

Allied health professionals themselves would argue that they meet the criteria for professional status by possessing an independent body of knowledge and expertise, by having university degrees as a minimum requirement, by achieving recognition of professional status by the state, and through ethical decision-making (also all characteristics of medicine). Arguments such as these are based on the **trait approach** to professions, which in turn reflects functionalist theory (outlined in chapter 2). The assumption is that professions perform necessary functions for society, and hence the criteria that define a profession represent essential characteristics. However, this reasoning fails to explain why allied health occupations, if they are professions according to these criteria, are still poorly paid, have low status, and are subordinated to medicine.

trait approach A general theory that assumes that professional status can be achieved by meeting a set of criteria (usually defined as specialised expertise and training), by having the exclusive right to practise in a particular field, by self-regulation (based on a code of ethics), and by charging a fee for service.

Not surprisingly, then, trait theory has itself come under criticism for obscuring the historical and political conditions under which occupations professionalise. In a review of the professionalisation of occupational therapy, Rob Irvine and Jenny Graham (1994) argue that, despite the fact that trait theory has failed to account for the historical rise of the professions, it is still accepted, relatively uncritically, by occupational therapy. (This is probably true of other allied health professions as well.) They argue that occupational therapists have limited themselves by defining their professional role according to this trait approach and advocate a critical approach as a more useful framework. This model emphasises social power, control, and monopoly of markets, and the authors conclude by suggesting that power is the only logical basis upon which to distinguish between dominant professions and other occupations. Witz (1992) also rejects a trait approach, but notes that those taking a critical approach have neglected the relationship between **gender** and professionalisation.

gender/sex This term refers to the socially constructed categories of feminine and masculine (the cultural values that dictate how men and women should behave), as opposed to the categories of biological sex (female or male).

Gender and profession in the case of allied health

Feminist theory (defined in chapter 2) describes how the production of labour by women can reduce economic costs. Just as women reduce the cost of domestic labour by performing household chores without financial remuneration, allied health professionals, who are predominantly female, cheapen the cost of labour in the acute care setting by being paid significantly less than doctors (Turner 1995). Marjorie DeVault (1995) asserts that the type of work done by predominantly female allied health professions is 'women's work' in that it consists of 'devalued tasks that connect the actualities of people's lives with more abstract, "governing" bodies of knowledge, in this case, the practical application of medical knowledge'.

Witz (1992) applies a feminist analysis of gender to the division of labour in the health system by viewing it within the context of **patriarchy**—the society-wide system of male dominance. Medical dominance, then, is also male dominance, since the majority of doctors are male and most allied health professionals are female (as illustrated in Table 17.3). This trend seems set to continue, with 69 per cent of 1998 enrolments in undergraduate health courses being female (AIHW, 2000).

patriarchy A system of power through which males dominate households. It is used more broadly by feminists to refer to society's domination by patriarchal power, which functions to subordinate women and children.

While some of these traditionally female professions are masculinising, Bryan Turner (1987, 1995) has noted that, rather than improving their status, this trend may divide the professions internally through the development of different career paths. In fact, there is some evidence that such a division is already operating within physiotherapy (du Toit 1995). Research on the career aspirations of health profession graduates by Lena Nordholm and Mary Westbrook (1981) found that female graduates were more likely to aspire to intermediate supervisory positions, while males aspired to leadership positions. Thus, as these professions masculinise, gender will increasingly play a role in determining the nature of work, with males having increasingly greater structural input into organisation within the health setting. It remains to be seen whether this masculinisation affects the status of the allied health professions. An examination of the way that the allied health occupations have tried to achieve professional status, and the extent to which they have been successful, is the subject of the next section.

Table 17.3 People employed in health occupations, by gender, Australia, for 1998–99

Occupation	Males	Females	Persons	Percentage female	Change in proportion of women compared with 1991 figures
General practitioner	21 600	10 000	31 600	32	1.7% increase
Medical specialist	11 200	2900	14 100	21	4.4% decrease
Dentist	6000	1400	7400	18	0.9% increase
Pharmacist	8200	5500	13 700	40.2	2.9% decrease
Occupational therapist	700	5700	6400	90	3.7% decrease
Optometrist	2000	1200	3200	37.5	8.2% increase
Dietitians	0	2100	2100	100	π
Physiotherapist	2800	8200	10 900	75	5.2% decrease
Speech pathologist	100	1700	1800	96	1.1% decrease
Podiatrist	300	800	1100	72.7	6.9% increase
Medical radiation scientist	3900	6400	10 300	62	4% decrease
Professional nurses (registered nurses)π	13 300	137 600	150 800	72.6	1% decrease
All health occupations	77 200	204 100	281 200	72.6	5% decrease

* Previously listed as radiography.

π These categories have changed since the last report; therefore gender comparisons are not possible.

Source: ABS 2000

Professionalisation strategies

Professionalisation has been described by Turner (1987, 1995) as a strategy of occupational control aimed at maintaining boundaries of practice. The setting of these boundaries around specified professional domains is known as **social closure**. Witz (1992) has conceptualised the search for professional recognition of specific occupations as the professionalising project of the group. Witz defines the professionalising projects as 'strategies of occupational closure, which aim for occupational monopoly over the provision of certain skills and competencies in a market for services' (Witz 1992, p. 5). (For further details of how the theories of Witz apply to female-dominated health professions, see chapter 15.)

Allied health professions and nursing have tended to adopt the professionalising project of medicine. Susan Roberts (1983) identifies this strategy as being typical of oppressed group behaviour and describes how the subordinate group internalises the **norms** of the dominant group. The subordinate group believes that if it can just be more like the dominant group it will achieve the same level of power and control. Professionalisation strategies that have been adopted by the subordinate allied health professions include:

- adopting a scientific body of knowledge and a code of professional conduct

social closure A term first used by Max Weber to describe the way that power is exercised to exclude outsiders from the privileges of social membership (in social classes, professions, or status groups).

norms Expectations about how people ought to act or behave.

- developing professional associations and accreditation of members
- establishing a university degree as the entry-level qualification.

These traits are all typical of the dominant group: medicine. The limitation of this trait approach is illustrated by the fact that, while medicine has achieved a high degree of autonomy and professional closure within its domain, sanctioned and maintained by the state, the same strategies will not work for the allied health professions. This is, first, because power that already existed within a privileged social **class** was used politically to achieve the professional status of medicine, rather than that power being conferred as a result of possessing the above-mentioned traits. Second, no government is likely ever again to deliver as much power to one profession as it did to medicine; indeed, the state is presently working to try to limit medicine's power.

So, given that allied health professions are likely to remain subordinate to medicine, there are few groups left within the health system over which allied health can exert power and control. This leads to conflicts between the constituent professions of the allied health grouping, and between allied health and nursing. These groups challenge each other since they cannot successfully challenge medicine.

Threats to professional domains

Willis conceptualises the division of labour in health care as 'a continuing struggle over appropriate occupational territories' (1989b, p. 4). (It should be noted that these groups engage in this struggle in order to enhance their power with the aim of strengthening their input into patient care.) Threats to the current boundaries of practice within allied health may come from three directions:

1 vertical **encroachment** from above
2 vertical encroachment from below
3 horizontal encroachment.

Vertical encroachment from above

This term refers to the possibility that the work of allied health professionals will be taken over by doctors. Physiotherapy may be at risk from doctors' use of electrotherapy or manipulative therapy (du Toit 1995), but otherwise, as long as allied health professionals continue to do the work that doctors are not interested in doing, doctors are unlikely to encroach upon their role. Allied health professionals see their own work as a specialised role that doctors are untrained to perform, while doctors largely perceive these tasks to be unchallenging or too time consuming.

class (or social class) A position within a system of structured inequality based on the unequal distribution of power, wealth, income, and status. Class membership is determined by three characteristics: ownership and control of scarce economic resources; ownership of marketable skills and qualifications; and wage labour. People who share a social-class position typically share similar life chances.

encroachment (vertical and horizontal) The threat to the occupational boundaries of professionals, which can take two forms: vertical and horizontal. Vertical encroachment can be from above (from medicine, for instance) or from below, whereby less qualified workers do some of the tasks previously done by a professional. Horizontal encroachment refers to the occupational take-over of one profession by another, where both have similar status and power.

Conversely, in cases in which allied health professionals encroached upon the work of doctors, the latter would act quickly either to exclude the allied health professionals from performing that role or to claim a superior skill in the task (Gardner & McCoppin 1995). For example, doctors are unlikely to be directly involved in the nourishment of hospital patients, leaving this role to dietitians, until patients are fed via a tube that is surgically inserted directly into the bloodstream (known as total parenteral nutrition). In this situation doctors take over the nutritional care of the patient, and the dietitian may or may not be consulted.

Vertical encroachment from below

The threat that is probably most underestimated by the allied health profession is that of encroachment from below. In 1992, following government policy of microeconomic reform, the New South Wales Health Department proposed to reorganise the system under what would be known as the 'structural efficiency principle' (Gardner & McCoppin 1995). A key feature of this plan was the encouragement of multi-skilling through the creation of generic health workers at the level of what were then known as enrolled nurses, who have only one year of post-secondary education. These health workers would undertake tasks that did not need to be conducted by more specialised professionals, while being paid substantially less. The allied health professions and nursing reacted strongly against this proposal at an individual, professional, professional association, and union level. The proposal was not implemented, but the threat has not disappeared. Other examples of encroachment from below are the encroachment of diversional therapists on occupational therapists (especially in States that do not require registration) and of physiotherapist aides on physiotherapists (du Toit 1995).

Horizontal encroachment

Allied health professionals also encroach on each other's territory as they vie for a better position within the system. For example, occupational therapy has expanded its role by encroaching on the work of both physiotherapists and nurses, and the treatment of hands (also conducted by physiotherapists) is a recognised specialty of occupational therapy. The model of the 'nurse-practitioner' also has the potential for horizontal encroachment on the work of the allied health practitioner, although the main threat is that nurses will vertically encroach on the role of doctors from below. The model includes the role of the nurse being expanded to take on some tasks traditionally provided by doctors (for example, an initiative currently under consideration is to give nurses prescribing rights). The impetus to trial the nurse–practitioner model came from the shortage of medical practitioners in rural and remote Australia, where there is often also a shortage of allied health specialisations. Thus the increased powers associated with this role would place nurses in a strong position for encroachment. In the next section we will see how systems such as registration and self-regulation are set up with the aim of protecting threatened professional domains.

Structural recognition of allied health occupations as professions: the role of the state and professional associations

In Australia, the state formally recognises allied health occupations as professions. There are three types of agencies that are responsible for this task:

1   Commonwealth government authorities
2   State and Territory government authorities
3   professional associations.

Commonwealth and State governments play a role in the recognition of the allied health occupations as professions by controlling the qualifications that people require in order to practise in Australia. This control is in the form of legislation that requires registration within the States and Territories. Thus the state legitimates the production and reproduction of professional status for these occupations (Willis 1989b).

In some cases, the government has devolved this responsibility to the professional associations in a system known as 'self-regulation'. This is consistent with a national move to establish self-regulation for professions that were previously registered in one or two of the States and Territories. Both dietetics and speech pathology were deregistered in this way in the 1990s (Gardner & McCoppin 1995). Some professional associations recognise anyone with association membership, whereas others have developed further systems of differentiation that involve compliance with continuing education requirements. Table 17.4 lists those health professions, including the allied health professions, that required registration and that were self-regulating in mid-2001 (National Office of Overseas Skills Recognition 2001).

Setting and examining the criteria for Australian recognition of overseas qualifications was previously the responsibility of the state, but this role has recently been devolved to bodies formed by professional associations. This will allow the professional associations more scope to practise exclusionary tactics, with the risk that overseas practitioners' access to job opportunities will be limited in a strictly controlled job market.

Table 17.4 Registration and self-regulation of health professions

Type of regulation	Occupation
State registration	Chiropractors and osteopaths
	Dentists
	Medical practitioners
	Medical radiation scientists (some States)
	Nurses
	Occupational therapists (some States)
	Optometrists
	Pharmacists
	Physiotherapists
	Podiatrists
	Psychologists
Self-regulation	Dietitians
Professional associations	Medical laboratory scientists
	Social workers
	Speech pathologists (registration required in Queensland only)
	Welfare workers

Source: National Office of Overseas Skills Recognition, 2001

Organisation of allied health within the hospital system: restructuring in an era of economic rationalism

As we have seen, the allied health professions arose to meet the need for increasing specialisation within the hospital system, and so it is worth considering how this group is located within such a system. Traditionally, in Australian hospitals, individual allied health departments were directly responsible to the medical superintendent or director of medical services. For example, in terms of lines of reporting, an occupational therapist would be responsible to the chief occupational therapist (or occupational therapist in charge), who would, in turn, be directly responsible to the medical superintendent (or the medical superintendent's deputy). The medical superintendent would thus be responsible for each individual allied health group, as well as for all the medical services. Nursing services were organised separately under a matron or director of nursing. A difficulty inherent in this system was that medical superintendents were, by definition, doctors, and so had limited understanding of the diverse professional groups in their charge. However, they did have a good understanding of the role of doctors, which had implications for the way in which they directed funding and resource allocation on behalf of both groups.

However, hospital restructuring during the 1990s, which has been driven by **economic rationalism**, has seen changes to this traditional structure. Two main alternatives are emerging for allied health in this restructuring:

economic rationalism or economic liberalism Terms used to describe a political philosophy based on 'small-government' and market-oriented policies, such as deregulation, privatisation, reduced government spending, and lower taxation.

1   the divisions of allied health model
2   the dispersed unit model (Boyce 1996).

The first model, where various allied health departments are grouped together in a single division, is generally favoured by allied health professions and their unions. In the era of cost-cutting and justification of service outcomes, allied health professionals are finding that they have more in common with other allied health professionals than they do with medicine. As a result, they grouped together to be responsible to hospital admin-istration through an allied health administrator. (Even if the group is not organised in this way in formal lines of responsibility, there is a tendency for the informal grouping of these professions to be recognised by management in lines of communication.) The advantages of the division of allied health system are that the allied health professions maintain discipline-specific units under the umbrella of allied health, and that they have the potential to achieve representation on the executive of hospital management. The potential disadvantages include the lack of an influential power-base for those professions not represented on the execu-tive, and the possibility of internal conflicts over who should manage the group, and which professions should be included in the allied health grouping.

In the other possible structure, the dispersed unit model, allied health professionals are responsible to either medical or nursing clinical units. Resistance to this model is based on concern about the destruction of established allied health career structures, lack of control over distribution of workloads, and lack of a united voice for allied health.

Whichever model is employed, doctors continue to have more administrative power than allied health professionals. This means medicine has survived the increased economic pressures imposed on the public health system in the late 1990s better than allied health.

Working within Medicare: how the state supports medical dominance and makes independent practice less lucrative for allied health professionals

One means of threatening the medical workforce is by granting non-physician health providers the right to independent practice. Physiotherapists have been successful in achieving the right to see patients in their own private practices without requiring a doctor's referral. They can even request specified X-rays, which will be funded by Medicare, without medical involvement in diagnosis. This has made the avenue of private practice a more viable option for the profession. Questioning of the other health professions shows that, in reality, few insist on referrals. However, the health funds have, in the past, colluded with medicine to keep allied health professionals subordinate. They have done so by specifying the need for a doctor's referral before they will pay the patient for a consultation with an allied health professional. This practice has decreased, although some key health funds, notably including that of the Australian Medical Association, continue to insist on this requirement.

The extent to which allied health practitioners will be able to achieve financially viable independent practice must be considered within the context of economic rationalism. If allied health practitioners choose to escape the medical dominance of the hospital system, they will doubtless find increased autonomy, but they are unlikely to receive increased power, status, or financial reward. This is because the state continues to reinforce medical dominance by financially rewarding doctors for working in a private setting. General practitioners and specialists receive Medicare rebates for consulting patients in the community, whereas allied health professionals do not. The only exceptions are optometrists, who receive a Medicare rebate directly for their services. Medical radiation scientists receive Medicare rebates, but all services are reported on by a radiologist (medical doctor) before being eligible; therefore a doctor is still involved in the process. Other health professions can also request a limited range of X-ray tests funded by Medicare, including occupational therapists, medical radiation scientists, and chiropractors.

The different earning capacities of doctors versus allied heatlh practitioners in private practice are illustrated in Table 17.5.

The allied health professional in private practice thus has a lower earning capacity than doctors, and patients usually bear the full cost

Table 17.5   Potential daily income of doctors compared with allied health practitioners in the community setting

Practitioner	Patients seen in an 8-hour day	Fee per patient	Amount paid by state	Amount paid by patient	Maximum income per day
General practitioner (standard consultation fee)	40	$30.00	$17.85	$12.15	$1200.00
General practitioner (bulk bills)	40	$17.85	$17.85	Nil	$714.00
Vocationally registered general practitioner	40	$27.00	$22.95	$4.05	$1080.00
Private dietitian	8 new patients	$66.00	Nil	$66.00	$528.00
Private physiotherapist	12 new patients	$40.00	Nil	$40.00	$480.00

These fees are averages of those charged in practice or recommended by professional associations, with the exception of the Medicare rebate of $17.85, which is set by the federal government. Rebates to the patients from private insurers have not been considered in these equations. Rates current as of January 2001.

of the consultation. The possible alternatives to this direct fee for allied health service are private health insurance or state-funded rebates. With the Commonwealth government initiatives of the late 1990s, aimed at halting the decline in private coverage, approximately eight million Australians at January 2001 had some private health cover. However only those who had some type of 'extras cover' were able to claim for a rebate for so-called 'ancillary services' (AIHW 1996a). For example, in 1994–95 the average amount of ancillary benefits paid in the category of 'other professional services' (which includes the allied health professions) was $30 per year for people privately insured. This amount is unlikely to cover the cost of even a single consultation (AIHW 1996a). Thus the 'out-of-pocket' expense for the patient is not significantly reduced by private insurance. In addition to lobbying public and private health insurance providers for increased rebates, allied health groups (including physiotherapists and dietitians) have lobbied the federal government for several years to establish a system of Medicare rebates that would improve the access of people on low incomes to their services. These attempts have met with no success, thus state-subsidised private allied health care is currently not an option.

A further consideration of the shift to private practice from the public health sector is the equity of access to available and affordable patient care. Deborah Schofield (1999) compared the fees of key allied health professions in private practice in terms of equity of patient access. She found no income barrier to the use of dietitian or physiotherapy services, on the basis of the predominance of access for free services through the public health system. However, this conclusion overlooks long waiting lists, and practices that restrict various categories of patient problems within the public system. So while there may be access to free services in theory, in reality those services may not be available.

Future directions: critical analysis of the allied health professions

Becoming allied with each other

The word 'allied', in the term 'allied health', has previously been understood to mean that these professions are allied to medicine. However, the term could be reinterpreted to mean that these professions form allegiances with each other as a group. Rosalie Boyce (1995) has suggested that for allied health to survive in this era of economic rationalism, the constituent professions must ally with each other, both inside and outside the health system. Allied health professionals have formed a variety of organisations in the attempt to represent the common interests of member professions.

In this way they have tried to counter the forces of medical dominance and of the sheer numbers of nurses.

It has been recognised that the Australian Council of Allied Health Professionals is not a significant lobby group (Gardner & McCoppin 1995). Part of this failure can be attributed to the difficulties experienced by a national association in dealing with health care systems and industrial conditions that are subject to the interests of the individual States. More recently, then, State-based organisations have been formed.

In New South Wales the professions have formed an allegiance with a more explicitly political purpose: The Allied Health Alliance NSW. The terms of reference of this body acknowledge that the Alliance was formed 'in recognition of the importance of having a single point of contact for organisations such as State government bodies, Area and District Health Boards etc'. The group, formed in October 1994, consists of representatives from the following professions: social work, speech pathology, radiography (both diagnostic and therapeutic), physiotherapy, podiatry, dietetics, occupational therapy, orthoptics, and pharmacy.

Other alliances have been formed for specific purposes—for example, the National Allied Health Casemix Committee and the Allied Health Best Practice Consortium (Boyce 1995). In grouping together for political and special purposes, allied health professions gain sufficient numbers to form an effective power bloc. The extent to which this strategy succeeds will depend on the ability of such groups to resist internal struggles between different professions.

Exploring options outside the acute-care setting

For as long as the majority of the health dollar funds acute care delivered in the hospital setting, doctors will continue to control the health system. However, with the current trend in hospital care towards decreasing the length of stay, health care delivery will increasingly be conducted in a community setting. Allied health professionals need to seize the opportunity to play a key role in discharge planning and in the continuity of patient care in the community.

Spiralling costs of medical treatment make prevention a more palatable option for decision-makers, and an emphasis on prevention has gained a stronger hold in health care (see chapter 10 for more detail). The Ottawa Charter for Health Promotion (1986) brought about international recognition of the need for a preventative approach to health care. Kenny and Adamson (1992) have identified **health promotion** as one of the broader social forces undermining medical power. Although medicine still has a strong input into health promotion and public health, it does not control it to the extent that it controls the hospital or illness system.

health promotion Any combination of education and related organisational, economic, and political interventions designed to promote behavioural and environmental changes conducive to good health. This promotion may cover a variety of strategies, including legislation, health education, community development, advocacy, and so on. Health promotion has usually, however, been restricted to interventions focusing on the behavioural end of the spectrum.

As such, allied health professionals who work in this area can potentially be freed from the dominance of the medical model. Dietetics is one example of a profession that is expanding in numbers by broadening in focus from acute care to apply its knowledge of nutrition in a preventative setting (Williams 1993). Other allied health professionals would perhaps do well to strengthen alternative avenues of employment along similar lines.

Focusing the professionalising projects

As we have seen, pursuit of power through the professionalising project of medicine is unlikely to yield the power and prestige sought by allied health professions. The fallacy of this approach is that it involves rejecting the cultural identity of the individual professions. This identity could be used instead to harness a different type of strength, which, as De Vault (1995) points out, is more practical and embodied. For example, most allied health professionals spend a significantly longer time in direct contact with patients than do doctors. The increased counselling role could be used to foster a model of patient empowerment, which medicine has failed to develop (despite rhetoric to the contrary).

Rather than trying to adopt the traits of medicine, allied health professionals should change the nature of their professionalising project and focus on changing the criterion of medical dominance that most affects the quality of patient care: the power of medicine to exert control over other professions. This would make the professional project of allied health one of seeking to increase professional autonomy. The right to independent practice—that is, the ability to see patients without a doctor's referral—is an important step in achieving this autonomy, as can be seen in the physiotherapists' increased strength in a private-practice setting. This then allows the allied health professional to focus their expertise and efforts on delivery of specialised patient care, which is, after all, the reason for their emergence.

Conclusion

Allied health practitioners have specialised contributions to make to patient care. The current position of allied health within the health system is characterised by a lack of autonomy, power, and prestige. While this perspective may seem negative, it is important to make a realistic appraisal of the current situation in order to move forward. Doctors are happy to coexist with other health professions in a system of medical dominance, until that dominance is challenged. It is up to the allied health professions to focus their professionalising projects in order to achieve a status that confers enough prestige for job satisfaction, and that results in optimal outcomes for patient care. One way to do this may be to ally with each other in forming a more substantial power bloc, provided that allied health can resist internal struggles between professions.

Summary of main points

- The allied health professions arose out of an increasing trend towards specialisation in the delivery of patient care within the health system.
- In working within the health system, allied health professions are subject to the forces that characterise it: the dominance of the medical profession (and consequent subordination of the allied health professions) and the current era of restructuring resulting from economic rationalism.
- Many of the allied health professions are following the professionalising project of medicine in trying to establish domains of practice, and obtain power and prestige.
- While some professions have made more gains than others, allied health remains largely subordinate to medicine. This subordination is gender related, since the predominantly female allied health professionals do 'women's work' within the health system.
- The extent to which the allied health professions will be successful in enhancing their status depends upon their ability to redevelop a professional project appropriate to their culture, present an allied front, and embrace continuity of care in the community and a shift to a preventative (rather than curative) approach to practice.

Discussion questions

1 Allied health professionals perform specialised tasks within the hospital system. What would the consequences be for patient care in a hospital setting if such professions were not there to fulfil that role?
2 Why is it that the allied health professions do not have total autonomy within the hospital system?
3 Discuss the role of gender in determining the nature of work done by allied health professionals, and the respect with which that work is regarded within the system.
4 Why is the organisation of allied health within the public hospital system important to the survival of these professions?
5 What opportunities exist for the allied health professions to strengthen their position?
6 What factors challenge, threaten, or undermine the role of allied health professions in the health system?

Further investigation

1 Choose one specific allied health profession. Identify the nature of the professionalising project of that profession by one or all of the following means:
   - Interview a professional currently working in the public or private health sector
   - Search the web site of the professional association (or obtain written information from that association)
   - Interview a final-year student of that profession (provided they have had significant practical experience).

2 Choose an allied health organisation and critique the strategies they are employing in terms of how successful they will be in improving the position of individual allied health professions within the health sector.

Further reading and web resources

Boyce, R. A. 1991, 'Hospital Restructuring: The Implications for Allied Health Professionals', *Australian Health Review*, vol. 14, pp. 147–54.

Duckett, S. J. 2000, *The Australian Health Care System*, Oxford University Press, Melbourne.

Gardner, H. & McCoppin, B. 1995, 'Struggle for Survival by Health Therapists, Nurses and Medical Scientists', in H. Gardner (ed.), *The Politics of Health*, 2nd edn, Churchill Livingstone, Melbourne.

Kenny, D. & Adamson, B. 1992, 'Medicine and the Health Professions: Issues of Dominance, Autonomy and Authority', *Australian Health Review*, vol. 15, p. 3.

Schofield, D. 1999, 'Ancillary and Specialist Health Services: The Relationship Between Income, User Rates and Equity of Access', *Australian Journal of Social Issues*, vol. 34, no. 1, pp. 79–96.

Turner, B. S. 1995, *Medical Power and Social Knowledge*, 2nd edn, Sage, London.

Web sites

Australian Association of Occupational Therapists:
Australian Association of Social Workers (AASW):
Australian Institute of Radiography:
Australian Physiotherapy Association (APA):
Australian Psychological Society (APS):
Dietitians Association of Australia (DAA):
National Office of Overseas Skills Recognition (NOOSR):
    <www.deet.gov.au/divisions/noosr/prof.htm>
Optometrists Association Australia:
Speech Pathology Australia:

18

Community Health Services in Australia[1]

Fran Baum

Overview

* *What are community health services and how did they develop in Australia?*
* *What are the philosophical underpinnings of community health services?*
* *What are some Australian examples of community health services in action?*

The community health sector in Australia first developed during the Whitlam Labor Government of the early 1970s. Community health services were conceived as a radically different means of structuring health services. They were designed as locally managed health centres operating on a social model of health and comprising multidisciplinary teams that would respond to all types of community health problems. The work of the centres was designed to include the provision of curative services, group work, community development, and social action. Despite the fact that the community health sector has considerable potential to contribute to improving population health in Australia, it is marginalised and under-funded. This chapter considers the historical development of community health services and examines some of the tensions that exist between community health services and the broader health system. It also describes the work typically undertaken by community health services. It concludes by arguing that the failure of successive Australian governments to support community health fully has been a lost opportunity.

Key terms

biomedicine/biomedical model
health promotion
Indigenous community-
controlled health services
new public health
positive health
primary health care
social model of health

---

1   Many thanks to Paul Laris, Clare Shuttleworth, and Frank Tesoriero, each of whom has contributed insights to this chapter, for their helpful comments.

Introduction: historical development of community health services in Australia

Policy frameworks

Australia had a nationally endorsed Community Health Policy for only three years, between 1973 and 1976. Initiated by the Whitlam Labor Government, this policy established the framework that led to the expansion of community health in Australia in the 1970s and 1980s. The Community Health Program (CHP) was formed following a recommendation of the Hospitals and Health Services Commission (HHSC), established in 1973, whose purpose was to be '[a] major community health program to develop facilities and services in a coordinated manner for the provision and planning of prevention, treatment, rehabilitation and related welfare aspects of community health' (HHSC 1973, p. 16).

The chief objective of the national program was 'to encourage the provision of high quality, readily accessible, reasonably comprehensive, coordinated and efficient health and welfare services at local, regional, State and national levels. Such services should be developed in consultation with, and where appropriate, the involvement of, the community to be served' (HHSC 1973, p. 4).

Raftery (1995, pp. 20–1) has summarised the key service components of the CHP as:

1   Programs of information and counselling to improve the habits, conditions and environment that may precede disorders of health.
2   Direct preventative action.
3   Disease detection procedures to discover incipient or pre-clinical phases of disease.
4   Information and counselling programs to motivate individuals to seek care once departure from normal health is perceived.
5   Specific diagnosis and treatment services.
6   Rehabilitation and supportive services for those with continuing disease and disability.
7   Provision of help for those with chronic disability who have to adapt to sheltered living or working conditions.

This program formed the basis for the subsequent development of community health services in Australia. The degree to which the program was radical in intent has been disputed. Alexander (1995) presented it as such and saw it as a forerunner of the Ottawa Charter for Health Promotion and the **new public health**. Raftery (1995, p. 23) interprets the 1973 program as more conservative and says it was unquestioning about certain **biomedical** assumptions: it was 'lacking in ideas about strategies to achieve its objectives; and it was vague and naïve about prevention of illness'.

new public health A social model of health linking 'traditional' public health concerns, which focus on physical aspects of the environment (clean air and water, safe food, occupational safety through legislation), with the behavioural, social, and economic factors that affect people's health. The model is supported by a social movement that emphasises primary prevention, participation, and primary health care.

biomedicine/biomedical model The conventional approach to medicine in Western societies. It diagnoses and explains illness as a malfunction of one of the body's biological mechanisms. The biomedical approach of most health services focuses on the treating of individuals, and generally ignores social, economic, and environmental factors.

She feels that the 1973 plan was a limited one that did not fore-shadow the new public health as has sometimes been supposed.

The CHP was reviewed on three occasions, in 1976, 1985 and 1992. Each of these reviews concluded that while it had not made a significant impact on the nature of the Australian health system, it had allowed some limited experimentation in styles of health care delivery. The main advances were seen in some experiment-ation with health education and with the provision of community-based services for diagnostic, therapeutic, and rehabil-itation services. But each review also noted that there continued to be a strong orientation to service provision and individual treat-ment, and to tertiary rather than primary or secondary prevention. The 1986 Review, conducted by the Australian Community Health Association, concluded that a community health program with 'some degree of coherence' and 'an established position within the overall mix of health services' had been established in all States and Territories. It went on to note that the program was marked by a 'degree of conservatism that was not in accord with the intentions of the original program' and that its core was 'essen-tially an illness-focused, paramedical, para-hospital, residual service, providing mainly secondary and tertiary prevention'. The review-ers also noted that the CHP had contributed to a broader understanding of health and had made the issue of community involvement more prominent in health debates. But it had had lit-tle impact on the overall priorities of the health system. Both Blewett (2000) and Milio (1983) have noted that the main politi-cal champions for more radical change in Australia invested most energy in the establishment of Medicare, Australia's universal health insurance scheme, rather than in the CHP.

The reviews of the CHP did note that its development was patchy across Australia. The Labor Governments in Victoria and South Australia during the 1970s and 1980s did most to establish a network of comprehensive community health services. In contrast, the CHP in Queensland made little progress within a traditional public service model characterised by central decision-making, slow responses to local decisions, and no political or bureaucratic com-mitment to community involvement. In Victoria and South Australia, however, community health development was at its peak during the 1980s. By this time these States had a network of centres that were developing innovative and creative approaches to com-prehensive **primary health care**. These States were acknowledged to have made far more significant progress in implementing com-munity health than any of the others. The 1992 ACHA review analysed the impact of different organisational structures on the ability of community health services to achieve their original aims. The review found that the independently incorporated community

primary health care Both the point of first contact with the health care system and a philos-ophy for delivery of that care.

health centres with their own Boards of Management and control over their own budgets were the most successful models. These States also established democratic forms of management for their centres whereby Boards of Management were elected (Victoria) or appointed (South Australia). These Boards were responsible for the overall management and direction-setting for the centres. This form of management is not without problems but during the 1980s and early 1990s the thinking about these challenges showed sophistication and a desire to improve its efficiency (see, for example, Laris 1992; Legge 1992; Laris 1995). Legge (1992, p. 96) noted:

> The achievements of community health over the last two decades have been huge and in large part are a consequence of the energy and direction gained from real community involvement. Having community members on committees is part of helping staff of the centre to understand the practical health problems that they deal with on a daily basis in the context of the more general concerns of the different communities in the locality.

Legge wrote this appreciation of community-driven community health during what turned out to be the golden period of the community health movement in Australia (the period approximately from 1985 to 1992). Since this time, however, the policy environment has been less favourable to community health and its development has stagnated and not been encouraged by policy at either federal or State level. Indeed Legge, in his article on community management, foreshadowed some of the key reasons for the decline in the fortunes of community health: 'The principles of community health run counter to how the mainstream health system works, although that is where many of our staff are trained and it is the conventional view of health that politicians and bureaucrats usually project. Community health principles also jar with new wave managerialism and the underlying ideology of economic rationalism' (Legge 1992, pp. 111–12).

It is worth considering what features of the policy environment during the 1970s and 1980s made the ground reasonably fertile for community health. The 1973 Community Health Program statement was crucial to the development. It provided a clear statement about the philosophy and styles of working in community health. When supported by a similarly strong commitment from a State government the situation for community health was positive. This is well exemplified by South Australia in the 1980s where both a Social Health Strategy and a Primary Health Care Policy were developed. These policy frameworks provided a strong endorsement of the principles of community health (as outlined earlier in this chapter) and so made it easier for the staff in the services to develop innovations that reflected these principles. Importantly also was the fact that both South Australia and Victoria during the 1980s provided sufficient resources to allow an expansion of community health services. This favourable local policy environment was supported by the policy direction of the World Health Organization which, through the Alma Ata Declaration and the Ottawa Charter for Health Promotion, led the development of the new public health in this period. This meant that the Australian community health movement was very much in step with the vanguard of health thinking at this time.

In the 1984 the active peak organisation, the Australian Community Health Association (ACHA), was formed, which engendered a sense of a national movement in community health. ACHA was a federated organisation with branches in each State. The work of the South Australian Community Health Association has been analysed by Broderick and Laris (1995) who they identified four key features of the Association:

- a focus on policy development in government and bureaucracy
- use of a small group of activists taking a vanguard role
- use of coalitions to focus on particular issues
- an appreciation of the importance of the association as a defence against threats to community health services.

Broderick and Laris describe the larrikin energy that was evident in the Association and demonstrate its effectiveness as a lobby group during the 1980s. But they also foreshadowed the weaknesses of community health that were to become prominent in the 1990s. Community health had developed a ghetto mentality and was increasingly seen in this light by the mainstream within the health system.

The 1990s were a distinctly difficult decade for community health. There was little sign of policy commitment from any State or federal government. The limited progress that had been made through the 1980s and early 1990s either stultified or was reversed during the remaining years of the century. The factors accounting for this reversal are discussed in the section below on community health in the 1990s.

What are community health services?

There is no simple definition of community health services. They have differed over time and also between States and Territories. At both national and at State level there are no comprehensive databases that describe the activities of community health services. In part this reflects the complexity of community health work but most significantly it reflects the lack of investment in information systems for community health services. There are, however, some common features of these services.

Philosophical underpinning

Community health services share a common philosophy with that espoused by the World Health Organization (WHO) in key documents such as the 1978 Alma Ata Health for All by the Year 2000 (HFA 2000) Declaration. This document set out a vision for a comprehensive primary health care driven health system. Grasping the philosophical underpinnings of the HFA 2000 strategy of the WHO is crucial to understanding the sort of comprehensive health service that community health in Australia has always strived for but never achieved. The Alma Ata Declaration established the following principles:

- Health is a fundamental human right and its achievement would reflect effort in many other social and economic sectors in addition to the health sector.
- Inequities in the health status between people in developed countries and those in developing countries, as well as within countries, are unacceptable, and the key to reducing these inequities and to achieving health for all lies in social and economic development.
- Community participation in planning and implementation of health care is seen as both a right and a duty.

Primary health care was defined as:

> ... essential health care based on practical, scientifically sound and socially acceptable methods and technologies made universally accessible to individuals and families in the community through their full participation and at a cost that the community and country can afford to maintain at every stage of their development in the spirit of self-reliance and self-determination. It forms an integral part both of the country's health system, of which it is the central function and main focus, and of the overall social and economic development of the community. It is the first level of contact of individuals, the family and community with the national health system bringing health care as close as possible to where people live and work, and constitutes the first element of a continuing health care process (WHO 1978).

The Ottawa Charter for Health Promotion, which in many ways translated the central messages of the HFA2000 Strategy into a language appropriate to developed countries, has also been used extensively by community health services in vision, goal and planning exercises (see, for example, Sanderson and Alexander 1995). The five strategies of the Ottawa Charter (develop healthy public policy, create supportive environments, encourage community action, develop personal skills, and re-orientate health services) provide a fairly accurate description of the work of community health services (as is shown in detail in the section describing their work below).

The jargon of official government and WHO documents can obscure the core philosophy of community health. This philosophy is well expressed through the story that portrays the mainstream health system as being concerned with pulling drowning bodies out of a river and then trying to revive them. By contrast the community health sector seeks to look upstream and discover why those people are falling in the river, consider how it can prevent them doing so, look at the communities from where the people come, and consider how they could be made more supportive so that people no longer fall in the river in the first place. Community health is firmly based on the premise that prevention is better than cure and that it takes a multidisciplinary team working closely with its community to effect this prevention and to go the step further and promote health in a positive way.

So the key features of the philosophy behind community health are:

- **Positive health** is a distinct concept from that of absence of disease. The latter is concerned more with a physical or psychological definition whereas a positive view of health is a holistic concept that takes into account culture, spirituality, community, and connectedness, as well as physical and behavioural factors. This means that community health services can be concerned with many aspects of the factors that affect health, and the areas they are concerned with will extend well-beyond the confines of health services.
- The comprehensiveness of services is crucial. Community health services should offer curative, rehabilitative disease prevention and **health promotion** interventions. Wherever possible the emphasis should be on disease prevention and health promotion.
- Multidisciplinary teams are preferable as the basis for community health work.
- Community involvement in the management and running of programs within community health services is an essential part of good practice. The aim of community health is to enable communities to take greater control of the social, economic, and physical environments that influence their health.
- Working in partnership with other sectors is a crucial part of community health work.
- Equity and a **social model of health** is fundamental to the operation and decision-making within the services. An

positive health A holistic view of health that focuses on wellness, rather than disease, and that it is culturally relative, incorporating notions of spirituality, community, and social support.

health promotion Any combination of education and related organisational, economic, and political interventions designed to promote behavioural and environmental changes conducive to good health. This promotion may cover a variety of strategies, including legislation, health education, community development, advocacy, and so on. Health promotion has usually, however, been restricted to interventions focusing on the behavioural end of the spectrum.

social model of health A model of health that focuses on social determinants such as the social production, distribution, and construction of health and illness, and the social organisation of health care. It directs attention to the prevention of illness through community participation and social reforms that address living and working conditions.

understanding of the social and economic determinants of health is fundamental to the logic of the work undertaken in community health services.

The vision of community health as a comprehensive underpinning of the entire health service has unfortunately never been realised. It has always remained marginalised to the mainstream system. While community health has provided a practical example of what could be possible if the model were to be adopted as the basis of the health system, there has never been the political will to implement the community health model in this way.

The main block to this has been the prevalence of fee-for–service general medical practice. This model has precluded the growth of community health because there has been no political will to provide the resources necessary to develop a strong salaried medical workforce within community health centres. There are some very real differences between the community health model and the form of health care practised by most general medical practitioners in Australia. Rogers and Veale (2000) have contrasted the two models. The key differences they have identified in services are that whereas a comprehensive model of primary health care stresses health promotion and rehabilitation and multidisciplinary team approaches, these are limited in general practice. They also argue that general practice does not address population-level needs-based planning, collaboration across sectors, and education. They also note that general practice does not adopt the philosophy advocated in the World Health Organization's description of primary health care (see above).

Primary medical care is not grounded in a social understanding of health in the way in which community health is. It is based primarily on the provision of one category of health services to individuals. While general practitioners have begun to do some group and community work through the Divisions of General Practice, this work is limited and is a long way from the vision of comprehensive primary health care offered by the Alma Ata Declaration.

What community health services do

Given the description of the philosophy underpinning community health, it is evident that the activities that these services undertake will be diverse, particularly between services in different States. There are three main areas of activity within community health services: one-to-one services; group programs; and community development and social action. The comprehensive nature of community health means that services would normally have some activities in each of these areas. The main service categories in community health have been defined in South Australia and these represent the range of work done by that community (see Box 18.1).

Box 18.1 Main service categories offered by community health services

Community development and capacity building

Working with community groups (e.g. suicide prevention, community gardens, urban re-generation), social action activities (environmental health action groups, health rights group, sexual abuse survivors), information and resources provision (e.g. Internet information provision, encouraging community participation).

Mental health

Counselling, support groups, information, advocacy.

Physical health

Medical and nursing, screening, health promotion to encourage healthy lifestyles.

Interpersonal violence

Child abuse, child sexual abuse, violence intervention, support groups, counselling.

Early childhood development

Speech pathology, nutrition, immunisation, information and education for parents, early intervention.

Drug and alcohol

Needle exchange, counselling, information and education, access to methadone program, community action, advocacy.

Sexual and reproductive health

Counselling, information and education, information about services and referral, screening for cancer.

Source: South Australian Department of Human Services, 2001

One-to-one services

Community health services offer a range of one-to-one services. These may include medical services but this is not the case in many community health services. Other services that may be offered are counselling, podiatry, physiotherapy, speech pathology, dietetics, and nutrition. The emphasis within these services is to encourage rehabilitation and prevent the likelihood of problems re-occurring in the future. Counselling of women experiencing domestic violence and/or sexual abuse is a service that is commonly provided.

Medical services offered within community health centres differ from those offered in most private general practitioner services. Studies of the work of medical practitioners within women's and community health centres indicate that the users of the centres identify the following advantages of medical practice within community health centres:

- Patients are able to spend more time with the doctor.
- Patients perceive that they are more likely to be treated as a 'whole' person.
- There is easy access to members of the multidisciplinary teams.
- People feel that they are encouraged to have more control of their own health and be involved in decisions about their health.
- Health promotion activities are easier to gain access to.
- Interpreters are readily available.
- The atmosphere at the centres is supportive and friendly, and is based on trusting relationships (Warin, Baum, Kalucy, Murray, & Veale 1998, pp. 87–9).

Box 18.2 contains some typical perceptions by the users of medical services within community health centres, which highlight the positive way in which these services are generally viewed.

Box 18.2 Users' perceptions of medical services within women's and community health centres in Adelaide, South Australia

I feel they like to know you as a person, you know. They see many people but they still have that time to talk to you as a person, whereas in general practice unless you're willing to pay X amount then you're rushed through and I feel it's like a factory production line, an assembly line (Warin, Baum et al. 1998, p. 56).

I don't like the concept of private practice, whereas at women's and community health centres there is access to other services and supports, and it's free … it's handy … it's easy to access, they're friendly … particularly over at Dale St … I know them and I've been in there sometimes in tears and they'll give me a hug—it's good … I don't feel like a total stranger (Warin and Baum 1998, p. 56).

The staff down there are absolutely wonderful—they are very pleasant people … it's not a depressing place to go to—you can always go down there and there's somebody you know … or even if you don't they strike up a conversation—that's why I prefer to go there (Warin, Baum et al. 1998, p. 59).

I think time would be the factor and they wouldn't be able to have that time to be able to give all that ... I'm not putting (down) all doctors in surgeries but the way that their surgeries are getting it is just fly by in and fly by out and it is all so quick—I felt so alien in a lot of normal doctor's surgeries. I just haven't felt as if I'm in control of my own health and somebody else is ... (Warin, Baum et al. p. 48).

There's kindness, openness and communication and it's just the way that she is a professional—she's a doctor but she doesn't put herself in that kind of hierarchical position—it's just a relationship between her and the community or the patient or the client ... it's very human—she puts human beings first before any other things ... she's like my friend (Warin, Baum et al. 1998, p. 79).

Table 18.1   Ottawa Charter planning framework: examples of doctors' roles

Ottawa Charter strategy	*Example of doctors' roles in strategy in community health centres (mostly done in collaboration with other workers)*
Healthy public policy	Advocacy for change in policies and practices of agencies which have an impact on health e.g. harm minimisation approach to drugs Assist in the development of asthma management procedures in schools
Creating supportive environments	Provision of supportive environment for those dependent on illicit drugs Lobbying public housing authority to assist patient to find better housing Education of private-practice GPs about domestic violence Training other health professionals
Community action	Supporting environmental action group by, for example, providing information of health effects of a particular type of pollution. Supporting community initiatives such as providing a home detoxification program
Personal skills	Support and education groups: advice and skill development (e.g. management of arthritis, asthma, diabetes, chronic pain, menopause)
Re-orientation of health services	Ensuring sufficient time is given to patients and that health promotion approaches are used whenever possible e.g. responsible use drugs, encouraging and supporting lifestyle change Applying personal problems from clinical practice to work for public solutions

Source: Adapted from Baum, Kalucy et al. (1996); Warin, Baum et al. (1998)

The service providers in community health services typically offer a range of services in addition to the one-to-one services. This is best illustrated by the role of medical practitioners and the ways in which working within a community health centre enable them to take on broader roles beyond one-to-one work. Table 18.1 uses the Ottawa Charter as a framework to describe the potential roles for doctors within community health. The studies on which this table is based show that doctors within the centres are more likely to take on these wider roles than are doctors in private practice.

Group programs

Community health services typically offer a range of group programs. The exact mix of groups offered by a particular community health service will depend on the needs of that community. Groups may focus on support for:

- a particular age-group (e.g. young gay people, older Indigenous women)
- people with the same chronic disease (e.g. diabetes, cancer, heart disease)
- people with the same social issue (e.g. domestic violence, sexual abuse, teenage parenthood, step-parenthood).

Usually the most important features of the groups are that they offer people new information about their situation and provide them with social support. Often the interaction with the other members of the group is as important as the input from the professional workers. These groups are typically offered on a no-fee or very low fee basis.

Groups are an important means by which practitioners within a community health centre can move away from a sole focus, as in one-to-one service provision, and be more creative in their work. An example of such creativity is the approach taken by podiatrists at the Port Adelaide and Parks Community Health Services in Adelaide where they sought to reduce the size of the waiting lists for their services by starting a group called Feet First. This group encourages members to do their own foot care and to care for the feet of others in the group, as well as providing support for those attending.

Centres have also developed drop-in groups for women experiencing domestic violence. Social workers talk to women before inviting them to join the groups. The groups reduce the waiting time for individual counselling and the women usually start to support one another and to offer each other practical ideas based on their own experiences.

Community development and social action

Many (though not all) community health services will become engaged in community development or social action campaigns.

Such campaigns have been a feature of generalist community health services in South Australia and Victoria and of Women's and Indigenous health services. At their best the local community in concert with the health service controls these initiatives. Community participation is a complex topic and an area in which there is considerable rhetoric about participation. In practice, examples of participation from within the health sector that are not driven by paid professionals are rare. Baum (1998, p. 326) defines four main types of participation that can be identified within the health sector:

- *Consultation*, which asks people to respond to set plans
- *Participation as a means*, which uses participation in an instrumental way to achieve an outcome defined by the health service
- *Substantive participation*, in which people are actively involved in determining priorities and implementation but the initiative remains externally controlled
- *Structural participation*, which is a fully engaged and developmental process in which the community control the initial agenda and process.

Community health services have been the most likely parts of the health sector to engage in substantive or structural participation. Even so, the examples of community-controlled health services are rare. The Aboriginal health movement was the first sector to develop the concept of community control and since 1970 **Indigenous community-controlled health services** have been established across Australia. Community development and social action programs are most likely to flourish in community-controlled or managed community health services. This principle is best illustrated through the examples discussed below.

Indigenous community-controlled health services
Independent local organisations, controlled and managed by indigenous people, that provide a range of services to meet the needs of their particular communities.

Example 1: Yarrabah—Suicide Prevention

Yarrabah, a small Aboriginal community in Far North Queensland, illustrates the potential of community control in solving health problems. From the mid-1980s Yarrabah experienced an increasing suicide rate. Analyses of approaches to reduce the increasing rate (Hunter et al. 1999; Mitchell 2000) in the community describe how the Yarrabah Community experienced a series of stages before entering into a state of full ownership of the suicide problem. Mitchell (2000, p. 17) comments, 'Full ownership is seen as stemming from an understanding that lasting solutions can only be found within the community itself and manifests as a widely shared political commitment to action. The process was slow and accompanied by much pain and grief over a long period.'

On the journey to full ownership of the problem the community established the Yarrabah Health Council, which adopted the framework of comprehensive primary health care for its work.

Eventually the community was able to move towards building sustainable structures for social, emotional, cultural, and spiritual well-being. Hunter et al. (1999) note that the big breakthrough for the community's response to suicide was when it moved from a focus on individual risk to a focus on community risk. The responses based on tackling individual risk factors were largely ineffective. On the other hand, the community-level risk approach appeared to have two main advantages. First, the approach acknowledges and addresses the true underlying causes of self-harming behaviour in Aboriginal communities. Second, it provides a conceptual and practice framework that accommodates the involvement of ordinary community members in a way that the individual risk focused approach does not (Mitchell 2000, p. 19).

Numerous strategies were used in the community approach. For example, a small group of women in the community worked with Anglican and Catholic churches and the Department of Family Services to organise a series of educational and practical activities. One of these considered the role of alcohol use and misuse in the community, including its role in self-harm. Links were established with, and visits were made by, Canadian Indigenous groups who had faced similar problems. Community meetings were held, which discussed issues such as the appropriateness of responses to attempted suicide and the social issues that people saw as contributing to suicides, such as authority over children, the situation at school, and local economic issues. The community also sought training in specific suicide-prevention skills, such as crisis intervention and counselling, which it believed were needed by community members. Mitchell notes that the Yarrabah story demonstrates that the 'capacity of the community to identify causes and solutions was associated with a long process of study and reflection' (2000, p. 20).

In the early 1990s the suicide rate in Yarrabah reached nine deaths. By the mid-1990s it stood at eight deaths. Yet, in 1997–98 there were no deaths from suicide. Hunter et al. (1999) attribute this reduction to the community-controlled process that was instituted. They note that this approach was particularly successful because suicide had been incorporated into the contemporary culture as a response to the ongoing dispossession, social inequity, and injustice experienced by Aboriginal people. A community-developed cultural response to counter these was essential.

Example 2: Parks Community Health Service, Adelaide[2]

The Parks Community Health Service is located in the northwest suburbs of Adelaide, an area that exhibits many indicators of low socioeconomic status and low health status. The Heath Service, whose staff consist of dedicated community development positions,

---

2   This section was written by Frank Tesoriero.

has been committed to a process approach to community development. In other words, it does not initiate community-based programs, but rather, works in partnership with groups who identify issues of concern to them. Over many years, the Health Service, largely through the work of its community development workers, has established a strong relationship with many parts of the community and with many individuals. It also has a reputation of supporting local groups in community development projects and social action campaigns. Two examples of the recent community development work of the Parks Community Health Service are described below.

Hoi Sinh Project

The Parks population is 29 per cent non-English-speaking background, and the majority of these are from Indo-China, including refugees. In 1978 the Health Service began to recruit Indo-Chinese health workers so that its services would be accessible to the Indo-Chinese communities. These workers engaged in one-to-one services, developed groups, and became involved in community development. Between 1978 and 1991, the Health Service and the Vietnamese community worked together in many ways and built a strong relationship.

In 1991 the Vietnamese Community Association brought its concern about illicit drug use among its young people to the Heath Service. The Health Service's philosophy led it to seek solutions that were sustainable by building the capacity of the Vietnamese community to support its young people. Accordingly, it was suggested that the Vietnamese Community Association and the Health Service identify the range of stakeholders and those with possible resources, and bring them together to discuss the plight of the community. In 1991 a Working Party was formed. In 1992 funding was received to employ a Vietnamese person to research the issue in the community. In 1994 a report of the action research was produced. From this, a committee was formed comprising different mainstream organisations and the Vietnamese Community Association, and the Hoi Sinh project was born. *Hoi Sinh* means 'regeneration' and encapsulates the hope of the Vietnamese community to arrest the escalating illicit drug use among its youth Since then, Hoi Sinh has employed a full-time street worker, supported a drug-peer education program, developed a convenience advertising campaign that has been adopted nationally, held community forums, and worked to inform and influence key community leaders, including the local Vietnamese doctors.

The process by which Hoi Sinh has achieved these things is critical to an understanding of the role of community development in health promotion in this case. From the view of the Vietnamese Community Association, it saw itself as having cultural competence but lacking the resources and technical expertise to address its concern. The ensuing partnership brought a range of expertise together and mobilised resources.

It has been generally acknowledged that the dominant response of the community to its drug problem was collective denial and that its professionals advocated total prohibition. Taking this as the starting point, it defined the community development role of the Health Service to help build an infrastructure in the Vietnamese community, through partnership, that would be supportive of its young people.

The Health Service community development worker engaged strategically and intensively with key people to support the action research and to ensure that the report of this research was used to influence mainstream systems to reorient resources towards this growing problem. The community development worker also brought a Heath Service doctor into the partnership. His medical status and influence in the community and among his Vietnamese colleagues have helped to change the view and practice of some leading Vietnamese doctors, who in turn have influenced other doctors to speak to the community about harm-minimisation strategies.

The key role of the Health Service throughout this process was building the capacity of the community to deal with its issue of concern by mobilising the relevant resources, harnessing them in a partnership, and reorienting many key stakeholders.

Parks Urban Redevelopment

The Parks Urban Redevelopment is a response to the South Australian government decision to sell its decaying assets to private developers. These developers are creating a housing estate aimed at the young, upwardly mobile market, with the objective of reducing public housing from around 85 per cent to 15 per cent over 15 years and the relocation of public housing tenants throughout the State.

The Parks is largely a public housing estate. Billed as government's social contribution to the industrial and economic development of South Australia, it was built originally to house workers. New migrants to South Australia also found cheap housing at the Parks. For many low-income families, single-parent families, and non-English-speaking background communities, the Parks has been an affordable place to live and has developed a strong and supportive identity. When the South Australian government announced its plans for the redevelopment of the Parks—the biggest urban renewal project in Australia to date—as a strategy to get rid of the 'ghetto', many local people were outraged. In their anger, they came to their Health Service. Together, they and the Health Service organised a public meeting between local people and officials of the

Housing Trust (the South Australian Government's public housing authority). Following this meeting, the local people, with the assistance of the Health Service, formed a community action group called the Voice.

In the meantime, the Housing Trust, the private developer, and local government had formed a partnership. Over a period of time, the Voice lobbied to be included as a partner in the project. As a result of much discussion within the community, it decided its stance would not be to halt the development. Rather, it would fight to ensure that no local resident would be worse off as a result of the redevelopment.

Somewhat grudgingly, local representation was accepted by the Housing Trust partnership, and a committee comprising the legal partners and local community representation, including the Voice and the Health Service, was formed—the Community Consultative Team. This team was bound by a community charter, outlining mutual roles, expectations, and responsibilities. The partnership is characterised by intense negotiation, lobbying, influencing, conflict, differing levels of trust, and very fluid alliances (Tesoriero 2001). In many ways, the community is the least powerful partner, so their competence in social action strategies and their partnership with the Health Service and its workers is critical to them in achieving their purpose.

Since the campaign began, the Health Service's role has changed. As the Voice becomes more capable in its social action, the Health Service's role has diminished to a more supportive, silent role in the relationship. The Voice has been successful in changing practices and policies in the urban renewal agenda. For example, it was instrumental in having a relocation policy adopted, not just for the Parks, but for all future urban renewal projects in South Australia. It is noteworthy that many of the professionals and bureaucrats involved have developed an appreciation of the local people's expertise and competence that comes from their lived experience.

The Parks residents have had many fights and have engaged in much social action on such issues as industrial pollution, and the loss of their high school and community centre. Some of these fights they have won; some they have lost, at great cost. However, each social action campaign has served to strengthen their resolve to insist on being included in major issues. The urban redevelopment project is no exception. It is clear to the Parks residents that the urban redevelopment means the destruction of their community, the dispersion of poverty, and the rendering of their disadvantage as invisible. They have chosen to fight for a social justice principle that no one ought to be any worse off. The project is 15 years old, and the Voice, with the assistance of the Health Service, will continue to influence processes that affect local people.

Lost opportunities in the 1990s

Primary health care

There were some significant changes to thinking about primary health care in Australia in the 1990s but the potential of these changes to advance a new public health agenda were unclear. The report *Improving Australia's Health: the Role of Primary Health Care* (1992) was commissioned under the National Better Health Program. It reported on the range of health promotion initiatives being conducted around Australia and recommended that the primary health care infrastructure should be strengthened. It saw a role for health promotion in the full range of primary health care settings, including hospitals and workplaces (NCEPH 1992). The agenda set by this report was based on a comprehensive view of primary health care. Unfortunately for the community health movement, its recommendations have not been implemented.

Coordinated care trials

An important innovation in primary health care in the 1990s was a series of federally funded coordinated care trials. Twelve trials were established across Australia and each was evaluated thoroughly (Silagy 2000). These trials aimed to test the proposition that services for people with complex and chronic conditions could be improved for no additional cost by improving the coordination of services. This coordination was to be done by pooling funds and having care planners to manage the coordination. From the viewpoint of community health the trials were disappointing because little attempt was made to incorporate community health services within the trials beyond domiciliary and aged care services. Most of the care coordination was done by GPs and while they are well suited to providing primary medical care, they are generally neither trained nor experienced in assisting clients to gain access to a range of community services and supports. By contrast this is exactly the kind of work in which community health services excel. An explicit attempt to involve community health services in care coordination may have improved the outcomes of the trials.

General practice reform strategy

Instead of a strengthened primary health care sector as a whole, the federal government established a General Practice Reform Strategy, which injected considerable resources into one part of the primary health care sector. This may well have been a missed opportunity to establish a stronger and more effective primary health care system that could have had a new public health mandate with an emphasis on community participation, multidisciplinary team work, a focus on communities rather than individuals, work across sectors, and health promotion. The main initiative of the General Practice Strategy was the establishment of Divisions of General Practice and a project grants program to encourage GPs to become involved in cooperative activities and improve their integration with the health system (Commonwealth Department of Health and Family Services 2001).

The Divisions have given GPs the opportunity to develop a range of preventive programs and to take a more population-based approach in their work. By 1995/96 the budget for the General Practice Strategy was $238 million (Commonwealth Department of Health and Family Services 2001). The strategy has focused on general practitioners and so does not encourage the multidisciplinary teamwork, which is at the heart of community health work. When resources flow to one profession, the power imbalances created almost certainly undermine attempts at effective multidisciplinary teamwork. However, the General Practice Strategy does offer some potential. For the first time in Australia it has encouraged GPs to come together and take a population view of the community they serve. This has also opened opportunities for them to integrate more effectively with hospitals and community-based health services. Furthermore, it has offered GPs a chance to move away from an exclusive focus on fee-for-service, if they wish. Both these features are potentially supportive of community health.

Community health sector
The community health sector, because of its philosophy and funding model, has been able to take a broader, population view of health and put more emphasis on health promotion and disease prevention. Frustration has been expressed by some community health workers that the style of health promotion undertaken by many GPs represents that which is typical of the lifestyle and behaviour-change era of the late 1970s and early 1980s. So while the General Practice Strategy does offer potential for changing general practice in a direction more compatible with community health, the failure to encourage greater integration with community health services must represent a lost opportunity. A policy more favourable to community health, encouraging integration between general practice and community health, would have been a program that established Divisions of Primary Health Care. These Divisions would have been better placed to take on the mantle of the community health movement. It would also have meant that the significant sums of money invested in primary health care would have been directed at strengthening a comprehensive model

rather than being used to support one part of the primary health care matrix. An encouraging sign in 2000 was that at least one Division of General Practice changed its name to a Division of Primary Health Care. What is less clear is whether the renamed Division can operate in a truly multidisciplinary manner and be open to leadership from all the professions involved in primary health care, not just medicine, and develop comprehensive models of planning and priority setting.

A further way in which general practice and community health services could have been integrated is through a program to fund salaried GPs within community health services. These GPs would then have the experience of working within a multi-disciplinary team within a service focusing on a social perspective of health. Such a program could offer significant national benefits by allowing a move away from private practice fee-for-service general practice and encouraging a community model for the provision of general practitioner services.

There were also cut-backs in funding to community health centres and services during the 1990s, particularly in Victoria and South Australia, where they were encouraged to concentrate on service delivery to the detriment of advocacy and community development (Baum 1996; Lewis and Walker 1997). Community health has always been somewhat marginalised and neglected but it has done more than any other part of the health sector to implement comprehensive primary health care. To have built on its strengths and provided the sector with sufficient resources to have capitalised on the promising work done would have been a sound investment.

Additionally in the 1990s community health lost the leader-ship offered by the Australian Community Health Association. The Association advocated on behalf of the sector to government, organised a series of national community health conferences, coordinated the activities of State community health associations, provided the auspice for innovative projects such as Healthy Cities Australia, and developed management tools such as the Community Health Accreditation and Standards Program (CHASP). In 1997 the Association lost its meagre government grant and had to close its secretariat. The demise of this Association was a loss to primary health care and public health in Australia and demonstrated a lack of commitment to community health from the federal government.

A recent review of general practice and community health concluded that if collaboration is to be encouraged (and the reviewers saw this as desirable) then it would be important to fund programs that explicitly encourage multidisciplinary team-work (Fry and Furler 2000). The collaboration will not happen without such incentives. A Victorian study (Swerrison et al. 2000) reviewed collaborative models between GPs and community health and recommended a range of strategies that could increase collaboration including funding, information provisions, and the removal of structural barriers to improved relations.

Hope in the twenty-first century

The most promising sign for community health in the early twenty-first century is a development in Victoria called Primary Care Partnerships. These partnerships aim to improve the health of Victorians by engaging consumers, carers, and communities in the planning and evaluation of services; improving health promotion, early intervention, and continuity of care; reducing the use of hospital services; and creating 'an identifiable and coordinated primary care service system underpinned by a social model of health' (Department of Human Services, Victoria 2001). These partnerships hold promise because they are bringing together all the key players in primary health care, including general practitioners and community health services, in a manner that does not privilege one group above another. The main means of implementing the strategy will be through community health plans. These plans will map the partnerships that need to be forged, and the service systems and infrastructures that need to be better integrated, and will be based on the needs of the population.

The Victorian Department of Human Services has also re-introduced the concept of direct election to Boards of community health centres. A majority of the board members will be elected. This restores the concept of community involvement being central to the governance of community health—a crucial step if these services are to be responsive to their community.

Conclusion

The community health sector in Australia is closer to a comprehensive model of primary health care than any other in Australia. The services are planned according to a population health model and develop interventions provided by multidisciplinary teams that focus on individuals, groups and populations. The philosophy underpinning the services draws on a comprehensive model of primary health care. Most significantly the services put emphasis on the importance of achieving health equity and plan their services to do this. The community health model was first supported federally during the 1970s and then continued to be strongly supported only by the Victorian and South Australian governments during the 1980s and early 1990s. Given this, it is true to say that community health has never received sustained long-term commitment from Australian health systems.

If Australian governments were to make a sustained investment in community health these services could form the backbone of a more sustainable health system that would be focused on health promotion and disease prevention. This system promises to be cost-effective and to offer considerable benefits in terms of population health, especially for low-income and otherwise disadvantaged communities. What is needed to capitalise on the promise of the community health sector is a national primary health care policy and strategy that makes a significant investment in the community health sector and puts community health at the centre of a health promoting health system.

Summary of main points

- Community health services offer the most comprehensive primary health care services in Australia by putting into practice the philosophy of the World Health Organization's Health for All Strategy.
- Community health services offer a wide range of services to individuals, including medicine, counselling, and a variety of physical therapies. They offer group support to help people to deal with a variety of diseases and social stresses, as well as engaging in social action and community development. Their approach to services is based on the use of multidisciplinary teams.
- Community health services have never been adequately funded and remain marginal to the mainstream health system.
- If community health services were adequately funded they could offer a way of underpinning the Australian health system with a focus on health promotion, disease prevention, and a better means of meeting the primary health care needs of the population.

Discussion questions

1   What features of community health services make them different from other parts of the health services?
2   What are the main differences between medical practice within community health services and within private general practice?
3   What dilemmas do you think community health services encounter when they use community development and social action strategies?
4   What do you see as the advantages and disadvantages of community management of community health services?
5   In whose interests do current community health care policies serve?
6   What do you think would be the benefits for Australia if its health system were based on a network of well-funded community health services?

Further investigation

1 The community health services never received a 'sustained long-term commitment' in the Australian health system. Discuss
2 Choose a specific area of community health services (Indigenous community-controlled health services, Divisions of General Practice, coordinated care trails) and examine its operation in terms of the principles of primary health care promoted by the World Health Organization.

Further reading and web resources

Baum, F. 1998, *The New Public Health: An Australian Perspective*, Oxford University Press, Melbourne.

Butler, C., Rissel, C., & Khavarpour, F. 1999, 'The Context for Community Participation in Health Action in Australia', *Australian Journal of Social Issues*, vol. 34, no. 3, pp. 253–65.

Butler, P. (ed.) 1994, *Innovation and Excellence in Community Health*, Centre for Innovation and Development in Health, Northcote.

Fry, D. & Furler, J. 2000, 'General Practice, Primary Health Care and Population Health Interface', in Commonwealth Department of Health and Aged Care (ed.), *General Practice in Australia 2000*, Commonwealth Department of Health and Aged Care, Canberra, pp. 385–424.

Legge, D., Wilson, G. et al. 1996, *Best Practice in Primary Health Care*, Centre for Development and Innovation in Health, La Trobe University, Melbourne.

Smith, J. 1999, 'Shifts in Community Care', in L. Hancock (ed.), *Health Policy in the Market State*, Allen & Unwin, Sydney, pp. 169–84.

Smith, J. 2000, 'Community Nursing and Health Care in the Twenty-first Century', *Australian Health Review*, vol. 23, no. 1, pp. 114–21.

Web sites

Carer's Association—a site with information for carers of people with chronic illness and disability. Contains a lot of information directed to carers as well as policies and research information: <www.carers.asn.au/index.html>. See also: ChronicillNet: <www.chronicillnet.org>

Commonwealth Department of Family and Community Services, Community Branch—describes a range of community programs run by this Department, including a description of Indigenous community programs: <www.facs.gov.au/internet/facsinternet.nsf/ aboutfacs/programs/community.htm>

Commonwealth Department of Health and Aged Care—a site with links to current Commonwealth Department of Health and Aged Care programs of relevance to community health. Demonstrates the lack of national commitment to community health in terms of a coherent program, policy, or funding scheme: <www.australiahealth.com/ Community%20Health/Community%20section.htm>

Community health in low-income countries—this Community Aid Abroad site contains descriptions of community health projects in low-income countries that concentrate on clean water provision, HIV/AIDs prevention and preventing violence against women: <www.caa.org.au/world/health/index.html>

Health Canada—Wired health—this site provides an electronic journal. A recent edition contained an article on community development and how health is promoted through empowerment and participation: <www.hc-sc.gc.ca/hppb/wired/community.html>

Human Rights and Equal Opportunities Commission, Healthy Communities—the HREOC web site contains a Healthy Communities section, which contains details of community projects in rural and remote Australia: <www.hreoc.gov.au/human_rights/ rural_health/index.html>

Primary Health Knowledge Bank—this Department of Human Services web site contains a Primary Health Knowledge bank that describes their Primary Care Partnerships and includes a range of useful information and resources relevant to community health: <www.dhs.vic.gov.au/phkb>

South Australian Community Health Research Unit (SACHRU)—produces a range of research reports on community health. The web site contains details of reports and current projects. It also contains a Project Evaluation Wizard, which allows users to plan evaluations of community health programs: <www.sachru.sa.gov.au/default.htm>

Conclusion

Future Directions in the Social Model of Health

... in creating its way of life, each society creates its way of death.

D. Eckholm 1987, p. 19

This book began with the premise that health sociology offers a second opinion to medical approaches by exploring the social determinants of health and illness. Throughout the chapters of this book we have attempted to expose the limitations of viewing health solely through the lens of biological determinism. However, in doing this we must be careful to avoid the similar sin of sociological determinism, that is, the view that we are merely 'puppets on strings' responding to unstoppable social forces. In the Conclusion to this book we highlight the potential of human agency and social action to create 'alternative futures' that foster a qualitatively healthier life for all. Specifically, the Conclusion consists of two chapters:

* Chapter 19 uses the concept of citizenship rights to reassert the notion that the right to health is a universal entitlement.
* Chapter 20, the concluding chapter, reviews the social model of health and provides some hints on how to continue to develop your own sociological imagination.

19

Citizenship and Health as a Scarce Resource

Bryan S. Turner

Overview

* *What is social citizenship?*
* *Is health a basic right of citizenship?*
* *Are health outcomes an effective measure of citizenship?*

Citizenship is a collection of rights and obligations that regulates access to scarce resources. It also confers identity and expresses notions of civic virtue. Citizenship therefore demarcates the moral boundaries of society in terms of insiders and outsiders. This chapter argues that societies have to manage two contradictory pressures: scarcity and solidarity. Citizenship provides a form of secular solidarity as a response to social scarcities. The chapter develops a model of citizenship in order to explore health as a desirable, but scarce, resource in the context of political changes to the welfare state, including the rise of economic rationalism.

Key terms

capabilities approach	epidemiology	pluralism
capitalism	feminisation of poverty	risk
citizenship	Fordism	social capital
class	gender	social closure
communism	Keynesianism	social contract theory
consumerism	neo-liberalism	social institutions
cultural capital	market	state
economic rationalism	patriarchy	

Introduction

gender This term refers to the socially constructed categories of feminine and masculine (the cultural values that dictate how men and women should behave), as opposed to the categories of biological sex (female or male).

class (or social class) A position within a system of structured inequality based on the unequal distribution of power, wealth, income, and status.

economic rationalism or economic liberalism Terms used to describe a political philosophy based on 'small-government' and market-oriented policies, such as deregulation, privatisation, reduced government spending, and lower taxation.

citizenship A collection of social rights and obligations that determine legal identity and membership of a nation state, and function to control access to scarce resources.

Human societies exist in the context of the impact of two contradictory social forces. First, they are confronted by systematic scarcities, which are produced by, and result in, exclusionary structures such as **gender** divisions, social **classes**, and generations. Second, they must also secure social solidarity in order to manage the social conflicts that are produced by scarcity. In the social sciences, these contradictory principles are described as the allocative and integrative requirements of social systems. The argument of this chapter is that health is a crucial example of a scarce resource ('a good') and that, especially where social inequality is intensified by **economic rationalism**, social **citizenship** functions as a basis of social solidarity. It does so by alleviating the genetic legacy of disease and mitigating the social causes of illness. Health results from the adequate institutionalisation of the social rights of citizenship rather than from technical medical interventions. For example, because preventative health measures and social security measures improve the social environment of individuals, their health characteristics will also improve. The history of infections suggests that the health of populations improved as a result of improvements in the social environment before vaccination measures had a significant impact. This historical assertion that disease is a social product of poor housing, inadequate food, and low standards of education raises important policy questions about how a government should allocate funding between conventional medical practice and social policies that are designed to improve the social environment.

In modern sociology, there has been an extensive analysis of citizenship (Andrews 1991; Beiner 1995; Blumer & Rees 1996; Roche 1992; Turner & Hamilton 1994). In this chapter, I discuss citizenship in terms of the legacy of T. H. Marshall (1893–1982), but I conclude by claiming that an adequate understanding of social rights in modern societies must go well beyond the Marshallian framework (Marshall 1950; 1981). Welfare citizenship is examined as a particular type of social right, and this chapter examines the sociology of health and illness from the perspective of welfare citizenship. More specifically, it provides an understanding of health issues in terms of the scarcity/solidarity distinction.

Models of citizenship

Citizenship is a collection of rights and obligations that gives individuals and social groups a formal legal identity. For example, citizens have a legal right to a passport and a legal obligation to pay taxes. These legal rights and obligations are constituted historically

social institutions Formal structures within society—such as health care, government, education, religion, and the media—that are organised to address identified social needs.

and sociologically as **social institutions** (for example, the jury system, parliaments, and welfare states). From a sociological point of view, we are interested in those social institutions that articulate the formal rights and obligations of individuals as members of a political community. Citizenship can be said to create the individual as a legal entity within the nation state. Figure 19.1 summarises the key components of contemporary citizenship.

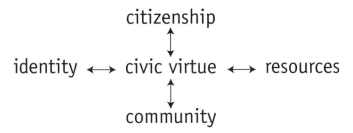

Figure 19.1 A sociological model of citizenship

This sociological approach is concerned with the social institutions of citizenship, including social identity, the nature of inequality, and access to socioeconomic resources. Sociologists attempt to understand how the institutions of citizenship protect individuals and groups from the negative consequences of the **market** in a **capitalist** society. This focus on the redistributive functions of citizenship institutions (the allocative processes) provide the basis for sociological approaches to questions about redistributive justice, as advocated by John Rawls (1970). Rawls equates justice with fairness; social arrangements are fair if there are no insupportable or unjustifiable grounds for discrimination among members of a society (Rawls 1970). The achievement of equality will require some redistribution of existing wealth from the very rich to the very poor. Such a redistribution may conflict with individual rights (to inheritance, for instance). Social arrangements are just if the basic liberties of individuals are compatible with the individual liberties of other members of society, and socioeconomic inequality may exist only if it can be reasonably expected to benefit the position of the least advantaged. The institution of citizenship attempts to reconcile individual rights (rights to free speech, for example) with collective rights (such as freedom from racial discrimination) within a democratic framework. In terms of health rights in a democracy, individual liberties (personal sexual preferences, for instance) have to be reconciled with collective health safeguards (from the unanticipated spread of AIDS). The right to health care must be negotiated within these parameters of redistributive justice. While most commentators (Daniels 1985) have concentrated on the right to health care, I want to treat health itself as a scarce resource, in the same way that we might treat housing as a scarce good.

market Any institutional arrangement for the exchange of goods according to economic demand and supply. This term is often used to describe the basic principle underlying the capitalist economy.

capitalism An economic system based on the private ownership of the means of production.

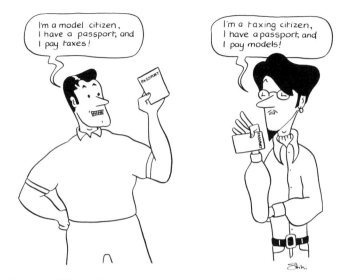

Models of citizenship

Citizenship, as a set of institutional mechanisms, controls the access of individuals and groups to scarce resources in society because it determines both membership and eligibility. Social rights and obligations, once they are institutionalised as formal status positions in a political community, give people entitlements to scarce resources. I approach the issue of scarcity from the perspective of Max Weber's political sociology, in which the principal variable is power. By 'resources' we mean primarily economic resources, such as property and liquid assets, but 'resources' can also include access to culturally desirable goods such as education. Cultural goods are **cultural capital** (Bourdieu 1984). Political resources themselves are related to access to the media of influence and authority in society: rights to vote, rights to participate politically, and so forth. Health is a scarce good that is unequally distributed in society along the fissures of social stratification and which, from an individual's point of view, diminishes inevitably with the wear and tear of ageing and the vicissitudes of the lifecycle.

It is conceptually useful to think of three generic types of resources (or power): economic, cultural, and political. Alongside these resources, we typically find three forms of rights: economic rights relating to the basic needs for food and shelter; the cultural rights of cultural capital (primarily education); and finally, political rights of liberal philosophy (such as freedom of assembly). These rights may be collectively designated as social rights, as distinct from human rights, because they presuppose membership of a political community—namely a nation state (James 1996).

The first thing to emphasise about citizenship is that it controls access to the scarce resources of society, and as a result, this allocative function is the basis of a profound conflict in modern societies

cultural capital This term refers primarily to the status that results from educational qualifications such as degrees and diplomas. It suggests that culture operates like economic goods to create hierarchies in society.

over citizenship membership criteria. Morbidity and mortality rates can be treated as an index of citizenship. For example, certain complaints relating to industrialisation such as 'miner's lung', repetitive strain injury, asbestosis, or hypertension are indicative of the quality of industrial relations legislation and the economic rights of workers. To take an extreme example, the health of slaves and servants may not be taken seriously where the supply of labour is elastic and where slaves and domestic servants, as in classical Greece, are not fully regarded as members of society. Social membership is obviously a precondition for sharing in social resources. The process of, and conditions for, naturalisation and denaturalisation tell us a great deal about the character of democracy in society, because these processes relate fundamentally to the basic notions of inclusion and exclusion. The willingness or otherwise of communities to share access to health care is a sensitive measure of the universalism of citizenship values. In legislative terms, nation states are generally reluctant to embrace new citizens without some checks of their age, health status, and health histories. These inclusionary and exclusionary processes mark both the political and moral boundaries of society. Moral panic about the international spread of AIDS through tourism and other means is an indicator of cultural **risk** in global societies (O'Neill 1990). In Australia, limitations on migration have historically been related to attempts to control access to resources by selective control of migration and naturalisation. The 'White-Australia' policy is a typical illustration of citizenship as a form of **social closure** (Parkin 1979).

Social closure is an elementary form of group solidarity, producing both social bonding and an inevitable alienation and stigmatisation of 'outsiders'. The boundaries of the state produce an enduring crisis of belonging for marginal communities in an ethnically plural society, and in this negative sense, citizenship is about the policing of normative borders (Connolly 1995). Any benchmark of citizenship would have to include some notion of egalitarian openness to difference and otherness as an essential ingredient of liberal democracy. Who gets citizenship clearly indicates the prevailing formal criteria of inclusion and exclusion within a political community, and how these resources are allocated and administered following citizenship membership largely determines the economic fate of individuals and families. From a historical perspective, the normative boundaries of society are, in practice, defined by tolerance of 'otherness'—a tolerance that is typically limited and in which otherness is often defined by reference to disease categories. In the medieval period, this boundary was determined by bubonic plague; the risks of modern society are indicated by the spread of new 'superbugs' and old infections, such as malaria, by global tourism. Other illustrations

risk or risk discourse 'Risk' refers to 'danger'. Risk discourse is often used in health promotion messages warning people that the lives they lead involve significant risks to their health.

social closure A term first used by Max Weber to describe the way that power is exercised to exclude outsiders from the privileges of social membership (in social classes, professions, or status groups).

of risk in modern technological societies would include 'mad cow disease' and thalidomide children (Beck 1992).

The next important aspect of citizenship is that it confers, in addition to a legal status, a particular cultural identity on individuals and groups. The notion of the 'politics of identity' indicates an important change in the nature of contemporary politics. In the early stages of industrialisation, much of the conflict over citizenship was related to class membership and class struggle in the labour market, where battles were fought over retirement, health insurance, and health benefits. Citizenship struggles in contemporary society, however, are often about claims to cultural identity. These struggles have been about sexual identity, gay rights, gender equality, and Aboriginality. Many debates about citizenship in contemporary political theory are about the question of contested collective identity in a context of radical pluralisation (Mouffe 1992). The health status of individuals is also related to their identity and membership. For example, disability often determines one's social identity, and struggles over the definition of 'disability' indicate the cultural and historical relativity of disease categories. Disability is ultimately about difference and personhood, and is shaped by political contestation that articulates the underlying values of society—that is, what society respects (Ingstad & Whyte 1995). This cultural dimension of citizenship also includes the notion of 'civic virtue', of which obligation, or 'the principle of duty' (Selbourne 1994), is the cornerstone. In a context of economic rationalism, there is a growing assumption that we are responsible for our own health and that we should not depend, as Mrs Thatcher argued, on the 'Nanny State'. Preventative-health philosophy now includes the assumption that we should practise 'safe sex', especially with strangers, and that we should avoid behaviours such as smoking or excessive dependence on alcohol, which have a negative impact on our health. With the increasing longevity of the populations of Western societies, the burden of dependency (the ratio of young and elderly to the working population) has a major impact on national budgets. These changes in public-health philosophy have encouraged 'voluntarism' and inevitably promote the idea that the family should be more involved in the care of its members (especially as health costs increase with the ageing of the population). This preventative ethic places, however, an increasing burden on private health care, in which those providing the care are often unemployed women and single mothers. Against such a trend, some sociologists argue that we have a right not to depend on the traditional charity of the family (Finch 1996).

This question of family obligation raises a particular issue to do with the changing forms of social involvement: the early stages in

Fordism The production processes of society that are based on the creation of the Ford motor car, which gave rise to a model of efficient and cheap production of mass goods. In a more general sense, it refers to a society that is dominated by Fordist production methods and values.

social contract theory Refers to the notion, prevalent in the works of Thomas Hobbes and Baruch Spinoza, that society is based on a contractual agreement regarding the collective exercise of power (typically by the state).

patriarchy A system of power through which males dominate households. It is used more broadly by feminists to refer to society's domination by patriarchal power, which functions to subordinate women and children.

feminisation of poverty Refers to the process whereby poverty is increasingly concentrated in households where women are single parents.

the development of citizenship appeared to depend on the unrecognised contributions of women, who were outside the formal labour market but involved in domestic labour. Feminist political theory notes that conventional patterns of citizenship depend upon **Fordism**, which assumes that men go to work to generate an income to sustain their own domestic arrangements and also to provide, through superannuation, for the future of their household. According to this model, women were assumed to be domestic labourers who serviced their men and reproduced society through child-bearing within the nuclear family. **Social contract theory** reproduced the dominant assumptions of **patriarchy**, which reproduced the public/private division (Pateman 1988). Women's unpaid domestic labour was thus essential to the maintenance of the external political structures of citizenship. These Fordist assumptions have been transformed by changes in the labour market (such as flexibilisation), by the increase in female employment, by changes to the family (which have often been associated with the **feminisation of poverty** with the growth in single-parent families), and by changes to retirement legislation. The conventional and simple division between the private and public realms has been transformed by changes to both. For feminist political theory, the historical relegation of women to the private domain of the nuclear family creates permanent dependency (Pateman 1989).

The final component of this sociological model of citizenship is the idea that a political community is the basis of citizenship; this political community is typically the nation state. When individuals become citizens, they not only enter into a set of institutions that confer upon them rights and obligations, they not only acquire a social identity, they are not only socialised into the civic virtues of duty, but they also become members of a political community with a particular territory and history. In order to have citizenship one has to be, at least in most modern societies, a bona fide member of a political community. Generally speaking, it is unusual for people to acquire citizenship if they are not simultaneously members of a political community—that is, a nation state. One should notice here an important difference between human rights and citizenship. Human rights are typically conferred upon people as humans, irrespective of whether they are Australian, British, Chinese, Indonesian, or whatever. But, because human rights legislation has been accepted by the nations of the world, people can claim human rights, even when they are stateless people or dispossessed refugees. Children, including unborn children, are believed to have human rights before they are recognised as members of a state. In general, citizenship is a set of rights and obligations that attach to members of formally recognised nation states within the system of nations, and hence citizenship corresponds to legal membership of a nation state. Now this relationship between nation state and citizenship is historical; it can be said to have its origins in the Napoleonic period, following the American and French revolutions. This close tie between nationality and citizenship can help us to understand some of the difficulties and issues that have surrounded Aboriginal health in Australia. Racial exclusion from the dominant political community has produced cultural exclusion, resulting in poor education, and inadequate housing and welfare provision. The low and problematic health status of Aboriginal communities is a clear reflection of their inadequate citizenship status in Australia (see chapter 6).

Scarcity and solidarity

One can conceptualise all human societies as divided or organised along two contradictory principles: solidarity and scarcity. All human societies, in order to exist, have to find some common basis, some form of solidarity, which—while it will not overcome them—will at least cope with the problems of difference, diversity, and conflict. All human societies must have some basis in solidarity in order to exist, but precisely because they are human societies, they are also characterised by scarcity. What do I mean by scarcity? The resources of society can never be wholly or systematically distributed to everybody in an egalitarian fashion because there are fundamental scarcities of an economic, cultural, and political nature. Scarcity is a very difficult notion to define. It is the basis of all economic theory; economics is about the management of scarce resources in matching means to ends, but it is wrong to think that scarcity exists in only primitive or simple societies. Indeed Marshall Sahlins (1974) argues in his economic anthropology that scarcity is institutionalised in modern economies, whereas so-called primitive economies were ones of abundance. One can easily imagine a hunter-gatherer society in which access to food was limited by the actual difficulties of hunting wild animals and gathering natural produce. But scarcity is always relative to demand as well as to need, and thus scarcity is a fundamental element of the most advanced and prosperous societies.

This argument is brilliantly analysed in Nicholas Xenos's *Scarcity and Modernity* (1989). Scarcity in wealthy societies is a function of growing expectations about assets, wealth, and success, and hence it is possible to date this form of scarcity to the rise of mass **consumerism**. Scarcity is as much a function of prosperity and wealth as it is of poverty. Scarcity is manifest in social inequality, and the typical forms of social inequality that we experience in modern societies are, obviously, differences of social class or access to wealth. However, scarcity also follows the contours of gender, age, and ethnicity. This tension between scarcity

consumerism The processes and institutions by which individuals satisfy their needs by purchasing goods and services in a market. Mass consumerism refers to postwar consumer practices, whereby the reduction of the cost of commodities and the extensive use of advertising and new credit arrangements created a mass market. It is often argued that consumerism has less to do with the satisfaction of wants than with the desire to be different and distinctive.

pluralism A theory whereby state power is shared with a large number of pressure or interest groups.

of perceived means to desired ends and the need for social solidarity in a context of **pluralism** is the focal point of citizenship.

Having outlined a general model of citizenship, we will now look more specifically at the issue of health as a scarce resource and at health care as a social right. In employing health as an index of social rights, we need to distinguish between morbidity (the statistics on illness and disease, in both acute and chronic conditions) and mortality rates (the pattern and causes of death over time). There is a strong sociological argument that the improvement in mortality rates (especially from infectious diseases among children) in the nineteenth and early twentieth centuries was a result of improvements in the standard of living (diet, water supply, education, and housing), rather than a consequence of medical intervention (McKeown 1979; Turner & Samson 1995). Population growth in the industrial societies resulted from a decline in infant mortality, which was in turn followed by a reduction in family size through increased control of reproduction, made possible by improvements in contraception. These historical illustrations can be used to argue that an increase in life expectancy from birth is a general index of citizenship, because we know that an improvement in the social environment reduces infant mortality. These debates are part of the legacy of the work of nineteenth-century health reformers such as Rudolf Virchow, whose work on typhus epidemics in the 1840s brought him to the conclusion that democracy is the best social response to disease (Gerhardt 1989). In other words, he concluded that improvements in social conditions were the most significant lasting basis for good health.

There is a significant amount of sociological research on the relationship between social class and health to confirm this general argument (Navarro & Berman 1977). In the United Kingdom, the Black Report in 1980 (Townsend & Davidson 1982) and *The Health Divide* (Whitehead 1988) demonstrated an almost perfect match between socioeconomic position and mortality. Similar data demonstrate the relations between class and health in Australia (see chapter 4). The research of Richard Wilkinson (1986, 1996) has been important for showing the persistence of class inequalities and illness, and the comparative importance of the welfare state in explaining better health outcomes in Scandinavian societies. There is a broad consensus that social class is crucial in understanding inequalities in morbidity and mortality, but there has been considerable debate about how this relationship between socioeconomic deprivation and illness should be understood. For example, it can be argued that this relationship is produced over time by the downward mobility of the physically and mentally sick. In this regard, it has been asserted that the over-representation of schizophrenia in the lowest social class is a product of downward mobility. The second alternative is that illness is a result of personal behaviour; for example, the high rates of lung cancer among working-class men result from their excessive use of tobacco. Against these arguments, sociologists have favoured a materialist explanation, which accounts for illness in terms of poor housing, inadequate education, dangerous working conditions, industrial pollution, and low incomes (Turner & Samson 1995, pp. 189–90).

Of course, these class and health relationships are complicated by gender and age structures. Women generally live longer than men but experience higher levels of morbidity (see chapter 5). There are important gender divisions in terms of both physical and mental health; these differences are primarily connected to different patterns of employment and lifestyle. Some differences between men and women may be related to variations in sickness-reporting behaviour, but feminist theory also points to the role of patriarchy in explaining such phenomena as anorexia nervosa. Improvements in female health have been associated with a decline in female fertility, improvements in the management of reproduction, and changes in education. In short, health in women is associated with the women's movement and the achievement of social rights. However, there is also evidence that, as women enter the labour force in significant numbers and leave traditional nurturing roles, they acquire the health profile of men. There is a convergence of lifestyles; one illustration of these changes would be the increasing use of alcohol and tobacco among employed women.

A similar set of arguments applies to ageing. There has been a significant increase in life expectancy for both men and women in Australia throughout this century. These improvements point to a general expansion of social-welfare provision through the institutions of citizenship. However, the paradox is that, while we live longer, morbidity data show a corresponding increase in patterns of chronic illness. There is a significant increase in the prevalence of disability for men and women over the age of 65 years, and in America 22 per cent of this age group require some form of assistance to accomplish daily tasks (Albrecht 1992). There is also a significant change in the **epidemiological** profile of society, with a distinctive increase in deaths from degenerative disease (in particular from cancers, strokes, and heart failure). Whether an improvement in citizenship alone can extend life expectancy and reduce chronic morbidity is a crucial question for public health in the next century. Epidemiological research suggests that, once a certain level of affluence has been achieved, then genetic legacy plays a crucial role in individual experiences of illness and disease. There are also puzzling and persistent inter-ethnic variations in terms of disease prevalence. For example, prostate and breast cancers are much lower in Japan than in the USA and Australia. These

epidemiology/ social epidemiology The statistical study of patterns of disease in the population. Originally focused on epidemics, or infectious diseases, it now covers non-infectious conditions such as stroke and cancer. Social epidemiology is a sub-field aligned with sociology that focuses on the social determinants of illness.

variations may be accounted for by differences in living conditions, dietary practices, and genetic legacy.

We have seen that citizenship provides access to resources that are important in protecting individuals and families from illness. The relationship between health, well-being and social resources has been expressed by Martha Nussbaum (2000, pp. 78–80) in terms of 'central human functional capabilities'. The basic idea behind this model is that we should be able to develop universal criteria to make judgments about justice in terms of basic human functions. She provides a list of ten such capabilities. These functional capabilities include: the ability to live a life of normal length; the enjoyment of good health, including reproductive health; the enjoyment of bodily integrity (such as freedom from sexual assault); the use of the senses (for imagination and reasoning); the emotional ability to form relationships with other humans; the capability to engage in critical reflection on one's life; the ability to form effective and rewarding affiliations with other people; the capacity to sympathise with other species and exercise stewardship over their lives; the ability to engage in play and to enjoy leisure; and finally the capability to exercise some control over one's political and material environment. Nussbaum believes that these capabilities are universal and that they form the basis of human rights—that is, a range of rights that universally protect and enhance these capabilities. Recognition of these fundamental capabilities provides a moral framework for democratic governance and the dignity of human beings. This **capabilities approach** throws further light on the importance of citizenship as a collection of social rights, and hence as the framework within which people can expect a basic level of good health. Those governments that fail to respect basic capabilities will necessarily undermine the health and well-being of their citizens. Her theory of capabilities has also been used to establish a basic legal framework for the protection of women and to insure that women's capabilities are given equal respect by society. Where extreme forms of social inequality exist in a class or caste society, the capabilities of individuals cannot be equally achieved. Nussbaum has developed this approach to provide a general set of values that can direct policy and strategy for development, but her criteria of capability would be equally valuable in assessing the success or failure of social policies designed to enhance social citizenship.

capabilities approach A moral framework of justice and universal human rights based on human functions or capabilities such as the ability to live to a normal life expectancy and be free from assault.

Conclusion: future directions

These historical relationships between health and citizenship—which were established by the expansion of welfare in the postwar period and by a general expansion of the economies of postwar industrial societies—have been challenged since the early 1980s by economic rationalism, privatisation, commodification, and changes in electoral philosophy. It is no longer assumed by the contemporary governments in Australia, for example, that full employment is the principal goal of economic policy. It is also increasingly assumed that:

- individuals will pay for welfare services (the 'user-pays' doctrine)
- the voluntary sector (such as the large charities) will contribute significantly to the national welfare effort
- there will be a significant level of privatisation in welfare and education
- welfare will be subject to the same controls and philosophy as industry itself (in the use of quality-control processes, 'out-sourcing', and competitive funding models).

It is unclear how great the impact of these changes on social rights will be in the long term, but it is clear that state provision of welfare will be increasingly relocated to the private sector.

We have seen that in the postwar period in the majority of industrial societies, there was a period of social reconstruction. After the ravages of warfare, many governments adopted social **Keynesian** policies for stimulating the economy through invest-ments in health, education, housing, and other so-called infra-structural expenditure. Following the social policies of J. M. Keynes (1883–1945), governments attempted to control the level of unemployment through investments in public works such as road building. Keynesianism can be seen as part of a more general phi-losophy arguing that the state rather than the market should be pivotal in providing for the needs of its citizens. In Britain, for exam-ple, the Beveridge reports such as *Full Employment in a Free Society* (1944) provided a framework for the development of a health sys-tem that would cover the health needs of the nation as a right. In the USA, there were similar developments in the twentieth century in the New Deal and Progressive Era, when American governments attempted to regulate industry and to improve the health of work-ers through legislation on social security measures (Eisner, 19993). In the 1970s and 1980s the Keynesian philosophy of public support for health and welfare became unpopular with governments who sought to reduce public expenditure, reduce personal taxation, and rely on market competition to drive down inflation. These policies, which have been adopted in the USA, United Kingdom, and Australia, are generally referred to as '**neo-liberalism**'.

The idea behind neo-liberalism is to increase the profitability of economic corporations by reducing their tax burden and removing legal constraints on their activities. At the same time, neo-liberal policies argue that individuals should take more responsibility for their own health care and in particular provide for their own retirement needs through personal investments. Because these policies attempted to reduce state expenditure, there has been a variety of experiments to transfer responsibility for the

Keynesianism A general philos-ophy based on the work of J. M. Keynes (1883–1945) that views the state as having prim-ary responsibility for meeting the needs of its citizens such as welfare provision, public works, and public services.

neo-liberalism A general philosophy based on the primacy of individual rights and minimal state intervention. Sometimes used interchangeably with economic rationalism/liberalism.

provision of health and welfare services to community groups and voluntary associations. Although these partnerships between the voluntary and state sectors can reduce welfare bureaucracy and bring services directly to the client, the voluntary sector cannot produce a uniform or universal service, and many critics have argued that the voluntary sector is driven by the same logic as the market, namely by the principle of resource maximisation (Brown, Kenny, & Turner 2000). Neo-liberalism arose because of fears that corporate profitability had been eroded by taxation and government regulation of the economy and by the greying of the population. It has been estimated, for example in Germany and Italy, that by 2030 for every person in employment there will be one person who is retired (Peterson 1999). Partnerships between the voluntary sector and the state are often promoted, not because they will create 'active citizenship', but because some measure of voluntarism will reduce the public cost of welfare services. The burden of voluntarism tends to fall primarily on women.

The consequences of neo-liberalism are thought to be incompatible with the values of social equality that underpinned the creation of the postwar welfare state. We have already noted that, while welfare improved the health of the population as a whole, it did not eradicate social class differences (the 'class gradient') in mortality and morbidity. In fact social class differences as measured by infant mortality rates and standardised mortality rates remained remarkably constant. While the health benefits of welfare state expenditure were often disappointing insofar as they failed to remove the effects of class inequality, it has been argued that neo-liberalism will have profoundly negative consequences for health.

The negative features of global neo-liberalism were spelt out in an influential article by David Coburn (2000) on 'income inequality, social cohesion and health status'. Coburn has argued that neo-liberalism diminishes the authority of the state, and makes it difficult for governments to achieve their welfare priorities. At the same time, it increases social inequality and reduces the level of social cohesion (or **social capital**) in society. These structural changes lower the level of social trust in a society and diminish self-respect among those sectors of the community that are exposed to growing social inequality. Low self-respect and declining social trust have a direct effect on health by lowering immunity to illness. Coburn's approach is important because it allows us to make a direct connection between the global growth of neo-liberalism, the decline in social cohesion, and the erosion of the health of individuals.

These changes suggest an important insight into the history of citizenship: social rights are not evolutionary and cumulative. Because Marshall argues that the rights of citizenship are cumulative, he also assumes that, once one has achieved legal rights, won

social capital A term used to refer to social relations, networks, norms, trust, and reciprocity between individuals that facilitate cooperation for mutual benefit.

the political battles of parliamentary democracy, and won social welfare rights, then these rights will not be eroded by subsequent social struggles. Marshall asserts that each of these historical stages represents a successful accumulation of citizenship. This is a very optimistic picture of the historical evolution of rights. One of the important debates emerging in contemporary democracies is whether previous rights can be sustained in a society that is increasingly dominated by the needs of the market-place and the rhetoric of economic rationalism. In a market-driven society, young people find it very difficult to enter the labour market and gain access to resources because of the nature of the modern economy. If we regard full employment as an entitlement, social rights may be obliterated or at least weakened as a consequence of economic rationalism. One can identify many societies that have highly developed social and economic rights, but they do not have adequate legal and political rights. In traditional debates about **communism** and capitalism, one criticism of the former communist regimes of Eastern Europe was that, while they had institutionalised social and economic forms of citizenship, these societies were often weak in terms of legal and political rights. They had economic rights without a comprehensive civil society, because they had achieved industrialisation without a liberal-bourgeois revolution against feudal privilege.

It is not clear how societies will manage the social conflicts that result from a failure to respect rights entitlements. Citizenship provides a form of solidarity—a kind of social glue, if you like—that binds societies that are divided by social class, by gender, by ethnicity, and by age. The solidarity of the political community of modern societies is provided by citizenship, which works as a form of civic religion. This model of the history of citizenship has either optimistic or pessimistic implications. The optimistic view is that, through the United Nations, and through agreements about human rights, modern societies can manage the problem of interstate violence, terrorism, and conflict. The alternative view is that we do not, in fact, have cumulative citizenship; what we have is a breakdown of citizenship. Nation states no longer adequately provide citizenship for their members, and instead we can observe an escalating war in which mega-cities and mega-economies are pitted against each other. Human rights will not be protected, because the so-called 'new world order' operates in the interests of a small number of powerful economies through the mechanisms of the World Bank, the International Monetary Fund, and the World Trade Agreement. The pessimistic outlook is that societies such as China will break down into mega-cities at war with each other. International economic links will undermine

communism/socialism Political ideology with numerous variations, but generally refers to the creation of societies in which private property and wealth accumulation are replaced by state ownership and distribution of economic resources. Communism represents a utopian vision of society based on communal ownership of resources, cooperation, and altruism to the extent that social inequality and the state no longer exist. Both terms are often used interchangeably to refer to societies ruled by a communist party.

traditional notions of citizenship, and the political future will be a much more insecure and uncertain environment. The future of health in Australia, therefore, depends on how citizenship rights survive in a global economy and cope with a partial erosion of national sovereignty.

Summary of main points

- T. H. Marshall's theory of citizenship—in terms of legal, political, and social rights—is a valuable framework for approaching health inequalities.
- To Marshall's model, we can add the notions of access to scarce resources (as forms of power), cultural identities, the political community as a product of social closure, and civic virtues (as obligation).
- Health can be analysed as a desirable good (that is, as a scarce resource).
- The health resource is distributed along the contours of social class, gender, and generations (or age cohorts).
- The notion of functional capabilities can provide a universalistic framework for evaluating citizenship programs.
- It is possible to use data on health as a measure of effective citizenship.
- Recent shifts in public policy reflect post-Fordism, and a new emphasis on preventative health and voluntarism in welfare delivery.
- These changes on a macro or global level can be collectively referred to as 'neo-liberalism'.

Discussion questions

1 What are the main criticisms of T. H. Marshall's theory of citizenship?
2 What are the social and economic consequences of the 'greying of the population' for government policies on health, retirement, and pensions?
3 What do you understand by the notion of 'social closure'? Can it help us to understand health inequalities?
4 Is illness best explained by 'material factors' (such as social class differences) or by 'cultural factors' (such as lifestyle) or by a combination of both types of factors?
5 Assume that people understand, through anti-smoking cam-paigns, that smoking causes lung cancer and various respiratory diseases. Can continuing to smoke be explained by rational models of economic behaviour such as consumer preference?
6 Discuss the right of individuals not to depend on the family for welfare services.

Further investigation

1 'The most significant cause of illness is poverty.' Discuss.
2 'There are no such things as universal human rights or capabilities.' Discuss.
3 Having read this chapter, what do you think are the crucial problems facing the government in terms of reducing class differences in health?
4 How successful has the advance of citizenship been in reducing class differences in health?
5 Compare and contrast Australian and Swedish data on mortality. Can you draw any conclusions about citizenship in the two societies?
6 'Despite advances in citizenship for White Australians, Aboriginal health statistics show that the enjoyment of citizenship rights is uneven.' Discuss.
7 'Infant mortality data are the best guide to the effectiveness of citizenship.' Discuss with special reference to Australian social trends.

Further reading and web resources

Barbalet, J. M. 1988, *Citizenship*, Open University Press, Milton Keynes.
Brown, K., Kenny, S., & Turner, B. S. 2000, *Rhetorics of Welfare. Uncertainty, Choice and Voluntary Associations*, Macmillan, Basingstoke.
Culpitt, I. 1992, *Welfare and Citizenship: Beyond the Crisis of the Welfare State?*, Sage, London.
Esping-Andersen, G. 1990, *The Three Worlds of Welfare Capitalism*, Polity, Cambridge.
Hindess, B. (ed.) 1990, *Reactions to the Right*, Routledge, London.
Turner, B. S. (ed.) 1993, *Citizenship and Social Theory*, Sage, London.
Turner, B. S. & Hamilton, P. (eds) 1994, *Citizenship: Critical Concepts*, 2 vols, Routledge, London.
Wilkinson, R. G. 1996, *Unhealthy Societies: The Afflictions of Inequality*, Routledge, London.

Web sites

Australian Human Rights Centre (AHRIC):
    <www.austlii.edu.au/au/other/ahric>
Centre for Citizenship and Human Rights:
    <www.arts.deakin.edu.au/cchr>
Center for Economic and Social Rights (USA): <www.cesr.org>
Human Rights Council of Australia: <www.hrca.org.au>
Human Rights and Equal Opportunity Commission: <www.hreoc.gov.au>
Human Rights Watch: <www.hrw.org>
Human Rights Web: <www.hrweb.org/resource.html>
World Health Organization—Human Rights:
    <www.who.int/m/topics/human_rights/en/index.html>

20

Health Sociology and Your Sociological Imagination

John Germov

Overview

* *What does the future hold for the social model of health?*
* *Is sociology beyond criticism?*
* *How can you further develop your sociological imagination?*

This book has served as an introduction to the key aspects of a social model of health. With the four features of the sociological imagination in mind, we have provided a template for understanding health and illness as social issues. This chapter summarises the main themes of the book in terms of what a social model of health entails. It also provides hints on how to develop your own sociological imagination further so that you continue to apply a second (sociological) opinion in examining and confronting health issues.

Key terms

agency
biomedicine/biomedical model
research methods
social model of health
social structure
sociological determinism
sociological imagination
structure/agency debate
theory

Introduction: sociology—the whole truth and nothing but ... ?

research methods Procedures used by researchers to collect and investigate data.

Throughout this book we have attempted to provide an overview of key areas of the health sociology field as the basis for you to make an objective evaluation of the strengths and weaknesses of the **research methods**, concepts, theories, and proposed solutions to the problems under study. In this attempt we have introduced you to the social model of health as an alternative to the conventional notions of health and illness drawn from biomedical approaches. We have also introduced you to the four features of a **sociological imagination** as an effective way of understanding and applying a sociological perspective to health issues.

sociological imagination A term coined by Charles Wright Mills to describe the sociological approach to analysing issues. We see the world through a sociological imagination, or think sociologically, when we make a link between personal troubles and public issues.

Therefore, it should be no surprise to you that sociology can be controversial. It may even challenge some of your own views. Sociology's critical approach seeks to challenge orthodox views and official positions. This is what sociological analysis is all about—taking nothing for granted and questioning the status quo—and thus it implies the need for organisational, political, and social change. However, as you've experienced through the chapters in this book, this does not mean there is only one way to apply sociology or one sociological solution to health problems. In fact, one of the benefits of sociology is that it regularly holds itself up for analysis of its theories and research findings— sociology itself is not beyond critique.

Despite the benefits of a sociological approach to health and illness, concepts and explanations have changed over time as some theories have been proven to be wrong or biased and new areas of investigation have emerged. Moreover, various authors continue to disagree about which are the most appropriate sociological explanations or solutions to the social and health problems we face.

structure/agency debate A key debate in sociology over the extent to which human behaviour is determined by social structure.

At this point it is worth returning briefly to the **structure/agency debate** first introduced in chapter 1. Health sociology critiques approaches to health and illness that rely primarily on individualistic explanations and biological determinism. In its place, health sociology advocates a focus on social determinants, social contexts, and social relations as the basis of understanding the complexity of illness-inducing and health-enhancing environments. In making this case, sociologists tend to highlight the structural factors that influence an individual's experience of health, illness, and health care. While a sociological imagination places individual behaviour, beliefs, and experiences in a social context, it is important to avoid **sociological determinism**, whereby individuals are viewed as 'puppets on strings' and 'society is to blame'. The potential of people to exert **agency**

sociological determinism A term used to describe the view that people's behaviour and beliefs are entirely shaped or determined by the social structure.

agency The ability of people, individually and collectively, to influence their own lives and the society in which they live.

at an individual and collective level should not be underestimated or dismissed. The structure/agency debate and sociology in general make us aware of the interdependence of individuals and their social environment. **Social structures** can be constraining or enabling, but the most important thing of all is that they are human creations—they are produced, reproduced, and changed by our actions or inactions. By raising awareness of the social context of health and illness, and by proposing reforms to identified problems, change is possible. Sociology offers this potential.

social structure The recurring patterns of social interaction through which people are related to each other, such as social institutions and social groups.

'Curiouser and curiouser ... '

The writing of *Second Opinion* has been underpinned by a desire to communicate the benefits of a sociological perspective *per se* and spark your intellectual curiosity for future sociological journeys. The philosopher Socrates is recorded as saying that he was sure of only one thing: that he knew nothing. What he meant was that it is useless to pretend that you always have the answers. In sociology too it is best to start from the humble position of assuming that there are things you know nothing about—issues you may not have considered. Even though the subject matter of sociology is often familiar, we need to be wary of assuming that we already know all there is to know about the society in which we live. The twentieth-century philosopher Bertrand Russell called this the constant need for 'constructive doubt'. In other words, we can benefit from adopting that child-like curiosity that always asks 'why?' When we ask why something is the way it is, we require an answer. Often what we are really asking is 'how could it be otherwise?' In sociology we seek alternative views and possible solutions to the issues under analysis. To help you further develop your sociological imagination, the next section provides some reflective questions and tips for constructing your own sociological theories and solutions.

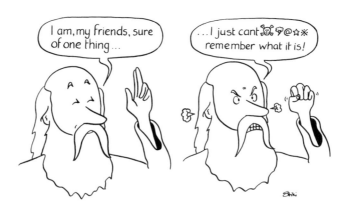

Future directions: developing your sociological imagination

Sociological analysis involves more than simply applying the four features of the sociological imagination template. It is based on an acceptance that some things may contradict and challenge what we believe, even though it is much more comfortable for us to believe that our opinions are right rather than wrong. Adopting a sociological imagination involves questioning our own views and assumptions about the world. Vincent Ruggiero (1996) suggests that one way to do this is by asking yourself the following questions:

1   How do you react to an idea you have never heard of before?
2   How do you react to change? Do you wholeheartedly embrace or resist it?
3   How do you deal with controversy? Do you evaluate each side of an argument, or do you immediately agree with one side?
4   How do you form views on particular issues? Does your view depend on where it came from (for instance, from the media, the government, your parents, your favourite celebrities)?
5   How flexible are you about changing your views? When was the last time you changed your opinion about a significant issue? Why did you change your mind?

William Shakespeare wrote, 'to thine own self be true', and in many ways these questions ask you to be true to yourself by consciously reflecting on and questioning your beliefs. Keeping these questions in mind will help you to think independently, ask penetrating questions, support what you say with knowledge of the available research findings, and hence reach sound conclusions.

Developing your own social theories

Ruggiero (1996) also provides a helpful approach to developing your own social **theories** or explanations. This entails following three steps to develop a sociological explanation of the issue you are studying:

theory A system of ideas that uses researched evidence to explain certain events and to show why certain facts are related.

1   *Reflective thinking*—this refers to reading, listening, and observing with curiosity so that you can identify issues requiring analysis. Being reflective means that no topic is off-limits or taken for granted. Everything, including every sociological theory and research finding, is open to further investigation. Such investigation starts by asking simple questions such as: Why are things as they are? What relationships exist between the various parts? What alternative views exist? How could things be improved?
2   *Creative thinking*—this refers to the production of ideas in order to resolve issues. This involves the use, adaptation, or creation of concepts and theories to help explain what you are investigating.

3   *Critical thinking*—this refers to the evaluation of the concepts and theories that you or others use. For example, do they fit the evidence? Are there any limitations? Do they account for alternative explanations?

Furthermore, Ruggiero (1996) outlines a number of techniques to help analyse theories, two of which are:

- brainstorming the 'pros' and 'cons' of various explanations and the evidence that you have gathered. The easiest way to start is to divide a page in two, with one section labelled, for example, 'It is', and the other 'It isn't'.

- deciding on the most appealing explanation and playing the 'devil's advocate'. Make a list of all the arguments that are used against your preferred view. Can such arguments be addressed or accommodated? If so, you should state how your preferred explanation stands up to criticisms. If you find that your preferred theory cannot answer all the criticisms, but on balance it remains your preferred explanation, then you still need to acknowledge the deficiencies of the argument that you have adopted.

This last point represents an important consideration: the need to resist adopting an 'either/or' position (Ruggiero 1996). It is possible to favour one argument while acknowledging or even accommodating some of the merits of opposing views, which is the case in most sociological theories. We are often presented with 'either/or' choices, but such choices tend to oversimplify social life, which is rarely that black and white. It is folly to adopt one position blindly and completely while rejecting all others automatically as being without foundation.

Conclusion

By studying the injustices and inequities of society, by gaining understanding and tolerance, and by promoting social change, sociology can help us to envision and ultimately produce a qualitatively better and healthier life for all. Perhaps Karl Marx summed it up best when he said, '[t]he philosophers have only interpreted the world in different ways; the point is to change it' (Marx 1859/1963, p. 84). In a world where we are constantly bombarded with glib media images and simplistic political slogans, the perspective of sociology provides a sounding board for the critical analysis of health issues. We have endeavoured to make your journey through the sociological landscape as stimulating as possible, but remember: no intellectual journey is worth taking if you already know what you will find. While it takes effort to scale the peaks of sociology, and even though the terrain may be rocky in patches, it is the journey itself that makes it all worthwhile. So persevere; the new and the unknown are exciting places to visit. Let sociology be your guide, and enjoy the view.

Discussion and further investigation questions

1   How can the issue of agency be addressed in the social model of health?
2   Are individuals or society to blame for health inequalities? Focus on one or two examples of health inequality and address the structure/agency debate in your answer.
3   'Health and illness are social constructions.' Discuss.
4   'The risk-factor approach displays an individualistic bias and ignores the social determinants of health.' Discuss.

Further reading and web resources

See Appendix 1 for information on key web sites, books, and journals related to health sociology. See Appendix 2 for tips on using and referencing the web, and how to reference this book.

Appendix 1: Key Web Sites, Books, and Journals

Web sites

Please note that web addresses tend to change often. An up-to-date list of weblinks is provided on the *Second Opinion* web site: <**www.oup.com.au/cws/germov**>

Health sociology professional associations

eSocHealth—Health Section of The Australian Sociological Association:
　　<www.latrobe.edu.au/telehealth/esohealth/>
Medical Sociology Group of the British Sociological Association:
　　<www.britsoc.org.uk/about/medsoc.htm>
Medical Sociology Section of the American Sociological Association:
　　<http://dept.kent.edu/sociology/asamedsoc>

Government and non-government agencies

Australian Bureau of Statistics: <www.abs.gov.au>
Australian Department of Health and Aged Care: <www.health.gov.au>
Australian Institute of Health & Welfare: <www.aihw.gov.au>
Australian Medical Workforce: <http://amwac.health.nsw.gov.au>,
　　see also: <www.health.gov.au/workforce/index.htm>
Australia New Zealand Food Authority: <www.anzfa.gov.au>
Centre for Clinical Governance Research in Health: <www.med.unsw.edu.au/clingov>
CNN Health Pages: <www.cnn.com/HEALTH>
Consumers' Health Forum: <www.chf.org.au>
Health Insurance Commission: <www.hic.gov.au>
Health Issues Centre: <http://avoca.vicnet.net.au/~hissues>
Health Report, ABC Radio National: <www.abc.net.au/rn/talks/8.30/helthrpt/default.htm>
National Centre for Epidemiology and Population Health: <www-nceph.anu.edu.au/>
National Health and Medical Research Council (NHMRC): <www.nhmrc.gov.au>
National Institutes of Health (NIH): <www.nih.gov>
National Library of Medicine (USA): <www.nlm.nih.gov/nlmhome.html>
Reuters Health: <www.reutershealth.com>
World Health Organization: <www.who.org>

Health professions

Australian Association of Occupational Therapists: <www.ausot.com.au>
Australian Association of Social Workers (AASW): <www.aasw.asn.au>
Australian Divisions of General Practice: <www.adgp.com.au>
Australian General Practice Accreditation Limited (AGPAL): <www.agpal.com.au/site/index.asp>
Australian Institute of Radiography: <www.a-i-r.com.au>
Australian Medical Association (AMA): <www.ama.com.au>
Australian Nursing Federation (ANF): <www.anf.org.au>
Australian Physiotherapy Association (APA): <www.physiotherapy.asn.au>
Australian Psychological Society (APS): <www.psychsociety.com.au>

Dietitians Association of Australia (DAA): <www.daa.asn.au>
Doctors Reform Society (DRS): <www.drs.org.au/drshome.htm>
National Office of Overseas Skills Recognition (NOOSR):
    <www.deet.gov.au/divisions/noosr/prof.htm>
NSW Health Department: <www.health.nsw.gov.au>
NSW Nurse Practitioners: <www.health.nsw.gov.au/nursing/npract.html>
NSW Nurses' Association: <www.nswnurses.asn.au>
Optometrists Association Australia: <www.optometrists.asn.au>
Royal Australian College of General Practitioners: <www.racgp.org.au>
Speech Pathology Australia: <www.speechpathologyaustralia.org.au>

Health politics and policy

Australian Democrats (AD): <www.democrats.org.au>
Australian Electoral Commission: <www.aec.gov.au>
Australian Greens: <www.greens.org.au>
Australian Labor Party (ALP): <www.alp.org.au>
Australian Parliamentary Library: <www.aph.gov.au/library>
Friends of Medicare: <www.pha.org.au/friends_of_medicare/frame_friends_of_medicare.html>
Liberal Party of Australia (LPA): <www.liberal.org.au>
National Party of Australia (NPA): <www.npa.org.au>

Aboriginal health

Australian Indigenous HealthInfoNet: <www.healthinfonet.ecu.edu.au>
Central Australian Aboriginal Congress: <http://caac.mtx.net/>
Indigenous Net: <www.indiginet.com.au>
National Aboriginal Community Controlled Health Organisation:
    <www.cowan.edu.au/chs/nh/clearinghouse/naccho/>
National Drug Research Institute: Indigenous Australian Alcohol and Other Drugs Databases:
    <www.db.ndri.curtin.edu.au>
Office for Aboriginal and Torres Strait Islander Health: <www.health.gov.au/oatsih/cont.htm>

Gender

Body Icon: http://nm-server.jrn.columbia.edu/projects/masters/bodyimage/
Body Image & Health Inc: <www.rch.unimelb.edu.au/BIHInc>
Eating disorders links: <www.uq.net.au/eda/documents/links.html>
Gender & Health Equity (Harvard University):
    <www.hsph.harvard.edu/grhf/HUpapers/gender/index.html>
Global Reproductive Health Forum (Harvard University):
    <www.hsph.harvard.edu/Organizations/healthnet/frame1/frame1.html>
Men's Bibliography by Michael Flood:
    <www.anu.edu.au/~a112465/mensbiblio/mensbibliomenu.html>
Mirror Mirror: <www.mirrormirror.com.au>
Women's Health Australia—the Australian Longitudinal Study on Women's Health:
    <www.newcastle.edu.au/centre/wha>
Women's Health Initiative (US): <www.nhlbi.nib.gov/whi/index.html>

Health promotion, public health, and social determinants

Healthy Cities Illawarra: <www.healthycitiesill.org.au>
International Public Health Watch: <www.ldb.org/iphw/index.htm>
Médecins Sans Frontières: <www.msf.org>
Noarlunga Healthy Cities project: <www.softcon.com.au/nhc>
Public Health Association of Australia: <www.phaa.net.au>

Public Health Virtual Library: <www.ldb.org/vl/index.htm>
Public Health Resources: <www.health.usyd.edu.au/research/index.html>
Public Health Resources on the Internet: <www.hlth.qut.edu.au/ph/phlinks/useful.htm>
Social Determinants of Health—The Solid Facts: <www.who.dk/healthy-cities/determ.htm>
Social Health Atlas of Australia: <www.publichealth.gov.au/atlas.htm>
Society for Medical Anthropology: <www.cudenver.edu//sma/>
Society for Social Medicine: <www.socsocmed.org.uk>
UK Health Equity Network: <www.ukhen.org.uk>
United Nations Report on the Global HIV/AIDS Epidemic:
       <www.unaids.org/epidemic_update/report/index.html>
WHO Health Promotion Declarations: <www.phs.ki.se/whoccse/Declarations.htm>
WHO World Health Report 2000: <www.who.int/whr/2000/en/report.htm>

Community health, carers associations and chronic illness groups
Carer's Association: <www.carers.asn.au/index.html>
Chronic Illness Net: <www.chronicillnet.org>
Commonwealth Department of Family and Community Services: Community Branch:
       <www.facs.gov.au/internet/facsinternet.nsf/aboutfacs/programs/community.htm>
Commonwealth Department of Health and Aged Care
       <www.australiahealth.com/Community%20Health/Community%20section.htm>
Community health in low income countries: <www.caa.org.au/world/health/index.html>
Disability Scholars Society (Queensland):
       <http://groups.yahoo.com/group/disabilityscholarssociety_qld>
Health Canada—Wired Health: <www.hc-sc.gc.ca/hppb/wired/community.html>
Human Rights and Equal Opportunities Commission—Healthy Communities:
       <www.hreoc.gov.au/human_rights/rural_health/index.html>
Primary Health Knowledge Bank: <www.dhs.vic.gov.au/phkb>
South Australian Community Health Research Unit: <www.sachru.sa.gov.au/default.htm>

New genetics
Centre for Law and Genetics: <www.lawgenecentre.org>
Council for Responsible Genetics: <www.gene-watch.org>
National Human Genome Research Institute: <www.nhgri.nih.gov>

Alternative therapies
Complementary health studies at University of Exeter: <www.exeter.ac.uk/chs>
Complementary Therapies in Medicine (journal):
       <www.harcourt-international.com/journals/ctim>
Complementary Therapies in Nursing & Midwifery (journal):
       <www.harcourt-international.com/journals/ctnm/default.cfm>
Guild of Complementary Practitioners (UK): <www.gcpnet.com>
Society of Homeopaths: <www.homeopathy-soh.org>

General sociology sites
Contemporary Philosophy, Critical Theory and Postmodern Thought
       <http://carbon.cudenver.edu/~mryder/itc_data/postmodern.html>
Dead Sociologists Society: <http://raven.jmu.edu/~ridenelr/DSS/INDEX.HTML>
Social Theory and Popular Culture: <www.Theory.org.uk>
Sociology Timeline from 1600 by Ed Stephan: <www.ac.wwu.edu/~stephan/timeline.html>
Sociosite: <www.pscw.uva.nl/sociosite/>
TASA: The Australian Sociological Association: <www.tasa.org.au>

Books

Essay and study skills

Germov, J. 2000, *Get Great Marks for Your Essays*, 2nd edn, Allen & Unwin, Sydney.
Germov, J. & Williams, L. 1999, *Get Great Information Fast*, Allen & Unwin, Sydney.
Williams, L. & Germov, J. 2001, *Surviving First Year Uni*, Allen & Unwin, Sydney.

Sociology dictionaries

Abercrombie, N., Hill, S., & Turner, B. S. 1998, *The Penguin Dictionary of Sociology*, 4th edn, Penguin, Melbourne.
Marshall, G. (ed.) 1998, *Oxford Dictionary of Sociology*, 2nd edn, Oxford University Press, Oxford.

General introductions to sociology

Beilharz, P. & Hogan, T. (eds) 2002, *Social Self, Global Culture: An Introduction to Sociological Ideas*, 2nd edn, Oxford University Press, Melbourne.
Bessant, J. & Watts, R. 2002, *Sociology Australia*, 2nd edn, Allen & Unwin, Sydney.
Giddens, A. 2001, *Sociology*, 4th edn, Polity Press, Cambridge.
Jureidini, R. & Poole, M. (eds) 2000, *Sociology: Australian Connections*, 2nd edn, Allen & Unwin, Sydney.
Najman, J. M. & Western, J. S. (eds) 2000, *A Sociology of Australian Society*, 3rd edn, Macmillan, Melbourne.
van Krieken, R., Smith, P., Habibis, D., McDonald, K., Haralambos, M., & Holborn, M., 2000, *Sociology: Themes and Perspectives*, 2nd Australian edn, Longman, Sydney.
Willis, E. 1999, *The Sociological Quest*, 3rd edn, Allen & Unwin, Sydney.

Health sociology texts

Albrecht, G. L., Fitzpatrick, R., & Scrimshaw, S. C. (eds) 2000, *Handbook of Social Studies in Health and Medicine*, Sage, London.
Annandale, E. 1998, *The Sociology of Health and Medicine: A Critical Introduction*, Polity Press, Cambridge.
Berkman, L. F. & Kawachi, I. (eds) 2000, *Social Epidemiology*, Oxford University Press, New York.
Bird, C., Conrad, P., & Fremont, A. M. (eds) 2000, *Handbook of Medical Sociology*, 5th edn, Prentice Hall, New Jersey.
Bury, M. 1997, *Health and Illness in a Changing Society*, Routledge, London.
Charmaz, K. & Paterniti, D. A. (eds) 1999, *Health, Illness and Healing: Society, Social Context and Self—An Anthology*, Roxbury Publishing, Los Angeles, Calif.
Cheek, J., Shoebridge, J., Willis, E., & Zadoroznyj, M. 1996, *Society and Health: Social Theory for Health Workers*, Longman, Melbourne.
Clarke, A. 2001, *The Sociology of Healthcare*, Prentice-Hall, Essex.
Cockerham, W. C., Glasser, M., & Heuser, L. S. (eds) 1998, *Readings in Medical Sociology*, Prentice Hall, New Jersey.
Conrad, P. & Kern, R. (eds) 2001, *The Sociology of Health and Illness: Critical Perspectives*, 6th edn, St Martin's Press, New York.
Conrad, P. & Schneider, J. 1992, *Deviance and Medicalisation: From Badness to Sickness*, 2nd edn, Temple University Press, Philadelphia.
Daly, J., Guillemin, M., & Hill, S. (eds) 2001, *Technologies and Health: Critical Compromises*, Oxford University Press, Melbourne.
Davey, B., Gray, A., & Seale, C. (eds) 2001, *Health and Disease: A Reader*, 3rd edn, Open University Press, Buckingham.
Davis, P. & Dew, K. (eds) 1999, *Health and Society in Aotearoa New Zealand*, Oxford University Press, Auckland.
Doyal, L. 1979, *The Political Economy of Health*, Pluto, London.
Eckersley, R., Dixon, J., & Douglas, J. (eds) 2001, *The Social Origins of Health and Well-being*, Cambridge University Press, Melbourne.
Field, D. & Taylor, S. (eds) 1998, *Sociological Perspectives on Health, Illness, and Health Care*, Blackwell Science, Oxford.
Fox, N. J. 1993, *Postmodernism, Sociology and Health*, Open University Press, Buckingham.
Freund, P. E. S. & McGuire, M. B. 1999, *Health, Illness, and the Social Body: A Critical Sociology*, 3rd edn, Prentice Hall, Englewood Cliffs, NJ.

George, J. & Davis, A. 1998, *States of Health: Health and Illness in Australia*, 3rd edn, Addison Wesley Longman, Melbourne.

Germov, J and Williams, L. (eds) 1999, *A Sociology of Food and Nutrition: The Social Appetite*, Oxford University Press, Melbourne.

Grbich, C. (ed.) 1999, *Health in Australia: Sociological Concepts and Issues*, 2nd edn, Longman, Sydney.

Heller, T., Muston, R., Sidell, M., & Lloyd, C. (eds) 2001, *Working for Health*, Open University Press/Sage, London.

Higginbotham, N., Albrecht, G., & Connor, L. 2001, *Health Social Science: A Transdisciplinary and Complexity Perspective*, Oxford University Press, Melbourne.

Lupton, G. M. & Najman, J. M. (eds) 1995, *Sociology of Health and Illness: Australian Readings*, 2nd edn, Macmillan, Melbourne.

Matcha, D. A. 2000, *Medical Sociology*, Allyn and Bacon, Boston.

Morris, D. 1998, *Illness and Culture in the Postmodern Age*, University of California Press, Berkeley.

Petersen, A. & Bunton, R. (eds) 1997, *Foucault, Health and Medicine*, Routledge, London.

Petersen, A. & Waddell, C. (eds) 1998, *Health Matters*, Allen & Unwin, Sydney.

Roach Anleu, S. L. 1999, *Deviance, Conformity and Control*, 3rd edn, Longman, Melbourne.

Samson, C. (ed.) 1999, *Health Studies: A Critical and Cross-Cultural Reader*, Blackwell, Oxford.

Scambler, G. 2002, *Health and Social Change: A Critical Theory*, Open University Press, Buckingham.

Scambler, G. & Higgs, P. (eds) 1998, *Modernity, Medicine and Health*, Routledge, London.

Seymour, W. 1998, *Remaking the Body: Rehabilitation and Change*, Allen & Unwin, Sydney

Turner, B. 1995, *Medical Power and Social Knowledge*, 2nd edn, Sage, London.

Weitz, R. 2001, *The Sociology of Health, Illness, and Health Care: A Critical Approach*, 2nd edn, Wadsworth, Calif.

White, K. 2001, *An Introduction to the Sociology of Health and Illness*, Sage, London.

Health statistics—key sources

ABS (various years) 1995, *National Nutrition Survey*, ABS, Canberra.

—— (various years) 1995, *National Health Survey*, ABS, Canberra.

AIHW 2002, *Australia's Health 2002*, Australian Institute of Health & Welfare, Canberra.

Lee, C. (ed.) 2001, *Women's Health Australia: What do we Know? What do we Need to Know?* Australian Academic Press, Brisbane.

Prometheus Information 1998, *HealthWiz*, Prometheus Information Pty Ltd, Canberra.

WHO 2000, *World Health Report 2000*, World Health Organization, Geneva.

—— 2000, *Healthy Life Expectancy Rankings*, World Health Organization, Geneva.

Health inequalities, social determinants, and occupational health

Acheson, D. 1998, *Independent Inquiry into Inequalities in Health*, Stationery Office, London.

Andarín, C. 1998, *Public Health Policies and Social Inequality*, New York University Press, New York.

Bartley, M., Blane, D., & Davey-Smith, G. (eds) 1998, *The Sociology of Health Inequalities*, Blackwell, Oxford (also published in *Sociology of Health & Illness*, vol. 20, no. 5).

Benzeval, M., Judge, K., & Whitehead, M. (eds) 1995, *Tackling Inequalities in Health: An Agenda or Action*, King's Fund, London.

Berkman, L. F. & Kawachi, I. (eds) 2000, *Social Epidemiology*, Oxford University Press, New York.

Blane, D., Brunner, E., & Wilkinson, R. G. (eds) 1996, *Health and Social Organisation: Towards a Health Policy for the Twenty-first Century*, Routledge, London.

Dahlgren, G. & Whitehead, M. 1992, *Policies and Strategies to Promote Equity in Health*, WHO, Copenhagen.

Daykin, N. & Doyal, L. (eds) 1999, *Health and Work: Critical Perspectives*, Macmillan, London.

Graham, H. (ed.) 2000, *Understanding Health Inequalities*, Open University Press, Buckingham.

Marmot, M. & Wilkinson, R. G. (eds) 1999, *Social Determinants of Health*, Oxford University Press, Oxford.

Mayhew, C. & Peterson, C. L. (eds) 1999, *Occupational Health and Safety in Australia*, Allen & Unwin, Sydney.

National Advisory Committee on Health and Disability 1998, *The Social, Cultural and Economic Determinants of Health in New Zealand*, National Advisory Committee on Health and Disability, Wellington.

Navarro, V. (ed.) 2001, *Political Economy of Social Inequalities: Consequences for Health and Quality of Life*, Baywood, Amityville.

Peterson, C. L. 1999, *Stress at Work: A Sociological Perspective*, Baywood Press, Amityville.

Royal Australasian College of Physicians 1999, *For Richer, For Poorer, In Sickness and in Health: The Socioeconomic Determinants of Health*, RACP.

Townsend, P., Davidson, N., & Whitehead, M. (eds) 1992, *Inequalities in Health: the Black Report and the Health Divide*, Penguin, London.

Turrell, G., Oldenburg, B., McGuffog, I., & Dent, R. 1999, *Socioeconomic Determinants of Health: Towards a National Research Program and a Policy and Intervention Agenda*, Centre for Public Health Research, School of Public Health, Queensland University of Technology, Brisbane.

Whitehead, M. 1987, *The Health Divide: Inequalities in Health in the 1980s*, Health Education Council, London.

Wilkinson, R. G. 1996, *Unhealthy Societies: The Afflictions of Inequality*, Routledge, London.

Wilkinson, R. & Marmot, M. (eds) 1998, *The Solid Facts: Social Determinants of Health*, World Health Organization, Copenhagen.

World Health Organization 1998, *Taskforce on Equity: Key Issues for the World Health Organization*, Draft Discussion Paper, WHO, Geneva.

—— 2000, *Health for All (HFA) in the 21st Century*, WHO, Geneva.

Gender and health

Albury, R. 1999, *The Politics of Reproduction*, Allen & Unwin, Sydney.

Annandale, E. & Hunt, K., 2000, *Gender Inequalities and Health*, Open University Press, Buckingham.

Berger, G. E. 1999, *Menopause and Culture*, Pluto Press, Sydney.

Broom, D. H. 1991, *Damned if We Do: Contradictions in Women's Health Care*, Allen & Unwin, Sydney.

Connell, R. W. 1995, *Masculinities*, Allen & Unwin, Sydney.

Doyal, L. 1995, *What Makes Women Sick: Gender and the Political Economy of Health*, Macmillan, London.

Ehrenreich, B. & English, D. 1973, *Witches, Midwives and Nurses*, Old Westbury Feminist Press, New York.

—— 1979, *For Her Own Good: 150 Years of Experts' Advice*, Pluto Press, London.

Fee, E. & Krieger, N. (eds) 1994, *Women's Health, Politics, and Power: Essays on Sex/Gender, Medicine, and Public Health*, Baywood, New York.

Kane, P. 1991, *Women's Health: From Womb to Tomb*, Macmillan, London.

Kent, J. 1999, *Social Perspectives on Pregnancy and Childbirth for Nurses and the Caring Professions*, Open University Press, London.

Lee, C. (ed.) 2001, *Women's Health Australia: What do we Know? What do we Need to Know?*, Australian Academic Press, Brisbane.

Lorber, J. 1997, *Gender and the Social Construction of Illness*, Sage, Thousand Oaks, Calif.

Oakley, A. 1980, *Women Confined*, Martin Robertson, Oxford.

Pringle, R. 1998, *Sex and Medicine: Gender, Power and Authority in the Medical Profession*, Cambridge University Press, Cambridge.

Riska, E. & Wegar, K. (eds) 1993, *Gender, Women and Medicine: Women and the Medical Division of Labour*, Sage, London.

Sabo, D. & Gordon, D. F. (eds) 1995, *Men's Health and Illness: Gender, Power and the Body*, Sage, Thousand Oaks, Calif.

Schur, E. 1983, *Labelling Women Deviant: Gender, Stigma, and Social Control*, Temple University Press, Philadelphia.

Wicks, D. 1999, *Nurses and Doctors at Work: Rethinking Professional Boundaries*, Allen & Unwin, Sydney.

World Health Organization 1998, *Gender and Health: Technical Paper, Women's Health and Development*, Geneva.

Aboriginal health

Hunter, E. 1993, *Aboriginal Health and History*, Cambridge University Press, Melbourne

Langton, M. 1993, 'Rum, Seduction and Death: "Aboriginality" and Alcohol', *Oceania*, vol. 63, no. 3, pp. 195–206.

McLennan, W. & Madden, R. 1999, *The Health and Welfare of Australia's Aboriginal and Torres Strait Islander Peoples*, ABS & Australian Institute of Health and Welfare, Canberra.

Reid, J. & Trompf, P. (eds) 1991, *The Health of Aboriginal Australia*, Harcourt Brace Jovanovich, Sydney.

Saggers, S. & Gray, D. 1991, *Aboriginal Health and Society: The Traditional and Contemporary Struggle for Better Health*, Allen & Unwin, Sydney.

—— 1998, *Dealing with Alcohol: Indigenous Usage in Australia, Canada and New Zealand*, Cambridge University Press, Melbourne.

Ethnicity and health

Castles, S., Foster, W., Iredale, R., & Withers, G. 1998, *Immigration and Australia: Myths and Realities*, Allen & Unwin, Sydney.

Donovan, J., d'Espaignet, E., Merton, C., & van Ommeren, M. (eds) 1992, *Immigrants in Australia: A Health Profile,* Ethnic Health Series, no. 1, Australian Institute of Health and Welfare & AGPS, Canberra.

Fadiman, A. 1997, *The Spirit Catches You and You Fall Down*, Farrar, Straus and Giroux, New York.

Ferguson, B. & Pittaway, E. (eds) 1999, *Nobody Wants to Talk About It: Refugee Women's Mental Health*, Transcultural Mental Health Centre, Sydney.

Jayasuriya, L., Sang, D., & Fielding, A. 1992, *Ethnicity, Immigration and Mental Illness: A Critical Review of Australian Research*, AGPS, Canberra.

Jupp, J. 1999, *Immigration*, 2nd edn, Oxford University Press, Melbourne.

National Health Strategy 1993, *Removing Cultural and Language Barriers to Health*, Issues Paper no. 6, AGPS, Canberra.

Reid, J. & Trompf, P. (eds) 1990, *The Health of Immigrant Australia: A Social Perspective*, Harcourt Brace Jovanovich, Sydney.

Rowland, D. T. 1991, *Pioneers Again: Immigrants and Ageing in Australia*, Bureau of Immigration Research & AGPS, Canberra.

Deviance, mental health and medicalisation

Aneshensel, C. S. & Phelan, J. C. (eds) 1999, *Handbook of the Sociology of Mental Health*, Kluwer Academic Publishers, Dordrecht.

Busfield, J. (ed.) 2000, Special Issue—Rethinking the Sociology of Mental Health, *Sociology of Health & Illness*, vol. 22, pp. 543–719.

Conrad, P. & Schneider, J. 1992, *Deviance and Medicalization: From Badness to Sickness*, 2nd edn, Temple University Press, Philadelphia.

Department of Health and Aged Care 1998, *National Mental Health Report 1997*, AGPS, Canberra.

Foucault, M. 1988, *Madness and Civilization: A History of Insanity in the Age of Reason*, trans. R. Howard, Vintage Books, New York.

Horwitz, A.V. & Scheid, T. L. (eds) 1999, *A Handbook for the Study of Mental Health*, Cambridge University Press, Cambridge.

Pilgrim, D. & Rogers, A. 1999, *A Sociology of Mental Health and Illness*, Open University Press, Buckingham.

Roach Anleu, S. L. 1999, *Deviance, Conformity and Control*, 3rd edn, Longman, Melbourne.

Schur, E. 1983, *Labelling Women Deviant: Gender, Stigma, and Social Control*, Temple University Press, Philadelphia.

Sociology of the body

Featherstone, M., Hepworth, M., & Turner, B. (eds) 1991, *The Body: Social Process and Cultural Theory*, Sage, London.

Hancock, P., Hughes, B., Jagger, E., Paterson, K., Russell, R., Tulle-Winton, E., & Tyrler, M. (eds) 2000, *The Body, Culture and Society: An Introduction*, Open University Press, Buckingham.

Nettleton, S. & Watson, J. (eds) 1998, *The Body in Everyday Life*, Routledge, London.

Petersen, A. 1998, *Unmasking the Masculine: 'Men' and 'Identity' in a Sceptical Age*, Sage, London.

Scott, S. & Morgan, D. (eds) 1993, *Body Matters: Essays on the Sociology of the Body*, Falmer Press, London.

Shilling, C. 1993, *The Body and Social Theory*, Sage, London.

Turner, B. 1996, *The Body and Society*, 2nd edn, Sage, London.

Weitz, R. (ed.) 1998, *The Politics of Women's Bodies: Sexuality, Appearance and Behavior*, Oxford University Press, New York.

Health promotion and public health

Ashton, J. & Seymour, H. 1988, *The New Public Health: The Liverpool Experience*, Open University Press, Milton Keynes.

Ashton, J. (ed.) 1992, *Healthy Cities*, Open University Press, Buckingham.

Baum, F. 1998, *The New Public Health: An Australian Perspective*, Oxford University Press, Melbourne.

Beaglehole, R. & Bonita, R. 1997, *Public Health at the Crossroads*, Cambridge University Press, Cambridge.

Blaxter, M. 1990, *Health and Lifestyles*, Routledge, London.

Bunton, R., Nettleton, S., & Burrows, R. (eds) 1995, *The Sociology of Health Promotion*, Routledge, London.

Hamilton, M., Kellehear, A., & Rumbold, G. (eds) 1998, *Drug Use in Australia: A Harm Minimisation Approach*, Oxford University Press, Melbourne.

Legge, D., Wilson, G. et al. 1996, *Best Practice in Primary Health Care*, Centre for Development and Innovation in Health, La Trobe University, Melbourne.

Lupton, D. 1995, *The Imperative of Health: Public Health and the Regulated Body*, Sage, London.

O'Connor-Fleming, M. L. & Parker, E. 2001, *Health Promotion*, 2nd edn, Allen & Unwin, Sydney.

Petersen, A. & Lupton, D. 1996, *The New Public Health: Health and Self in the Age of Risk*, Allen & Unwin, Sydney.

Health policies

Bloom, A. L. 2000, *Health Reform in Australia and New Zealand*, Oxford University Press, Melbourne.

Davis, P. & Ashton, T. (eds) 2001, *Health and Public Policy in New Zealand*, Oxford University Press, Auckland.

Duckett, S. J. 2000, *The Australian Health Care System*, Oxford University Press, Melbourne.

Gardner, H.(ed.) 1995, *The Politics of Health: The Australian Experience*, 2nd edn, Churchill Livingstone, Melbourne.

—— (ed.) 1997, *Health Policy in Australia*, Oxford University Press, Melbourne.

Gillespie, J. A. 1991, *The Price of Health: Australian Governments and Medical Politics 1910–1960*, Cambridge University Press, Melbourne.

Hancock, L. (ed.)1999, *Health Policy in the Market State*, Allen & Unwin, Sydney.

Leeder, S. R. 2000, *Healthy Medicine: Challenges Facing Australia's Health Services*, Allen & Unwin, Sydney.

Lumby, J. 2001, *Who Cares?*, Allen & Unwin, Sydney.

Mooney, G. & Scotton, R. (ed.) 1998, *Economics and Australian Health Policy*, Allen & Unwin, Sydney.

Powell, D. D & Wessen, A. F. (eds) 1999, *Health Care Systems in Transition: An International Perspective*, Sage, Thousand Oaks, Calif.

Sax, S. 1984, *A Strife of Interests: Politics and Policies in Australian Health Services*, Allen & Unwin, Sydney.

Scott, C. 1999, *Public–Private Interfaces in Health Care Systems*, Open University Press, London.

Health professions

Abbott, A. 1988, *The System of Professions: An Essay on the Division of Expert Labor*, University of Chicago Press, Chicago.

Exworthy, M. & Halford, S. (eds) 1999, *Professionals and the New Managerialism in the Public Sector*, Open University Press, Buckingham.

Freidson, E. 2001, *Professionalism: The Third Logic*, Polity Press, Cambridge.

—— 1994, *Professionalism Reborn: Theory, Prophecy and Policy*, Polity Press, Cambridge.

Gabe, J., Kelleher, D., & Williams, G. (eds) 1994, *Challenging Medicine*, Routledge, London.

Pringle, R. 1998, *Sex and Medicine: Gender, Power and Authority in the Medical Profession*, Cambridge University Press, Cambridge.

Salmon, J. W. (ed.) 1990, *The Corporate Transformation of Health Care: Issues and Directions*, vol. 1, Baywood, New York.

—— (ed.) 1994, *The Corporate Transformation of Health Care: Perspectives and Implications*, vol. 2, Baywood, New York.

Walby, S. & Greenwell, J. 1994, *Medicine and Nursing: Professions in a Changing Health Service*, Sage, London.

Walton, M. 1998, *The Trouble with Medicine: Preserving the Trust Between Patients and Doctors*, Allen & Unwin, Sydney.

Willis, E. 1989, *Medical Dominance*, revised edn, Allen & Unwin, Sydney.

Witz, A. 1992, *Professions and Patriarchy*, Routledge, London.

History of medicine

Duffin, J. 1999, *History of Medicine*, University of Toronto Press, Toronto.

Le Fanu, J. 1999, *The Rise and Fall of Modern Medicine*, Abacus, London.

Porter, R. 1997, *The Greatest Benefit to Mankind: A Medical History of Humanity from Antiquity to the Present*, HarperCollins Publishers, London.

New genetics

Conrad, P. & Gabe, J. (eds) 1999, *Sociological Perspectives on the New Genetics*, Blackwell, Malden.

Hubbard, R. & Wald, E. 1997, *Exploding the Gene Myth*, revised edn, Beacon Press, Boston.

Nelkin, D. & Lindee, S. 1995, *The DNA Mystique: The Gene as a Cultural Icon*, Freeman and Co., New York.

Wilkie, T. 1994, *Perilous Knowledge: The Human Genome Project and Its Implications*, Faber & Faber, London.

Ageing, death and dying

Arber, S. & Ginn, J. (eds) 1995, *Connecting Gender and Ageing: A Sociological Approach*, Oxford University Press, Oxford.

Chapman, S. & Leeder, S. 1995, *The Last Right?*, Mandarin, Melbourne.

Kellehear, Allan (ed.) 2000, *Death and Dying in Australia*, Oxford University Press, Melbourne.

—— 1999, *Health Promoting Palliative Care*, Oxford University Press, Melbourne.

McNamara, B. 2001, *Fragile Lives: Death, Dying and Care*, Allen & Unwin, Sydney.

Poole, M. & Feldman, S. (eds) 1999, *A Certain Age: Women Growing Older*, Allen & Unwin, Sydney.

Alternative therapies

Cant, S. & Sharma, U. (eds) 1996, *Complementary and Alternative Medicines: Knowledge in Practice*, Free Association Press, London.

Easthope, G. 1986, *Healers and Alternative Medicine*, Gower, Aldershot.

Goldstein, M. S. 1999, *Alternative Health Care: Medicine, Miracle, or Mirage?*, Temple University Press, Philadelphia.

Healey, K. (ed.) 1998, *Alternative Medicine: Issues in Society*, vol. 100, Spinney Press, Sydney.

Salmon, J. W. (ed.) 1984, *Alternative Medicines: Popular and Policy Perspectives*, Tavistock, New York.

Vincent C. & Furnham A. 1998, *Complementary Medicine: A Research Perspective*, Wiley, Chichester.

General social theory books

Abbott, P. & Wallace, C. 1997, *An Introduction to Sociology: Feminist Perspectives*, 2nd edn, Routledge, London.

Adam, B., Beck, U., & van Loon, J. (eds) 2000, *The Risk Society and Beyond: Critical Issues for Social Theory*, Sage, London.

Alexander, J. C. 1998, *Neofunctionalism and After*, Blackwell, Oxford.

Barrett, M. & Phillips, A. (eds) 1992, *Destabilizing Theory: Contemporary Feminist Debates*, Polity Press, Cambridge.

Beasley, C. 1999, *What is Feminism Anyway?*, Allen & Unwin, Sydney.

Beck, U. 1992, *Risk Society: Towards a New Modernity*, Sage, Thousand Oaks, Calif.

Berger, P. & Luckmann, T. 1967, *The Social Construction of Reality*, Penguin, Harmondsworth.

Butler, J. 1990, *Gender Trouble: Feminism and the Subversion of Identity*, Routledge, London.

Connell, R. W. 1987, *Gender and Power*, Allen & Unwin, Sydney.

Craib, I. 1992, *Modern Social Theory*, 2nd edn, Harvester Wheatsheaf, London.

—— 1997, *Classical Social Theory*, Oxford University Press, Oxford.

Cuff, E. C., Sharrock, W. W., & Frances, D. W. 1998, *Perspectives in Sociology*, 4th edn, Routledge, London.

Danaher, G., Schirato, T., & Webb, J. 2000, *Understanding Foucault*, Allen & Unwin, Sydney.

Hepworth, J. 1999, *The Social Construction of Anorexia Nervosa*, Sage, Thousand Oaks, Calif.

Lemert, C. (ed.) 1997, *Social Theory: The Multicultural and Classic Readings*, Westview, Oxford.

Lupton, D. 1999, *Risk*, Routledge, New York.

May, T. 1996, *Situating Social Theory*, Open University Press, Buckingham.

McNay, L. 1992, *Foucault and Feminism*, Polity Press, Cambridge.

Pateman, C. 1988, *The Sexual Contract*, Polity Press, Cambridge.

—— 1996, *Sociological Theory*, 4th edn, McGraw-Hill, New York.

Ritzer, G. 1997, *Postmodern Social Theory*, McGraw-Hill, New York.

Tong, R. P. 1998, *Feminist Thought: A Comprehensive Introduction*, 2nd edn, Allen & Unwin, Sydney.

Walby, S. 1990, *Theorizing Patriarchy*, Blackwell, Oxford.

Wearing, B. 1996, *Gender: The Pain and Pleasure of Difference*, Addison Wesley Longman, Melbourne.

Weedon, C. 1987, *Feminist Practice and Poststructuralist Theory*, Blackwell, Oxford.

Research methods

Alasuutari, P. 1995, *Researching Culture: Qualitative Method and Cultural Studies*, London, Sage.

Crotty, M. 1998, *The Foundations of Social Research: Meaning and Perspective in the Research Process*, Allen & Unwin, Sydney.

Daly, J., Kellehear, A., & Glicksman, M. 1997, *The Public Health Researcher*, Oxford University Press, Melbourne.

Denzin, N. 1997, *Interpretive Ethnography*, London, Sage.

Ezzy, D. 2001, *Qualitative Analysis*, Allen & Unwin, Sydney.

Grbich, C. 1999, *Qualitative Research in Health: An Introduction*, Allen & Unwin, Sydney.

Rice, P. & Ezzy, D. 1999. *Qualitative Research Methods: A Health Focus*, Oxford University Press, Melbourne.

Relevant journals

Alternative Health Practitioner
Australian and New Zealand Journal of Public Health
Australian Health Review
Body & Society
Complementary Therapies in Medicine
Complementary Therapies in Nursing & Midwifery
Critical Public Health
Health: An Interdisciplinary Journal for the Social Study of Health, Illness and Medicine
Health Promotion Journal of Australia
Health Sociology Review (formerly *Annual Review of Health Social Sciences*)
Healthy Weight Journal
International Journal of Health Services
Journal of Allied Health
Journal of Alternative and Complementary Medicine
Journal of Health Politics, Policy and Law
Journal of Health Services Research & Policy
Journal of Sociology
Milbank Quarterly
Public Health
Qualitative Health Research
Social History of Medicine
Social Science & Medicine
Sociology of Health & Illness
Women and Health

Appendix 2: Tips on Web Use, and Referencing the Web and this Book

This Appendix provides some handy tips on how to critically assess the information found on web sites you may use in your research for assignments. It also shows you how to reference web sources as well as how to correctly reference chapters and information from this book.

How to evaluate the credibility of web sites: not all web sites are created equal

Because anyone can publish what they like on the web, it is important to exercise caution when obtaining information from a web site. You need to evaluate the credibility of a web site, before using it as a source of information for assignments. Ask yourself the following questions to help evaluate the credibility of the information contained on a web site:
- Can an author be identified?
- Is a date and title supplied?
- Are contact details for the author or publisher provided?
- How objective is the information provided? Does it represent the interests of a particular organisation, political party, or pressure group? How might this bias the information presented?
- If the source is an academic one, is it properly referenced and is the material self-published or has it been peer reviewed, such as articles published in online academic journals?

The general point to remember is not to take anything on the web at face value and to ensure that the source is a credible one. Often the easiest way to judge credibility is to ask yourself whether you would use the source if you had found it in hard copy form on your library shelves.

How to reference the web

To reference information from a web site, aim to include as much information as possible where it is available, such as:
- the author of the information (a person or organisation)
- date (sometimes found at the bottom of a web page)
- the title of the site or specific page you used
- the URL (web address)
- the date you accessed the web site (as web sites often change, or revise their information, and sometimes cease to exist).

In the text of your assignment you would reference your information in the usual way, noting the author and date. If no author is given, then the title of the web site can be used instead (avoid including the URL as this is included in the details you provide in your reference list at the end of your assignment). In your reference list, the complete reference would appear as:

Germov, J. 2002, *Second Opinion* web [web page], http://www.oup.com.au/cws/germov, date accessed: 01 January 2002.

If the web site you use is an online journal or publication that you can download, your reference list entry would appear as for hard copy publication, with the addition of the web site URL and the date you accessed the site. For example:

Harris, P. 2001, 'From Relief to Mutual Obligation: Welfare Rationalities and Unemployment in 20th-century Australia', *Journal of Sociology*, vol. 37, no. 1, pp. 5–26, [online version: http://www.sagepub.co.uk/journals/details/j0366.html], date accessed: 01 January 2002.

How to reference this book

A common mistake in referencing an edited book is to reference the editor rather than the chapter author. The first rule to remember when referencing content from an edited book such as *Second Opinion* is to reference the author of the chapter from which you obtained information. For example, let's say you need to reference information in your assignment that you found in the chapter by Lauren Williams entitled: 'In Search of Profession: A Sociology of Allied Health'. In the text of your assignment, you would reference the chapter author, that is, you would reference Williams, so that in your assignment it might appear as:

Williams (2002) argues that allied health professions are subordinate to the medical profession …

Note that the year is obtained from the date of publication of the book in which the chapter appears. In your reference list at the end of your assignment, the complete reference would appear as:

Williams, L. 2002, 'In Search of Profession: A Sociology of Allied Health', in J. Germov (ed.), *Second Opinion: An Introduction to Health Sociology*, 2nd edn, Oxford University Press, Melbourne.

The above entry provides the reader with specific details about where you got your information from, by identifying the chapter author and chapter title, as well as the book it appeared in. Some referencing systems may require you to include the first and last page numbers of the chapter in your reference list, which are usually placed at the end of the reference. While the formatting of your references will depend on which system you employ, you will generally need to include the above information no matter which referencing system you use.

Even when the chapter author and the editor are the same person, the same rules apply, so that a chapter by Germov, would appear in your reference list as:

Germov, J. 2002, 'Challenges to Medical Dominance', in J. Germov (ed.), *Second Opinion: An Introduction to Health Sociology*, 2nd edn, Oxford University Press, Melbourne.

If you need to reference a section of the book, such as the glossary, you can do so in the following way:

Germov, J. 2002, 'Glossary', in J. Germov (ed.), *Second Opinion: An Introduction to Health Sociology*, 2nd edn, Oxford University Press, Melbourne.

Further information

You can get further help on study skills, particularly on how to reference, write essays and assignments and how to effectively use the web, from the following books I have published:

Germov, J. 2000, *Get Great Marks for Your Essays*, 2nd edn, Allen & Unwin, Sydney.
Germov, J. & Williams, L. 1999, *Get Great Information Fast*, Allen & Unwin, Sydney.
Williams, L. & Germov, J. 2001, *Surviving First Year Uni*, Allen & Unwin, Sydney.

Glossary

accident-proneness

A term invented by industrial psychologists to 'explain' workplace injury and illness. It is based on the false and unproven assumption that workers are careless and malingering, and are therefore solely responsible for accidents.

ageism

A term, like 'sexism' and 'racism', that denotes discrimination, in this case, discrimination based on age.

agency

The ability of people, individually and collectively, to influence their own lives and the society in which they live.

alcohol misuse

Excessive consumption of alcohol leading to health and/or social problems.

allopathy

A descriptive name often given to orthodox medicine. Allopathy is the treatment of symptoms by opposites.

assimilation/assimilationism

A policy term referring to the expectation that indigenous people and migrants will 'shed' their culture and become indistinguishable from the Anglo–Australian majority.

autoethnography

An ethnography that focuses on the experience of the researcher.

biological determinism

The unproven belief that people's biology determines their social, economic, and health statuses.

biomedicine/biomedical model

The conventional approach to medicine in Western societies. It diagnoses and explains illness as a malfunction of one of the body's biological mechanisms. The biomedical approach of most health services focuses on the treating of individuals, and generally ignores social, economic, and environmental factors.

biopsychosocial model

This model is an extension of the biomedical model. It is a multi-factorial model of illness that takes into account the biological, psychological, and social factors implicated in a patient's condition. Like the biomedical model, it focuses on the individual patient for diagnosis, explanation, and treatment.

biotechnology

The use of molecular biology and genetic engineering to modify plants and animals, including humans, at the molecular level.

capabilities approach

A moral framework of justice and universal human rights based on human functions or capabilities such as the ability to live to a normal life expectancy and be free from assault.

capitalism

An economic system based on the private ownership of the means of production.

Cartesian dualism

Also called mind/body dualism and named after the philosopher Descartes, it refers to a belief that the mind and body are separate entities. This assumption underpins medical approaches that view disease in physical terms and thus ignore the psychological and subjective aspects of illness.

citizenship

A collection of social rights and obligations that determine legal identity and membership of a nation state, and function to control access to scarce resources.

class (or social class)

A position within a system of structured inequality based on the unequal distribution of power, wealth, income, and status. Class membership is determined by three characteristics: ownership and control of scarce economic resources; ownership of marketable skills and qualifications; and wage labour. People who share a social-class position typically share similar life chances.

clinical gaze

A term originally used by Michel Foucault (1975) to refer to a doctor's direct focus on a patient's body. It is a characteristic feature of doctor–patient interaction, and tends to ignore the patient's emotions, psychology, and personality.

clinical governance

A term to describe a range of quality assurance measures that control doctors' clinical decision-making through standardised work protocols and performance measurement at the clinical level.

collective conscience

A term used to describe shared moral beliefs that act to unify society.

colonisation/colonialism

A process by which one nation imposes itself economically, politically, and socially upon another.

commodification of health care

Treating health care as a commodity to be bought and sold in the pursuit of profit maximisation.

commodity culture

The world of advertising and commercial marketing.

complementary medicine

A term used to describe those alternative medical practitioners and practices that do not stand in opposition to orthodox medicine but that collaborate with orthodox practice.

consumerism

The processes and institutions by which individuals satisfy their needs by purchasing goods and services in a market. Mass consumerism refers to postwar consumer practices, whereby the reduction of the cost of commodities and the extensive use of advertising and new credit arrangements created a mass market. It is often argued that consumerism has less to do with the satisfaction of wants than with the desire to be different and distinctive.

convergence

The process, which may or may not be occurring, whereby orthodox medicine adopts many of the practices of alternative medicine, and alternative medicine acts to become more orthodox by, for example, seeking to license practitioners and make practitioners subject to training.

cultural capital

This term refers primarily to the status that results from educational qualifications such as degrees and diplomas. It suggests that culture operates like economic goods to create hierarchies in society.

cultural diversity

A term used to refer to the existence of a range of different cultures in a single society. In popular usage, it typically refers to ethnic diversity, but sociologically the term can equally refer to differences based on gender, social class, age, disability, and so on.

cultural stereotypes

Shared images of the members of an ethnic group that are often negative and are based on a simplistic, overgeneralised, and homogenous view of an 'ethnic' culture.

deinstitutionalisation

A trend in mental health treatment whereby individuals are admitted for short periods of time, rather than undergoing lifetime hospitalisation. In theory, such policies are meant to be supported by extensive community resources, to 'break down the barriers' and integrate the mentally ill into the community. However, in practice, this has not occurred on a wide scale because of the lack of funding of community services.

deprofessionalisation

A general theory predicting the decline of medical status and power because of increasing health education of the population and because of decreasing public trust as a result of negative media stories of medical fraud and negligence.

deviance

Behaviour or activities that violate social expectations about what is normal.

discourse

A domain of language-use that is characterised by common ways of talking and thinking about an issue (for example, the discourses of medicine, madness, or sexuality).

discourses about health

A domain of language-use that is characterised by common ways of talking and thinking about health.

dispossession

The removal of people from land they regard as their own.

doctor/nurse game

A concept that derives from an article by L. Stein (1967), who describes a 'game' that, he claims, is played out between doctors and nurses. The main feature of this game is that the nurse must be assertive and make positive suggestions regarding patient care while not appearing to do so. In other words, nurses must couch suggestions regarding patient care in such a way that doctors can pick them up and act on them as though they were their own initiatives.

ecological model

A model of health, derived from the field of human ecology, that suggests that the environmental impacts of urban and rural settlements, including industry, technology, education, and culture, are linked to quality of life.

economic rationalism or economic liberalism

Terms used to describe a political philosophy based on 'small-government' and market-oriented policies, such as deregulation, privatisation, reduced government spending, and lower taxation.

embodiment

The lived experience of both being a body and having a body.

emotional labour

Refers to the use of feelings by employees as part of their paid work. In health care, a key part of nursing work is caring for patients, often by providing emotional support.

empirical

Describes observations or research that is based on evidence drawn from experience. It is therefore distinguished from something based only on theoretical knowledge or on some other kind of abstract thinking process.

encroachment (vertical and horizontal)

The threat to the occupational boundaries of professionals, which can take two forms: vertical and horizontal. Vertical encroachment can be from above (from medicine, for instance) or from below, whereby less qualified workers do some of the tasks previously done by a professional. Horizontal encroachment refers to the occupational take-over of one profession by another, where both have similar status and power.

epidemiology/social epidemiology

The statistical study of patterns of disease in the population. Originally focused on epidemics, or infectious diseases, it now covers non-infectious conditions such as stroke and cancer. Social epidemiology is a sub-field aligned with sociology that focuses on the social determinants of illness.

essentialism

An approach based on the assumption that there is an essential core or essence to identity that is inevitable and stable over time (for example, that women are essentially caring and nurturing).

ethnic communities

Those ethnic groups that have established a large number of ethnic organisations, thus providing a shared context for interaction between members. Only some ethnic groups develop the institutional structure that enables them to become ethnic communities.

ethnic group

A group of people who not only share an ethnic background but also interact with each other on the basis of their shared ethnicity.

ethnicity

Sociologically, the term refers to a shared cultural background, which is a characteristic of all groups in society. As a policy term, it is used to identify migrants who share a culture that is markedly different from that of Anglo-Australians. In practice, it often refers only to migrants from non-English-speaking backgrounds (NESB migrants).

ethnic minorities

Ethnic groups that are not the dominant ethnic group in a society. Unlike the term 'ethnic group', it highlights the power differences between different ethnic groups in society.

ethnocentric

Viewing others from one's own cultural perspective. Implied is a sense of cultural superiority based on an inability to understand or accept the practices and beliefs of other cultures.

ethnography

A research method that is based on direct observation of a particular social group's social life and culture—of what the people actually do.

ethnospecific services

Services established to meet the needs of specific ethnic groups or a number of ethnic groups. Members of the ethnic group(s) are the targeted clientele, so that these services are distinct from, and often run parallel with, mainstream services.

eugenics

The study of human heredity based on the unproven assumption that selective breeding could improve the intellectual, physical, and cultural traits of a population.

euthanasia

Meaning 'gentle death', the term is used to describe voluntary death, often medically assisted, as a result of incurable and painful disease.

evidence-based medicine (EBM)

An approach to medicine arguing that all clinical practice should be based on evidence from randomised control trials (RCTs) to ensure the effectiveness and efficacy of treatments.

feminisation

A shift in the gender base of a group from being predominantly male to increasingly female.

feminisation of poverty

Refers to the process whereby poverty is increasingly concentrated in households where women are single parents.

feminism/feminist

A broad social and political movement based on a belief in equality of the sexes and the removal of all forms of discrimination against women. A feminist is one who makes use of, and may act upon, a body of theory that seeks to explain the subordinate position of women in society.

Fordism

The production processes of society that are based on the creation of the Ford motor car, which gave rise to a model of efficient and cheap production of mass goods. In a more general sense, it refers to a society that is dominated by Fordist production methods and values.

functional pre-requisites

A debated concept based on the assumption that all societies require certain functions to be performed for them to survive and maintain social order. Also known as functional imperatives.

gender/sex

This term refers to the socially constructed categories of feminine and masculine (the cultural values that dictate how men and women should behave), as opposed to the categories of biological sex (female or male).

gendered health

A term used to acknowledge the different experiences and exposures to health and illness that result from gender.

geneism

A form of discrimination—like racism, sexism, and ageism—in which people are judged on their ascribed, rather than achieved, status. In this case, their genetic make-up is used as the basis for determining access to social rewards such as employment or health insurance.

genetic manipulation

Alteration of the genetic material of living cells to perform new functions (by rearranging or deleting existing genes), including the transferral of genetic information from one species to another.

genetic reductionism

An assumption that people are simply the sum of their individual genes, so that the causes of disease are reduced to an individual's genes rather than the social, economic, and political context in which they live. See 'biological determinism'.

globalisation

Political, social, economic, and cultural developments—such as the spread of multinational companies, information technology, and the role of international agencies—that result in people's lives being increasingly influenced by global, rather than national or local, factors.

gross domestic product (GDP)

The market value of all goods and services that have been sold during a year.

health promotion

Any combination of education and related organisational, economic, and political interventions designed to promote behavioural and environmental changes conducive to good health. This promotion may cover a variety of strategies, including legislation, health education, community development, advocacy, and so on. Health promotion has usually, however, been restricted to interventions focusing on the behavioural end of the spectrum.

healthism

The extreme preoccupation with personal health that is evident within the general population.

horizontal violence

A concept derived from Paolo Friere that describes a behaviour common to all oppressed groups, whereby, because of their powerlessness, the oppressed are unable to direct their anger towards their oppressor and so turn it towards each other, with various degrees of violence and negativity.

ideal type

A concept originally devised by Max Weber to refer to the abstract or pure features of any social phenomenon.

ideology

In a political context, ideology refers to those beliefs and values that relate to the way in which society should be organised, including the appropriate role of the state.

immigrants

The overseas-born population in a society. The term is sometimes extended to refer to the descendants of immigrants through the terms 'second-generation' and 'third-generation immigrants'. However, this usage tends to confuse the term, as it obscures the important fact that those born overseas have a set of immigrant experiences that their descendants do not.

Indigenous community-controlled health services

Independent local organisations, controlled and managed by indigenous people, that provide a range of services to meet the needs of their particular communities.

individualism/individualisation

A belief or process supporting the primacy of individual choice, freedom, and self-responsibility.

individualist health promotion (IHP)

IHP is a set of programs that provide health education about health risks to persuade people to change their lifestyles. A wide group of professionals are involved in these programs, including doctors, nurses, allied health professionals, psychologists, educators, and media and marketing experts.

institutionalisation

A process by which the lives of individuals are regulated in every way, and which creates dependent relationships between the institutionalised person and authority figures.

Keynesianism

A general philosophy based on the work of J. M. Keynes (1883–1945) that views the state as having primary responsibility for meeting the needs of its citizens such as welfare provision, public works, and public services.

labelling

Labelling theory focuses on the effect that social institutions (such as the police, the courts, and psychiatry) have in labelling (or defining) what is deviant.

liberalism

An ideology that regards the interests of individuals and their place in the market-place as being of primary importance.

life chances

A term derived from Max Weber that refers to the opportunities available to people in society. People with different social-class locations have different life chances, including different opportunities with regard to education, wealth, and health.

lifestyle choices/factors

The decisions people make that are likely to impact on their health such as diet, exercise, smoking, alcohol, and other drugs. The term implies that people are solely responsible for choosing and changing their lifestyle.

McDonaldisation

A term coined by George Ritzer to refer to the standardisation of work processes by rules and regulations. It is based on increased monitoring and evaluation of individual performance, akin to the uniformity and control measures used by fast-food chains.

mainstreaming

A policy term that refers to the provision of services to all members of the community through the same institutional structure. In Australia, it refers to a structure of service provision that is contrasted with that of ethnospecific services.

managerialism

The introduction of private-sector management techniques into the public sector.

market

Any institutional arrangement for the exchange of goods according to economic demand and supply. This term is often used to describe the basic principle underlying the capitalist economy.

materialist analysis

An analysis that is embedded in the real, actual, material reality of everyday life.

medical dominance

A general term used to describe the power of the medical profession in terms of its control over its own work, over the work of other health workers, and over health resource allocation, health policy, and the way that hospitals are run.

medical-industrial complex

The growth of profit-oriented medical companies and industries, whereby one company may own a chain of health services, such as hospitals, clinics, and radiology and pathology services.

medicalisation

The process by which non-medical problems become defined and treated as medical issues, usually in terms of illnesses, disorders, or syndromes.

men's health

Running parallel to women's health initiatives, the men's health movement recognises that certain elements of masculine identity and behaviour can be hazardous to health.

meta-analysis and meta-narratives

The 'big picture' analysis that frames and organises observations and research on a particular topic.

modernism

A view of the possibilities and direction of social life that is grounded in a faith in rational thought. From a modernist perspective, truth, beauty, and morality exist as objective realities that can be discovered and understood through rational and scientific means. These themes are rejected by postmodernists.

multiculturalism

A policy term referring to the expectation that all members of society have the right to equal access to services, regardless of 'race', ethnicity, culture, or religion. It is based on the recognition that all people have the right to maintain their cultural beliefs and identity while adhering to the laws of the nation state.

negotiated order

A symbolic interactionist concept that refers to any form of social organisation in which the exercise of authority and the formation of rules are outcomes of human interaction and negotiation.

neo-liberalism

A general philosophy based on the primacy of individual rights and minimal state intervention. Sometimes used interchangeably with economic rationalism/liberalism.

new public health

A social model of health linking 'traditional' public health concerns, which focus on physical aspects of the environment (clean air and water, safe food, occupational safety through legislation), with the behavioural, social, and economic factors that affect people's health. The model is supported by a social movement that emphasises primary prevention, participation, and primary health care.

norms

Expectations about how people ought to act or behave.

nurse-practitioner

The title given to nurses with an enhanced and extended role, such as the ability to prescribe certain drugs and undertake procedures such as Pap smears and minor surgery. In some countries (such as the USA) it may also refer to the nurse's ability to charge a fee for service.

occupational welfare

Welfare provision—such as tax relief for business expenses and superannuation investment—that benefits higher paid workers.

orthodox medicine

The medical practices and institutions developed in Europe during the nineteenth and twentieth centuries that are legally recognised by the state. Central to these practices is the teaching hospital, where all new doctors are inducted into laboratory science, clinical practice, and allopathic biomedicine. These practices and institutions are now dominant in all parts of the world.

patriarchy

A system of power through which males dominate households. It is used more broadly by feminists to refer to society's domination by patriarchal power, which functions to subordinate women and children.

phenomenology

Its main aim is the analysis and description of everyday life. It is the study of the ways in which individuals construct the daily realities of their social world through interaction with others.

placebo/placebo effect

Any therapeutic practice that has no clear clinical effect. In practice it usually means giving patients an inert substance to take as a medication. When a patient reacts to a placebo in a way that is not clinically explicable, this is called the 'placebo effect'.

pluralism

A theory whereby state power is shared with a large number of pressure or interest groups.

positive health

A holistic view of health that focuses on wellness, rather than disease, and that it is culturally relative, incorporating notions of spirituality, community, and social support.

positivism

Research methods that attempt to study people in the same way that physical scientists study the natural world by focusing on quantifiable and directly observable events.

postmodern society

A disputed term to refer to a society in which many of the central institutions, including the state, have lost their power to determine social outcomes. There are no longer clear paths for the individual to influence events by participating in such institutions as political parties, unions, or professional bodies.

postmodernity

A hotly debated term in sociology that broadly refers to a social condition following modernity, in which society becomes fragmented as a result of a high level of social differentiation and cultural diversity.

post-structuralism (and postmodernism)

Often used interchangeably with postmodernism, it refers to a perspective that is opposed to the view that social structure determines human action, and that emphasises the local, the specific, and the contingent in social life.

primary health care

Both the point of first contact with the health care system and a philosophy for delivery of that care.

professional bureaucracy

Mintzberg's (1979) term for an organisation that relies on staff with specialised knowledge and expertise to deliver complex services that require decision-making autonomy at the point of service delivery.

professionalisation (professional project)

The process of becoming a profession, whereby an occupational group attains publicly recognised and government-legitimated monopoly and autonomy over its area of work. Professional status is usually associated with certain traits (see 'trait approach').

proletarianisation

A theory that predicts the decline of medical power as a result of deskilling and the salaried employment of medical practitioners. This results in a loss of economic independence, whereby doctors lose control over their work because of managerial authority and bureaucratic regulations.

public health/public health infrastructure

Public policies and infrastructure to prevent the onset and transmission of disease among the population, with a particular focus on sanitation and hygiene such as clean air, water, and food, and immunisation. Public health infrastructure refers specifically to the buildings, installations, and equipment necessary to ensure healthy living conditions for communities and populations.

purposive sampling

Refers to the selection of units of analysis to ensure that the processes involved are adequately studied, and where statistical representativeness is not required.

qualitative research

Research that focuses on the meanings and interpretations of the participants.

quantitative research

Research that focuses on the collection of statistical data.

'race'

A term without scientific basis that uses skin colour and facial features to describe allegedly biologically distinct groups of humans. It is a social construction that is used to categorise groups of people and usually infers assumed (and unproven) intellectual superiority or inferiority.

racism

Beliefs and actions used to discriminate against a group of people because of their physical and cultural characteristics.

randomised control trials (RCTs)

A biomedical research procedure used to evaluate the effectiveness of particular medications and therapeutic interventions. 'Random' refers to the equal chance of participants being in the experimental or control group (the group to which nothing is done and is used for comparison), and 'trial' refers to the experimental nature of the method. It is often mistakenly viewed as the best way to demonstrate causal links between factors under investigation, but privileges biomedical over social responses to illness.

rationalisation

The standardisation of social life through rules and regulations (see also McDonaldisation).

reductionism

The belief that all illnesses can be explained and treated by reducing them to biological and pathological factors.

research methods

Procedures used by researchers to collect and investigate data.

rigour

A term used by qualitative researchers to describe trustworthy research that carefully scrutinises and describes the meanings and interpretations given by participants.

risk or risk discourse

'Risk' refers to 'danger'. Risk discourse is often used in health promotion messages warning people that the lives they lead involve significant risks to their health.

risk factors

Conditions that are thought to increase an individual's susceptibility to illness or disease such as abuse of alcohol or smoking.

risk society

A term coined by Ulrich Beck (1992) to describe the centrality of risk calculations in people's lives in Western society, whereby the key problem of society today is unanticipated hazards, such as the risks of pollution and environmental degradation.

ruling class

This is a hotly debated term used to highlight the point that the upper class in society has political power as a result of its economic wealth. The term is often used interchangeably with 'upper class'.

self-determination

A government policy designed to ensure that Indigenous communities decide the pace and nature of their future development.

sexism in medicine

Refers to discriminatory and harmful treatment of women by doctors in terms of ignoring women's health concerns in medical research and intervention, not informing women about alternative treatments or the side effects of drugs/therapies, and labelling women's problems as 'psychosomatic' rather than 'real'.

sexual division of labour

This refers to the nature of work performed as a result of gender roles. The stereotype is that of the male breadwinner and the female home-maker.

sick role

A concept used by Talcott Parsons to describe the social expectations of how sick people are expected to act and of how they are meant to be treated.

social capital

A term used to refer to social relations, networks, norms, trust, and reciprocity between individuals that facilitate cooperation for mutual benefit.

social closure

A term first used by Max Weber to describe the way that power is exercised to exclude outsiders from the privileges of social membership (in social classes, professions, or status groups).

social cohesion

A term used to refer to the social ties that are the basis for group behaviour and integration.

social construction/constructionism

Refers to the socially created characteristics of human life based on the idea that people actively construct reality, meaning it is neither 'natural' nor inevitable. Therefore, notions of normality/abnormality, right/wrong, and health/illness are subjective human creations that should not be taken for granted.

social contract theory

Refers to the notion, prevalent in the works of Thomas Hobbes and Baruch Spinoza, that society is based on a contractual agreement regarding the collective exercise of power (typically by the state).

social control

Mechanisms that aim to induce conformity, or at least to manage or minimise deviant behaviour.

social Darwinism

The incorrect application of Charles Darwin's theory of animal evolution to explain social inequality by transferring his idea of 'survival of the fittest' among animals to 'explain' human inequality.

social death

The marginalisation and exclusion of elderly people from everyday life, resulting in social isolation.

social epidemiology, *see* epidemiology

social institutions

Formal structures within society—such as health care, government, education, religion, and the media—that are organised to address identified social needs.

socialism/communism

Political ideology with numerous variations, but generally refers to the creation of societies in which private property and wealth accumulation are replaced by state ownership and distribution of economic resources. Communism represents a utopian vision of society based on communal ownership of resources, cooperation, and altruism to the extent that social inequality and the state no longer exist. Both terms are often used interchangeably to refer to societies ruled by a communist party.

social justice

A belief system that gives high priority to the interests of the least advantaged.

social liberalism

An ideology that is based on individual freedom but that acknowledges the need for state intervention to overcome the inadequacies of the market, which can act to limit the freedom of individuals to fully participate in society.

social model of health

A model of health that focuses on social determinants such as the social production, distribution, and construction of health and illness, and the social organisation of health care. It directs attention to the prevention of illness through community participation and social reforms that address living and working conditions.

social structure

The recurring patterns of social interaction through which people are related to each other, such as social institutions and social groups.

social support

The support provided to an individual by being part of a network of kin, friends, or colleagues.

social wage

Government spending on health, social security, education, and housing (often referred to as welfare spending).

socialisation

The process of learning the culture of a society (its language and customs), which shows us how to behave and communicate.

sociobiology

A theory of evolutionary biology, associated with E. O. Wilson, that seeks to explain the evolution of social organisation and social behaviour as based on biological characteristics.

sociological determinism

A term used to describe the view that people's behaviour and beliefs are entirely shaped or determined by the social structure.

sociological imagination

A term coined by Charles Wright Mills to describe the sociological approach to analysing issues. We see the world through a sociological imagination, or think sociologically, when we make a link between personal troubles and public issues.

state

A term used to describe a collection of institutions, including the parliament (government and Opposition political parties), the public-sector bureaucracy, the judiciary, the military, and the police.

stigma

A physical or social trait, such as a disability or a criminal record, that results in negative social reactions such as discrimination and exclusion.

'stolen children'

Children who were forcibly removed from their families during the nineteenth and twentieth centuries by the agents of government in order to assimilate them into mainstream Australia.

structural explanations

Explanations that locate causality outside of the individual. For instance, these may include one's social class position, age, or gender.

structuralist-collectivist health promotion (SCHP)

SCHP encompasses a wide range of interventions, including participatory community programs, legislation, and bureaucratic interventions. The latter range from needle exchanges to the enactment of laws restricting industrial pollution, fireworks, flammable nightwear, cigarette advertising, and smoking in public places.

structure/agency debate

A key debate in sociology over the extent to which human behaviour is determined by social structure.

terra nullius

A Latin term used by the British to legally define Australia as an unoccupied land belonging to no one and therefore open to colonisation.

theodicy

An explanation of suffering, evil, and death.

theory

A system of ideas that uses researched evidence to explain certain events and to show why certain facts are related.

total institutions

A term used by Erving Goffman to refer to institutions such as prisons and asylums in which life is highly regulated and subjected to authoritarian control to induce conformity.

traditional medical system

Indigenous beliefs and practices about health and illness.

trait approach

A general theory that assumes that professional status can be achieved by meeting a set of criteria (usually defined as specialised expertise and training), by having the exclusive right to practise in a particular field, by self-regulation (based on a code of ethics), and by charging a fee for service.

trickle down

The theory that everyone benefits by allowing the upper class to prosper relatively unfettered. If wealthy capitalists are allowed and encouraged to maximise their profits, it is believed that this increased wealth will eventually 'trickle down' to the workers.

victim-blaming

The process whereby social inequality is explained in terms of individuals being solely responsible for what happens to them in relation to the choices they make and their assumed psychological, cultural, and/or biological inferiority.

women's health movement

A term used broadly to describe attempts to address sexism in medicine by highlighting the importance of gender in health research and treatment. Achievements include women's health centres and the National Women's Health Policy.

References

Abbott, A. 1988, *The System of Professions: An Essay on the Division of Expert Labor*, University of Chicago Press, Chicago.

Abbott, P. & Wallace, C. 1997, *An Introduction to Sociology: Feminist Perspectives*, 2nd edn, Routledge, London.

Abel-Smith, B. 1960, *A History of the Nursing Profession*, Heinemann, London.

Abercrombie, N., Hill, S., & Turner, B. 1988, *Dictionary of Sociology*, Penguin, London.

Aboriginal Health Development Group 1989, *Report to Commonwealth, State and Territory Ministers for Aboriginal Affairs and Health*, AGPS, Canberra.

Aboriginal and Torres Strait Islander Commission 1994, *The National Aboriginal Health Strategy: An Evaluation*, ATSIC, Canberra.

—— 1998, *As A Matter of Fact: Answering the Myth and Misconceptions about Indigenous Australians*, ATSIC, Canberra.

ABS, see Australian Bureau of Statistics.

Acheson, D. 1998, *Independent Inquiry into Inequalities in Health*, Stationery Office, London.

Acton, T. & Chambers, D. 1990, 'Where Was Sociology in the Struggle to Re-establish Public Health?', in P. Abbott & G. Payne (eds), *New Directions in the Sociology of Health*, Falmer, London, pp. 165–74.

Adam, B. & Sears, A. 1996, *Experience HIV*, Columbia University Press, New York.

Adler, S. R. 1996, 'Refugee Stress and Folk Belief: Hmong Sudden Deaths', *Social Science and Medicine*, vol. 40, no. 12, pp. 1623–9.

AIHW, see Australian Institute of Health and Welfare.

Alasuutari, P. 1995, *Researching Culture: Qualitative Method and Cultural Studies*, Sage, London.

Albrecht, G. L. 1992, *The Disability Business. Rehabilitation in America*, Sage, London.

Alcorso, C. & Schofield, T. 1991, *The National Non-English Speaking Background Women's Health Strategy*, AGPS, Canberra.

Alexander, J. C. 1998, *Neofunctionalism and After*, Blackwell, Oxford.

Alexander, J. C. (ed.) 1985, *Neofunctionalism*, Sage, Beverly Hills.

Alford, R. R. 1975, *Health Care Politics: Ideological and Interest Group Barriers to Reform*, University of Chicago Press, Chicago.

Allied Health Alliance NSW 1996, *Allied Health Alliance NSW: Terms of Reference*, unpublished document.

American Psychiatric Association 1952, *Diagnostic and Statistical Manual of Mental Disorders*, APA, Washington, DC.

—— 1987, *Diagnostic and Statistical Manual of Mental Disorders*, 3rd edn, APA, Washington, DC.

—— 1994, *Diagnostic and Statistical Manual of Mental Disorders*, 4th edn, APA, Washington, DC.

Ames, D. 1991, 'Geriatric Psychiatry in a Culturally Diverse Society', in I. H. Minas (ed.), *Cultural Diversity and Mental Health*, Royal Australian and New Zealand College of Psychiatrists—Victorian Transcultural Psychiatry Unit, Melbourne, pp. 115–24.

Andarin, C. 1998, *Public Health Policies and Social Inequality*, New York University Press, New York.

Anderson, B. 1983, *Imagined Communities: Reflections on the Origin and Spread of Nationalism*, Verso, London.

Anderson, P., Bhatia, K., & Cunningham, J. 1996, *Occasional Paper: Mortality of Indigenous Australians*, Cat. no. 3315.0, ABS & Australian Institute of Health and Welfare, Canberra.

Andrews, G. (ed.) 1991, *Citizenship*, Lawrence & Wishart, London.

Aneshensel, C. S., Rutter, C., & Lachenbruch, P. A. 1991, 'Social Structure, Stress, and Mental Health: Competing Conceptual and Analytic Models', *American Sociological Review*, vol. 56, pp. 166–78.

Annandale, E. & Clarke, J. 1996, 'What is Gender? Feminist Theory and the Sociology of Human Reproduction', *Sociology of Health and Illness*, vol. 18, no. 1, pp. 17–44.

Annandale, E. & Hunt, K., 2000, *Gender Inequalities and Health*, Open University Press, Buckingham.

Arber, S. 1991, 'Class, Paid Employment and Family Roles: Making Sense of Structural Disadvantage, Gender and Health Status', *Social Science and Medicine*, vol. 32, no. 4, pp. 425–36.

Archer, J.1995, *Bad Medicine*, Simon & Schuster, Sydney.

Aries, P. 1981, *The Hour of Our Death*, trans. H. Weaver, Knopf Publishers, New York.

Armstrong, D. 1983, *Political Anatomy of the Body: Medical Knowledge in Britain in the Twentieth Century*, Cambridge University Press, Cambridge.

—— 1984, 'The Patient's View', *Social Science and Medicine*, vol. 18, no. 9, pp. 737–44.

Ashton, J. 1990, 'Public Health and Primary Care: Towards a Common Agenda', *Public Health*, vol. 104, pp. 387–98.

—— (ed.) 1992, *Healthy Cities*, Open University Press, Buckingham.

Ashton, J. & Seymour, H. 1988, *The New Public Health: The Liverpool Experience*, Open University Press, Milton Keynes.

Astin, J. A. 1998, 'Why Patients use Alternative Medicine: Results of a National Study', *Journal of the American Medical Association*, vol. 279, no. 19, pp. 1548–53.

Astin J. A., Marie A., Pelletier K. R., Hansen E., & Haskell W. L. 1998, 'A Review of the Incorporation of Complementary and Alternative Medicine by Mainstream Physicians', *Archives of Internal Medicine*, vol. 158, pp. 2303–10.

ATSIC, see Aboriginal and Torres Strait Islander Commission.

Audit Commission 1991, *The Virtue of Patients: Making the Best Use of Ward Resources*, HMSO, London.

Auditor-General 1992, *Medifraud and Excessive Servicing*, Audit Report no. 17, Health Insurance Commission, Canberra.

Auditor-General of Victoria 1993, *Visiting Medical Officer Arrangements*, Special Report. no. 21, April, Victorian Department of Health, Melbourne.

Australian Bureau of Statistics 1992, *1989–90 National Health Survey: Health Related Actions*, Australia, Cat no. 43750, ABS, Canberra.

—— 1993, *Characteristics of Persons Employed in Health Occupations, Australia 1991*, Cat. no. 4346.0, ABS, Canberra.

—— 1994, 'Household and Family Trends in Australia', *Year Book Australia, 1994*, ABS, Canberra.

—— 1994, *Women's Health*, Cat. no. 4365.0, ABS, Canberra.

—— 1995, *Australian Women's Yearbook 1995*, Cat. no. 4124.0, ABS, Canberra.

—— 1996a, *Projections of the Populations of Australia, States and Territories*, Cat. no. 3222.0, ABS, Canberra.

—— 1996b, *Women's Safety Australia*, Cat. no. 4128.0, ABS, Canberra.

—— 1997, *National Health Survey: Summary of Results*, Cat. no. 4364.0, ABS, Canberra.

—— 1997, *National Health Survey 1995*, AGPS, Cat. no. 4368.0, ABS, Canberra.

—— 1998, *National Survey of Mental Health and Wellbeing: Profile of Adults, Summary of Results*, Cat. no. 4326.0, ABS, Canberra.

—— 1998, 'Experimental Estimates of the Aboriginal and Torres Strait Islander Population, 30 June 1971 – 30 June 1996', Cat. no. 3230.0, ABS, Canberra.

—— 1998, *Women's Health*, Cat. no. 4365.0, ABS, Canberra.

—— 1999a, 'Australia's Older Population: Past, Present and Future', Population Feature Article, *Australian Demographic Statistics*, Cat. no. 3101.0, ABS, Canberra.

—— 1999b, 'Deaths of Older Persons', Population Feature Article, *Australian Demographic Statistics*, Cat. no. 3101.0, ABS, Canberra.

—— 1999c, 'Housing—Housing Assistance: Home Care, Hostels and Nursing Homes', *Australian Social Trends 1999*, ABS, Canberra.

—— 1999d, 'International Comparisons—Population', *Australian Social Trends 1999*, ABS, Canberra.

—— 1999e, 'Older People, Australia: A Social Report 1999', Cat. no. 4109.0, ABS, Canberra.

—— 1999f, 'Population—Population Projections: Our Ageing Population, *Australian Social Trends*, ABS, Canberra

—— 2000, AusStats: Health Workforce [web site], ABS, <www.abs.gov>, date accessed: 17 January, 2001.

Australian Health Ministers 1995, *National Mental Health Policy*, AGPS, Canberra.

Australian Institute of Health and Welfare 1992, *Australia's Health 1992*, AGPS, Canberra.

—— 1994, *Australia's Health 1994*, AGPS, Canberra.

—— 1996a, *Australia's Health 1996*, AGPS, Canberra.

—— 1996b, *Health Expenditure Bulletin*, no. 12, December.

—— 1996c, *Tobacco Use and its Health Impact in Australia*, AIHW, Canberra.

—— 1996d, *Female Participation in the Australian Medical Workforce*, AIHW, Canberra.

—— 1998, *Australia's Health 1998*, AIHW, Canberra.

—— 1999a, *The Burden of Disease and Injury in Australia*, AIHW, Canberra.

—— 1999b, *Older Australia at a Glance*, AIHW, Canberra.

—— 2000, *Australia's Health 2000*, AIHW, Canberra.

Australian Medical Association 1993, *Position Statement on Women's Health*, AMA, Canberra.

Ayanian, J. Z. & Epstein, A. M. 1991, 'Differences in the Use of Procedures between Men and Women', *National Men's Health Conference*, AGPS, Canberra, pp. 100–11.

Bagenal, F. S. et al. 1990, 'Survival of Patients with Breast Cancer Attending Bristol Cancer Help Centre', *Lancet*, 8 September, pp. 606–10.

Barnett, J. R., Barnett, P., & Kearns, R. A. 1998, 'Declining Professional Dominance? Trends in the Proletarianisation of Primary Care in New Zealand', *Social Science and Medicine*, vol. 46, no. 2, pp. 193–207.

Barraclough, S. 1992, 'Policy through Legislation: Victoria's Tobacco Act', in H. Gardner (ed.), *Health Policy: Development, Implementation and Evaluation in Australia*, Churchill Livingstone, Melbourne, pp. 183–210.

Barrett, B., Kiefer, D., & Rabago, D. 1999, 'Assessing the Risks and Benefits of Herbal Medicine: An Overview of Scientific Evidence', *Alternative Therapies in Health and Medicine*, vol. 5, no. 4, pp. 40–50.

Barrett, M. 1991, *The Politics of Truth: From Marx to Foucault*, Polity Press, Cambridge.

Barrett, M. & Phillips, A. 1992, *Destabilizing Theory: Contemporary Feminist Debates*, Polity Press, Cambridge.

Barrett, M. & Roberts, H. 1978, 'Doctors and their Patients', in C. Smart & B. Smart (eds), *Women, Sexuality and Social Control*, Routledge, London, pp. 41–52.

Bartky, S. L. 1998, 'Foucault, femininity, and the modernization of patriarchal power', in R. Weitz (ed.), *The Politics of Women's Bodies: Sexuality, Appearance and Behavior*, Oxford University Press, New York.

Bartley, M., Ferrie, J., & Scott, S. M. 1999, 'Living in a High-unemployment Economy: Understanding the Health Consequences', in M. Marmot & R. G. Wilkinson (eds), *Social Determinants of Health*, Oxford University Press, Oxford, pp. 81–104.

Bates, E. 1983, *Health Systems and Public Scrutiny: Australia, Britain and the United States*, Croom Helm, London.

Bates, E. & Lapsley, H. 1985, *The Health Machine*, Penguin, Melbourne.

Batt, S. 1994, *Patient No More: The Politics of Breast Cancer*, Scarlet Press, London.

Baum, F. 1990, 'The New Public Health: Force for Change or Reaction?', *Health Promotion International*, vol. 5, no. 2, pp. 145–50.

—— (ed.) 1995, *Health For All: The South Australian Experience*, Wakefield Press, Adelaide.

—— 1996, 'Community Health Services and Managerialism', *Australian Journal of Primary Health*, vol. 2, no. 4, pp. 31–41.

—— 1998, *The New Public Health: An Australian Perspective*, Oxford University Press, Melbourne.

Baum, F., Fry, D., & Lennie, I. (eds) 1992, *Community Health: Policy and Practice in Australia*, Pluto Press, Sydney.

Baum, F., Kalucy, E. et al. 1996, *Medical Practice and Women's and Community Health Centres in South Australia*, SACHRU, Adelaide.

Baum, F., Palmer, C., Modra, C., Murray, C., & Bush, R. 2000, 'Families, Social Capital and Health', in I. Winter (ed.), *Social Capital and Public Policy in Australia*, Australian Institute of Family Studies, Melbourne, pp. 250–75.

Baum, F. & Sanders, D. 1995, 'Can Health Promotion and Primary Health Care Achieve Health for All without a Return to their More Radical Agenda?', *Health Promotion International*, vol. 10, no. 2, pp. 149–60.

Bauman, A., Harris, E., Leeder, S., Nutbeam, D., & Wise, M. 1993, *Goals and Targets for Australia's Health in the Year 2000 and Beyond*, AGPS, Canberra.

Bauman, Z. 1991, *Mortality, Immortality and Other Life Strategies*, Polity Press, Cambridge.

Baume, P. 1994, *A Cutting Edge: Australia's Surgical Workforce 1994*, report of the Inquiry into the Supply of, and Requirements for, Medical Specialist Services in Australia, AGPS, Canberra.

—— 1995, 'Voluntary Euthanasia—Mercy or Sin?', *New Doctor*, vol. 63, pp. 13–14.

Beaglehole, R. & Bonita, R. 1997, *Public Health at the Crossroads*, Cambridge University Press, Cambridge.

Beardshaw, V. & Robinson, R. 1990, *New for Old? Prospects for Nursing in the 1990s*, King's Fund Institute, London.

Beardsley, T. 1996, 'Trends in Human Genetics', *Scientific American*, March, pp. 25–7.

Beasley, C. 1999, *What is Feminism Anyway?*, Allen & Unwin, Sydney.

Beattie, A. 1991, 'Knowledge and Control in Health Promotion: A Test Case for Social Policy and Social Theory', in J. Gabe, M. Calnan, & M. Bury (eds), *The Sociology of the Health Service*, Routledge, London, pp. 162–202.

Beauchamp, T. L. & Faden, R. R. 1979, 'The Right to Health and the Right to Health Care', *The Journal of Medicine and Philosophy*, vol. 4, no. 2, pp. 118–31.

Beck, U. 1992, *Risk Society: Towards a New Modernity*, Sage, London.

Becker, H. S. 1963, *Outsiders: Studies in the Sociology of Deviance*, Free Press, New York.

Beckwith, J. 1991, 'Foreword: The Human Genome Initiative: Genetics', *Lightning Rod American Journal of Law and Medicine*, vol. 17, nos 1–2, pp. 1–13.

Beilharz, P., Considine, M., & Watts, R. 1992, *Arguing about the Welfare State: The Australian Experience*, Allen & Unwin, Sydney.

Beiner, R. (ed.) 1995, *Theorizing Citizenship*, State University of New York Press, Albany, NY.

Bennett, C. & Shearman, R. 1989, 'Maternity Services in New South Wales: Childbirth Moves towards the 21st Century', *Medical Journal of Australia*, vol. 150, pp. 673–6.

Bennett, P. & Hodgson, R. 1992, 'Psychology and Health Promotion', in R. Bunton & G. Macdonald (eds), *Health Promotion: Disciplines and Diversity*, Routledge, London, pp. 23–41.

Benzeval, M., Judge, K., & Whitehead, M. (eds) 1995, *Tackling Inequalities in Health: An Agenda or Action*, King's Fund, London.

Berger, P. L. 1966, *Invitation to Sociology: A Humanistic Perspective*, Penguin, Harmondsworth.

Berger, P. & Luckmann, T. 1967, *The Social Construction of Reality*, Penguin, Harmondsworth.

Berliner, H. S. 1984, 'Scientific Medicine since Flexner', in J. W. Salmon (ed.), *Alternative Medicines: Popular and Policy Perspectives*, Tavistock, New York.

Bensoussan, A. & Myers, S. P. 1996, *Towards a Safer Choice: The Practice of Traditional Chinese Medicine in Australia*, Faculty of Health, University of Western Sydney, Sydney.

Berman, B. M., Swyers, J. P., Hartnoll, M., Sigh, B. B, & Bausell, B. 2000, 'The Public Debate over Alternative Medicine: The Importance of Finding a Middle Ground', *Alternative Therapies in Health and Medicine*, vol. 6, no. 1, pp. 98–101.

Bessant, J. & Watts, R. 1999, *Sociology Australia*, Allen & Unwin, Sydney.

—— 2001, *Sociology Australia*, 2nd edn, Allen & Unwin, Sydney.

Better Health Commission 1986, *Looking Forward to Better Health*, AGPS, Canberra.

Bevan, K. 2000, 'Young People, Culture, Migration and Mental Health: A Review of the Literature', in M. Bashir & D. Bennett (eds), *Deeper Dimensions: Culture, Youth and Mental Health*, NSW Transcultural Mental Health Centre, Sydney, pp. 1–63.

Beveridge, W. H. 1944, *Full Employment in a Free Society*, Allen & Unwin, London.

Bicknell, N. A., Pieper, K. S., Lee, K. L., Mark, D. B., Glower, D. D., Pwor, D. B. et al. 1992, 'Referral Patterns for Coronary Artery Disease Treatment: Gender Bias or Good Clinical Judgment?', *Annals of Internal Medicine*, vol. 116, pp. 791–7.

Biggins, D. 1995, 'Occupational Health in Australia: Issues in the 1990s', *Annual Review of Health Social Sciences*, vol. 5, pp. 115–36.

Billings, P., Kohn, M., de Cuevas, M., Beckwith, J., Alper, J., & Natowicz, M. 1992, 'Discrimination as a Consequence of Genetic Testing', *American Journal of Human Genetics*, vol. 50, pp. 476–82.

Bittman, M. 1991, *Juggling Time: How Australian Families Use Time*, Office of the Status of Women, Canberra.

Blaxter, M. & Paterson, E. 1982, *Mothers and Daughters: A Three Generational Study of Health Attitudes and Behaviour*, Heinemann, London.

Blewett, N. 2000, 'The Politics of Health', *Australian Health Review*, vol. 23, no. 2, pp. 10–19.

—— 2000, 'Community Health Services', Speech given at Annual Public Health Association Conference, Canberra, December.

Bloom, A. L. 2000, *Health Reform in Australia and New Zealand*, Oxford University Press, Melbourne.

Blumer, M. & Rees, A. M. 1996, *Citizenship Today: The Contemporary Relevance of T. H. Marshall*, UCL Press, London.

BMA, see British Medical Association.

Bombardieri D. & Easthope G. 2000, 'Convergence between Orthodox and Alternative Medicine: A Theoretical Elaboration and Empirical Test', *Health*, vol. 4, no. 4, pp. 479–94.

Bordo, S. 1993, *Unbearable Weight: Feminism, Western Culture, and the Body*, University of California Press, Berkeley, Calif.

Borland, R., Donaghue, N., & Hill, D. 1994, 'Illnesses that Australians Most Feared in 1986 and 1993', *Australian Journal of Public Health*, vol. 18, pp. 366–9.

Bourdieu, P. 1984, *Distinction: A Social Critique of the Judgement of Taste*, Routledge & Kegan Paul, London.

—— 1986, 'The Forms of Capital', in J. Richardson (ed.), *Handbook of Theory and Research for the Sociology of Education*, Greenwood Press, New York, pp. 241–58.

Boyce, R. A. 1991, 'Hospital Restructuring: The Implications for Allied Health Professionals', *Australian Health Review*, vol. 14, pp. 147–54.

—— 1995, 'The Business of Economic Reform in Health: What's Allied Health Got to do with It?', *Proceedings of the South-West Pacific Regional Dietitians Conference*, 11–13 May 1995, Brisbane, Dietitians Association of Australia, Canberra.

—— 1996, 'Researching the Organisation of Allied Health Professions: Sorting Fact from Fantasy', paper presented at the Second National Allied Health Conference, 15–16 November, Sydney.

Brady, M. 1990, 'Indigenous and Government Attempts to Control Alcohol Use among Australian Aborigines', *Contemporary Drug Problems*, vol. 17, no. 2, pp. 195–220.

—— 1991, 'Drug and alcohol use among Aboriginal people' in J. Reid & P. Trompf, *The Health of Aboriginal Australia*, Harcourt Brace Jovanovich, Sydney.

Braithwaite, J. 1984, *Corporate Crime in the Pharmaceutical Industry*, Routledge & Kegan Paul, London.

Bray, F. & Chapman, S. 1991, 'Community Knowledge, Attitudes and Media Recall about AIDS, Sydney 1988 and 1989', *Australian Journal of Public Health*, vol. 15, pp. 107–13.

British Medical Association 1993, *Complementary Medicine: New Approaches to Good Practice*, Oxford University Press, Oxford.

Broadhead, P. 1985, 'Social Status and Morbidity in Australia', *Community Health Studies*, vol. 9, no. 2, pp. 87–98.

Brock, P. 1993, *Outback Ghettos: Aborigines, Institutionalisation and Survival*, Cambridge University Press, Melbourne.

Broderick, D. & Laris, P. 1995, 'The South Australian Community Health Association', in F. Baum (ed.), *Health For All: The South Australian Experience*, Wakefield Press, Adelaide, ch. 14, pp. 230–41.

Bromberger, B. & Fife-Yeomans, J. 1991, *Deep Sleep: Harry Bailey and the Scandal of Chelmsford*, Simon & Schuster, Sydney.

Broom, D. 1984, 'The Social Distribution of Illness: Is Australia More Equal?', *Social Science and Medicine*, vol. 18, no. 11, pp. 909–17.

—— 1986, 'The Occupational Health of Houseworkers', *Australian Feminist Studies*, vol. 2, pp. 15–34.

—— 1991, *Damned if We Do: Contradictions in Women's Health Care*, Allen & Unwin, Sydney.

—— 1994, 'Taken Down and Used against Us', in C. Waddell & A. R. Petersen (eds), *Just Health: Inequality in Illness, Care and Prevention*, Churchill Livingstone, Melbourne, pp. 397–405.

—— 1997, *There Should Be More: Women's Use of Community Health Facilities*, National Centre for Epidemiology and Population Health, Canberra.

Broom, D. H. & Woodward, R. V. 1996, 'Medicalisation Reconsidered: Toward a Collaborative Approach to Care', *Sociology of Health and Illness*, vol. 18, no. 3, pp. 57–78.

Broom-Darroch, D. 1978, 'Power and Participation: The Dynamics of Medical Encounters', PhD thesis, Australian National University, Canberra.

Brown, E. R. 1979, *Rockefeller Medicine Men*, University of California Press, Berkeley, Calif.

Brown, K., Kenny, S., & Turner, B. S. 2000, *Rhetorics of Welfare: Uncertainty, Choice and Voluntary Associations*, Macmillan, Basingstoke.

Brown, S. & Owen, N. 1992, 'Self-help Smoking Cessation Materials', *Australian Journal of Public Health*, vol. 16, pp. 188–91.

Brown, W., Bryson, L., Byles, J., Dobson, A., Manderson, L., Schofield, M. et al. 1996, 'Women's Health Australia: Establishment of the Australian Longitudinal Study on Women's Health', *Journal of Women's Health*, vol. 5, no. 5, pp. 467–72.

Brown, W. & Redman, S. 1995, 'Setting Targets: A Three-stage Model for Determining Priorities for Health Promotion', *Australian Journal of Public Health*, vol. 19, pp. 263–9.

Brownlea, A. 1987, 'Participation, Myth, Realities and Prognosis', *Social Science and Medicine*, vol. 25, pp. 605–14.

Brundtland Report 1987, see World Commission on Environment and Development.

Bryson, L. 1991, 'Education for Public Sector Management', *Australian Journal of Public Administration*, vol. 50, no. 2, pp. 191–8.

Bumiller, K. 1987, 'Victims in the Shadow of the Law: A Critique of the Model of Legal Protection', *Signs: Journal of Women in Culture and Society*, vol. 12, pp. 421–39.

Burdess, N. 1996, 'Class and Health', in C. Grbich (ed.), *Health in Australia: Sociological Concepts and Issues*, Prentice Hall, Sydney, pp. 163–87.

Bury, M. & Gabe, J. 1990, 'Hooked? Media Responses to Tranquilizer Dependence', in P. Abbott & G. Payne (eds), *New Directions in the Sociology of Health*, Falmer, London, pp. 87–103.

Bury, M. R. 1986, 'Social Constructionism and the Development of Medical Sociology', *Sociology of Health and Illness*, vol. 8, no. 3, pp. 137–69.

Busfield, J. 1988, 'Mental Illness as Social Product or Social Construct: A Contradiction in Feminists' Arguments?', *Sociology of Health and Illness*, vol. 10, no. 4, pp. 521–42.

—— 1989, 'Sexism and Psychiatry', *Sociology*, vol. 23, pp. 343–64.

Butler, J. 1990, *Gender Trouble: Feminism and the Subversion of Identity*, Routledge, London.

Button, V. 2000, 'Genetic Testing: Call for Reform', *Age*, 21 July: <www.theage.com.au/news/20000721/A19870-2000Jul20.html>

Byde, P. 1995, 'Contexts and Communication for Health Promotion', in G. M. Lupton & J. Najman (eds), *Sociology of Health and Illness: Australian Readings*, 2nd edn, Macmillan, Melbourne, pp. 301–24.

Bytheway, B. 1995, *Ageism*, Open University Press, Buckingham.

Callahan, D. 1990, *What Kind of Life: The Limits of Medical Progress*, Simon & Schuster, New York.

Caplan, A. 1992, *When Medicine Went Mad: Bioethics and the Holocaust*, Humana, New Jersey.

Caplan, A. & Merz, J. 1996, 'Patenting Gene Sequences: Not in the Best Interests of Science or Society' (editorial), *British Medical Journal*, vol. 44 p. 7036.

Capra, F. 1982, *The Turning Point: Science, Society and the Rising Culture*, Simon & Schuster, Great Britain.

Cashman, P. 1989, 'The Dalkon Shield', in P. Grabosky & A. Sutton (eds), *Stains on a White Collar*, Hutchinson, Sydney.

Cassileth, B. R., Lusk, E. J., Miller, D. S., Brown, L. L., & Miller, C. 1985, 'Psychosocial Correlates of Survival in Advanced Malignant Disease?', *New England Journal of Medicine*, vol. 312, no. 24, pp. 1551–5.

Castel, R. 1991, 'From Dangerousness to Risk', in G. Burchell, C. Gordon, & P. Miller (eds), *The Foucault Effect: Studies in Governmentality with Two Lectures and an Interview with Michel Foucault*, Harvester Wheatsheaf, London.

Castles, S. 1992, 'Australian Multiculturalism: Social Policy and Identity in a Changing Society', in G. Freeman & J. Jupp (eds), *Nations of Immigrants: Australia, the United States, and International Migration*, Oxford University Press, Melbourne, ch. 11, pp. 184–201.

Castles, S. & Davidson, A. 2000, *Citizenship and Migration*, Macmillan, London.

Castles, S., Foster, W., Iredale, R., & Withers, G. 1998, *Immigration and Australia: Myths and Realities*, Allen & Unwin, Sydney.

Castles, S. & Miller, M. 1998, *The Age of Migration*, 2nd edn, Macmillan, London.

Castles, S., Kalantzis, M., & Cope, B. 1986, 'W(h)ither Multiculturalism?', *Australian Society*, October, pp. 15–18.

Causer, G. & Exworthy, M. 1999, 'Professionals as Managers Across the Public Sector', in M. Exworthy & S. Halford (eds), *Professionals and the New Managerialism in the Public Sector*, Open University Press, Buckingham.

CDHSH, see Commonwealth Department of Human Services and Health.

Chapman, S. 1998, 'Postmodernism and public health', *Australian and New Zealand Journal of Public Health*, vol. 22, no. 3, pp. 403–5.

Charlesworth, M. 1992, *Distributing Health Care Resources: Ethical Assumptions*, Australian Health Ethics Committee, Canberra.

Charmaz, K. 1994, 'Identity dilemmas of chronically ill men', *The Sociological Quarterly*, vol. 35, pp. 269–88.

Clarke, J., Gewirtz, S., & McLaughlin. E. (eds) 2000, *New Managerialism, New Welfare?*, The Open University and Sage, London.

Clarke, J. & Newman, J. 1997, *The Managerial State: Power, Politics and Ideology in the Remaking of Social Welfare*, Sage, London.

Coburn, D. 1988, 'Canadian Medicine: Dominance or Proletarianization?', *The Milbank Quarterly*, vol. 62, no. 2, pp. 92–116.

—— 1992, 'Freidson Then and Now: An Internalist Critique of Freidson's Past and Present Views of the Medical Profession', *International Journal of Health Services*, vol. 22, no. 3, pp. 497–512.

—— 2000, 'Income Inequality, Social Cohesion and the Health Status of Populations: The Role of Neoliberalism', *Social Science and Medicine*, vol. 51, no. 1, pp. 135–46.

Coburn, D., Rappolt, S., & Bourgeault, I. 1997, 'Decline vs. Retention of Medical Power Through Restratification: An Examination of the Ontario Case', *Sociology of Health & Illness*, vol. 19, no. 1, pp. 1–22.

Coburn, D. & Willis, E. 2000, 'The Medical Profession: Knowledge, Power, and Autonomy', in G. L. Albrecht, R. Fitzpatrick, & S. C. Scrimshaw (eds), *Handbook of Social Studies in Health and Medicine*, Sage, London, pp. 377–93.

Cocozza, J. J. & Steadman, H. J. 1978, 'Prediction in Psychiatry: An Example of Misplaced Confidence in Experts', *Social Problems*, vol. 25, pp. 265–76.

Coleman, J. 1988, 'Social Capital in the Creation of Human Capital', *American Journal of Sociology*, vol. 94, pp. 95–120

Coleman, V. 1994, 'Betrayal of Trust', *British Medical Journal*, vol. 42, p. 9602.

Collins, J. 1991, *Migrant Hands in a Distant Land*, 2nd edn, Pluto Press, Sydney.

—— 1996, 'The changing political economy of Australian racism', in E. Vasta & S. Castles (eds), *The Teeth are Smiling: The Persistence of Racism in Multicultural Australia*, Allen & Unwin, Sydney, pp. 73–96.

Collins, R. 1975, *Conflict Sociology: Towards an Explanatory Science*, Academic Press, New York.

Comaroff, J. 1993, 'The Diseased Heart of Africa: Medicine, Colonialism, and the Black Body', in S. Lindenbaum, S. Lock, & M. Lock (eds), *Knowledge, Power and Practice: The Anthropology of Medicine and Everyday Life*, University of California Press, Berkeley, Calif.

Comeau, P. & Santin, A. 1995, *The First Canadians: A Profile of Canada's Native People Today*, James Lorimer & Co., Toronto.

Commission of the European Communities 1989, *Modified Proposal for a Council Decision, Adopting a Specific Research and Technological Development Program in the Field of Health (1990–1991)*, 13 November, CEC, Brussels.

Commonwealth of Australia, Senate Community Affairs References Committee, 2000, *First Report—Public Hospital Funding and Options for Reform*, Commonwealth of Australia, Canberra, [web site] <www.aph.gov.au/senate/committee/clac_ctte/phealth_first/contents.htm>

Commonwealth Department of Community Services and Health 1989, *National Women's Health Policy: Advancing Women's Health in Australia*, AGPS, Canberra.

Commonwealth Department of Health and Aged Care 2000, Health Financing Series Occasional Papers [web site] <http://www.health.gov.au/pubs/hfsocc/occpdf.htm>, Commonwealth Department of Health and Aged Care, Canberra, date accessed: 30 November 2001.

Commonwealth Department of Health and Aged Care 2000, New Series Occasional Papers [web site] <http://www.health.gov.au/pubs/hfsocc/occpdf.htm>, Commonwealth Department of Health and Aged Care, Canberra, date accessed: 30 November 2001.

Commonwealth Department of Health and Aged Care 2001, First Series Occasional Papers [web site] <http://www.health.gov.au/pubs/hfsocc/occpdf.htm>, Commonwealth Department of Health and Aged Care, Canberra, date accessed: 30 November 2001.

Commonwealth Department of Health and Family Services 2001, *General Practice in Australia: 1996*, Canberra; General Practice Branch, Commonwealth Department of Health and Family Services.

Community and Public Service Union 1995, CPSU Policy Position on Allied Health Management Structures, unpublished document.

Coney, S. 1988, *The Unfortunate Experiment*, Penguin, Melbourne.

Connell, R. W. 1977, *Ruling Class, Ruling Culture*, Cambridge University Press, Cambridge.

—— 1983, *Which Way is Up? Essays on Sex, Class and Culture*, Allen & Unwin, Sydney.

—— 1987, *Gender and Power*, Allen & Unwin, Sydney.

—— 1988, 'Class Inequalities and "Just Health"', *Community Health Studies*, vol. 12, no. 2, pp. 212–17.

—— 1995, *Masculinities*, Allen & Unwin, Sydney.

Connell, R. W. & Irving, T. H. 1992, *Class Structure in Australian History: Poverty and Progress*, 2nd edn, Longman Cheshire, Melbourne.

Connolly, E. 2000, 'Court Criticises Doctors Over Coma Patient', *Sydney Morning Herald*, 30 December, p. 1.

Cooley, C. H. 1964/1906, *Human Nature and the Social Order*, Scribner's, New York.

Connolly, W. E. 1995, *The Ethos of Pluralisation*, University of Minnesota Press, Minneapolis.

Conrad, P. 1992, 'Medicalization and Social Control', *Annual Review of Sociology*, vol. 18, pp. 209–32.

—— 1997, 'Public Eyes and Private Genes: Historical Frames, News Constructions and Social Problems', *Social Problems*, vol. 44, no. 2, pp. 139–54.

Conrad, P. & Gabe, J. 1999, 'Introduction: Sociological Perspectives on the New Genetics: An Overview', *Sociology of Health and Illness*, vol. 21, no. 5, pp. 505–16

Conrad, P. & Schneider, J. 1992, *Deviance and Medicalisation: From Badness to Sickness*, 2nd edn, Temple University Press, Philadelphia.

Considine, M. 1988, 'The Corporate Management Framework as Administrative Science: A Critique', *Australian Journal of Public Administration*, vol. 47, no. 1, pp. 36–45.

—— 1990, 'Managerialism Strikes Out', *Australian Journal of Public Administration*, vol. 49, no. 2, pp. 166–78.

Consumers' Health Forum 1994, 'A Landmark Case in South Australia on Overcharging by Doctors', *Health Forum*, no. 30, July, p. 3.

Cook-Deegan, R. 1994, *The Gene Wars: Science, Politics and the Human Genome*, Norton, New York.

Cooper, N., Stevenson, C., & Hale, G. (eds) 1996, *Integrating Perspectives on Health*, Open University Press, Buckingham.

Coote, A. (ed.) 1992, *The Welfare of Citizens: Developing New Social Rights*, Rivers Oram Press, London.

Cormack, M. & Hindle, D. 1999, 'In Strife Again: The Next Great Health Debate', *Australian Health Review*, vol. 22, no. 3, pp. 3–6.

Cowlishaw, G. 1988, *Black, White or Brindle: Race in Rural Australia*, Cambridge University Press, Melbourne.

Cox, D. R. 1989, *Welfare Practice in a Multicultural Society*, Prentice Hall, Sydney.

Cox, E. 1995, *A Truly Civic Society: Boyer Lectures 1995*, ABC Books, Sydney.

Cox, S. & McKellin, S. 1999, 'There's This Thing in Our Family: Predictive Testing and the Construction of Risk for Huntington Disease', *Sociology of Health and Illness*, vol. 21, no. 5, pp. 622–46.

Craib, I. 1992, *Modern Social Theory*, 2nd edn, Harvester Wheatsheaf, London.

Crawford, R. 1980, 'Healthism and the Medicalisation of Everyday Life', *International Journal of Health Services*, vol. 10, no. 3, pp. 365–88.

—— 1984, 'A Cultural Account of "Health": Control Release and the Social Body', in J. McKinlay (ed.), *Issues in the Political Economy of Health Care*, Tavistock, London, pp. 60–103.

Crichton, A. 1990, *Slowly Taking Control? Australian Governments and Health Care Provision 1788–1988*, Allen & Unwin, Sydney.

Crompton, R. 1998, *Class and Stratification: An Introduction to Current Debates*, 2nd edn, Polity Press, Cambridge.

Crowley, S., Dunt, D., & Day, N. 1995, 'Cost-effectiveness of Alternative Interventions for the Prevention and Treatment of Coronary Heart Disease', *Australian Journal of Public Health*, vol. 19, pp. 336–46.

Cunningham, J., Sibthorpe, B., & Anderson, I. 1997, *Self-assessed Health Status, Indigenous Australians, 1994*, Australian Bureau of Statistics, National Centre for Epidemiology & Population Health, Canberra.

Dalton, T., Draper, M., Weeks, W., & Wiseman, J. 1996, *Making Social Policy in Australia: An Introduction*, Allen & Unwin, Sydney.

Daly, J., Kellehear, A., & Glicksman, M. 1997, *The Public Health Researcher*, Oxford University Press, Melbourne.

Daniel, A. 1990, *Medicine and the State*, Allen & Unwin, Sydney.

—— 1995, 'The Politics of Health: Medicine Versus the State', in G. M. Lupton & J. M. Najman (eds), *Sociology of Health and Illness: Australian Readings*, 2nd edn, Macmillan, Melbourne, pp. 57–76.

—— 1998, *Scapegoats for a Profession: Uncovering Procedural Injustice*, Harwood Academic, Amsterdam.

Daniels, N. 1985, *Just Health Care*, Cambridge University Press, Cambridge.

Davies, C. 1977, 'Continuities in the Development of Hospital Nursing in Britain', *Journal of Advanced Nursing*, vol. 2, pp. 479–93.

Davis, L. 1995, *Enforcing Normalcy: Disability, Deafness, and the Body*, Verso, London.

Davison, C., Finkel, S., & Davey Smith, G. D. 1992, '"To Hell with Tomorrow": Coronary Heart Disease Risk and the Ethnography of Fatalism', in S. Scott et al. (eds), *Private Risks and Public Dangers*, Aldershot, Avebury, pp. 95–111.

Day, R. & Day, J.V. 1977, 'A Review of the Current State of Negotiated Order Theory: An Appreciation and a Critique', *The Sociological Quarterly*, vol. 18, Winter, pp. 126–42.

De Vault, M. L. 1995, 'Between Science and Food: Nutrition Professionals in the Health Care Hierarchy', in J. J. Kronenfeld (ed.), *Research in the Sociology of Health Care: Patients, Consumers, Providers and Caregivers*, vol. 12, JAI Press, Connecticut, pp. 60–75.

Deeble, J. 1991, *Medical Services Through Medicare*, Background Paper no. 2, AGPS, Canberra.

Deeble, J., Mathers, C., Smith, L. et al. 1998, *Expenditures on Health Services for Aboriginal and Torres Strait Islander People*, Australian Institute for Health and Welfare, Department of Health & Family Services and National Centre for Epidemiology and Population Health, Canberra.

Dent, M. 1998, 'Hospitals and New Ways of Organisation of Medical Work in Europe: Standardisation of Medicine in the Public Sector and the Future of Medical Autonomy', in P. Thompson & C. Warhurst (eds), *Workplaces of the Future*, Macmillan, London.

—— 1993, 'Professionalism, Educated Labour and the State: Hospital Medicine and the New Managerialism', *The Sociological Review*, vol. 41, no. 2, pp. 244–73.

Denzin, N. 1997, *Interpretive Ethnography*, Sage, London.

Department of Health and Aged Care 1998, *National Mental Health Report 1997*, AGPS Canberra.

—— 1999, *Mental Health Information Development*, AGPS, Canberra.

—— 2000, *Annual Report*, Department of Health and Aged Care, Canberra: <www.health.gov.au/pubs/annrep/ar2000/index.htm>

Department of Health and Social Security 1980, *Inequalities in Health*, Report of a Working Group Chaired by Sir Douglas Black, DHSS, London.

Department of Human Services and Health 1994, *Better Health Outcomes for Australians: National Goals, Targets and Strategies for Better Health Outcomes into the Next Century*, AGPS, Canberra.

—— 1995, *Mental Health Statement of Rights and Responsibilities*, AGPS, Canberra.

—— 1996, *National Drug Strategy Household Survey: Urban Aboriginal and Torres Strait Islander Peoples Supplement 1994*, Australian Government Publishing Service, Canberra.

Derkley, K. 1998, 'Easing the Pressure Points', *Age*, 19 June, p. 21.

Dew, K. 2000, 'Apostasy to Orthodoxy: Debates Before a Commission of Inquiry into Chiropractic', *Sociology of Health and Illness*, vol. 22, no. 3, pp. 310–30.

Dewdney, J. C. H. 1972, *Australian Health Services*, John Wiley & Sons, Sydney.

DHSH, see Department of Human Services and Health.

DHSS, see Department of Health and Social Security.

Dickson, D. 1974, *Alternative Technology and the Politics of Technological Change*, Fontana, Glasgow.

Dilnot, A. 1990, 'From Most to Least: New Figures on Wealth Distribution', *Australian Society*, July, pp. 14–17.

Dingwall, R., Rafferty, A. M., & Webster, C. 1988, *An Introduction to the Social History of Nursing*, Routledge, London.

'The Doctors versus the Nurses' 1962, *Nursing Times*, 15 June, pp. 783–4.

Donaldson, L. J. 2000, 'Clinical Governance—a Mission to Improve', *British Journal of Clinical Governance*, vol. 5, no. 1, pp. 1–8.

—— 1998, 'Clinical Governance and Service Failure in the NHS', *Public Money and Management*, vol. 18, no. 4, pp. 10–11.

Doran, B. 1999, The Growth of Alternative Therapies as a Challenge to Medical Dominance, unpublished honours thesis, School of Sociology and Social Work, University of Tasmania.

Doyal, L. 1979, *The Political Economy of Health*, Pluto, London.

—— 1995, *What Makes Women Sick: Gender and the Political Economy of Health*, Rutgers University Press, New Brunswick, NJ.

Draper, E. 1991, *Risky Business: Genetic Testing and Exclusionary Practice in Hazardous Workplaces*, Cambridge University Press, Cambridge.

Driscoll, T. & Mayhew, C. 1999, 'Extent and Cost of Occupational Injury and Illness', in C. Mayhew & C. L. Peterson (eds), *Occupational Health and Safety in Australia*, Allen & Unwin, Sydney, pp. 28–51.

Dubos, R. 1959, *Mirage of Health: Utopias, Progress, and Biological Change*, Harper & Row, New York.

—— 1968, *Man, Medicine, and Environment*, Pall Mall Press, London.

Duckett, S. J. 1984, 'Structural Interests and Australian Health Policy', *Social Science and Medicine*, vol. 18, no. 11, pp. 959–66.

—— 1995, 'The Australian Health Care System: An Overview', in G. M. Lupton & J. M. Najman (eds), *Sociology of Health and Illness: Australian Readings*, 2nd edn, Macmillan, Melbourne.

—— 1996, 'The New Market in Health Care: Prospects for Managed Care in Australia', *Australian Health Review*, vol. 19, no. 2, pp. 7–22.

—— 2000, *The Australian Health Care System*, Oxford University Press, Melbourne.

Duffin, J. 1999, *History of Medicine*, University of Toronto Press, Toronto.

Durkheim, É. 1951/1897, *Suicide*, Free Press, New York.

—— 1893/1984, *The Division of Labor in Society*, trans. W. Halls, Free Press, New York.

Duster, T. 1990, *Backdoor to Eugenics*, Routledge, New York.

du Toit, D. 1995, 'The Allied Health Professionals in Australia: Physio, Occupational and Speech Therapy Professions', in G. M. Lupton & J. M. Najman (eds), *Sociology of Health and Illness: Australian Readings*, 2nd edn, Macmillan, Melbourne.

Easteal, P. 1996, *Shattered Dreams: Marital Violence Against Overseas-born Women in Australia*, AGPS, Canberra.

Easteal, P. W. 1993, *Killing the Beloved: Homicide Between Adult Sexual Intimates*, Australian Institute of Criminology, Canberra.

Easthope, G. 1985, 'Marginal Healers', in K. Jones (ed.), *Sickness and Sectarianism*, Gower, Aldershot, pp. 51–71.

—— 1986, *Healers and Alternative Medicine*, Gower, Aldershot.

—— 1993, 'The Response of Orthodox Medicine to the Challenge of Alternative Medicine in Australia', *Australian and New Zealand Journal of Sociology*, vol. 29, no. 3, pp. 289–301.

Easthope, G., Beilby, J., Gill, G., & Tranter, B. 1998, 'Acupuncture in Australian General Practice: Practitioner Characteristics, *Medical Journal of Australia*, vol. 169, no. 4, pp. 197–200.

Easthope, G., Gill, G., Beilby, J., & Tranter, B. 1999, 'Acupuncture in Australian General Practice: Patient Characteristics', *Medical Journal of Australia*, vol. 170, no. 6, pp. 259–62.

Easthope, G. & Julian, R. 1996, 'Mental Health and Ethnicity', in M. Clinton & S. Nelson (eds), *Mental Health and Nursing Practice*, Prentice Hall, Sydney, ch. 7, pp. 121–37.

Easthope, G., Tranter, B., & Gill, G. 2001, 'The Incorporation of an Alternative Therapy by Australian General Practitioners: the Case of Acupuncture', *Australian Journal of Primary Health-Interchange*, vol. 7, no. 1.

—— 2000a, 'General Practitioners' Attitudes Toward Complementary Therapies', *Social Science and Medicine*, vol. 51, pp. 1555–61.

—— 2000b 'The Normal Medical Practice of Referring Patients for Complementary Therapies Among Australian General Practitioners', *Journal of Complementary Therapies in Medicine*, vol. 8, no. 4, pp. 241–7.

Eastwood, H. 2000, 'Why are Australian GPs Using Alternative Medicine? Postmodernisation, Consumerism and the Shift Towards Holistic Health', *Journal of Sociology*, vol. 36, no. 2, pp. 133–56.

Eccleston, B. 1997, 'Bad Medicine', *The Weekend Australian*, 21–22 June, p. 1.

Eckerman, E. 1999, 'Towards a New Gendered and "Differentiated" Social Epidemiology', in L. Hancock (ed.), *Analysing Health Policy*, Allen & Unwin, Sydney.

Eckholm, D. 1987, *The Picture of Health: Environmental Sources of Disease*, W. W. Norton, New York.

Eder, K. 1993, *The New Politics of Class: Social Movements and Cultural Dynamics in Advanced Societies*, Sage, London.

Edwards, A. 1988, *Regulation and Repression*, Allen & Unwin, Sydney.

Ehrenreich, B. & English, D. 1973, *Witches, Midwives and Nurses*, Old Westbury Feminist Press, New York.

—— 1974, *Complaints and Disorders: The Sexual Politics of Sickness*, Compendium, London.

—— 1979, *For Her Own Good: 150 Years of Experts' Advice*, Pluto Press, London.

Eisenberg, D. M., Davis, R. B., Ettner, S. L., Appel, S., Wilkey, S., Van Rompay, M., & Kessler, R. C. 1998, 'Trends in Alternative Medicine use in the United States, 1990–1997, *JAMA*, vol. 289, no. 18, pp. 1569–75.

Eisner, M. A. 1993, *Regulatory Politics in Transition*, John Hopkins University Press, Baltimore.

Elkin, A. P. 1977, *Aboriginal Men of High Degree*, University of Queensland Press, St Lucia.

Elliott, H. 1995, 'Community Nutrition Education for People with Coronary Heart Disease: Who Attends?', *Australian Journal of Public Health*, vol. 19, pp. 205–10.

Ellis, C. 1995, *Final Negotiations: A Story of Love, Loss, and Chronic Illness*, Temple University Press, Philadelphia.

—— 1998, 'Exploring Loss through Autoethnographic Inquiry', in J. Harvey (ed.), *Perspectives on Loss: A Sourcebook*, Mazel, Brunner.

Elston, M. A. 1991, 'The Politics of Professional Power: Medicine in a Changing Health Service', in J. Gabe, M. Calnan, & M. Bury (eds), *The Sociology of the Health Service*, Routledge, London, pp. 58–88.

Encel, S. 1970, *Equality and Authority*, Cheshire, Melbourne.

Engel, G. L. 1977, 'The need for a new medical model: A challenge for biomedicine', *Science*, vol. 196, pp. 129–36.

—— 1980, 'The Clinical Application of the Biopsychosocial Model', *American Journal of Psychiatry*, vol. 137, no. 5, pp. 535–44.

Engels, F. 1958/1845, *The Condition of the Working Class in England*, trans. W. O. Henderson & W. H. Chaloner, Basil Blackwell, Oxford.

Engleman, S. & Forbes, J. 1986, 'Economic Aspects of Health Education', *Social Science and Medicine*, vol. 22, no. 2, pp. 443–58.

Ernst, E. 1996, 'Complementary Medicine: Doing More Good than Harm?', *British Journal of General Practice*, vol. 46, no. 403, pp. 60–1.

Ernst, E. & White, A. 2000, 'The BBC Survey of Complementary Medicine use in the UK', *Journal of Complementary Therapies in Medicine*, vol. 8, no. 1, pp. 32–6.

Estroff, S. 1995, 'Whose story is it anyway? Authority, voice, and responsibility in narratives of chronic illness', in S. Toombs, D. Barnard, & R. Carson (eds), *Chronic Illness: From Experience to Policy*, Indiana University Press, Bloomington.

Evatt Foundation 1996, *The State of Australia*, Evatt Foundation, Sydney.

Ewer, P., Hampson, I., Lloyd, C., Rainford, J., Rix, S., & Smith, M. 1991, *Politics and the Accord*, Pluto Press, Sydney.

Exworthy, M. & Halford, S. (eds) 1999, *Professionals and the New Managerialism in the Public Sector*, Open University Press, Buckingham.

Ezzy, D. 2000a, 'Illness narratives: time, hope and HIV', *Social Science and Medicine*, vol. 50, pp. 605–17.

—— 2000b, 'Fate and Agency in Job Loss Narratives', *Qualitative Sociology*, vol. 23, no. 1, pp. 121–34.

—— 2001, *Qualitative Analysis*, Allen & Unwin, Sydney.

—— 2002 'Finding Life through Facing Death', in B. Rumbold (ed.), *Spirituality and Palliative Care*, Oxford University Press, Melbourne.

Fadiman, A. 1997, *The Spirit Catches You and You Fall Down*, Farrar, Straus and Giroux, New York.

Famighetti, R. 1995, *The World Almanac and Book of Facts*, Funk & Wagnalls Corporation, New York.

Featherstone, M. 1991, 'The Body in Consumer Culture', in M. Featherstone, M. Hepworth, & B. Turner, *The Body: Social Process and Cultural Theory*, Sage, London, pp. 170–96.

Featherstone, M. & Hepworth, M. 1995, 'Images of Positive Aging: A Case Study of Retirement Choice Magazine', in M. Featherstone & A. Wernick (eds), *Images of Aging: Cultural Representations of Later Life*, Routledge, London, pp. 182–95.

Featherstone, M. Hepworth, M., & Turner, B. S. (eds) 1991, *The Body: Social Process and Cultural Theory*, Sage, London.

Fee, E. & Krieger, N. (eds) 1994, *Women's Health, Politics, and Power: Essays on Sex/Gender, Medicine, and Public Health*, Baywood, New York.

Feibach, N. H., Viscoli, C. M., & Horwitz, R. I. 1990, 'Differences between Women and Men in Survival after Myocardial Infarction', *Journal of the American Medical Association*, vol. 263, no. 8, pp. 1092–6.

Feinstein, A. 1985, *Clinical Epidemiology*, W. B. Saunders Co., Philadelphia.

Ferguson, B. & Pittaway, E. (eds) 1999, *Nobody Wants to Talk About It: Refugee Women's Mental Health*, Transcultural Mental Health Centre, Sydney.

Finch, J. 1996, 'Family Responsibilities and Rights', in M. Bulmer & A. M. Rees (eds), *Citizenship Today*, UCL Press, London, pp. 170–83.

Fine, G. A. 1984, 'Negotiated Orders and Organizational Cultures', *Annual Review of Sociology*, vol. 10, pp. 239–62.

Fine, M. 1988, 'A Continuum of Care? Thinking About Services for the Aged', in T. McDonald (ed.), *Ageing in Perspective, Conference Proceedings*, School of Health Sciences, University of Wollongong, Wollongong, pp. 206–22.

Finnegan, L. P. 1996, 'The NIH Women's Health Initiative: Its Evolution and Expected Contributions to Women's Health', *American Journal of Preventive Medicine*, vol. 12, no. 5, pp. 292–3.

Fisher, A. 1996, 'The Brave New World of Genetic Screening: Ethical Issues', in J. Flader (ed.), *Death or Disability?* University of Tasmania, Hobart, pp. 22–46.

Fitzgerald, M. H., Ing, V., Ya, T. H., Hay, S. H., Yang, T., Duong, H. L., Barnett, B., Matthey, S., Silove, D., Mitchell, P., & McNamara, J. 1998, *Hear Our Voices: Trauma, Birthing and Mental Health Among Cambodian Women*, Transcultural Mental Health Centre, Sydney.

Flaherty, B., Homel, P., & Hall, W. 1991, 'Public Attitudes Towards Alcohol Policies', *Australian Journal of Public Health*, vol. 15, pp. 301–6.

Fletcher, R. 1995, *An Introduction to the New Men's Health*, University of Newcastle, Newcastle, NSW.

Flood, J. 1999, *Archaeology of the Dreamtime: The Story of Prehistoric Australia and Its People*, revised edn, HarperCollins, Sydney.

Flynn, R. 2001, 'Clinical Governance and Governmentality', paper presented to the BSA Medical Sociology Conference, 21–23 September, University of York.

Forder, A., Caslin, T., Ponton, G., & Walklate, S. 1984, *Theories of Welfare*, Routledge & Kegan Paul, London.

Foucault, M. 1975, *The Birth of the Clinic: An Archaeology of Medical Perception*, trans. A. M. Sheridan, Vintage Books, New York.

—— 1978, 'About the Concept of the "Dangerous Individual" in 19th Century Legal Psychiatry', trans. A. Baudot & J. Couchman, *International Journal of Law and Psychiatry*, vol. 1, pp. 1–18.

—— 1979, *Discipline and Punish*, Penguin, Harmondsworth.

—— 1988, *Madness and Civilization: A History of Insanity in the Age of Reason*, trans. R. Howard, Vintage Books, New York.

Fox, N. J. 1993, *Postmodernism, Sociology and Health*, Open University Press, Buckingham.

Fox, T. 1963, 'The Antipodes: Private Practice Publicly Supported', *Lancet*, vol. 20 April, pp. 875–9; 27 April, pp. 933–9; 4 May, pp. 988–94.

Frankfort, E. 1972, *Vaginal Politics*, Bantam Publishers, New York.

Franzway, S., Court, D., & Connell, R. W. 1989, *Staking a Claim*, Allen & Unwin, Sydney.

Freidson, E. 1970, *Profession of Medicine*, Harper & Row, New York.

—— 1986, *Professional Powers: A Study of the Institutionalisation of Formal Knowledge*, University of Chicago Press, Chicago.

—— 1988, *Profession of Medicine: A Study of the Sociology of Applied Knowledge*, University of Chicago Press, Chicago.

—— 1994, *Professionalism Reborn: Theory, Prophecy and Policy*, Polity Press, Cambridge.

Friends of Medicare 1999, Fact Sheet 5: Myth Busting: <www.phaa.net.au/friends_of_medicare/factsheet5.html>

Fry, D. & Furler, J. 2000, 'General Practice, Primary Health Care and Population Health Interface', in Commonwealth Department of Health and Aged Care (ed.), *General Practice in Australia 2000*, Commonwealth Department of Health and Aged Care, Canberra, pp. 385–424.

Gabe, J., Kelleher, D., & Williams, G. (eds) 1994, *Challenging Medicine*, Routledge, London.

Galton, F. 1883, *Inquiries into Human Faculty*, Macmillan, London.

Gamarnikow, E. 1978, 'Sexual Division of Labour: The Case of Nursing', in A. Kuhn & A. M. Wolpe (eds), *Feminism and Materialism*, Routledge & Kegan Paul, London, pp. 96–123.

Game, A. & Pringle, R. 1983, *Gender at Work*, Allen & Unwin, Sydney.

Gamson, J. 1989, 'Silence, Death, and the Invisible Enemy: AIDS Activism and Social Movement "newness"', *Social Problems*, vol. 36, pp. 351–67.

Gardner, H. (ed.) 1995, *The Politics of Health: The Australian Experience*, 2nd edn, Churchill Livingstone, Melbourne.

Gardner, H. (ed.) 1997, *Health Policy in Australia*, Oxford University Press, Melbourne.

Gardner, H. & McCoppin, B. 1995, 'Struggle for Survival by Health Therapists, Nurses and Medical Scientists', in H. Gardner (ed.), *The Politics of Health*, 2nd edn, Churchill Livingstone, Melbourne, pp. 371–427.

Garfinkel, H. 1967, *Studies in Ethnomethodology*, Prentice Hall, Englewood Cliffs.

Gatens, M. 1991, 'A Critique of the Sex/Gender Distinction', in S. Gunew (ed.), *A Reader in Feminist Knowledge*, Routledge, London, pp. 139–57.

George, V. & Wilding, P. 1976, *Ideology and Social Welfare*, Routledge & Kegan Paul, London.

Gerhardt, U. 1989, *Ideas about Illness: An Intellectual and Political History of Medical Sociology*, Macmillan, London.

Germov, J. 1993, 'The Waiting List Bypass', Health Forum, vol. 27, October, pp. 23–4.

—— 1994, 'Medi-fraud: The Systemic Infection', *Australian Journal of Social Issues*, vol. 28, no. 3, pp. 301–4.

—— 1995a, 'Duty of Disclosure: Medical Negligence and New Patient Rights', *Australian Journal of Social Issues*, vol. 30, no. 1, pp. 95–7.

—— 1995b, 'Equality before the Law: The Limits of Legal Aid and the Cost of Social Justice', *Australian Journal of Social Issues*, vol. 30, no. 2, pp. 162–78.

—— 1995c, 'Medifraud, Managerialism and the Decline of Medical Autonomy: Proletarianisation and Deprofessionalisation Reconsidered', *Australia and New Zealand Journal of Sociology*, vol. 31, no. 3, pp. 51–66.

Germov, J. & Williams, L. 1996, 'The Epidemic of Dieting Women: The Need for a Sociological Approach to Food and Nutrition', *Appetite*, vol. 27, pp. 97–108.

Gibson, D. & Allen, J. 1993, 'Phallocentrism and Parasitism: Social Provision for the Aged', *Policy Sciences*, vol. 26, pp. 79–98.

Giddens, A. 1983, *Sociology: A Brief but Critical Introduction*, Macmillan, London.

—— 1984, *The Constitution of Society: Outline of the Theory of Structuration*, Polity Press, Cambridge.

—— 1986, *Sociology: A Brief but Critical Introduction*, 2nd edn, Macmillan, London.

—— 1991, *Modernity and Self-identity: Self and Society in the Late Modern Age*, Stanford University Press, Stanford, Calif.

—— 1996, *In Defence of Sociology*, Polity Press, Cambridge.

—— 1997, *Sociology*, 3rd edn, Polity Press, Cambridge.

Gillespie, J. A. 1991, *The Price of Health: Australian Governments and Medical Politics 1910–1960*, Cambridge University Press, Melbourne.

Gillespie, R. & Gerhardt, C. 1995, 'Social Dimensions of Sickness and Disability', in G. Moon & R. Gillespie (eds), *Society and Health: An Introduction to Social Science for Health Professionals*, Routledge, London, pp. 79–94.

Gillett, S. & Katauskas, E. 1993, *Waiting Lists: A Look at the Literature*, Australian Institute of Health and Welfare, AGPS, Canberra.

Girgis, A., Doran, C. M., Sanson-Fisher, R. W., & Walsh, R. A. 1995, 'Smoking by Adolescents: Large Revenue but Little for Prevention', *Australian Journal of Public Health*, vol. 19, pp. 29–33.

Glik, D. 1990, 'The Redefinition of the Situation: The Social Construction of Spiritual Healing Experiences', *Sociology of Health and Illness*, vol. 12, no. 2, pp. 151–68.

Glover, J. & Woolacott, T. 1992, *A Social Atlas of Australia*, Cat. no. 4385.0, ABS, Canberra.

Glover, J., Harris, K., & Tennant, S. 1999, *A Social Health Atlas of Australia*, vol. 1, 2nd edn, Public Health Informational Development Unit, Adelaide.

Goffman, E. 1961, *Asylums: Essays on the Social Situation of Mental Patients and Other Inmates*, Penguin, Harmondsworth.

—— 1963, *Stigma: Notes on the Management of Spoiled Identity*, Simon & Schuster, New York.

Goldbeck-Wood, S., Dorozynski, A., Lie, G. L., Yamauchi, M., Zinn, C., Josefson, D. et al. 1996, 'Complementary Medicine is Booming Worldwide', *British Medical Journal*, no. 313, 20 July, pp. 131–3.

Goldberg, D. 1993, *Racist Culture*, Blackwell, Oxford.

Goldthorpe, J. 1996, 'Class and Politics in Advanced Industrial Societies', in D. J. Lee & B. S. Turner (eds), *Conflicts About Class*, Longman, London.

Good, B. 1994, *Medicine, Rationality, and Experience: An Anthropological Perspective*, Cambridge University Press, Cambridge.

Goodall, H. 1996, *Invasion to Embassy*, Allen & Unwin, Sydney.

Gordon, D. 1976, *Health, Sickness and Society. Theoretical Concepts in Social and Preventive Medicine*, University of Queensland Press, Brisbane.

Gore, C. J., Owen, N., Pederson, D., & Clarke, A. 1996, 'Educational and Environmental Interventions for Cardiovascular Health Promotion in Socially Disadvantaged Primary Schools', *Australian Journal of Public Health*, vol. 20, pp. 188–94.

Graetz, B. 1993, 'Health Consequences of Employment and Unemployment: Longitudinal Evidence for Young Men and Women', *Social Science and Medicine*, vol. 36, pp. 715–24.

Graetz, B. & McAllister, I. 1994, *Dimensions of Australian Society*, 2nd edn, Macmillan, Melbourne.

Grant, C. & Lapsley, H. M. 1993, *The Australian Health Care System 1992*, School of Health Services Management, Sydney.

Gray, D., Drandish, M., Moore, L., Wilkes, T., Riley, R., & Davies, S. 1995, 'Aboriginal Wellbeing and Liquor Licensing Legislation in Western Australia', *Australian Journal of Public Health*, vol. 19, pp. 177–85.

Gray, D., Morfitt, B., Williams, S., Ryan, K., & Coyne, L. 1996, *Drug Use and Related Issues among Young Aboriginal People in Albany*, National Centre for Research into the Prevention of Drug Abuse, Perth.

Gray, D. & Saggers, S. 1994, 'Aboriginal Ill Health: The Harvest of Injustice', in C. Waddell & A. Petersen (eds), *Just Health: Inequality in Illness, Care and Prevention*, Churchill Livingstone, Melbourne.

Gray, D., Saggers, S., Drandich, M., Wallam, D., & Plowright, P. 1995, 'Evaluating Government Health and Substance Abuse Programs for Indigenous Peoples: A Comparative Review', *Australian Journal of Public Health*, vol. 19, pp. 567–72.

Gray, D., Saggers, S., Sputore, B., & Bourbon, D. 2000 'What Works?: A Review of Alcohol Misuse Interventions Among Aboriginal Australians', *Addiction*, vol. 95, no.1, pp.11–22

Gray, G. 1991, *Federalism and Health Policy: The Development of Health Systems in Canada and Australia*, University of Toronto Press, Toronto.

Gray, J. A. 1999, 'Postmodern Medicine', *Lancet*, vol. 354, October, pp. 1550–3.

Green, D. G. & Cromwell, L. G. 1984, *Mutual Aid or Welfare State: Australia's Friendly Societies*, Allen & Unwin, Sydney.

Green, J. 1998, 'Commentary: Grounded Theory and the constant comparative method', *British Medical Journal*, vol. 316, no. 7137, pp. 1064–5.

Green, R. 1992, *Productivity and Nurses' Pay*, NSW Nurses' Association, Sydney.

Greer, G. 1967, *The Female Eunuch*, Angus & Robertson, Sydney.

Haebich, A. 2000, *Broken Circles. Fragmenting Indigenous Families 1800–2000*, Fremantle Arts Centre Press, Perth.

Hall, J. 1992, 'Economics and Public Health', *Choice and Change: Ethics, Politics and Economics of Public Health*, Public Health Association, Canberra, pp. 15–24.

Hall, K. & Giles-Corti, B. 2000, 'Complementary Therapies and the General Practitioner: A Survey of Perth GPs, *Australian Family Physician*, vol. 29, no. 6, pp. 602–6.

Hallowell, N. 1999, 'Doing the Right Thing: Genetic Risk and Responsibility', *Sociology of Health and Illness*, vol. 21, no. 5, pp. 597–621.

Ham, C. 1992, *Health Policy in Britain: The Policies and Organisation of the National Health Service*, 3rd edn, Macmillan, London.

Ham, C. & Hill, M. 1984, *The Policy Process in the Modern Capitalist State*, Wheatsheaf Books, Brighton.

Ham, C., Robinson, R., & Benzeval, M. 1990, *Health Check: Health Care Reforms in an International Context*, King's Fund Institute, London.

Hancock, L. (ed.) 1999, *Health Policy in the Market State*, Allen & Unwin, Sydney.

Hancock, T. 1985, 'The Mandala of Health: A Model of the Human Ecosystem', *Family and Community Health*, November, pp. 1–10.

Haralambos, M. & Holborn, M. 1991, *Sociology: Themes and Perspectives*, 3rd edn, Collins Educational, London.

Harding, A. & Greenwell, H. 2001, 'Trends in Income and Expenditure Inequality in the 1980s and 1990s', *Paper Presented to the 30th Annual Conference of Economists*, 24 September.

Harrison, S. & Pollitt, C. 1994, *Controlling Health Professionals: The Future of Work and Organization in the NHS*, Open University Press, Buckingham.

Hart, B. 1989, 'Community Health Promotion Programs', in H. Gardner (ed.), *The Politics of Health: The Australian Experience*, Churchill Livingstone, Melbourne, pp. 414–32.

Haug, M. R. 1973, 'Deprofessionalisation: An Alternative Hypothesis for the Future', *Sociological Review Monograph*, no. 20, pp. 195–211.

—— 1988, 'A Re-examination of the Hypothesis of Physician Deprofessionalisation', *Milbank Quarterly*, vol. 66, no. 2, pp. 48–56.

Hawe, P. 1994, 'Measles Control: A Best-Practice Challenge in Public Health', *Australian Journal of Public Health*, vol. 18, pp. 241–3.

Hay, I. 1992, *Money, Medicine and Malpractice in American Society*, Praeger, New York.

Hazleton, M. 1990, 'Medical Discourse on Contemporary Nurse Education: An Ideological Analysis', *Australian and New Zealand Journal of Sociology*, vol. 26, no. 1, pp. 107–25.

Healey, E. 1996, 'Welfare Benefits and Residential Concentrations amongst Recently Arrived Migrant Communities', *People and Place*, vol. 4, no. 2, pp. 20–31.

Healey, K. (ed.) 1998, *Alternative Medicine*: Issues in Society vol. 100, Spinney Press, Sydney.

Health Insurance Commission 1993, 'Medicare Fraud and Over-Servicing: What the Health Insurance Commission Proposes', *Health Issues*, vol. 36, September, p. 20.

—— 1994, *Financial Statements and Report on Operations: 1993–94*, AGPS, Canberra.

Health Issues Centre 1988, *What's Wrong with the Health System?*, HIC, Melbourne.

Health Ministers' Advisory Council 1988, *Continuing Education for Primary Health Care in Australia*, AGPS, Canberra.

Hehir, J. B. 1996, 'Justice and Healthcare', *Chicago Studies*, vol. 35, no. 3, pp. 238–48.

Henderson, L. & Kitzinger, J. 1999, 'The Human Drama of Genetics: Hard and Soft Media Representations of Inherited Breast Cancer', *Sociology of Health and Illness*, vol. 21, no. 5, pp. 560–78.

Hepworth, M. 1995, 'Positive Ageing: What is the Message?', in R. Bunton, S. Nettleton, & R. Burrow (eds), *The Sociology of Health Promotion*, Routledge, London.

Hepworth, M. & Turner, B. S. 1982, *Confession: Studies in Deviance and Religion*, Routledge & Kegan Paul, London.

Herdman, E. 1995, 'Professionalisation, Rationalisation and Policy Change: The Transfer of Pre-registration Nurse Education to the University Sector', *Annual Review of Health Sciences, Health Policy*, University of NSW, Sydney.

Hertzel, B. 1995, 'From Papua New Guinea to the United Nations', *Australian Journal of Public Health*, vol. 19, pp. 231–34.

Herzlich, C. & Pierret, J. 1987, *Illness and Self in Society*, Johns Hopkins University Press, Baltimore.

Higginbotham, N., Heading, G., Pont, J., Plotnikoff, R., Dobson, A. J., Smith, E. 1993, 'Community Worry about Heart Disease: A Needs Survey in the Coalfields and Newcastle Areas of the Hunter Region', *Australian Journal of Public Health*, vol. 17, pp. 314–21.

Higgins, K., Cooper-Stanbury, M., & Williams, P. 2000, *Statistics on Drug use in Australia*, Australian Institute of Health and Welfare, Canberra.

Hill, D. & White, V. 1995, 'Australian Adult Smoking Prevalence in 1992', *Australian Journal of Public Health*, vol. 19, pp. 305–8.

Hill, D., White, V., & Segan, C. 1995, 'Prevalence of Cigarette Smoking among Australian Secondary School Students in 1993', *Australian Journal of Public Health*, vol. 19, pp. 445–9.

Hilmer, F. G., Rayner, M. R., & Taperell, G. Q. 1993, *National Competition Policy: Report by the Independent Committee of Inquiry: Executive Overview*, AGPS, Canberra.

Himmel, W., Schulte, M., & Kochen, M. M. 1993, 'Complementary Medicine: Are Patients' Expectations Being Met by Their General Practitioners?', *British Journal of General Practice*, vol. 43, pp. 232–5.

Hindess, B. 1987, *Freedom, Equality, and the Market: Arguments on Social Policy*, Tavistock, London.

Hirschauer, S. 1991, 'The Manufacture of Bodies in Surgery', *Social Studies of Science*, vol. 21, pp. 279–319.

Hoffenburg, R. 1996, 'Live and Let Die', in J. Morgan (ed.), *An Easeful Death?*, Federation Press, Annandale, NSW.

Holloway, G. 1994, 'Susto and the Career Path of the Victim of an Industrial Accident: A Sociological Case Study', *Social Science and Medicine*, vol. 38, no. 7, pp. 989–97.

Holstein, J. & Gubrium, J. 1995, *The Active Interview*, Sage, Beverly Hills, Calif.

Horin, Adele 2000, 'Exposed: Nursing Homes from Hell', *Sydney Morning Herald*, 4 March, p. 1.

Hospital and Health Services Commission 1974, *A Community Health Program for Australia*, AGPS, Canberra.

Hothschild, A. R. 1979, 'Emotion work, feeling rules and social structure', *American Journal of Sociology*, vol. 85, no. 3, pp. 551–75.

House, J. S., Landis, K. R., & Umberson, D. 1988, 'Social Relationships and Health', *Science*, no. 241, pp. 121–4.

House of Representatives Standing Committee on Aboriginal Affairs 1979, *Aboriginal Health*, AGPS, Canberra.

Howden-Chapman, P. & Tobias, M. (eds) 2000, *Social Inequalities in Health: New Zealand 1999*, New Zealand Ministry of Health, Wellington.

Howson, A. 1998, 'Embodied Obligation: The Female Body and Health Surveillance', in S. Nettleton & J. Watson (eds), *The Body in Everyday Life*, Routledge, London, pp. 218–40.

Hubbard, R. & Wald, E. 1997, *Exploding the Gene Myth*, revised edn, Beacon Press, Boston.

Hughes, D. 1988, 'When Nurse Knows Best: Some Aspects of Nurse/Doctor Interaction in a Casualty Department', *Sociology of Health and Illness*, vol. 10, no. 1, pp. 51–63.

Human Rights and Equal Opportunity Commission 1997, *Bringing Them Home: Report of the National Inquiry into the Separation of Aboriginal and Torres Strait Islander Children from their Families*, Human Rights and Equal Opportunity Commission, Canberra.

Hunter, E. 1989, 'Changing Patterns of Aboriginal Mortality in the Kimberley Region of Western Australia', *Aboriginal Health Information Bulletin*, vol. 11, pp. 27–32.

Hunter, E., Reser, J., Baird, M., & Reser, P. 1999, *An Analysis of Suicide in Indigenous Communities of North Queensland: The Historical, Cultural and Symbolic Landscape*, Department of Social and Preventive Medicine, University of Queensland.

Hupalo, P. & Herden, K. 1999, *Health Policy and Inequality*, Occasional Papers, New Series, no. 5, Commonwealth Department of Health and Aged Care, Canberra.

Hurst, D. 1996, 'Men's Violence and Men's Health: Some Recent Worldwide Trends', in Commonwealth Department of Human Services and Health (ed.), *Proceedings of the National Men's Health Conference*, AGPS, Canberra, pp. 125–32.

Industry Commission 1994, *Workers' Compensation in Australia*, AGPS, Canberra.

Ingleby, D. 1985, 'Mental Health and Social Order', in S. Cohen & A. Scull (eds), *Social Control and the State*, Basil Blackwell, Oxford, pp. 52–75.

Ingstad, B. & Whyte, S. R. (eds) 1995, *Disability and Culture*, University of California Press, Berkeley, Calif.

Illich, I. 1977, *Limits to Medicine, Medical Nemesis: The Exploration of Health*, Penguin, Harmondsworth.

Irvine R. & Graham J. 1994, 'Deconstructing the Concept of Profession: A Prerequisite to Carving a Niche in a Changing World', *Australian Occupational Therapy Journal*, vol. 41, pp. 9–18.

Jackson, T. 1993, 'Consumer Support for Casemix: Walking the Fine Line', *Health Issues*, vol. 37, December, pp. 5–6.

Jaensch, D. 1984, *An Introduction to Australian Politics*, 2nd edn, Longman Cheshire, Melbourne.

James, P. 1996, *Nation Formation*, Sage, London.

Jamison, J. 1995, 'Australian Dietary Targets in 1995: Their Feasibility and Pertinence to Dietary Goals for 2000', *Australian Journal of Public Health*, vol. 19, pp. 522–4.

Jamrozik, A., Boland, C., & Urquhart, R. 1995, *Social Change and Cultural Transformation in Australia*, Cambridge University Press, Melbourne.

Jarvis, M. J. & Wardle, J. 2000, 'Social patterning of individual health behaviours: the case of cigarette smoking', in M. Marmot & R. G. Wilkinson (eds), *Social Determinants of Health*, Oxford University Press, Oxford.

Jayasuriya, L. 1992, 'The Facts, Policies and Rhetoric of Multiculturalism', in T. Jagtenberg & P. D'Alton (eds), *Four Dimensional Social Space: Class, Gender, Ethnicity and Nature*, 2nd edn, Harper Educational, Sydney, pp. 215–20.

Jayasuriya, L., Sang, D., & Fielding, A. 1992, *Ethnicity, Immigration and Mental Illness: A Critical Review of Australian Research*, AGPS, Canberra.

Johanson, M., Larsson, U. S., Säljö, R, & Svärdsudd, K. 1996, 'Addressing Life Style in Primary Health Care', *Social Science and Medicine*, vol. 43, no. 3, pp. 389–400.

Johnson, T. 1972, *Professions and Power*, Macmillan, London.

Joint Committee of Public Accounts 1982, *Medical Fraud and Overservicing: Progress Report*, Report no. 203, AGPS, Canberra.

—— 1985, *Report on Pathology*, Report no. 2363, AGPS, Canberra.

Jones, W. K. 1996, 'Centres for Disease Control and Prevention', *American Journal of Preventive Medicine*, vol. 12, no. 5, p. 410.

Judge, K., Mulligan, J., & Benzenval, M. 1998, 'Income Inequality and Population Health', *Social Science and Medicine*, vol. 46, nos 4–5, pp. 567–79.

Julian, R. & Easthope, G. 1996, 'Migrant Health', in C. Grbich (ed.), *Health in Australia: Sociological Concepts and Issues*, Prentice Hall, Sydney, ch. 6, pp. 103–25.

Jupp, J. 1999, *Immigration*, 2nd edn, Oxford University Press, Melbourne.

Jupp, J., McRobbie, A., & York, B. 1991, *Metropolitan Ghettoes and Ethnic Concentration*, Working Papers on Multiculturalism, Office of Multicultural Affairs, AGPS, Canberra.

Kane, P. 1991, *Women's Health: From Womb to Tomb*, Macmillan, London.

Kaplan, G. A., Pamuk, E., Lynch, J. W., Cohen, R. D., & Balflour, J. L. 1996, 'Income Inequality and Mortality in the United States', *British Medical Journal*, vol. 312, pp. 999–1003.

Kaplan, R. M. 1988, 'The Value Dimension in Studies of Health Promotion', in S. Spacapan & S. Oskamp (eds), *The Social Psychology of Health*, Sage, Newbury Park, Calif., pp. 207–36.

Kassulke, D., Stenner-Day, K., Coory, M., & Ring, I. 1993, 'Information-Seeking Behaviour and Sources of Health Information: Associations with Risk Factor Status in an Analysis of Three Queensland Electorates', *Australian Journal of Public Health*, vol. 17, pp. 51–7.

Kavanagh, A. & Broom, D. 1997, 'Women's understanding of abnormal cervical smear test results: A qualitative interview study', *British Medical Journal* , vol. 314, pp. 1388–92.

Kawachi, I. & Berkman, L. 2000, 'Social Cohesion, Social Capital, and Health', in L. F. Berkman & I. Kawachi (eds), *Social Epidemiology*, Oxford University Press, New York, pp. 174–90.

Keating, M. 1990, 'Managing For Results in the Public Interest', *Australian Journal of Public Administration*, vol. 49, no. 4, pp. 387–98.

Kellehear, A. 1993, *The Unobtrusive Researcher*, Allen & Unwin, Sydney.

—— 1999, *Health Promoting Palliative Care*, Oxford University Press, Melbourne.

Kelly, K. & Van Vlaenderen, H. 1996, 'Dynamics of Participation in a Community Health Project', *Social Science and Medicine*, vol. 43, no. 8, pp. 1235–46.

Kelly, S. 2001, 'Trends in Australian Wealth—New Estimates for the 1990s', Paper Presented to the 30th Annual Conference of Economists, University of Western Australia, 26 September.

Kendall, I. 1995, 'The founding of the NHS', in G. Moon & R. Gillespie (eds), *Society and Health: An Introduction to Social Science for Health Professionals*, Routledge, London, pp. 143–61.

Kennedy, B. P., Kawachi, I., & Prothrow-Stith, D. 1996, 'Income Distribution and Mortality: Cross-sectional Ecological study of the Robin Hood Index in the United States', *British Medical Journal*, vol. 312, pp. 1004–7.

Kennedy, M. 1990, *Borne a Half-Caste*, Aboriginal Studies Press, Canberra.

Kenny, D. & Adamson, B. 1992, 'Medicine and the Health Professions: Issues of Dominance, Autonomy and Authority', *Australian Health Review*, vol. 15, no. 1, p. 3.

Kevles, D. & Hood, L. 1992, 'Reflections', in D. Kevles & L. Hood (eds), *The Code of Codes: Scientific and Social Issues in the Human Genome Project*, Harvard University Press, Cambridge, Mass, pp. 210–22.

Kickbusch, I. 1989, 'Approaches to an Ecological Base for Public Health', *Health Promotion*, vol. 4, no. 4, pp. 265–8.

King, A., Walker, A., & Harding, A. 1999, *Social Security, Ageing and Income Distribution in Australia*, Natsem Discussion Paper no. 44, University of Canberra, Canberra.

Kittrie, N. N. 1971, *The Right to be Different: Deviance and Enforced Therapy*, Penguin, Baltimore.

Kleinman, A. 1980, *Patients and Healers in the Context of Culture*, University of California Press, Berkeley, Calif.

—— 1988, *The Illness Narrative: Suffering, Healing and the Human Condition*, Basic Books, New York.

Klimidis, S. & Minas, I. H. 1995, 'Migration, culture and mental health in children and adolescents', in C. Guerra & R. White (eds), *Minority Youth in Australia*, National Clearing House for Youth Studies, Hobart, pp. 85–99.

Kolberg, B. 2000, *Gene Therapy: Status and Prospects in Clinical Medicine*, SMM report 1\2000, Norwegian Center for Health Technology Assessment: <www.oslo.sintef.no/smm/News/FramesetNews.htm>

Koshland, D. 1989, 'Sequences and Consequences of the Human Genome', *Science*, no. 246, p. 246.

Krupinski, J. & Burrows, G. 1986, *The Price of Freedom: Young Indochinese Refugees in Australia*, Pergamon Press, Sydney.

Kunkel, S. R. & Atchley, R. C. 1996, 'Why Gender Matters: Being Female is Not the Same as Not Being Male', *American Journal of Preventive Medicine*, vol. 12, no. 5, pp. 294–6.

Kymlicka, W. 1990, *Contemporary Political Philosophy: An Introduction*, The Clarendon Press, Oxford.

Labonté, R. 1991, 'Econology: Integrating Health and Sustainable Development', *Health Promotion International*, vol. 6, no. 1, pp. 49–63.

La Follette, M. C. 1992, *Stealing into Print: Fraud, Plagiarism and Misconduct in Scientific Publishing*, University of California Press, Berkeley, Calif.

Langer, B. 1998, 'Globalisation and the Myth of Ethnic Community: Salvadoran refugees in multicultural states', in D. Bennett (ed.), *Multicultural States: Rethinking Difference and Identity*, Routledge, London, pp. 163–77.

Langton, M. 1992, 'Too Much Sorry Business', *Aboriginal and Islander Health Worker Journal*, vol. 16, no. 2, pp. 10–23.

—— 1993, 'Rum, Seduction and Death: "Aboriginality" and Alcohol', *Oceania*, vol. 63, no. 3, pp. 195–206.

Laris, P. 1992, 'The way of the Manager: The Context and Roles of Community Health Management', in F. Baum, D. Fry, & I. Lennie (eds), *Community Health: Policy and Practice in Australia*, Pluto Press in association with the Australian Community Health Association, Sydney, pp. 64–76.

—— 1995, 'Boards of Directors of Community Health Services', in F. Baum (ed.), *Health For All: The South Australian Experience*, Wakefield Press, Adelaide, ch. 5, pp. 82–93.

Larkin, G. 1983, *Occupational Monopoly and Modern Medicine*, Tavistock, London.

Larson, M. S. 1977, *The Rise of Professionalism: A Sociological Analysis*, University of California Press, Berkeley.

Laslett, A. 1989, 'The Demographic Scene: An Overview', in J. Eekelaar & D. Pearl (eds), *An Aging World*, Clarendon Press, Oxford, pp. 1–10.

Lawler, J. 1991, *Behind the Screens: Nursing, Somology, and the Problem of the Body*, Churchill Livingstone, Melbourne.

Lawson, J. S. 1991, *Public Health Australia: An Introduction*, McGraw-Hill, Sydney.

Lawson, J. S. & Forde, K. 1995, 'Medicare Related Payments to Australian Medical Practitioners', *Australian Health Review*, vol. 18, no. 4, pp. 353–70.

Le Fanu, J. 1986, 'Diet and Disease: Nonsense and Non-science', in D. Anderson (ed.), *A Diet of Reason: Sense and Nonsense in the Healthy Eating Debate*, The Social Affairs Unit, London, pp. 109–24.

—— 1999, *The Rise and Fall of Modern Medicine*, Abacus, London.

Lee, A., Bailey, A. P., Yarmirr, D., O'Dea, K., & Mathews, J. D. 1994, 'Survival Tucker: Improved Diet and Health Indicators in an Aboriginal Community', *Australian Journal of Public Health*, vol. 18, pp. 277–85.

Lee, A., Bonson, A. P. V., & Powers, J. R. 1996, 'The Effect of Retail Store Managers on Aboriginal Diet in Remote Communities', *Australian Journal of Public Health*, vol. 20, pp. 212–14.

Lee, C. (ed.) 2001, *Women's Health Australia: What do we Know? What do we Need to Know?*, Australian Academic Press, Brisbane.

Legge, D. 1992, 'Community Management: Open Letter to a new Committee Members', in F. Baum, D. Fry, & I. Lennie (eds), *Community Health: Policy and Practice in Australia*, Pluto Press in association with the Australian Community Health Association, Sydney, pp. 95–114.

Legge, D., McDonald, D., & Benger, C. 1993, *Improving Australia's Health: The Role of Primary Health Care*, Final Report, National Centre for Epidemiology and Population Health, Australian National University, Canberra.

Lewis, B. & Walker, R. 1997, *Changing Central-Local Relationships in Health Services Provision: Final Report*, School of Health Systems Science, La Trobe University, Melbourne.

Lewis, M. 1992, *A Rum State: Alcohol and Public Policy in Australia 1788–1988*, AGPS, Canberra.

Lewith, G. 1999, 'The Homeopathic Conundrum Revisited', *Alternative Therapies in Health and Medicine*, vol. 5, no. 5, pp. 32–5.

—— 2000, 'Complementary and Alternative Medicine: An Educational, Attitudinal and Research Challenge', *Medical Journal of Australia*, vol. 172, pp. 102–3.

Lien, O. 1992, 'The Experience of Working with Vietnamese Patients Attending a Psychiatric Service', *Journal of Vietnamese Studies*, vol. 5, pp. 95–105.

Light, D. W. 1993, 'Countervailing Power: The Changing Character of the Medical Profession in the United States', in F. W. Hafferty & J. B. McKinlay (eds), *The Changing Medical Profession: An International Perspective*, Oxford University Press, New York.

—— 2000, 'The Medical Profession and Organizational Change: From Professional Dominance to Countervailing Power', in C. Bird, P. Conrad & A. M. Fremont (eds), *Handbook of Medical Sociology*, 5th edn, Prentice Hall, New Jersey.

Lin, V. & Pearse, W. 1990, 'A Workforce at Risk', in J. Reid & P. Trompf (eds), *The Health of Immigrant Australia: A Social Perspective*, Harcourt Brace Jovanovich, Sydney, pp. 66–82.

Lincoln, Y. 1995, 'Emerging criteria for quality in qualitative and interpretive research', *Qualitative Inquiry*, vol. 1, pp. 275–89.

Link, B. & Phelan, J. 1995, 'Social Conditions as Fundamental Causes of Disease', *Journal of Health and Social Behaviour*, extra issue, pp. 80–94.

Lloyd, P., Lupton, D., & Donaldson, C. 1991, 'Consumerism in the Health Care Setting: An Exploratory Study of Factors Underlying the Selection and Evaluation of Primary Medical Services', *Australian Journal of Public Health*, vol. 15, pp. 194–201.

Lloyd, P., Lupton, D., Wiesner, D., & Hasleton, S. 1993, 'Choosing Alternative Therapy: An Exploratory Study of Sociodemographic Characteristics and Motives of Patients Resident in Sydney', *Australian Journal of Public Health*, vol. 17, pp. 135–44.

Lock, M. 1993, 'The Politics of Mid-life and Menopause: Ideologies for the Second Sex in North America and Japan', in S. Lindenbaum & M. Lock (eds), *Knowledge, Power and Practice: The Anthropology of Medicine and Everyday Life*, University of California Press, Berkeley, pp. 330–63.

López, J. & Scott, J. 2000, *Social Structure*, Open University Press, Buckingham

Lowenberg, J. S. & Davis, F. 1994, 'Beyond Medicalisation–Demedicalisation: The Case of Holistic Health', *Sociology of Health and Illness*, vol. 16, no. 5, pp. 579–600.

Lukes, S. 1974, *Power: A Radical View*, Macmillan, London.

Lumby, J. 1996, 'Nurses, Doctors: Sacred Cows', guest editorial, *Australian Health Review*, vol. 19, no. 2, pp. 1–6.

Lupton, D. 1994, *Medicine as Culture: Illness, Disease and the Body in Western Societies*, Sage, London.

—— 1995, *The Imperative of Health: Public Health and the Regulated Body*, Sage, London.

—— 1996, *Food, the Body and the Self*, Sage, London.

—— 1998, 'A postmodern public health?', *Australian and New Zealand Journal of Public Health*, vol. 22, no. 2, pp. 3–5.

Lynch, J. 2000, 'Income Inequality and Health: Expanding the Debate', *Social Science & Medicine*, vol. 51, no. 3, pp. 1001–5.

Lyon, P. 1990, *What Everybody Knows about Alice: A Report on the Impact of Alcohol Abuse on the Town of Alice Springs*, Tangentyere Council, Alice Springs, NT.

McClelland, A. 1991, *In Fair Health? Equity and the Health System*, Background Paper no. 3, AGPS, Canberra.

MacDonald, J. 1992, *Primary Health Care: Medicine in its Place*, Earthscan, London.

McDonald, R. & Steel, Z. 1997, *Immigrants and Mental Health: An epidemiological analysis*, Transcultural Mental Health Centre, Sydney.

McGuinness, P. 1996, 'Aboriginal Health a Vicious Circle', *Sydney Morning Herald*, 19 September.

McGuinness, S. 1999, *The Australian Health Care System: An Outline* [web site], Commonwealth Department of Health and Aged Care, Canberra, <www.health.gov.au/haf/pubs/ozhealth/ozsys299.htm>, date accessed: 31 November 2001.

McGuire, L. 1994, 'Service Delivery Agreements: Experimenting with Casemix Funding and Schools of the Future', in J. Alford & D. O'Neill (eds), *The Contract State: Public Management and the Kennett Government*, Centre for Applied Social Research, Deakin University, Geelong, pp. 74–100.

McInerney, Fran 2000, '"Requested death": A New Social Movement', *Social Science and Medicine*, vol. 50, no. 1, 147–54.

Macintyre, M. 1994, 'Migrant Women from El Salvador and Vietnam in Australian Hospitals', in C. Waddell & A. R. Petersen (eds), *Just Health: Inequality in Illness, Care and Prevention*, Churchill Livingstone, Melbourne, ch. 10, pp. 159–68.

Macintyre, S. 1997, 'The Black Report and Beyond: What are the Issues?', *Social Science and Medicine*, vol. 44, no. 6, pp. 723–45.

Macintyre, S., Hunt, K., & Sweeting, H. 1996, 'Gender Differences in Health: Are Things Really as Simple as They Seem?', *Social Science and Medicine*, vol. 42, no. 4, pp. 617–24.

Mackay, L. 1993, *Conflicts in Care: Medicine and Nursing*, Chapman & Hall, London.

McKeown, T. 1976, *The Role of Medicine: Dream, Mirage or Nemesis?*, Nuffield Hospital Trust, London.

—— 1979, *The Role of Medicine: Dream, Mirage or Nemesis?*, Basil Blackwell, Oxford.

—— 1988, *The Origins of Human Disease*, Basil Blackwell, Oxford.

McKinlay, J. B. 1994, 'A Case for Refocussing Upstream: The Political Economy of Illness', in P. Conrad & R. Kern (eds), *The Sociology of Health and Illness: Critical Perspectives*, 4th edn, St Martin's Press, New York, pp. 509–23.

—— 1996, 'Some Contributions from the Social System to Gender Inequalities in Heart Disease', *Journal of Health and Social Behaviour*, vol. 37, pp. 1–26.

McKinlay, J. B. & Arches, J. 1985, 'Towards the Proletarianization of Physicians, *International Journal of Health Services*, vol. 15, no. 2, pp. 161–95.

McKinlay, J. B. & McKinlay, S. M. 1977, 'The questionable effect of medical measures on the decline of mortality in the United States in the twentieth century', *Milbank Memorial Fund Quarterly*, vol. 55, pp. 405–28.

McKinlay, J. B. & Stoeckle, J. D. 1988, 'Corporatization and the Social Transformation of Doctoring', *International Journal of Health Services*, vol. 18, no. 2, pp. 191–205.

Macklin, J. 1990, *Setting the Agenda for Change*, Background Paper no. 1, AGPS, Canberra.

MacLennan, A. H., Wilson, D. H., & Taylor, A. W. 1996, 'Prevalence and Cost of Alternative Medicine in Australia', *Lancet*, no. 347, pp. 569–73.

McLennan, W. & Madden, R. 1999, *The Health and Welfare of Australia's Aboriginal and Torres Strait Islander Peoples*, ABS & Australian Institute of Health and Welfare, Canberra.

McLeod, K. S. 2000, 'Our Sense of Snow: The Myth of John Snow in Medical Geography', *Social Science and Medicine*, vol. 50, pp. 923–35.

MacMahon, B. & Pugh, T. F. 1970, *Epidemiological Principles and Methods*, Little Brown, Boston.

McMasters, A. 1996, 'Research from an Aboriginal Health Worker's Point of View', *Australian Journal of Public Health*, vol. 20, pp. 319–20.

McMichael, A. J. 1985, 'Social Class (as Estimated by Occupational Prestige) and Mortality in Australian Males in the 1970s', *Community Health Studies*, vol. 9, no. 3, pp. 220–30.

—— 1991, 'Food, Nutrients, Health and Disease: A Historical Perspective on the Assessment and Management of Risks', *Australian Journal of Public Health*, vol. 15, pp. 7–13.

McNamara, Beverley, Waddell, Charles and Colvin, Margaret 1994, 'The Institutionalization of a Good Death', *Social Science and Medicine*, vol. 39, no. 11, 1501–9.

McNay, L 1992, *Foucault and Feminism*, Polity Press, Cambridge.

MacSween, M. 1993, *Anorexic Bodies: A Feminist and Sociological Perspective on Anorexia Nervosa*, Routledge, London.

Madden, R. 1995, *National Aboriginal and Torres Strait Islander Survey 1994: Detailed Findings*, Australian Government Publishing Service, Canberra.

Manderson, L. & Mathews, M. 1981, 'Vietnamese Attitudes towards Maternal and Infant Health', *Medical Journal of Australia*, vol. 1, pp. 69–72.

—— 1985, 'Care and Conflict: Vietnamese Medical Beliefs and the Australian Health Care System', in I. Burnley, S. Encel, & G. McCall (eds), *Immigration and Ethnicity in the 1980s*, Longman Cheshire, Melbourne, pp. 248–60.

Manderson, L. & Reid, J. C. 1994, 'What's Culture Got to Do with It?', in C. Waddell & A. R. Petersen (eds), *Just Health: Inequality in Illness, Care and Prevention*, Churchill Livingstone, Melbourne, ch. 1, pp. 7–25.

Mann, C. 1994, 'Behavioural Genetics in Transition', *Science*, no. 264, pp. 1686–9.

Manning, N. 2000, 'Psychiatric Diagnosis Under Conditions of Uncertainty: Personality Disorder, Science and Professional Legitimacy', *Sociology of Health & Illness*, vol. 22, pp. 621–39.

Markens, S. 1996, 'The Problematic of "Experience": A Political and Cultural Critique of PMS', *Gender and Society*, vol. 10, pp. 42–58.

Marmot, M. 1999, 'Introduction', in M. Marmot & R. G. Wilkinson (eds), *Social Determinants of Health*, Oxford University Press, Oxford.

—— 2000, 'Social Determinants of Health: From Observation to Policy', *Medical Journal of Australia*, vol. 172, 17 April, pp. 379–82.

Marmot, M., Siegrist, J., Theorell, T., & Feeney, A. 1999, 'Health and the Psychosocial Environment at Work', in M. Marmot & R. G. Wilkinson (eds), *Social Determinants of Health*, Oxford University Press, Oxford.

Marmot, M. & Wilkinson, R. G. (eds) 1999, *Social Determinants of Health*, Oxford University Press, Oxford.

Marmot, M. G., Bosma, H., Hemingway, H., Brunner, E., Stansfeld, S., 1997, 'Contribution of Job Control and Other Risk Factors to Social Variations in Coronary Heart Disease Incidence', *Lancet*, July 26, vol. 350, no. 9073, pp. 235–9.

Marmot, M. G., Davey Smith, G., Stansfield, S., Patel, C., North, F., Head, J., White, I., Brunner, E., & Feeney, A. 1991, 'Health Inequalities among British Civil Servants: the Whitehall II Study', *Lancet*, vol. 337, no. 8754, pp. 1387–93.

Marmot, M. G., Rose, G., Shipley, M., & Hamilton, P. J. S. 1978, 'Employment Grade and Coronary Heart Disease in British Civil Servants', *Journal of Epidemiology and Community Health*, vol. 32, pp. 244–9.

Marshall, T. H. 1950, *Citizenship and Social Class and Other Essays*, Cambridge University Press, Cambridge.

—— 1981, *The Right to Welfare and Other Essays*, Heinemann, London.

Martin, E. 1987, *The Woman in the Body: A Cultural Analysis of Reproduction*, Beacon Press, Boston.

—— 1998, 'Immunology on the Street: How Nonscientists see the Immune System', in S. Nettleton & J. Watson (eds), *The Body in Everyday Life*, Routledge, London, pp. 45–63.

Martin, J. 1978, *The Migrant Presence: Australian Responses 1847–1977*, Allen & Unwin, Sydney.

Martin, K. A. 1993, 'Gender and Sexuality: Medical Opinion on Homosexuality, 1900–1950', *Gender and Society*, vol. 7, pp. 246–60.

Martyr, P. 1994, The Professional Development of Rehabilitation in Australia, 1870–1981, PhD thesis, the University of Western Australia and Phillipa Martyr, Internet <www.healthsci.utas.edu.au/~pmartyr/thesis10.html> 2 January 1997.

Marx, K. 1859/1963, 'A Contribution to the Critique of Political Economy', in T. Bottomore & M. Rubel (eds), *Karl Marx: Selected Writings in Sociology and Social Philosophy*, 2nd edn, Penguin, Harmondsworth.

Mason, M. & Winslow, L. R. 1994, 'Professional Roles of Dietitians: Do Dietitians and Physicians Agree?', *Nutrition Review*, vol. 52, no. 9, pp. 315–17.

Mathers, C. D 1994, *Health Differentials Among Adult Australians Aged 25–64 Years*, Australian Institute of Health and Welfare, Canberra.

Mathers, C. D. & Schofield, D. 1998, 'The Health Consequences of Unemployment: The Evidence', *Medical Journal of Australia*, vol. 168, pp. 178–82.

Mathers, C., Vos, T., & Stevenson, C. 1999, *The Burden of Disease and Injury: Summary Report*, Australian Institute of Health and Welfare, Canberra.

Matthews, J. J. 1984, *Good and Mad Women: The Historical Construction of Femininity in Twentieth Century Australia*, Allen & Unwin, Sydney.

Maunsell, E., Brisson, J., & Deschenes, L. 1995, 'Social Support and Survival Among Women with Breast Cancer', *Cancer*, vol. 76, no. 4, pp. 631–7.

May, C. 1992, 'Nursing Work, Nurses' Knowledge, and the Subjectification of the Patient', *Sociology of Health and Illness*, vol. 14, no. 4, pp. 472–87.

Mayhew, C. & Peterson, C. L. (eds) 1999, Occupational Health and Safety in Australia, Allen & Unwin, Sydney.

Mechanic, D. 1994, 'Promoting Health: Implications for Modern and Developing Nations', in L. Chen, A. Kleinman, & N. Ware (eds), *Health and Social Change in International Perspective*, Harvard University Press, Cambridge, Mass., pp. 471–89.

Meier, R. F. 1982, 'Perspectives on the Concept of Social Control', *Annual Review of Sociology*, vol. 8, pp. 35–55.

Meischke, H., Eisenberg, M. S., & Larsen, M. P. 1993, 'Prehospital Delay Interval for Patients Who Use Emergency Medical Services', *Annals of Emergency Medicine*, vol. 22, no. 10, pp. 1597–601.

Melbourne District Health Council 1990, *A Sliver—Not Even a Slice*, District Health Councils of Victoria, Melbourne.

Mercury 2000, 2 June, p. 5.

Merrill Lynch and Cap Gemini Ernst & Young 2001, World Wealth Report 2001, [web site], <www.ir.ml.com/news/ML051401.pdf>, Merrill Lynch and Cap Gemini Ernst & Young, date accessed: 3 November.

Metherall, M. 2000, 'Scanner doctors won't be charged', *Sydney Morning Herald*, September 28, p. 1.

Milio, N. 1983, 'Next Steps in Community Health Policy: Matching Rhetoric with Reality', *Community Health Studies*, vol. 2, no. 2, pp. 185–92.

Millet, K. 1977, *Sexual Politics*, Virago, London.

Mills, C. W. 1959, *The Sociological Imagination*, Oxford University Press, New York.

Milner, N. 1989, 'The Denigration of Rights and the Persistence of Rights Talk: A Cultural Portrait', *Law and Social Inquiry*, vol. 14, pp. 631–75.

Minas, I. H. 1990, 'Mental Health in a Culturally Diverse Society', in J. Reid & P. Trompf (eds), *The Health of Immigrant Australia: A Social Perspective*, Harcourt Brace Jovanovich, Sydney, pp. 250–87.

Minas, I. H., Lambert, T. S. R., Kostov, S., & Borangh, G. 1996, *Mental Health Services for NESB Immigrants: Transforming Policy into Practice*, AGPS, Canberra.

Mintzberg, H. 1979, *The Structuring of Organizations*, Prentice Hall, Englewood Cliffs, New Jersey.

Mitchell, P. 2000, 'Yarrabah: A Success Story in Community Empowerment', *Youth Suicide Prevention Bulletin*, no. 4, October, Australian Institute of Family Studies.

Moodie, P. M. 1973, *Aboriginal Health*, Australian National University Press, Canberra.

Mooney, G. & Scotton, R. (eds) 1998, *Economics and Australian Health Policy*, Allen & Unwin, Sydney.

Morgan, J. 1996, 'Easeful Death: Culture and Medicine in the Debate on Death, Dying and Euthanasia', in John Morgan (ed.), *An Easeful Death?*, The Federation Press, Annandale.

Morgan, M., Calnan, M., & Manning, N. 1985, *Sociological Approaches to Health and Medicine*, Croom Helm, London.

Morris, B. 1989, *Domesticating Resistance: The Dhan-Gadi Aborigines and the Australian State*, Berg, Oxford.

Morrissey, M., Mitchell, C., & Rutherford, A. 1991, *The Family in the Settlement Process*, AGPS, Canberra.

Mouffe, C. (ed.) 1992, *Dimensions of Radical Democracy*, Verso, London.

Mulkay, M. 1993, 'Social Death in Britain', in D. Clark (ed.), *The Sociology of Death*, Blackwell, Cambridge, pp. 31–49.

Mulvany, J. 2000, 'Disability, Impairment or Illness? The Relevance of the Social Model of Disability to the Study of Mental Disorder', *Sociology of Health and Illness*, vol. 22, pp. 582–601.

Muntaner, C. & Lynch, J. 1999, 'Income Inequality, Social Cohesion, and Class Relations: A Critique of Wilkinson's Neo-Durkheimian Research Program', *International Journal of Health Services*, vol. 29, no. 1, pp. 59–81.

Muntaner, C., Lynch, J., & Davey Smith, G. 2001, 'Social Capital, Disorganized Communities and the Third Way: Understanding the Retreat from Structural Inequalities in Epidemiology and Public Health', *International Journal of Health Services*, vol. 31, no. 2, pp. 213–37.

Muntaner, C., Lynch, J., & Oates, G. L. 1999, 'The Social Class Determinants of Income Inequality and Social Cohesion', *International Journal of Health Services*, vol. 29, no. 4, pp. 699–732.

Murray, J. & Shepherd, S. 1993, 'Alternative or Additional Medicine? An Exploratory Study in General Practice', *Social Science and Medicine*, vol. 37, no. 8, pp. 983–8.

Najman, J. 1980, 'Theories of disease causation and the concept of general susceptibility', *Social Science and Medicine*, vol. 14A, pp. 231–7.

—— 1993, 'Health and poverty: past, present and prospects for the future', *Social Science and Medicine*, vol. 36, pp. 157–66.

Najman, J. M. & Davey Smith, G. 2000, 'The Embodiment of Class-related and Health Inequalities: Australian Policies', *Australian and New Zealand Journal of Public Health*, vol. 24, no. 1, pp. 3–4.

Nash, H. 1989, The History of Dietetics in Australia, Dietitians Association of Australia, Canberra.

Nash, M. 1992, 'Dangerousness Revisited', *International Journal of the Sociology of Law*, vol. 20, pp. 337–49.

National Aboriginal Health Strategy Working Party 1989, *A National Aboriginal Health Strategy*, AGPS, Canberra.

National Aboriginal Community Controlled Health Organisation 1999, *Report on the Implementation of the Framework Agreements on Aboriginal and Torres Strait Islander Health*, National Aboriginal Community Controlled Health Organisation, Canberra: <www.cowan.edu.au/chs/nh/clearinghouse/naccho/>

National Advisory Committee on Health and Disability 1998, *The Social, Cultural and Economic Determinants of Health in New Zealand*, National Advisory Committee on Health and Disability, Wellington.

National Centre for Epidemiology and Population Health 1992, *Improving Australia's Health: the Role of Primary Health Care*, Final Report of the Review of the Role of Primary Health Care in Health Promotion in Australia, NCEPH, Australian National University, Canberra.

National Centre for Social and Economic Modelling 1995, *Income Distribution Report*, Faculty of Management, University of Canberra, Canberra.

National Commission of Audit 1996, Report to the Commonwealth Government, AGPS, Canberra.

National Drug Research Institute 2000, *Indigenous Australian Alcohol and Other Drugs Databases*, National Drug Research Institute, Curtin University of Technology, Perth: <http://db.ndri.curtin.edu.au>

National Health Strategy 1991, *The Australian Health Jigsaw: Integration of Health Care Delivery*, Issues Paper no. 1, AGPS, Canberra.

—— 1992, *Enough to Make You Sick: How Income and Environment Affect Health*, AGPS, Canberra.

—— 1993a, *Healthy Participation: Achieving Greater Public Participation and Accountability in the Australian Health Care System*, Issues Paper no. 12, AGPS, Canberra.

—— 1993b, *Removing Cultural and Language Barriers to Health*, Issues Paper no. 6, AGPS, Canberra.

National Nursing Organisations 2000, 'Nurse Practitioner Positions a Reality at Last', Australian Nursing Federation [web site], <www.anf.org.au/>, accessed: 13 November.

National Office of Overseas Skills Recognition (NOOSR) 2001, [web site], <www.deet.gov.au/divisions/noosr/prof.htm>, date accessed: 17 January.

Navarro, V. 1986, *Crisis, Health and Medicine: A Social Critique*, Tavistock, London.

—— 1976, *Medicine Under Capitalism*, Prodist, New York.

—— 1988, 'Professional Dominance or Proletarianisation? Neither', *Milbank Quarterly*, vol. 66, no. 2, pp. 57–75.

—— 1992, *Why the United States Does Not Have a National Health Program*, Baywood Publishing, New York.

—— 1998, 'Book Review of Private Medicine and Public Health: Profits, Politics and Prejudice in the American Health Care Enterprise by Lawrence D. Weiss', *Contemporary Sociology*, vol. 27, no. 4, pp. 419–20.

Navarro, V. & Berman, D. M. 1977, *Health and Work: An International Perspective*, Baywood Publishing, New York.

NEB, see Nurses Education Board of NSW.

Neff, J. A., McFall, S. L., & Cleaveland, T. D. 1987, 'Psychiatry and Medicine in the US: Interpreting Trends in Medical Specialty Choice', *Sociology of Health and Illness*, vol. 9, no. 1, pp. 45–61.

Nelkin, D. & Lindee, S. 1995, *The DNA Mystique: The Gene as a Cultural Icon*, Freeman, New York.

Nettleton, S. 1995, *The Sociology of Health and Illness*, Polity Press, Cambridge.

NHS, see National Health Strategy.

Nordholm, L. A. & Westbrook, M. T. 1981, 'Career Selection, Satisfaction and Aspirations among Female Students in Five Health Professions', *Australian Psychologist*, vol. 16, p. 1.

Norman, J. 1998, 'Physician Heal Thyself', *Australian Magazine*, 4–5 April, p. 30.

Northcott, H. C. & Bachynsky, J. A. 1993, 'Concurrent Utilisation of Chiropractic, Prescription Medicines, Non Prescription Medicines and Alternative Health Care', *Social Science and Medicine*, vol. 37, no. 3, pp. 431–5.

Nozick, R. 1975, *Anarchy, State, and Utopia*, Blackwell, Oxford.

NSW Department of Health 1995, Final Report of the Steering Committee into the Nurse Practitioner Project Stage 3, NSW Department of Health, Sydney.

—— 2000, NSW Nurse Practitioners [web site], <www.health.nsw.gov.au/nursing/npract.html>, accessed: 13 November.

Nuckolls, C. 1997, 'Allocating Value to Gender in Official American Psychiatry, Part I: The Cultural Construction of the Personality Disorder Classification System', *Anthropology & Medicine*, vol. 4, pp. 45–66.

Nurses Education Board of NSW 1980, *Report of the Committee Established to Consider the Future Organisation of Nursing Education in the Sydney Metropolitan Area*, NEB (NSW), Sydney.

Nussbaum, M. C. 2000, *Women and Human Development: The Capabilities Approach*, Cambridge University Press, Cambridge.

Oakley, A. 1972, *Sex, Gender and Society*, Sun Books, Melbourne.

—— 1980, *Women Confined*, Martin Robertson, Oxford.

O'Connor, M. L. & Parker, E. 1995, *Health Promotion: Principals and Practice in the Australian Context*, Allen & Unwin, Sydney.

Office of the Status of Women. 1999, *Women in Australia*, Office of the Status of Women, Canberra.

O'Malley, P. 1996, 'Risk and Responsibility', in A. Barry, T. Osborne, & N. Rose (eds), *Foucault and Political Reason: Liberalism, Neo-liberalism and Rationalities of Government*, UCL Press, London.

O'Neill, A. 1994, *Enemies Within and Enemies Without: Educating Chiropractors, Osteopaths and Traditional Acupuncturists*, La Trobe University Press, Melbourne.

—— 1995, 'Daylight at Noon: Alternative Health Battles', in H. Gardner (ed.), *The Politics of Health*, 2nd edn, Churchill Livingstone, Melbourne, pp. 428–52.

O'Neill, J. 1990, 'AIDS as a Globalizing Panic', *Theory, Culture and Society*, vol. 7, nos 2–3, pp. 329–42.

Orona, C. 1990, 'Temporality and identity loss due to Alzheimer's disease', *Social Science and Medicine*, vol. 30, no. 11, pp. 1247–56.

Ornish, D. 1990, *Reversing Heart Disease*, Century, London.

Ornish, D., Brown, S. E., Scherwitz, L. W., Billings, J. H., Armstrong, W. T. Ports, T. A. et al. 1990, 'Can Lifestyle Changes Reverse Coronary Heart Disease?', *Lancet*, no. 336, pp. 129–33.

Orwell, G. 1945, *Animal Farm*, Secker & Warburg, London.

OSW, see Office of the Status of Women

Ottawa Charter for Health Promotion 1986, *Conference Proceedings of an International Conference on Health Promotion, 17–21 November*, Ottawa, Canada, World Health Organization and Health and Welfare, Canada.

Outram, S. 1989, *Social Policy*, Longman, London.

Pakulski, J. & Waters, M. 1996, *The Death of Class*, Sage, London.

Palmer, G. R. & Short, S. D. 1994, *Health Care and Public Policy*, 2nd edn, Macmillan, Melbourne.

Parkin, F. 1979, *Marxism and Class Theory: A Bourgeois Critique*, Tavistock, London.

Parsons, T. 1951a, 'Illness and the Role of the Physician: A Sociological Perspective', *American Journal of Orthopsychiatry*, vol. 21, pp. 452–66.

—— 1951b, *The Social System*, Free Press, New York.

—— 1971, *The System of Modern Societies*, Prentice-Hall, Englewood Cliffs, NJ.

Pateman, C. 1970, *Participation and Democratic Theory*, Cambridge University Press, Cambridge.

—— 1988, *The Sexual Contract*, Polity Press, Cambridge.

—— 1989, *The Disorder of Women*, Polity Press, Cambridge.

Paterson, J. 1988, 'A Managerialist Strikes Back', *Australian Journal of Public Administration*, vol. 47, no. 4, pp. 287–95.

Peale, S. & De Grandpre, R. 1995, 'My Genes Made Me Do It', *Psychology Today*, July/August, pp. 50–68.

Pearson, A. (ed.) 1988, *Primary Nursing: Nursing in Burford and Oxford Nursing Development Units*, Croom Helm, London.

Pearson, N. 1999, *Our Right to take Responsibility*, Noel Pearson & Associates, Ainslie, ACT.

Perron, M. 1995, untitled contribution, in S. Chapman & S. Leeder (eds), *The Last Right?*, Mandarin, Melbourne, pp. 45–57.

Petersen, A. 1996, 'Risk and the Regulated Self: The Discourse of Health Promotion as Politics of Uncertainty', *Australian and New Zealand Journal of Sociology*, vol. 32, pp. 44–57.

—— 1997, 'The Portrayal of Research into Genetic-based Research into Sex and Sexual Orientation: A Study of Popular Science Journals; 1980 to 1997', *Journal of Communication Inquiry*, vol. 23, no. 2, pp. 163–82.

—— 1998, 'The New Genetics and the Politics of Public Health', *Critical Public Health*, vol. 8, no. 1, pp. 59–71.

—— 2001, 'Biofantasies: Genetics and Medicine in the Print News Media', *Social Science and Medicine*, vol. 52, no. 8, pp. 1255–68.

Petersen, A. & Bunton, R. (eds) 1997, *Foucault, Health and Medicine*, Routledge, London.

Petersen, A. & Lupton, D. 1996, *The New Public Health: Health and Self in the Age of Risk*, Allen & Unwin, Sydney, and Sage, London.

Peterson, P. G. 1999, 'Gray Dawn. The Global Aging Crisis', *Foreign Affairs*, vol. 78, no. 1, pp. 42–56.

Phillips, D. L. & Segal, B. E. 1969, 'Sexual Status and Psychiatric Symptoms', *American Sociological Review*, vol. 34, pp. 58–72.

PIAC, see Public Interest Advocacy Centre.

PHIAC 2002: <www.phiac.gov.au>

Pinell, P. 1996, 'Modern Medicine and the Civilising Process', *Sociology of Health and Illness*, vol. 18, no. 1, pp. 1–16.

Pirotta, M. V., Cohen, M. M., Kotsirilos, V., & Farish, S. J. 2000, 'Complementary Therapies: Have They Become Accepted in General Practice?', *Medical Journal of Australia*, vol. 172, pp. 105–9.

Pittaway, E. 1999, 'Refugee Women—The Unsung Heroes', in B. Ferguson & E. Pittaway (eds), *Nobody Wants to Talk About It: Refugee Women's Mental Health*, Transcultural Mental Health Centre, pp. 1–20.

Pollitt, C. 1993, *Managerialism and the Public Services*, 2nd edn, Blackwell, Oxford.

Porter, R. 1997, *The Greatest Benefit to Mankind: A Medical History of Humanity from Antiquity to the Present*, HarperCollins, London.

Porter, R. & Porter, D. 1988, *In Sickness and In Health: the British Experience 1650–1850*, Fourth Estate, London.

Porter, S. 1992, 'The Poverty of Professionalization: A Critical Analysis of Strategies for the Occupational Advancement of Nursing', *Journal of Advanced Nursing*, vol. 17, pp. 720–6.

—— 1995, *Nursing's Relationship with Medicine*, Avebury, Aldershot.

Poovey, M. 1988, 'Feminism and deconstruction', *Feminist Studies*, vol. 14, no. 1, pp. 51–65.

Precope, J. 1961, *Iatro Philosophers of the Hellenic States*, Heinemann, London.

Primary Health Care Group 1996, Draft National Men's Health Policy, Commonwealth Department of Human Services and Health, Canberra.

Pringle, R. 1988, *Secretaries Talk: Sexuality, Power and Work*, Allen & Unwin, Sydney.

—— 1995, 'Destabilising Patriarchy', in B. Caine & R. Pringle (eds), *Transitions: New Australian Feminisms*, Allen & Unwin, Sydney, pp. 198–211.

—— 1998, *Sex and Medicine: Gender, Power and Authority in the Medical Profession*, Cambridge University Press, Cambridge.

Putnam, R. 1993, *Making Democracy Work: Civic Traditions in Modern Italy*, Princeton University Press, Princeton.

—— 2000, *Bowling Alone: The Collapse and Revival of American Community*, Simon & Schuster, New York.

Pyke, K. D. 1996, 'Class-based Masculinities: The Interdependence of Gender, Class and Interpersonal Power', *Gender & Society*, October, pp. 527–49.

Quinlan, M. 1988, 'Psychological and Sociological Approaches to the Study of Occupational Illness: A Critical Review', *Australia and New Zealand Journal of Sociology*, vol. 24, no. 2, pp. 189–206.

—— (ed.) 1993, *Work and Health*, Macmillan, Melbourne.

Radley, A. (ed.) 1993, *Worlds of Illness: Biographical and Cultural Perspectives on Health and Disease*, Routledge, London.

Raftery, J. 1995, 'The Social and Historical Context', in F. Baum (ed.), *Health for All: The South Australian Experience*, Wakefield Press, Adelaide, ch. 1, pp. 19–37.

RAFI, see Rural Advancement Foundation International.

Ragg, M. 1997, 'Good Medicine', *Australian*, 11 November, p. 13.

Raskall, P. 1993, 'Widening Income Disparities in Australia', in S. Rees, G. Rodley, & F. Stilwell (eds), *Beyond the Market: Alternatives to Economic Rationalism*, Pluto Press, Sydney.

Ratcliffe, J., Wallack, L., Fagnani, F., & Rodwin, V. 1984, 'Perspectives on Prevention: Health Promotion vs Health Protection', in J. de Kervasdoue, J. R. Kimberley, & G. Rodwin (eds), *The End of an Illusion: The Future of Health Policy in Western Industrialized Nations*, University of California Press, Berkeley, Calif., pp. 56–84.

Rawls, J. 1970, *A Theory of Justice*, The Clarendon Press, Oxford.

Rayner, L. & Easthope, G. (in press) 'Postmodern Consumption and Alternative Medications, *Journal of Sociology*.

Redman, S., Booth, P., Smyth, H., & Paul, C. 1992, 'Preventive Health Behaviours among Parents of Infants Aged Four Months', *Australian Journal of Public Health*, vol. 16, pp. 175–81.

Redman, S., Hennrikus, D. J., Bowman, J. A., & Sanson-Fisher, R. W. 1988, 'Assessing Women's Health Needs', *Medical Journal of Australia*, no. 148, pp. 123–7.

Rees, S. & Rodley, G. (eds) 1995, *The Human Costs of Managerialism: Advocating the Recovery of Humanity*, Pluto Press, Sydney.

Rees, S., Rodley, G., & Stilwell, F. (eds) 1993, *Beyond the Market: Alternatives to Economic Rationalism*, Pluto Press, Sydney.

Reid, J. & Trompf, P. (eds) 1990, *The Health of Immigrant Australia: A Social Perspective*, Harcourt Brace Jovanovich, Sydney.

Reid, R., Maag, J., & Vasa, S. 1993, 'Attention deficit hyperactivity disorder as a disability category: a critique', *Exceptional Children*, vol. 60 pp. 198–215.

Reilly, D. T., Taylor, M. A., McSharry, C., & Aitchison, T. 1986, 'Is Homoeopathy a Placebo Response? Controlled Trials of Homoeopathic Potency, with Pollen in Hayfever as a Model', *Lancet*, vol. 333, no. 2, pp. 881–5.

Reiman, C. 2001, *The Gender Wage Gap in Australia*, Discussion Paper no. 54, March, NATSEN, Canberra.

Relman, A. S. 1980, 'The New Medical-Industrial Complex', *New England Journal of Medicine*, vol. 303, no. 2, pp. 963–70.

Renwick, M. & Sadkowsky, K. 1991, *Variations in Surgery Rates*, AGPS, Canberra.

Reynolds, C. 1995, *Public Health Law in Australia*, Federation Press, Leichhardt.

Reynolds, H. 1995, *Aboriginal Resistance to the European Invasion of Australia*, 2nd edn, Penguin, Melbourne.

Rhodes, R. A. W. 1991, 'Introduction', *Public Administration*, vol. 69, no. 1, pp. 1–12.

Rice, P. & Ezzy, D. 1999, *Qualitative Research Methods: A Health Focus*, Oxford University Press, Melbourne.

Rice, P. L. 2000, *Hmong Women and Reproduction*, Bergin & Garvey, Westport, CT.

Rice, P. L. (ed.) 1994, *Asian Mothers, Australian Birth, Pregnancy, Childbirth and Childrearing: The Asian Experience in an English-Speaking Country*, Ausmed Publications, Melbourne.

Rice, P. L., Ly, B., & Lumley, J. 1994, 'Childbirth and Soul Loss: The Case of a Hmong Woman', *Medical Journal of Australia*, vol. 160, pp. 577–8.

'Rich 200' 2001, *Business Review Weekly*, 18 May, vol. 23, no. 19.

Richards, E. 1988, 'The politics of Therapeutic Evaluation: The Vitamin C and Cancer Controversy', *Social Studies of Science*, vol. 18, pp. 653–701.

Richards, T. 1991, *The Commodity Culture of Victorian England*, Verso, London.

Richardson, J. 1998, 'The Health Care Financing Debate', in G. Mooney & R. Scotton (eds), *Economics and Australian Health Policy*, Allen & Unwin, Sydney, 192–213.

Richardson, L. 1994, 'Writing: A method of inquiry', in N. Denzin & Y. Lincoln (eds), *Handbook of Qualitative Research*, Sage, Thousand Oaks.

Richmond, C. 1990, 'Report on UK Cancer Survival Rates Raises Questions about Alternative Medicine', *Canadian Medical Association Journal*, vol. 143, no. 9, pp. 922–3.

Richmond, K. 1995, 'Knowledge, Attitudes, Beliefs and Behaviour of Women Factory Workers in Relation to Cardiovascular Disease', in R. Sorger (ed.), *Women Have a Heart Too*, Healthsharing Women's Health Resource Service, Melbourne, pp. 51–5.

Rieger, E. 1996, 'The Diet–Heart Disease Hypothesis: A Response to Atrens', *Social Science and Medicine*, vol. 42, no. 9, pp. 1227–33.

Riessman, C. 1993, *Narrative Analysis*, Sage, Newbury Park.

Riska, E. 1993, 'Introduction', in E. Riska & K. Wegar (eds), *Gender, Women and Medicine: Women and the Medical Division of Labour*, Sage, London.

Ritchie, J., Herscovitch, F., & Norfor, J. 1994, 'Beliefs of Blue Collar Workers Regarding Coronary Risk Behaviours', *Health Education Research*, vol. 9, pp. 95–103.

Ritzer, G. 1993, *The McDonaldization of Society*, Pine Forge Press, Thousand Oaks, Calif.

—— 1996, *Sociological Theory*, 4th edn, McGraw-Hill, New York.

—— 1997, *Postmodern Social Theory*, McGraw-Hill, New York.

Rixon, G., March, L., & Holt, D. A. 1994, 'Immunisation Practices of General Practitioners in Metropolitan Sydney', *Australian Journal of Public Health*, vol. 18, pp. 258–60.

Roach Anleu, S. L. 1993, 'Reproductive Autonomy: Infertility, Deviance and Conceptive Technology', *Law in Context*, vol. 11, pp. 17–40.

—— 1999, *Deviance, Conformity and Control*, 3rd edn, Longman, Melbourne.

Roberts, G. L. 1994, *Domestic Violence Victims in a Hospital Emergency Department*, University of Queensland, Department of Psychiatry.

Roberts, S. J. 1983, 'Oppressed Group Behaviour: Implications for Nursing', *Advances in Nursing Science*, vol. 5, no. 4, pp. 21–30.

Roche, M. 1992, *Rethinking Citizenship: Welfare, Ideology and Change in Modern Society*, Polity Press, Cambridge.

Rogers v. Whitaker (1992) ATR 81.

Rose, H. 1994, *Love, Power and Knowledge: Towards a Feminist Transformation of the Sciences*, Polity Press, Cambridge.

Rose, N. 1993, 'Government, Authority and Expertise in Advanced Liberalism', *Economy and Society*, vol. 22, no. 3, pp. 283–99.

Rosen, G. 1972, 'The evolution of social medicine', in H. E. Freeman, S. Levine, & L. G. Reeder (eds), *Handbook of Medical Sociology*, 2nd edn, Prentice-Hall, Englewood Cliffs, NJ, pp. 30–60.

Rosenhan, D. L. 1973, 'Being Sane in Insane Places', *Science*, no. 179, pp. 250–8.

Ross, B., Nixon, J., Snasdell-Taylor, J., & Delaney, K., 1999, *International Approaches to Funding Health Care*, Occasional Papers: Health Financing Series, vol. 2, Commonwealth of Australia, Canberra, [web site], <www.health.gov.au:80/hfs/pubs/hfsocc/ocpahfsv2.pdf>

Ross, B., Snasdell-Taylor, J., Cass, J., & Azmi, S., 1999, Occasional Papers: Health Financing Series, vol. 1, Commonwealth of Australia, Canberra, [web site], <www.health.gov.au/pubs/hfsocc/ocpahfsv1.pdf>

Rothman, B. K. 1986, *The Tentative Pregnancy: Prenatal Diagnosis and the Future of Motherhood*, Norton, New York.

—— 1998, *Genetic Maps and Human Imaginations*, Norton, New York.

Rowland, D. T. 1991, *Pioneers Again: Immigrants and Ageing in Australia*, Bureau of Immigration Research and AGPS, Canberra.

Rowley, C. D. 1970, *The Destruction of Aboriginal Society*, Australian National University Press, Canberra.

—— 1978, *A Matter of Justice*, Australian National University Press, Canberra.

Rowse, T. 1998, *White Flour, White Power: From Rations to Citizenship in Central Australia*, Cambridge University Press, Melbourne.

Royal Australasian College of Physicians 1999, *For Richer, For Poorer, In Sickness and in Health: The Socioeconomic Determinants of Health*, RACP.

Ruggiero, V. R. 1996, *A Guide to Sociological Thinking*, Sage, Thousand Oaks, Calif.

Rural Advancement Foundation International 1996, *Indigenous Person from Papua New Guinea Claimed in US Government Patent*, Internet <www.charm.net/~rafi/release01.html>, 12 December.

Russell, C. 1981, *The Ageing Experience*, Allen & Unwin, Sydney.

Russell, C. & Schofield, T. 1986, *Where it Hurts: An Introduction to Sociology for Health Workers*, Allen & Unwin, Sydney.

Ryan, W. 1971, *Blaming the Victim*, Vintage, New York.

Sabo, D. & Gordon, D. F. (eds) 1995, *Men's Health and Illness: Gender, Power and the Body*, Sage, Thousand Oaks, Calif.

Sackett, D. 1981, 'How to read clinical journals: V: To distinguish useful from useless or even harmful therapy', *Journal of the Canadian Medical Association*, vol. 124, pp. 1156–62.

Sackett, L. 1988, 'Resisting arrests: drinking, development and discipline in desert context', *Social Analysis*, no. 24, 66–77.

Saggers, S. & Gray, D. 1991a, *Aboriginal Health and Society: The Traditional and Contemporary Struggle for Better Health*, Allen & Unwin, Sydney.

—— 1991b, 'Policy and Practice in Aboriginal Health', in J. Reid & P. Trompf (eds), *The Health of Aboriginal Australia*, Harcourt Brace Jovanovich, Sydney.

—— 1998a, 'Alcohol, Risk and Liberty: An Analysis of Interventions in Indigenous Australian Communities', in A. Petersen & C. Waddell (eds), *Health Matters: A Sociology of Illness, Prevention and Care*, Allen & Unwin, Sydney.

—— 1998b, *Dealing with Alcohol: Indigenous Usage in Australia, Canada and New Zealand*, Cambridge University Press, Melbourne.

Sahlins, M. 1974, *Stone Age Economics*, Tavistock, London.

Saks, M. 1994, 'The Alternatives to Medicine', in J. Gabe, D. Kelleher, & G. Williams (eds), *Challenging Medicine*, Routledge, London, pp. 84–103.

Salmon, J. W. (ed.) 1990, *The Corporate Transformation of Health Care: Issues and Directions*, vol. 1, Baywood, New York.

—— (ed.) 1994, *The Corporate Transformation of Health Care: Perspectives and Implications*, vol. 2, Baywood, New York.

Salmond, C., Soljak, M. A., Bandaranayake, D. R., & Stehr-Green, P. 1994, 'Impact of a Promotion Program for Hepatitis B Immunisation', *Australian Journal of Public Health*, vol. 18, pp. 253–7.

Salvage, J. 1988, 'Professionalism—or Struggle for Survival? A Consideration of Current Proposals for the Reform of Nursing in the United Kingdom', *Journal of Advanced Nursing*, vol. 13, pp. 515–19.

—— 1992, 'The New Nursing: Empowering Patients or Empowering Nurses?', in A. Robinson, A. Gray, & R. Elkan (eds), *Policy Issues in Nursing*, Open University Press, Buckingham, pp. 9–23.

Sampson, A. 2000, 'How the Boomers Are Being Skinned', *Sydney Morning Herald* (Insight), 19 September, p. 7.

Sanderson, C. & Alexander, K. 1995, 'Community Health Services Planning for Health', in F. Baum (ed.), *Health For All: The South Australian Experience*, Wakefield Press, Adelaide, ch. 10, pp. 161–71.

Sansom, B. 1980, *The Camp at Wallaby Cross*, Australian Institute of Aboriginal Studies, Canberra.

Sanson-Fisher, R., Schofield, M. J., & Sia, M. 1992, 'Availability of Cigarettes to Minors', *Australian Journal of Public Health*, vol. 16, pp. 354–9.

Saunders, C. 1994, 'Acupuncture Gaining Popularity', *Australian Doctor*, 25 February, p. 16.

Saunders, P. 1996, *Poverty, Income Distribution and Health: An Australian Study*, Social Policy Research Centre, University of New South Wales, Sydney.

Savcigil, R. 1982, 'Migrant Women at Work: The Boss is Like a Dictator', *Migration Action*, vol. 6, no. 2, pp. 28–34.

Sawyer, M. G. et al. 1994, 'The Use of Alternative Therapies by Children with Cancer', *Medical Journal of Australia*, vol. 160, pp. 320–2.

Sax, S. 1984, *A Strife of Interests: Politics and Policies in Australian Health Services*, Allen & Unwin, Sydney.

—— 1990, *Health Care Choices and the Public Purse*, Allen & Unwin, Sydney.

Sayer-Jones, Moya 2000, 'Modern Guru', *Good Weekend*, 16 December, p. 13.

Scheff, T. J. 1966, *Being Mentally Ill: A Sociological Theory*, Aldine, Chicago.

Scheper-Hughes, N. & Lock, M. 1987, 'The Mindful Body: A Prolegomenon to Future Work in Medical Anthropology', *Medical Anthropology Quarterly*, vol. 1, pp. 6–41.

Schofield, D. 1999. 'Ancillary and specialist health services: the relationship between income, user rates and equity of access', *Australian Journal of Social Issues*, vol. 34, no. 1, pp. 79–96.

Schuessler, K. F. & Cressey, D. R. 1950, 'Personality Characteristics of Criminals', *American Journal of Sociology*, vol. 55, pp. 476–84.

Schur, E. 1983, *Labelling Women Deviant: Gender, Stigma, and Social Control*, Temple University Press, Philadelphia.

Schutz, A. 1972/1933, *The Phenomenology of the Social World*, Heinemann, London.

Schwartz-Cowan, R. 1992, 'Genetic Technology and Reproductive Choice', in D. Kevles & L. Hood (eds), *The Code of Codes: Scientific and Social Issues in the Human Genome Project*, Harvard University Press, Cambridge, Mass., pp. 244–63.

Scott, J., Begley, A. M., & Miller, M. R., & Binns, C. W. 1991, 'Nutrition Education in Supermarkets: The Lifestyle 2000 Experience', *Australian Journal of Public Health*, vol. 15, pp. 49–55.

Scotton, R. B. 1998, 'The Doctor Business', in G. Mooney & R. Scotton (eds), *Economics and Australian Health Policy*, Allen & Unwin, Sydney, pp. 72–92.

Scotton, R. B. & Macdonald, C. R. 1993, *The Making of Medibank*, School of Health Services Management, University of New South Wales, Sydney.

Scrimgeour, D., Rowse, T., & Knight, S. 1994, 'Food-purchasing in an Aboriginal Community: Evaluation of an Intervention', *Australian Journal of Public Health*, vol. 18, pp. 67–70.

Scull, A. T. 1975, 'From Madness to Mental Illness: Medical Men as Moral Entrepreneurs', *Archives Européennes de Sociologie*, vol. 16, pp. 218–61.

—— 1977, 'Madness and Segregative Control: The Role of the Insane Asylum', *Social Problems*, vol. 24, pp. 337–51.

Scull, A. T. & Favreau D. 1986, 'A Chance to Cut is a Chance to Cure: Sexual Surgery for Psychosis in Three Nineteenth-century Societies', *Research in Law, Deviance and Social Control*, vol. 8, London, pp. 3–39.

Seale, C & Pattison, S. (eds) 1994, *Medical Knowledge: Doubt and Certainty*, Open University Press, Buckingham.

Selbourne, D. 1994, *The Principle of Duty*, Sinclair-Stevenson, London.

Select Committee on Euthanasia 1995, Report of the Inquiry, Legislative Assembly of the Northern Territory, Darwin.

Self, P. 1993, *Government by the Market?*, Macmillan, London.

Shaw, G. B. 1908, *The Doctor's Dilemma*, Constable, London.

—— 1930, *Back to Methuselah*, Constable, London.

Sheehy, E. A., Stubbs, J., & Tolmie, J. 1992, 'Defending Battered Women on Trial: The Battered Woman Syndrome and its Limitations', *Criminal Law Journal*, vol. 16, pp. 369–94.

Sherrard, J., Ozanne-Smith, J., Brumen, I. A., Routley, V., & Williams, F. 1994, *Domestic Violence: Patterns and Indicators*, Monash University, Melbourne.

Short, S. D. & Sharman, E. 1995, 'The Nursing Struggle in Australia', in G. M. Lupton & J. Najman (eds), *Sociology of Health and Illness: Australian Readings*, 2nd edn, Macmillan, Melbourne, pp. 236–51.

Short, S. D., Sharman, E., & Speedy, S. 1993, *Sociology for Nurses: An Australian Introduction*, Macmillan, Sydney.

Siahpush, M. 1998, 'Postmodern Values, Dissatisfaction with Conventional Medicine and Popularity of Alternative Therapies, *Journal of Sociology*, vol. 34, pp. 58–70.

—— 1999, 'Why do People Favour Alternative Medicine?', *Australian and New Zealand Journal of Public Health*, vol. 23, no. 3, pp. 266–71.

Siegel, K. L. M., Brooks, C. M., & Kern, R. 1989, 'The Motives of Gay Men for Taking or Not Taking the HIV Antibody Test', *Social Problems*, vol. 36, pp. 368–83.

Silagy, C. 2000, 'Co-ordinated Care Trials', in Commonwealth Department of Health and Aged Care (ed.), *General Practice in Australia 2000*, Commonwealth Department of Health and Aged Care, Canberra, pp. 471–92.

Silove, D., Tarn, R., Bowles, R., & Reid, J. 1991, 'Psychotherapy for Survivors of Torture', in I. H. Minas (ed.), *Cultural Diversity and Mental Health*, Royal Australian and New Zealand College of Psychiatrists—Victorian Transcultural Psychiatry Unit, Melbourne, pp. 171–93.

Simon, J. 1993, *Poor Discipline: Parole and the Social Control of the Underclass, 1890–1990*, University of Chicago Press, Chicago.

Sindall, C. 1992, 'Health Promotion and Community Health in Australia', in F. Baum, D. Fry, & I. Lennie (eds), *Community Health: Policy and Practice in Australia*, Pluto Press, Sydney, pp. 277–95.

Singer 1994, *Rethinking Life and Death*, Text Publishing Company, Melbourne.

Singleton, V. 1996, 'Feminism, Sociology of Scientific Knowledge and Postmodernism: Politics, Theory and Me', *Social Studies of Science*, vol. 26, pp. 445–68.

Siskind, V., Copeman, R., & Najman, J. M. 1987a, 'Socioeconomic Status and Mortality: A Brisbane Area Analysis', *Community Health Studies*, vol. 11, no. 1, pp. 15–23.

—— 1987b, 'Infant Mortality in Socioeconomically Advantaged and Disadvantaged Areas of Brisbane', *Community Health Studies*, vol. 11, no. 1, pp. 24–30.

Siskind, V., Najman, J., & Veitch, C. 1992, 'Socioeconomic Status and Mortality Revisited: An Extension of the Brisbane Area Analysis', *Australian Journal of Public Health*, vol. 16, pp. 315–20.

Skolbekken, J. A. 1995, 'The Risk Epidemic in Medical Journals', *Social Science and Medicine*, vol. 40, no. 2, pp. 291–305.

Smaje, C. 1996, 'The Ethnic Patterning of Health: New Directions for Theory and Research', *Sociology of Health and Illness*, vol. 18, no. 2, pp. 139–71.

Smart, C. 1976, *Women, Crime and Criminology: A Feminist Critique*, Routledge & Kegan Paul, London.

Smith, J. P. 1981, *Sociology and Nursing*, Churchill Livingstone, Edinburgh.

Smith, R. 1987, *Unemployment and health: A Disaster and a Challenge*, Oxford University Press, Oxford.

Snell, J. 2000, 'Trading Places', *Health Service Journal*, vol. 110, no. 5716, August, pp. 26–9.

Snow, J. 1936/1855, *On the Mode of Communication of Cholera* [reprinted as *Snow on Cholera*], Hafner, New York.

Sonke, G. S., Beaglehold, R., Stewart, A. W., Jackson, R., & Stewart, F. M. 1996, 'Sex Differences in Case Fatality before and after Admission to Hospital after Acute Cardiac Events: Analysis of Community Based Coronary Heart Disease Register', *British Medical Journal*, vol. 313, pp. 853–5.

South Australian Department of Human Services 2001, *Community Health Service Review—Definition of Core Services*, Metropolitan Health Services Division, SA Department of Human Services, Adelaide.

'Special Report: A Critical Condition' 1996, *Age*, 8 October.

Stacey, M. 1991, 'The Potential of Social Science for Complementary Medicine', *Complementary Medical Research*, vol. 5, no. 3, pp. 183–6.

Stanway, A. 1979, *Alternative Medicine: A Guide to Natural Therapies*, Rigby, Adelaide.

Stark, E. & Flincraft, A. 1991, 'Spouse Abuse', in M. Rosenberg & A. Finley (eds), *Violence in America: A Public Health Approach*, Oxford University Press, New York, pp. 161–81.

Starr, P. 1982, *The Social Transformation of American Medicine: The Rise of a Sovereign Profession and the Making of a Vast Industry*, Basic Books, New York.

Stein, L. 1967, 'The Doctor–Nurse Game', *Archives of General Psychiatry*, vol. 16, pp. 699–703.

Steingart, R. M., Packer, M., Hamm, P., Colianese, M. E., Gersh, B., Geltman, E. M. et al. 1991, 'Sex Differences in the Management of Coronary Artery Disease', *New England Journal of Medicine*, vol. 325, no. 4, pp. 226–30.

Stilwell, F. 1993, *Economic Inequality: Who Gets What in Australia*, Pluto Press, Sydney.

Strasser, R. D. 1992, 'The Gatekeeper Role of General Practice', *Medical Journal of Australia*, vol. 156, pp. 108–10.

Strauss, A. 1978, *Negotiations: Varieties, Contexts, Processes, and Social Order*, Jossey-Bass, San Francisco.

Strauss, A. & Corbin, J. 1990, *Basics of Qualitative Research*, Sage, London.

Strauss, A., Schatzman, L., Ehrlich, D., Bucher, R., & Sabshin, M. 1963, 'The hospital and its negotiated order', in E. Freidson (ed.), *The Hospital in Modern Society*, Free Press, New York.

Stretton, H. & Orchard, L. 1994, *Public Goods, Public Enterprise, Public Choice*, Macmillan, London.

Strong, P. M. 1979, 'Sociological Imperialism and the Profession of Medicine: A Critical Examination of the Thesis of Medical Imperialism', *Social Science and Medicine*, vol. 13A, no. 2, pp. 199–215.

'Sugaring the Pill' 1996, *New Scientist*, 27 January, pp. 27–9.

Sullivan, F. 2000, 'Complaints will Continue Until Care is Funded', media release, *Catholic Health Australia*, 27 July.

Sutton, J. R. 1991, 'The Political Economy of Madness: The Expansion of the Asylum in Progressive America', *American Sociological Review*, vol. 56, pp. 665–78.

Svensson, R. 1996, 'The Interplay between Doctors and Nurses: A Negotiated Order Perspective', *Sociology of Health and Illness*, vol. 18, no. 3, pp. 379–98.

Swan, P. & Raphael, B. 1995, 'Ways Forward', National Consultancy Report on Aboriginal and Torres Strait Islander Mental Health, parts 1 & 2, AGPS, Canberra.

Sweet, M. 1996, 'Why Men are More Likely to Die Young', *Sydney Morning Herald*, 25 July.

Swerrissen, H. et al. 1998, *Community Health and General Practitioners: Partnerships in Care*, Primary Health Care Research and Development Centre, LaTrobe University, Melbourne.

Szasz, T. S. 1960, 'The Myth of Mental Illness', *The American Psychologist*, vol. 15, pp. 113–18.

—— 1961, *The Myth of Mental Illness*, Holber-Harper, New York.

—— 1970, *The Manufacture of Madness*, Harper and Row, New York.

—— 1973, *Ideology and Insanity: Essays on the Psychiatric Dehumanization of Man*, Colder & Boyars, London.

Szreter S. 1988, 'The Importance of Social Intervention in Britain's Mortality Decline c. 1850–1914: A Reinterpretation of the Role of Public Health', *Society for the Social History of Medicine*, vol. 1, no. 1, pp. 1–37.

Tannahill, A. 1992, 'Epidemiology and Health Promotion: A Common Understanding', in R. Bunton & G. Macdonald (eds), *Health Promotion: Disciplines and Diversity*, Routledge, London, pp. 86–107.

Taskforce on Quality in Australian Health Care 1996, *The Final Report of the Taskforce on Quality in Australian Health Care*, Australian Health Minister's Advisory Council, Canberra.

Taylor, R., Herrman, H., & Preston, G. 1983, *Occupation and Mortality in Australian Working Age Males, 1975–77*, Health Commission of Victoria and the Department of Social and Preventive Medicine, Monash University, Melbourne.

Taylor, R., Morrell, S., Slaytor, E., & Ford, P. 1998, 'Suicide in urban New South Wales, Australia 1985–94: Socio-economic and migration interactions', *Social Science and Medicine*, vol. 47, pp. 1677–86.

Taylor, R. & Salkeld, G. 1996, 'Health Care Expenditure and Life Expectancy in Australia: How Well Do We Perform?', *Australian and New Zealand Journal of Public Health*, vol. 20, no. 3, pp. 233–40.

Tesoriero, F. 2001, 'Partnerships in Health Promotion and the Place of Trust and Equality as Obstacles to Promoting Health', *Health Promotion Journal of Australia*, vol. 11, no. 1.

Thame, C. 1974, 'Health and the State: The Development of Collective Responsibility for Health Care in Australia in the First Half of the Twentieth Century', PhD thesis.

Thomas, K. J. et al. 1991, 'Use of Non-orthodox and Conventional Health Care in Great Britain', *British Medical Journal*, vol. 302, pp. 207–302.

Thomson, N. 1984, 'Australian Aboriginal Health and Health Care', *Social Science and Medicine*, vol. 18, pp. 939–48.

Thorogood, N. 1992, 'What is the Relevance of Sociology for Health Promotion', in R. Bunton & G. Macdonald (eds), *Health Promotion: Disciplines and Diversity*, Routledge, London, pp. 42–65.

Titmuss, R. M. 1974, *Social Policy: An Introduction*, Allen & Unwin, London.

Tobin, J. N., Wassertheil-Smoller, S., Wexler, J. P., Steingart, R. M., Budner, N., Lense, L. et al. 1987, 'Sex Bias in Considering Coronary Bypass Surgery', *Annals of Internal Medicine*, vol. 107, pp. 19–25.

Tong, R. P. 1998, *Feminist Thought: A Comprehensive Introduction*, 2nd edn, Allen & Unwin, Sydney.

Townsend, P. & Davidson, N. (eds) 1982, *Inequalities in Health: The Black Report*, Penguin, Harmondsworth.

Townsend, P., Davidson, N., & Whitehead, M. (eds) 1992, *Inequalities in Health: The Black Report and the Health Divide*, Penguin, London.

TQAHC, see Taskforce on Quality in Australian Health Care.

Tran, H. 1994, 'Antenatal and Postnatal Maternity Care for Vietnamese Women', in P. L. Rice (ed.), *Asian Mothers, Australian Birth—Pregnancy, Childbirth and Childrearing: The Asian Experience in an English-speaking Country*, Ausmed Publications, Melbourne, ch. 5, pp. 61–76.

Travers, K. 1996, 'The Social Organization of Nutritional Inequities', *Social Sciences and Medicine*, vol. 43, pp. 543–53.

Trevelyan, J. & Booth, B. 1994, *Complementary Medicine for Nurses, Midwives and Health Visitors*, Macmillan, London.

Tulloch, P. 1983, 'The Welfare State and Social Policy', in B. Head (ed.), *State and Economy in Australia*, Oxford University Press, Melbourne, pp. 252–71.

Turbet, P. 1989, *The Aborigines of the Sydney District Before 1788*, Kangaroo Press, Sydney.

Turnbull, D., Adelson, P., & Irwig, L. 1992, 'Evaluating the Impact of a Promotional Campaign for Screening Mammography: Women's Knowledge and Sources of Awareness', *Australian Journal of Public Health*, vol. 16, pp. 72–8.

Turner, B. S. 1982, 'The government of the body: medical regimes and the rationalisation of diet', *British Journal of Sociology*, vol. 33, no. 2, pp. 254–69.

—— 1986a, *Citizenship and Capitalism: The Debate over Reformism*, Allen & Unwin, London.

—— 1986b 'The Vocabulary of Complaints: Nursing Professionalism and Job Context', *Australian and New Zealand Journal of Sociology*, vol. 22, no. 3, pp. 368–86.

—— 1987, *Medical Power and Social Knowledge*, Sage, London.

—— 1989, 'Outline of a Theory of Citizenship', *Sociology*, vol. 24, pp. 189–217.

—— 1992, *Regulating Bodies: Essays in Medical Sociology*, Routledge, London.

Turner, B. S. & Hamilton, P. (eds) 1994, *Citizenship: Critical Concepts*, 2 vols, Routledge, London.

Turner, B. S. with Samson, C. 1995, *Medical Power and Social Knowledge*, 2nd edn, Sage, London.

Turrell, G. & Mathers, C. D. 2000, 'Socioeconomic Status and Health in Australia', *Medical Journal of Australia*, vol. 172, 1 May, pp. 434–8.

—— 2001, 'Socioeconomic Inequalities in All-cause and Specific-cause Mortality in Australia: 1985–1987 and 1995–1997', *International Journal of Epidemiology*, vol. 30, pp. 231–9.

Turrell, G., Oldenburg, B., McGuffog, I., & Dent, R. 1999, *Socioeconomic Determinants of Health: Towards a National Research Program and a Policy and Intervention Agenda*, Centre for Public Health Research, School of Public Health, Queensland University of Technology, Brisbane.

Tye, C. C. & Ross, F. M. 2000, 'Blurring Boundaries: Professional Perspectives of the Emergency Nurse Practitioner Role in a Major Accident and Emergency Department', *Journal of Advanced Nursing*, vol. 31, no. 5, May, pp. 1089–96.

Unwin, E., Thomson, N., & Gracey, M. 1994, *The Impact of Tobacco Smoking and Alcohol Consumption on Aboriginal Mortality and Hospitalisation in Western Australia: 1983–1991*, Health Department of Western Australia, Perth.

Valverde, M. & White-Mair, K. 1999, '"One Day at a Time" and Other Slogans for Everyday Life: The Ethical Practices of Alcoholics Anonymous', *Sociology*, vol. 33, pp. 393–410.

Van Bergen, J. 1996, 'Epidemiology and Health Policy: A World of Difference? A Case-study of a Cholera Outbreak in Kaputa District, Zambia', *Social Science and Medicine*, vol. 43, no. 1, pp. 93–9.

Van Beurden, E., James, R., Montague, D., Christian, J., & Dunn, T. 1993, 'Community-based Cholesterol Screening and Education to Prevent Heart Disease: Five Year Results of the North Coast Cholesterol Check Campaign', *Australian Journal of Public Health*, vol. 17, pp. 109–16.

Van Wijk, C. M. T. G., Van Vliet, K. P., & Kolk, A. M. 1996, 'Gender Perspectives and Quality of Care: Towards Appropriate and Adequate Health Care for Women', *Social Science and Medicine*, vol. 43, no. 5, pp. 707–20.

Vasta, E. & Castles, S. (eds) 1996, *The Teeth are Smiling: The Persistence of Racism in Multicultural Australia*, Allen & Unwin, Sydney.

Vaughan P. 1959, *Doctors' Commons: A Short History of the British Medical Association*, Heinemann, London.

Vedhera, K., Fox, J. D., & Wang, E. C. 1999, 'The Measurement of Stress-related Immune Dysfunction in Psychoneuroimmunology', *Neuroscience and Behavioral Review*, vol. 23, no. 5, pp. 699–715.

Verhoef, M. J., Sutherland, L. R., & Brkich, L. 1990, 'Use of Alternative Medicine by Patients Attending a Gastroenterology Clinic', *Canadian Medical Association Journal*, vol. 142, no. 2, pp. 121–5.

Verhoef, M. J. & Sutherland L. R. 1995, 'Alternative Medicine and General Practitioners', *Canadian Family Physician*, vol. 41, pp. 1005–11.

Vincent, C. & Furnham, A. 1998, *Complementary Medicine: A Research Perspective*, Wiley, Chichester.

Viviani, N. 1996, *The Indochinese in Australia—1975–1995: From Burning Boats to Barbeques*, Oxford University Press, Melbourne.

Viviani, N., Coughlan, J., & Rowland, T. 1993, *Indochinese in Australia: The Issues of Unemployment and Residential Concentration*, AGPS, Canberra.

Waddell, C. & Petersen, A. R. (eds) 1994, *Just Health: Inequality in Illness, Care and Prevention*, Churchill Livingstone, Melbourne.

Waitzkin, H. 1983, *The Second Sickness: Contradictions of Capitalist Health Care*, Free Press, New York.

—— 2000, *The Second Sickness: Contradictions of Capitalist Health Care*, 2nd edn, Rowman & Littlefield, Lanham.

Walby, S. 1990, *Theorising Patriarchy*, Blackwell, Oxford.

—— 1992, 'Post-post-modernism? Theorizing Social Complexity', in M. Barrett & A. Phillips (eds), *Destabilizing Theory: Contemporary Feminist Debates*, Polity Press, Cambridge, pp. 31–52.

Walby, S. & Greenwell, J. 1994, *Medicine and Nursing: Professions in a Changing Health Service*, Sage, London.

Waldby, C., Kippax, S., & Crawford, J. 1995, 'Epidemiological Knowledge and Discriminatory Practice: AIDS and the Social Relations of Biomedicine', *Australian and New Zealand Journal of Sociology*, vol. 31, pp. 1–14.

Waldron, I. 1995, 'Contributions of Changing Gender Differences in Behavior and Social Roles to Changing Gender Differences in Mortality', in D. Sabo & D. F. Gordon (eds), *Men's Health and Illness: Gender, Power and the Body*, Sage, Thousand Oaks, Calif., pp. 22–45.

Walker, A. 1990, 'The Economic "burden" of Ageing and the Prospect of Intergenerational Conflict', *Ageing and Society*, vol. 10, pp. 377–96.

Waller, L. & Williams, C. R. 1993, *Criminal Law: Texts and Cases*, 7th edn, Butterworths, Sydney.

Wardlow, H. & Curry, R. 1996, '"Sympathy for My Body": Breast Cancer and Mammography at Two Atlanta Clinics', *Medical Anthropology*, vol. 16, pp. 319–40.

Warin, M., Baum, F. et al. 1998, *Not Just a Doctor: Community Perspective on Medical Services in Women's and Community Health Centres*, SACHRU, Adelaide.

Watson, J. 2000, *Male Bodies: Health, Culture and Identity*, Open University Press, Buckingham.

Waxler-Morrison, N, Hislop T. G., Mears B., & Kan L. 1991, 'Effects of social relationships on survival for women with breast cancer: a prospective study', *Social Science & Medicine*, vol. 33, no. 2, pp. 177–83.

Wearing, B. 1996, *Gender: The Pain and Pleasure of Difference*, Addison Wesley Longman, Sydney.

Weber, M. 1968/1921, *Economy and Society*, Bedminster, New York.

—— 1981, *The City*, Free Press, New York.

Weedon, C. 1987, *Feminist Practice and Poststructuralist Theory*, Blackwell, Oxford.

Weiss, R. & Their, S. 1988, 'HIV Testing is the Answer—What's the Question?', *New England Journal of Medicine*, vol. 319, no. 5, pp. 1010–12.

Westergaard, J. 1995, *Who Gets What? The Hardening of Class Inequality in the Late Twentieth Century*, Polity Press, Cambridge.

Western, M. 2000, 'Class in Australia in the 1980s and 1990s', in J. M. Najman & J. S. Western (eds), *A Sociology of Australian Society*, 3rd edn, Macmillan, Melbourne, ch. 4, pp. 68–88.

Wharton, R. & Lewith, G. 1986, 'Complementary Medicine and the General Practitioner', *British Medical Journal*, vol. 292, no. 6534, pp. 1498–500.

Wheelwright, T. 1990, 'Are the Rich Getting Richer and the Poor Poorer? If So, Why?', in A. Gollan (ed.), *Questions for the Nineties*, Left Book Club, Sydney, pp. 199–215.

White, J. P. & Mulvaney, D. J. 1987, 'How Many People?' in D. J. Mulvaney & J. P. White (eds), *Australians to 1788*, Fairfax, Syme and Weldon, Sydney.

White, K. 1991, 'The sociology of health and illness: A trend report', *Current Sociology*, vol. 39, no. 2, pp. 1–115.

—— 2000, 'The State, the Market, and General Practice: The Australian Case', *International Journal of Health Services*, vol. 30, no. 2, pp. 285–308.

White, K. & Willis, E. 1998. 'Evidence Based Medicine and the Sociology of Medical Knowledge', Paper presented at the Annual National Conference of the Australian Sociological Association, Brisbane.

Whitehead, M. 1987, *The Health Divide: Inequalities in Health in the 1980s*, Health Education Council, London.

—— 1992, 'The Concepts and Principles of Equity and Health', *International Journal of Health Services*, vol. 22, pp. 429–45.

—— 1995, 'Tackling Inequalities: A Review of Policy Initiatives', in M. Benzeval, K. Judge, & M. Whitehead (eds), *Tackling Inequalities in Health: An Agenda or Action*, King's Fund, London.

Whitehead, M., Judge, K., Hunter, D. J., Maxwell, R., & Scheuer, M. A. 1993, 'Tackling Inequalities in Health: The Australian Experience', *British Medical Journal*, vol. 306, pp. 783–7.

Wicks, D. 1995a, 'Contested Femininity: Gender and Work at the Sydney Infirmary 1868–1875', *Journal of Interdisciplinary Gender Studies*, vol. 1, pp. 89–99.

—— 1995b, 'Nurses and Doctors and Discourses of Healing', *Australian and New Zealand Journal of Sociology*, vol. 31, no. 2, pp. 122–39.

—— 1999, *Nurses and Doctors at Work: Rethinking Professional Boundaries*, Allen & Unwin, Sydney.

Wicks, D., Bryson, L., & Mishra, G. 1997, *Health and Socio-economic Class: A Survey of a Cohort of Australian Women*, conference paper presented to the 29th Annual Conference of the Public Health Association, Melbourne, 5–8 October.

Wild, R. 1974, *Bradstow*, Angus & Robertson, Sydney.

—— 1978, *Social Stratification in Australia*, George Allen & Unwin, Sydney.

Wiley, K. 1979, *When the Sky Fell Down: The Destruction of the Tribes of the Sydney Region 1788–1850s*, Collins, Sydney.

Wilkie, T. 1994, *Perilous Knowledge: The Human Genome Project and Its Implications*, Faber & Faber, London.

Wilkinson, M. 2000, 'Negative Imaging', *Sydney Morning Herald*, May 13, p. 40.

Wilkinson, R. & Marmot, M. (eds) 1998, *The Solid Facts: Social Determinants of Health*, World Health Organization, Copenhagen.

Wilkinson, R. G. (ed.) 1986, *Class and Health: Research and Longitudinal Data*, Tavistock, London.

—— 1992, 'Income Distribution and Life Expectancy', *British Medical Journal*, vol. 304, pp. 165–8.

—— 1996, *Unhealthy Societies: The Afflictions of Inequality*, Routledge, London.

—— 1999, 'Putting the Picture Together: Prosperity, Redistribution, Health, and Welfare', in M. Marmot & R. G. Wilkinson (eds), *Social Determinants of Health*, Oxford University Press, Oxford, pp. 256–74.

Willcox, S. 1991, *A Health Risk? Use of Private Insurance*, Background Paper no. 4, AGPS, Canberra.

Williams, F. 1989, *Social Policy*, Polity Press, Cambridge.

Williams, L. & Germov, J. 1999, 'The thin ideal: Women, food and dieting', in J. Germov & L. Williams (eds), *A Sociology of Food and Nutrition: The Social Appetite*, Oxford University Press, Melbourne.

Williams, L. S. & McKenzie, F. 1996, *Understanding Australia's Population*, AGPS, Canberra.

Williams, P. 1993, 'Trends in the New South Wales Dietetic Workforce 1984–1991', *Australian Journal of Nutrition and Dietetics*, vol. 50, no. 3, pp. 116–19.

Williams, R. 1990, *A Protestant Legacy: Attitudes to Death and Illness among Older Aberdonians*, Oxford University Press, Oxford.

Williams, S. & Calnan, M. 1996, 'The "Limits" of Medicalization? Modern Medicine and the Lay Populace in "Late" Modernity', *Social Science and Medicine*, vol. 42, no. 12, pp. 1609–20.

Willis, E. 1983, *Medical Dominance*, Allen & Unwin, Sydney.

—— 1989a, 'Complementary Healers', in G. M. Lupton & J. Najman (eds), *Sociology of Health and Illness: Australian Readings*, Macmillan, Melbourne, pp. 259–79.

—— 1989b, *Medical Dominance*, revised edn, Allen & Unwin, Sydney.

—— 1994, *Illness and Social Relations*, Allen & Unwin, Sydney.

—— 1995, 'The Political Economy of Genes', *Journal of Australian Political Economy*, vol. 36, pp. 104–13.

—— 1999, *The Sociological Quest*, 3rd edn, Allen & Unwin, Sydney.

—— 1998, 'Public Health, Private Genes: The Social Context of Genetic Biotechnologies', *Critical Public Health*, vol. 8, no. 2, pp. 131–9.

Wilson, P. R. 1989, 'Medical Fraud and Abuse in Medical Benefit Programs', in P. Grabosky & A. Sutton (eds), *Stains on a White Collar*, Hutchinson, Sydney, pp. 76–91.

Wilson, P. R. & Gorring, P. 1985, 'Social Antecedents of Medical Fraud and Over-Servicing: What Makes a Doctor Criminal?', *Australian Journal of Social Issues*, vol. 20, no. 3, pp. 175–87.

Wilson, R. M., Gibberd, R., Hamilton, [?], & Harrison, B. 1999, 'Safety of healthcare in Australia: Adverse events to hospitalised patients', in M. M. Rosenthal, L. Mulcahy, & S. Lloyd-Bostock (eds), *Medical Mishaps: Pieces of the Puzzle*, Open University Press, Buckingham, pp. 95–106.

Winter, I. (ed.) 2000a, *Social Capital and Public Policy in Australia*, Australian Institute of Family Studies, Melbourne.

—— 2000b, 'Major Themes and Debates in the Social Capital Literature: The Australian Connection', in I. Winter (ed.), *Social Capital and Public Policy in Australia*, Australian Institute of Family Studies, Melbourne, pp. 7–42.

Wirthlin Worldwide Australasia Ltd 2000, *Quantitative Benchmark Research; May 15 2000*, a report presented to the RACGP.

Witz, A. 1992, *Professions and Patriarchy*, Routledge, London, pp. 23–45.

—— 1994, 'The Challenge of Nursing', in D. Kelleher, J. Gabe, & G. Williams (eds), *Challenging Medicine*, Routledge, London, pp. 23–45.

Wolf, N. 1990, *The Beauty Myth*, Vintage, London.

Wolf, Z. 1988, *Nurses' Work: The Sacred and the Profane*, University of Pennsylvania Press, Philadelphia.

Wooden, M., Holton, R., Hugo, G., & Sloan, J. 1994, *Australian Immigration: A Survey of the Issues*, 2nd edn, AGPS, Canberra.

Woolcock, M. 1998, 'Social Capital and Economic Development: Toward a Theoretical Synthesis and Policy Framework', *Theory & Society*, vol. 27, pp. 151–208.

'Work: A Major Health Hazard for Migrant Women' 1993, *Workplace News*, October, pp. 11–15.

World Bank 1993, *World Development Report 1993: Investing in Health*, Oxford University Press, New York.

World Commission on Environment and Development 1987, *Our Common Future*, Oxford University Press, Oxford.

World Health Organization 1946, *Constitution of the World Health Organization*, WHO, Geneva.

—— 1978, *Primary Health Care: Report of the International Conference on Primary Health Care*, Alma-Ata, USSR, 6–12 September, WHO, Geneva.

—— 1986, *Ottawa Charter for Health Promotion*, First International Conference on Health Promotion: The Move Towards a New Public Health, 17–21 November, Ottawa, Canada, and WHO, Geneva.

—— 1988, *Learning Together to Work Together for Health*, Technical Report Series, no. 769, WHO, Geneva.

—— 1996, *Traditional Medicine Fact Sheet 134*, WHO, Geneva.

—— 1998a, *The World Health Report 1998: Life in the 21st Century—A Vision for All*, World Health Organization, Geneva.

—— 1998b, *Gender and Health: Technical Paper*, Geneva, Women's Health and Development.

—— 1998c, *Taskforce on Equity: Key Issues for the World Health Organization*, Draft Discussion Paper, WHO, Geneva.

—— 1999, *The World Health Report 1999: Making a Difference*, World Health Organization, Geneva.

—— 2000, *Health for All (HFA) in the 21st Century*, World Health Organization, Geneva.

Wright, E. O. 1997, *Class Counts: Comparative Studies in Class Analysis*, Cambridge University Press, Cambridge.

Xenos, N. 1989, *Scarcity and Modernity*, Routledge, London.

Yates, P. M., Patsy, M., Beadle, G., Claravino, A., Najman, J. M., Thomson, D. et al. 1993, 'Patients with Terminal Cancer who use Alternative Therapies: Their Beliefs and Practices', *Sociology of Health and Illness*, vol. 15, no. 2, pp. 199–216.

Yeatman, A. 1987a, 'Administrative Reform and Management Improvement: A New Iron Cage?', *Flinders Studies in Policy and Administration*, no. 3, March, pp. 2–15.

—— 1987b, 'The Concept of Public Management and the Australian State in the 1980s', *Australian Journal of Public Administration*, vol. 46, no. 4, pp. 339–56.

—— 1990a, *Bureaucrats, Technocrats, Femocrats: Essays on the Contemporary Australian State*, Allen & Unwin, Sydney.

—— 1990b, 'Reconstructing Public Bureaucracies: The Residualisation of Equity and Access', *Australian Journal of Public Administration*, vol. 49, no. 1, pp. 17–21.

Yen, I. & Syme, S. L. 1999, 'The social environment and health: A discussion of the epidemiologic literature', *Annual Review of Public Health*, vol. 20, pp. 287–308.

Young, C. M. 1987, 'Migration and Mortality: The Experience of Birthplace Groups in Australia', *International Migration Review*, vol. 21, pp. 531–54.

Zola, I. K. 1972, 'Medicine as an Institution of Social Control', *Sociological Review*, vol. 20, pp. 487–504.

Zollman C. & Vickers A. 1999, 'Users and Practitioners of Complementary Medicine, *British Medical Journal*, vol. 319, pp. 836–8.

Index

Aboriginal Health Services
126, 377–8
Aboriginal people:
alcohol consumption
115–16, 122–3, 125
assimilation   113, 121–2
citizenship   398
class   118
death   97, 114
dispossession   119–20
health promotion   208
health status   54, 114–17,
127
life expectancy   5, 114, 234
mental health   116–17
missions and reserves   121
public policies   122, 125,
126–8
racism   119
self-determination   125
smoking   116, 118
stolen children   116
suicide   116
victim blaming   118–19
violence   116
accident-proneness   84, 144
ACTU   83
acupuncture   329
age   102, 141, 145–6, 188–9
aged-care facilities   242,
244–5, 261
ageing   234, 400
community care   245–6
defining 'old'   236
ethnicity   145–6
fourth age   244
pension   237, 238
population   234, 238
retirement   237
social burden   241–3
successful   244
third age   243
ageism   236, 239–41
agency   20, 31, 38, 44, 183, 303

AIDS *see* HIV/AIDS
alcohol consumption   105,
115–16, 122–3
Alcoholics Anonymous   168
Alford, R.   276
allied health   98, 284, 285, 286,
289, 302, 344
description   345, 347
economic rationalism   357,
359
gender   352
history   348
income   359
nature of work   346, 348
professional autonomy
349–50
professionalisation   350–3
role of the State   356–60
Allied Health Alliance, NSW
361
allopathy   326
Alma Ata Declaration   125, 197,
369, 370
ALP   124, 129, 269, 270, 275,
287, 296
alternative medicine   329–38
challenge to doctors   295
chronic and terminal treatment   251, 334–5
convergence   339
effectiveness   331–2, 335–6
and general practitioners
339
healer–patient relationship
333
popularity   329–30
types   332
AMA *see* Australian Medical
Association
Aries, P.   234
artefact explanation for health
inequality   79
assimilation   113, 121–2
asylums   161, 163

ATSIC   126, 127
Attention Deficit (Hyperactivity)
Disorder (AD(H)D)   53, 168
Australian Bureau of Statistics
74, 345
Australian Community Health
Association   367, 369, 384
Australian Council of Allied
Health Professionals   361
Australian Council of Trade
Unions   83
Australian Institute of Health and
Welfare   192, 241
Australian Labor Party *see* ALP
Australian Longitudinal Study on
Women's Health 74
Australian Medical Association
36, 263, 269, 287, 302, 359
autonomy *see* medical autonomy

battered woman syndrome   174
Baudrillard, J.   43
Beattie, A.   199
Beck, U.   200
Becker, H.   39
behavioural genetics   216, 222
Best Practice   299
Better Health Commission   197
Better Health Outcomes for
Australians   76
Biggins, D.   83
biological determinism   10, 42,
227, 310, 408
biological inferiority   80
biomedical model   7, 8–11, 16,
17, 36, 50, 52, 84, 137, 156,
166, 167, 168
biomedicine   326
biopsychosocial model of health
14
biotechnology   216, 217, 223
Black Report   74, 79, 80, 81,
84, 399
body   181

beliefs of body   182
body maintenance   188–9
body politic   182
body rituals   186
 health professionals   186, 187
 ideal body   189
 individual body   181
 men's bodies   191–2
 patients' bodies   184–5
 social body   182
 women's bodies   190–1
bourgeoisie   35
Broom, D.   15
Burden of Disease and Injury in
 Australia   77
Burdess, N.   204
Business Review Weekly (BRW)
 70, 71

Calwell, A.   139
cancer   51, 97, 99, 104, 226
Capra, F.   10, 11
cardiovascular disease   100–1,
 202
Cartesian dualism   8
Chadwick, E.   7, 74
Chifley government   268
chiropractors   329, 331
chronic fatigue syndrome   169,
 184
citizenship   151
 models of citizenship   392–8
 scarcity   394, 398
 and solidarity   398–401, 404
 states role   396, 397, 402–3
civic virtue   396
class, social class   6, 35, 37, 287,
 399
 and Aboriginal people
  117–18
 analysis   72–3, 85
 death of   72–3
 definition   68–9
 ethnicity   139
 and gender   102
 and health inequality   70,
  73–8
 and health promotion
  205–6
 middle   37, 69, 89, 204
 ruling   71, 273

upper   35, 68, 70–1, 89
 women   41
 working/lower   35, 69, 90,
  204, 273
clinical gaze   185
clinical governance   299–300
Coburn, D.   403
collective conscience   251
Collins, J.   140
Collins, R.   35
colonialism   119–20
commodification of health   36,
 297
commodity culture   188, 189
communism   404
Community Health Program
 (CHP)   366, 367
community health services   209,
 361, 366–85
 community participation
  377
 definition   369–72
 doctors' role   372, 375
 history   366–9
 lost opportunities   382–5
 marginalisation   372
 state, role of   368–9
 types of services   373–6
community mental-health
 services   177
complementary medicine   326
 see also alternative medicine
conflict theory *see* 'Marxism'
Connell, R.   287, 297, 310
consensus theory *see* 'structural
 functionism'
Constitution, Australian   259, 287
consumer culture   200
consumerism   201, 398
contraceptives   106
convergence   339
corporatisation   297
Crawford, R.   200, 206
criminal law   172–4
 see also law
critical sociology   408–9
critical theory   35
cultural capital   394
cultural diversity   139
culturalist explanation   138–9,
 147–8

cultural stereotypes   149

David, G.   174
death   75, 82–3, 97–8, 114,
 246–52
 social   241
deinstitutionalisation   165
demedicalisation   175–6
deprofessionalisation   291
Descartes, R.   8
deviance   34, 39, 156, 158–9,
 163–4, 166, 171, 172, 175, 188
*Diagnostic and Statistical Manual of
 Mental Disorders*   165, 168,
 171, 175
Dilnot, A.   70
disability   396
disciplinary power   185
discourse   147, 159, 169, 176,
 188, 206, 252, 313
discrimination   176–7, 188, 223,
 226
 geneism   226–7
 racism   119, 143, 145
 sexism   103, 106, 243, 290
 victim-blaming   118–19, 203
dispersed unit model   358
Division of Allied Health Model
 358
Divisions of Primary Health
 Care   383–4
doctor–patient relationship
 185, 266, 269, 295
doctor–nurse game   314
Doctors' Reform Society (DRS)
 302
domestic violence   100–1,
 144–5, 376
DSM-IV   168
dual closure   316
Dubos, R.   9
Duckett, S.   277
Durkheim, E.   4, 33, 87, 251,
 337

Easthope, G.   295
ecological model of health   14
economic rationalism   72, 87,
 88, 252, 274, 392
economism   72
Ehrenreich, B.   288, 309

Elston, M.   285
embodiment   182, 183, 187
emotional labour   41
empiricism   296, 314
employment   74, 81
encroachment:
    horizontal   355–6
    vertical   354–5
Engels, F.   6, 35, 74
English, D.   288, 309
Enlightenment   162, 234
epidemiology   50, 53–4, 172,
    175, 176, 199, 201–3, 400
essentialism   323
ethnic communities   140
ethnic group   137, 145, 149,
    219
ethnic minorities   88, 136
ethnicity:
    ageing   141, 143, 145–6
    cultural difference   136–7
    gender   140, 144–5, 146
    government policy   139–41,
        149–51
    health services   146–7,
        150–1
    mental health   142–3, 146
    mortality and morbidity
        142
    occupation   140–1
    occupational health   143–4
    refugees   140, 141, 143, 145
ethnocentrism   119, 138
ethnospecific services   150
eugenics   219
European Community   224
euthanasia   233, 249–51
Evatt, H.   269
evidence-based medicine   52–3,
    300

Family Planning clinics   106
Featherstone, M.   189
fee-for-service medicine   290,
    372
femininity   104
feminisation of poverty   397
feminist theory   30, 33, 40–2,
    44, 309–14, 352, 397
Fordism   397
Foucault, M.   43, 161, 172, 173,
    184, 185, 312–13

Fourth World Congress on
    Women   107
Fox, T.   258
Franzway, S.   320
Fraser government   270
Freidson, E.   158, 284, 285, 301,
    349, 350
Freud, S.   163
friendly societies   267
functionalism see 'structural
    functionalism'

Galton, F.   219
Gamson, J.   176
Garmarnikow, E.   309, 310
gays see homosexuality
GDP and health   86, 237, 266
gender   22, 40–2, 95–110, 400
    body   104, 190–2
    cancer 99, 104
    causes of death   97–8
    class   74–6, 102
    doctor consultations   98
    domestic violence   100–1
    eating disorders   100
    ethnicity   140, 144–5
    exercise   99–100
    experience of illness   98
    exposure to illness   99–100
    Fourth World Congress on
        Women   107
    government policy   104,
        107, 108
    life expectancy   97
    medical research   103–5
    medication   98
    medicine   103, 288
    men's health 104–5
    mental illness   170–2
    nursing   307, 313
    occupation   99, 102
    smoking   99–105
geneism   226–7
General Practice Reform
    Strategy   382–3
general practitioners   265, 384
genetic manipulation   224
genetic reductionism   224
genetic screening   222, 225, 226
germ theory   333
Giddens, A.   217, 232, 233, 252
Gillespie, J.   267

Goals and Targets for Australia's
    Health in the Year 2000 and
    Beyond   197
Goffman, E.   163
Goldthorpe, J.   68
Good, B.   182
grounded theory   58
Gross Domestic Product and
    health see GDP and health

health, as defined by WHO   13
health insurance   242, 263
    allied health   360
    alternative therapies   330–1
    financing   261
    government expenditure
        261–2
    history   259–60, 267–72
    international comparisons
        264
    private   264, 270, 271
    public   263, 264
    universal versus selective
        263, 264, 270
    see also Medibank; Medicare
Health Insurance Act 1983
    (NSW)   270
Health Insurance Commission
    292
healthism   200
health promotion   196, 361
    Aboriginal   208
    allied health   361
    diet   201, 203, 207–8
    elderly   243
    immunisation   208
    individualist   196, 198–203,
        204, 205, 211
    smoking   199, 207
    structural-collectivist   196,
        203–6, 210, 211
health sociology   3
healthy worker effect   142
Herdman, E.   320
Hirschauer, S.   186
HIV/AIDS   53, 57, 61–2, 105,
    175, 176, 177, 205
Home and Community Care
    (HACC)   245
homosexuality   18, 53, 105, 171,
    175, 177, 225
horizontal violence   308

Howard Government   278

Human Genome Project   167, 216–28

human rights *see* rights

hysteria   170, 184

ideology   219, 246, 258, 272, 287, 310

immigrants   4, 102, 136, 139–41, 219, 395

immigration *see* 'immigrants'

in vitro fertilisation   158

Index of Socioeconomic Disadvantage   74

indigenous health status   54, 114–17, 127

   see also Aboriginal people

individual community-controlled health services   377

individualisation   72

individualism   162, 273

individualistic explanations   12, 278

individualist health programs   199

industrial psychology   84

inequality:

   health   74–8, 79–87, 90, 114–17

   wealth   70–1, 86

   see also Aboriginal people; class; gender

infanticide   221

insanity defence   172

institutionalisation   40, 43, 121, 160

International Monetary Fund   404

interpreters   147, 210

intersectoral collaboration

Jayasuriya, L.   149

Keynes, J.   402

Koch, R.   7

   Koch's postulates   7

labelling theory   39–40, 156, 164

   see also deviance

Labor Party *see* ALP

Larson, M.   38

Laslett, A.   243, 244

law, and psychiatry   172–4

Lawler, J.   315

lay health beliefs   182

liberalism   273, 274, 278

Liberal–National Party   124, 129, 269, 270, 275, 278

life expectancy   4, 5, 10, 11, 73, 85, 97, 114, 232, 233–4, 244, 399, 400

   see also Aboriginal people; class; gender

life chances   68, 149, 275

lifestyle   149, 198, 199, 200–1, 335

lifetime community rating   271

Lloyd, P.   295

'looking-glass self'   39

Lukes, S.   276

Lumby, J.   321

Lupton, D.   198, 199

Lyotard, J.   43

McDonaldisation   38, 291, 298–301

Mcintyre, S.   79, 80, 81, 84

McKeown, T.   11, 12

McKinlay, J.   11, 202, 296

mainstreaming   150

managerialism   298–9, 300

managerial prerogative   83

mandala of health *see* ecological model

Marmot, M.   79, 85, 86, 89

Marshall, T.   392, 403, 404

Marx, K.   6, 35, 73, 411

Marxism   30, 32, 35–7

masculinity   55–6, 104, 108, 171, 191, 192, 352

materialist analysis   81, 204, 310, 400

Mathers, C.   76, 77, 81, 82

Mead, G.   38

Mechanic, D.   201

Medibank   269, 277

medical autonomy   285–6, 299

medical dominance   36, 57, 137, 185, 209, 235, 268, 284–303

   and allied health   349–50

   challenges to   106, 167, 270, 277, 184, 291–7

doctors' incomes   296, 359

exclusion   288

gender   288

history   286–8

incorporation   288

limitation   288, 289–90

Medicare   277

psychiatry   158, 160, 161, 162

re-stratification   302

State's role   286–7

subordination   288

medical encounter   187

medical fraud   292, 293

medical–industrial complex   36, 297

medicalisation   156, 157–60, 168, 169, 200

medical knowledge   185

medical model *see* biomedical model

medical negligence   293–4

Medicare   36, 124, 223, 242, 260, 261, 264, 265, 270, 271, 277, 298, 295, 296, 358, 359, 367

medicine:

   complementary   331, 339

   education   319

   orthodox   326–9, 334, 336

   profession   35–6

   professionalisation   285

   research   103–5

   sexism   290

   students   187

   see also alternative medicine; medical autonomy; medical dominance

menopause   183

men's health   108, 191–2

mental health policy   165, 166

mental illness   53, 55, 116–17, 142–3, 161–2

Menzies, R.   268, 269, 287

Merton, R.   33

meta-narratives   313

Mill, C.W.   20, 21

Millet, K.   41

modernism   224

moral entrepreneur   156

mortality and morbidity   11, 73

   class   74–8, 86, 399

   ethnicity   142

sex comparisons   97–9
see also Aboriginal people
MRI (medical resonance
   imaging)   292–3
multicultural   56
multiculturalism   149, 150, 151
multidisciplinary teams   346, 384

National Aboriginal Community
   Controlled Health
   Organisation (NACCHO)
   125
National Aboriginal Health
   Strategy (NAHS)   127
National Agenda for
   Multicultural Australia   149
National Alliance for the
   Mentally Ill   168
National Better Health Program
   382
National Health Strategy   54, 74
National Health Survey   76, 81,
   97, 329
National Inquiry into the
   Separation of Aboriginal and
   Torres Strait Islander
   Children and their Families
   116–17
National Mental Health Policy
   165
National Mental Health Strategy
   166
National Women's Health Policy
   107
Navarro, V.   36, 297
Nazis   219, 250
negotiated order   302
neo-functionalism   34, 87–8, 89
neo-liberalism   402–3
neo-Marxism   35
New Nursing   316–19, 320–1
New Public Health   14, 15, 16,
   17, 196, 197, 211, 366, 371
new social movements   72
non-English-speaking backgrounds (NESB)   141, 143,
   144, 146
normative work   168
Nurse Education Board   320
nurse-practitioner   314, 317,
   318, 321–2, 355

nursing   56, 187, 284, 286, 302
   'active' nursing   315
   autonomy   315
   enhanced role   319
   feminist theory   309–14
   gender   307
   handmaiden   308
   'Nightingale'   308, 309
   nurse–doctor interactions
      308, 310, 314
   professionalisation   315–16
   State's role   320
nursing development units   317
Nussbaum, M.   401

occupational disease   82
occupational health   82–3
occupational health and safety
   (OHS)   82–5, 99
occupational injuries   82
occupational welfare   72, 204
Office of Aboriginal & Torres
   Strait Islander Health
   (OATSIH)   128
One Nation   129
ontological insecurity   252
oppression   312
Ottawa Charter   197, 361, 366,
   369, 370, 275
overweight and obesity   189,
   221

Packer, K.   247
Page Plan   269
palliative care   248–9
panopticon   43
Parsons, T.   33, 34, 157
Pasteur, L.   7, 8, 327
patients' rights   294
   see also rights
patriarchy   41, 290, 310, 313,
   352, 397
personality disorder   165
Petersen, A.   199
Pharmaceutical Benefits Scheme
   (PBS)   261
phenomenology   311
Pinel, P.   161
placebo   336–7
pluralism   151, 276, 277
positive health   371

positivist research methodologies
   50
postmodern feminism   44
postmodernism 30, 33, 42–4, 309
postmodernity   151
postmodern society   335
post-structuralism   30, 33, 42–4,
   309
power   276, 291
premenstrual dysphoric disorder
   (PDD)   168–9
premenstrual syndrome (PMS)
   168–9, 174
preventative paradox   202
primary care partnerships   385
primary health care   124, 367,
   372, 382
primary nursing   318
Pringle, R.   312–13
private health insurance   124
professional bureaucracy   291
professionalisation   285, 350,
   351, 362
professionalising project   353–4,
   362
profit motive   35, 52, 83
Project 2000   317
proletarianisation   291, 295–6
proletariat   35
psychiatry   159–65, 167, 172,
   174, 177
   law   172–4
psychoanalysis   163, 171
psychology   39
psychoneuroimmunology (PNI)
   337
psychosocial factors   82, 85–7
psychotropic drugs   164
public health   5, 7, 12, 74, 124
Public Hospital Nurses (State)
   Award   321

qualitative and quantitative
   research   54–5
Quality in Australian Healthcare
   Study   293
Quinlan, M.   83

'race'   205
racism   119, 143, 145
   see also Aboriginal people

randomised controlled trials
  50–3, 104, 336, 338
rationalisation   38, 298
Rawls, J.   393
redistributive justice   393
reductionism   10
refugees   86, 140, 141, 143, 145
rehabilitative model   173
reliability   56
religion   162, 164, 251, 333
Relman, A. S.   297
Renaissance   162
repetitive strain injury (RSI)   84
research methods   319, 320
    gender   103–5
    positive methods   50–3
    qualitative   54–60
retirement   193
rights   166, 274, 294–5, 393, 397
risk   13, 50, 80, 85, 98, 99, 115,
  337, 175–6, 200, 201, 202,
  337
    discourse   199
    society   200, 330
risk-taking   100, 105, 108, 157,
  395
Ritzer, G.   298
Rogers v. Whitaker   294
Rosenhan, D.   160
RSI   84
Ruggiero, V.   410, 411
Russell, B.   409
Russell, C.   151

Sahlins, M.   398
Salvage, J.   318
Sax, S.   258
Scheff, T.   164
Schofield, T.   151
scientific testing *see* randomised
  controlled trials
Sex Discrimination Act 1984
  (Cwlth)   107
sexism   41–2, 103, 106, 243, 290
sexual division of labour   41,
  96, 99, 102, 310, 349
'sick role'   34, 157, 176
Singer, P.   216
smoking   99, 105, 116, 118, 207
Snow, J.   6
social capital   85, 87, 88

Social Health Atlas of Australia
  77, 78
social class *see* class
social closure   37, 353, 395
social cohesion   88, 89
social construction   39, 42, 113,
  158, 159, 200, 232
social context of health   4–5
social contract theory   397
social control   43, 158, 159, 163,
  164, 170, 201, 226, 290
social Darwinism   80, 224
social gradient   85, 86
social institutions   20, 309, 393
socialisation   276
socialism   275
social isolation   201
social justice   84, 90, 226
social liberalism   275
social model of health   14, 15,
  16, 17, 18
    see also New Public Health
social norm   95, 156, 160
social policy   163, 217, 225
social production of health and
  illness   5–7, 316
social solidarity   87, 337
social structure   10–11, 19, 69,
  71, 190, 223, 225, 240, 251,
  275 282, 409
social support   210, 336–7
social wage   71
sociobiology   224
socioeconomic status (SES)   69,
  86, 117–18
    difference from class   74–8
sociological analysis   410–11
sociological determinism   408
sociological imagination
  19–20, 21, 22, 410
sociological perspectives   32–3
Socrates   409
State   12, 239, 258, 269, 287,
  302
    and allied health   356–60
    and medical dominance
      286–7
    and nursing   320
status groups   37
Stein, L.   314
Stoeckle, J.   296

stolen children   116
structural functionalism   30, 32,
  33–5, 351
structuralist explanation   31,
  81–2, 84, 203
structure/agency debate   20, 31,
  88–9, 309, 408–9
subordination   349–50
suicide   4, 108, 116, 143, 377
Superannuation Guarantee
  Scheme   238–9
Sutton, J.   162
symbolic interactionism   30,
  32–3, 38–40
Szasz, T.   164
Szreter, S.   12

tax paid by Australian companies
  79
technology   218, 235
technophoria   228
terra nullius   119
thematic analysis   58
theodicy   336
theory   28–46
therapeutic model   173, 177
thin ideal   189
Total Quality Management
  (TQM)   299
trait approach   285, 351, 354
transformational capacity   73
trickle-down theory   72, 274
Turrell, G.   78

unemployment   55, 81–2, 89
unions   83, 88, 210
United Nations   166
United States health system
  264
universal health insurance   260,
  261, 263, 264
    see also health insurance;
      Medicare

validity of research   56, 57
victim-blaming   10–11, 13, 80,
  84, 89, 108, 118–19, 203
Victorian Government   301
Vietnamese Community
  Association   379
violence   116

Virchow, R.   6, 7, 74, 399
voluntarism   396–7, 403
Voluntary Euthanasia Society
    249

waiting lists   301
Walby, S.   313
Walker, L.   174
Watson, J.   225
wealth distribution   23, 24,
    70–1
web of causation   14
Weber, M.   37, 200, 394
Weberian theory   30, 32, 37–8
welfare services   84

'White Australia' policy   139, 395
Whitehall studies   85, 117
Whitehead, M.   90
Whitlam government   366
WHO *see* World Health
    Organisation
Wilkinson, R.   79, 80, 85, 86,
    89
Willis, E.   286, 287, 288, 349
Witz, A.   310, 316, 318, 348
Wolf, Z.   186
women's health centres   106
Women's Health Initiative   104
women's health movement   41,
    106–7, 290

women's liberation movement
    22, 106
    see also gender
working conditions   82–5
    careless worker myth   83
    see also class; occupational
        health and safety
World Bank   88
World Health Organisation   13,
    125, 197, 232, 369, 370
World Trade Agreement   404
World Wealth Report   71
Wright, E. O.   68

Xenos, N.   398